ENDORSEMENTS

"This wonderful book has assembled some 25 authors expressing well a view of qi *which entirely does justice to its nature. Meticulously referenced, it is a milestone to set beside Maciocia's* Foundations of Chinese Medicine *and Deadman's* Manual of Acupuncture. *Here at last are the beginnings of a true science of* qi.... *There is truly nothing like it in contemporary literature. Alone, it lays the foundation for the beginnings of a modern science of* qi."

Richard Bertschinger
Acupuncturist and translator, Somerset, UK.
Titles include *The Golden Needle* (Churchill Livingstone, 1991) and
The Secret of Everlasting Life (Singing Dragon, 2010)

"This book offers a timely and thorough examination of the experience and nature of qi, *including a series of fascinating philosophical discussions with a direct application to our patients. Required reading for acupuncture practitioners seeking to justify and clarify their clinical reasoning."*

Val Hopwood PhD FCSP
Physiotherapist, acupuncturist, researcher and educator
Course director, MSc Acupuncture, Coventry University, UK
Co-author, *Acupuncture in Neurological Conditions* (Churchill Livingstone, 2010) and
other acupuncture textbooks for physical therapists

"Over the last decade most books on Asian medicine paid tribute to the aura of evidence-based medicine – experience counted little, RCTs were convincing. This book, at last, returns to an old tradition of debate, opening up quite a few new horizons. Reading it, my striving for knowledge was married with enjoyment and happiness. This book made me happy!"

Thomas Ots MD PhD
Medical acupuncturist specialising in psychiatry, Graz, Austria
Editor-in-Chief, *Deutsche Zeitschrift für Akupunktur*
Author of 'The silenced body' (1994)

ENERGY
MEDICINE
East and West

Dedication

To those who have taught me to appreciate the energies of life, in particular Herbert L Weaver, Gerda Boyesen, J R Worsley and the Venerable Lama Chime Rimpoche.

David Mayor, MA, BAc

To the philanthropists of the Bravewell Collaborative for Integrative Medicine who taught me it is better to be their neighbor than their employee.

Marc S Micozzi, MD, PhD

Commissioning Editor: Claire Wilson
Development Editor: Catherine Jackson
Project Manager: Beula Christopher
Designer: Kirsteen Wright
Illustration Manager: Merlyn Harvey
Illustrator: Cactus

ENERGY MEDICINE
East and West
A NATURAL HISTORY OF QI

Edited by

David Mayor MA BAc
Acupuncturist, Welwyn Garden City, Hertfordshire
Research Associate, Department of Physiotherapy,
University of Hertfordshire, UK

Marc S Micozzi MD PhD
Adjunct Professor, Department of Medicine
University of Pennsylvania, Philadelphia, PA
Department of Physiology and Biophysics, Georgetown University,
Washington, DC, USA

Foreword by

James L Oschman PhD
President, Nature's Own Research Association
Dover, NH, USA
Author of *Energy Medicine: The scientific basis*

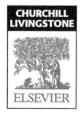

CHURCHILL
LIVINGSTONE

ELSEVIER

EDINBURGH LONDON NEW YORK OXFORD PHILADELPHIA ST LOUIS
SYDNEY TORONTO 2011

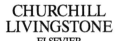

CHURCHILL
LIVINGSTONE
ELSEVIER

ISBN 978 0 7020 3571 5

British Library Cataloguing in Publication Data
A catalogue record for this book is available from the British Library

Library of Congress Cataloging in Publication Data
A catalog record for this book is available from the Library of Congress

CONTENTS

CONTENTS

A 21-page online glossary providing a useful resource for further reading can be found at
http://www.welwynacupuncture.co.uk/files/energymedicine_glossary.pdf

Abstracts to the chapters appear on this book's page on the Elsevier website

CONTENTS

FOREWORD AND SPECIAL CONTRIBUTION: THE LIVING MATRIX
James L Oschman

> *In every culture and in every medical tradition before ours,*
> *healing was accomplished by moving energy [1].*
> *Albert Szent-Györgyi*

The above quote inspires an exploration of two questions:

1. Why has modern medicine, with its powerful analytical tools, given so little attention to exploring the medicines of other cultures and other medical traditions before ours?
2. Exactly what is meant by 'healing accomplished by moving energy'?

Albert Szent-Györgyi (1893-1986) was regarded by many as one of the most insightful scientists of the twentieth century. He made three profoundly important discoveries: the synthesis of vitamin C, for which he received the Nobel Prize in 1937; the synthesis of actomyosin, the contractile protein of muscle, for which he received the Albert Lasker Award for Basic Medical Research in 1954; and the role of energy in biology, for which he received virtually no acknowledgement from the biomedical community.

Motivated by loss of his second wife and only daughter to cancer, Szent-Györgyi decided to focus his legendary scientific brilliance and instincts in a search for a cure for cancer. He quickly realized that there was something profoundly important that was being ignored by Western biomedicine, and that this missing piece was preventing us from understanding and treating the major health issues of our times: cancer and cardiovascular disease. The missing piece was *energy*.

The discoveries made by Szent-Györgyi and his colleagues have enabled us to make sense of a variety of energy therapies, including those that have come from Asia. When I say, 'make sense' I mean that the discoveries enable us to make an intelligent and detailed hypothesis about the underlying mechanisms involved in a variety of diseases and in a variety of therapeutic approaches.

These days many scientists are hesitant to make hypotheses for fear that they will be proven wrong, and thereby they will lose respect or, even worse, their grant funding. This concern is, of course, absurd, for true science does not progress without hypotheses that can be confirmed or refuted. In practice, refutation of hypotheses is an extremely important process. Moreover, it is in the process of testing hypotheses that major discoveries are made – often in areas remote from the original hypothesis. In the case of *qi*, we might look for hypotheses that integrate the successes of some of the most ancient and successful medical traditions with contemporary scientific medicine and, in this way, learn more about human structure and function in health and disease.

Discussing something like *qi* or vital energy poses some fascinating challenges. Asian medicine comprises a remarkably diverse set of techniques and theories. Some schools of thought attempt to apply acupuncture to the treatment of Western pathologies. Others seek to correct a single energetic condition that underlies all health problems: imbalance. As in any endeavor, practitioners are passionate about their particular theories and methods. Thus, any scientific statement about Asian medicine will elicit disapproval from at least some quarters in the therapeutic community. Some regard acupuncture as a complete and independent practice and philosophy that is incommensurate with modern science. The practice of acupuncture and related methods do, indeed, require that practitioners straddle competing and often paradoxical or irreconcilable perspectives. This conundrum may well hold true for any medical practice that relies on both art and science.

After giving a little more background, I will propose some hypotheses that I regard as worthwhile for consideration. These hypotheses bring together the effects of treatments with needles, touch, movement, magnets, electromagnets, electrical fields, electroacupuncture, light therapies, herbal remedies, aromatherapy, flower essences, homeopathy and intentionality. Such interactions fall into the discipline of biophysics.

I had the privilege of knowing Albert Szent-Györgyi and working across the hall from his Institute for Muscle Research at Woods Hole, Massachusetts, in the 1970s and 1980s. It was fascinating to watch close-up as he and his international team of scientists charted new ground by exploring the molecular, atomic and subatomic basis for biological energetics. It was also fascinating to see how the scientific community reacted (or failed to react) to this research. When I talked to colleagues about this line of investigation, many were prepared to reject it as unimportant – although, when pressed to explain the basis for their opinion, they usually said that they did not understand it. This just did not seem right, and inspired me to dig deeper to find out what this great man was talking about that nobody seemed able to follow. In retrospect, I can see how the biomedical community's attitude toward Szent-Györgyi's research on energy corresponded to the biomedical community's long-standing reaction to energy medicine. Until recently, the attitude could be characterized as hostility and skepticism. It is fortunate that this reaction is changing, and this volume, *Energy Medicine East and West*, is a tribute to the efforts of many thoughtful therapists and scientists who are helping to bring energy therapies to the people who need them.

Szent-Györgyi would celebrate the description of 'vital energy' (*prana* in India and *qi* in China) on page 3 of this book:

> The ancient Chinese ideogram for qi (氣) symbolized a cloudlike vapor, as when the breath is seen on a cold day.

Research in physics, quantum physics and materials sciences has provided an energetic picture of clouds of free, mobile, or delocalized electrons in living matter. These 'particles' are electrons that are not fixed in place, but rather belong to the whole system – they can give rise to holistic properties. By their nature, clouds of charged electrons are susceptible to external influences such as magnetism, heat, light, sound, vibration, electrical fields, pressure and so on. This observation is not to say that *qi* is identical with clouds of electrons. Instead of trying to make a definitive statement, we can say that clouds of electrons may be a partial representation of, or a partial correspondence to, one of the diverse forms of *qi*. Although such correspondences are interesting, they are certainly not essential to the wealth of diagnostic and treatment approaches found in Asian Medicine described in this book.

One image that comes to mind is the Tantric diagram of the energy circuits within and around the human body shown in Figure F.1. It is important to emphasize that this diagram is *not* a substitute for the acupuncture meridian system. Instead, the diagram shows that there are understandings from various traditions of circuits of energy flow within and around the human body. Modern biomedical science has obtained preliminary glimpses of this ancient wealth of information on bioenergetics, but much more work is needed for biomedicine to catch up with the concepts illustrated. I believe this work is profoundly important and will open new vistas to biology and medicine.

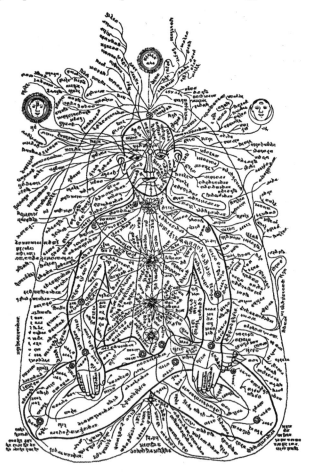

FIG F.1   **Diagram of the energetic pathways in and around the human body.** Attributed to the prophet Ratnasara, Tibet, *c.* nineteenth century. Published in Oscham, Energy Medicine in Therapeutics and Human Performance, 2003, published by Butterworth Heinemann. Reprinted with permission of Elsevier Ltd.

Biomedical research has demonstrated, for example, that the heart generates electrical currents that flow throughout the body (see Ch. 24 in this book). Science knows about one pathway for this energy flow, consisting of the blood and other conductive body fluids. As the most powerful electrical generator in the body, the electrical currents that the heart produces within the tissues create biomagnetic fields detectable in the space around the body [2]. Modern science, however, has yet to determine the details of other conductive pathways through the body represented by the various named circuits shown in Figure F.1, or by the meridian and flow systems as illustrated in Chapters 4, 17 and 19 in this book.

A clue about the conductive pathways within the body was provided by the intersection of the work of Albert Szent-Györgyi and his colleagues with a picture that was emerging at the same time in the field of cell biology. Szent-Györgyi had recognized that protein molecules and the structures made of proteins can be electronic semiconductors [3]. This observation meant that the protein frameworks found in cells and tissues are probably electronic 'circuits' that can silently and rapidly move energy and information throughout the organism. He suggested that chronic diseases arise when these circuits are not working properly. His picture of the cause of cancer was that of a *lack of flow* of electrons, a concept comparable to 'stagnant *qi*' in Oriental medicine.

At the time when this energetic picture was coming into focus, two key discoveries in cell biology led to the profound idea that the body contains a continuous molecular fabric that reaches into every nook and cranny of the organism. The first discovery was by Mark Bretscher at Cambridge University in England. He found that there are proteins extending across cell surfaces, which connect the cell interior with its surroundings. Eventually it was recognized that important molecules called *integrins* connect the cytoskeleton of every cell with that of neighboring cells and with the surrounding extracellular connective tissue matrix that pervades the body [4,5]. Secondly, Berezney and colleagues from Johns Hopkins University in Baltimore, Maryland found that there are also connections across the nuclear envelope, joining the cytoskeletal matrix with the nuclear matrix [6]. Taken together, these observations mean there is a continuous physical system or matrix that actually extends throughout the body and that reaches into every part, even into the nucleus and the DNA. Additional evidence from the Johns Hopkins laboratory revealed that the components of the living matrix network are capable of vibrating in a dynamic manner with measurable complex harmonics [7]. The language of this system is spoken in electrical oscillations and the information is encoded as frequencies – as described by Cyril Smith in Chapter 9 in this book. It is intriguing to consider this continuous system as the substrate for the energetic electronic regulatory system for which Szent-Györgyi was searching during the last part of his life. This body-wide continuum has been named the 'living matrix' (Fig. F.2) [8].

Stephen Birch and Kiiko Matsumoto, when writing their book *Hara Diagnosis: Reflections on the Sea* [9], discovered that the earliest Chinese medical classics, the *Su Wen, Ling Shu* and *Nan Jing*, all made reference to the location of the meridians or channels in 'fatty and greasy' tissue, the 'body lining', or the 'space between the organs, bones and flesh'. This image of shiny material was replicated in leading texts down through the ages, and had to be a reference to what we now know as the connective tissue and fascial systems that extend throughout the body, and are visible as the shiny coverings of muscles, tendons and ligaments. Moreover, the shiny or reflective aspect of

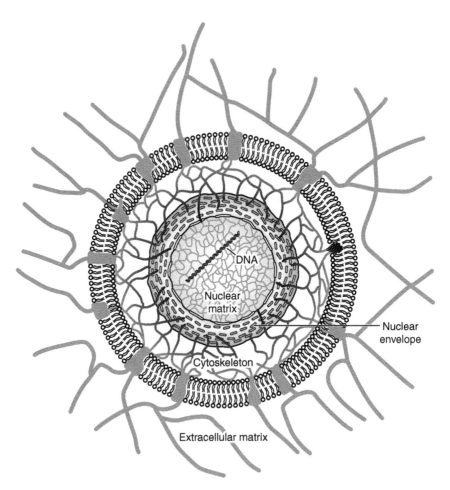

FIG F.2   The living matrix. Published in Oscham, Energy Medicine: The scientific basis, 2000, published by Churchill Livingstone. Reprinted with permission of Elsevier Ltd.

this material indicates the presence of free electrons – as in a metal. The living matrix concept shows how this continuous system extends across the surfaces of cells, through the cytoskeletons and into the nuclear matrices of every cell in the body.

Matsumoto and Birch have considered the possibility that the living matrix system and Szent-Györgyi's electronic biology could provide a basis for the Oriental medical perspective of a metasystem that links and influences every aspect of human physiology [9]. The concept of a fascial, connective tissue metasystem has been reiterated by Langevin [10].

Finando and Finando have recently written a thoughtful article suggesting that the properties of the fascia actually account for many, if not all, aspects of the mechanism of action of acupuncture therapy [11]. Their conclusions are based in part on the following:

- The fascia are involved in virtually all dysfunctions and diseases.
- The fascia are involved in the circulation of the blood and lymphatic fluids.
- The fascia connect the surface of the body with the viscera.

- The fascia react to stimuli wherever the latter are applied.
- The fascia are involved in the initial nonspecific immune response of the body to injury and pathogens.

The fascia, with its connections to the interior of cells and cell nuclei, and with its electronic conduction properties, could be a whole body regulatory system that works silently in the background – that is, below our conscious awareness, integrating and coordinating the functioning of all of the parts of the body. Perhaps this entity is the energetic system, the dysregulation of which gives rise to so many chronic diseases that have resisted treatment by Western biomedicine.

To this picture, we can add the discovery by Langevin and Yandow of the frequent relationship of acupuncture points and meridians to connective tissue planes [12], as summarized by Finando and Finando [11]:

> *Langevin and Yandow found an 80% correlation between acupuncture points and intermuscular or intramuscular septa, along fascial planes. The clue to the mechanism of acupuncture is therefore anatomical. Loci where maximum stimulation of the fascia may occur are the focus of treatment. Although any needle insertion, at virtually any point on the surface of the body provides stimulation of the fascia, acupuncture points and channels have a unique anatomical correlation to fascial anatomy.*

In considering the role of fascia, it is important to recognize that the connective tissue is a composite material; it consists of a strong fibrous protein core, collagen, embedded in a soft polymer gel known as the 'ground substance' (Fig. F.3A) [13]. The collagen is the conductor of electrons (it is actually a semiconductor) and the ground substance stores the negative electrons. A field or cloud of negative charge therefore surrounds the 'matrisome', which is the structural unit of the ground substance (Fig. F.3B) [14].

Another perspective emerges from considering the vital role of water in the body [15,16]. Each collagen molecule has a helical shell of water molecules intimately associated with it. Taken together the various layers of fascia form the largest organ system in the body, and the only system that touches all of the other systems [14]. The highly regular and nearly crystalline arrays of collagen molecules organize equally regular arrays of water molecules, which tend to have a particular orientation with respect to the collagen because of interactions between the repeating charges on the collagen and the electrically polar water molecules (i.e. water molecules line up in an electric field). For further details, see Oschman [17]. I suspect that this 'water system' in the body acts as an antenna, which is very sensitive to resonant interactions with chemicals or signals in the environment. This sensitivity arises because the water forms a coherent phase-correlated system (see Smith's discussion of the work of Herbert Fröhlich in Chapter 9, page 110; also see the work of Stephen Strogatz on the tendency of oscillating systems to become synchronized [18]). This property can explain the way vibrational frequencies from therapeutic devices, herbal remedies, essential oils and homeopathic remedies can all interact so sensitively with the living system – as discussed by Cyril Smith in Chapter 9. Smith has pointed out that a homeopathic remedy, or a toxic molecule, need not be taken internally to have an effect, as substances emit electromagnetic fields that can have an influence at a distance.

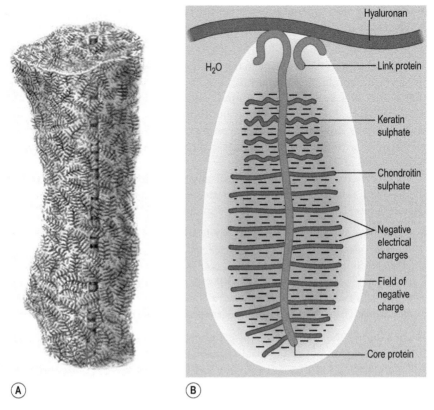

FIG F.3 **(A) Collagen fibril embedded in the ground substance gel. From Matrix-Center-Munchen. (B) The way the 'matrisome' or unit of ground substance stores negative charges, creating a cloud or field of negative charge in the surrounding space. Published in Lee, Interface: mechanisms of spirit in osteopathy, 2005. Reprinted from Stillness Press LLC.**

The semiconduction of electrons through the collagen matrix, the migration of protons through the water matrix, and the clouds of mobile electrons described above are just a few of the possible biophysical mechanisms that could account for aspects of *vital energy*, *prana* or *qi* in living systems.

It has now been demonstrated that electrons are indeed moving about within the body. Barefoot contact with the earth, sometimes referred to as 'earthing', allows mobile electrons from the surface of our planet – nature's own antioxidants [19] – to enter our bodies and migrate to sites of inflammation. The process can often be felt as a warming or tingling in the legs by a person who has not been in contact with the earth for a long time and who then stands barefoot on it. These feelings are caused by the dilation of blood vessels in the legs, and thinning of the blood brought about by the increase in negative charge on the surfaces of the blood cells and vascular walls. This negativity (the 'zeta potential') increases as electrons from the earth enter the body through the feet or any other part of the body in contact with the earth (Chevalier et al, submitted for publication, 2010). The process can also be monitored with medical infrared imaging, which reveals areas of inflammation because they are warmer than surrounding tissues. Parts of the body that have been inflamed for a long time, such as muscles or joints, will warm dramatically within minutes of conductive contact with the earth [20]. It is only in recent times that our shoes, with their insulating soles made of plastic or rubber, and our contemporary homes and buildings have disconnected us from the earth. This seemingly harmless or even beneficial change in our lifestyle has had a dramatic impact on the incidence of chronic diseases associated with inflammation.

Earthing has now become the topic of careful study by more than a dozen scientists from the USA and Canada [21], and has recently been confirmed by an entirely independent group in Poland [22]. Chevalier and Mori [23], for example, have found that the bottoms of the feet are especially conductive at the region around the point known in the acupuncture literature as Kidney 1 (*yongquan*, KI-1), allowing electrons from the earth to pass through the skin there. They are then distributed throughout the human body from this point, which connects to the Kidney and Bladder meridians and thence to all of the other meridians via the *luo* meridians that traverse the whole body and that spirally wrap the internal organs by coursing through their fascial envelopes [12] (and [9, p 142]). Electrons can thus be conducted from the Kidney meridian to a site of injury or inflammation anywhere in the body.

The electronic properties of the living matrix allow electrons from the earth, or from electron 'reservoirs' in the body (the ground substance), to protect healthy tissue from damage by reactive oxygen species (ROS, sometimes referred to as 'free radicals') that can occur as a result of normal metabolism, injury, or exposure to toxins or pollutants. When charged with electrons from the earth, the ground substance can thus keep the body in a state of *inflammatory preparedness*. This is a whole system condition that enables the immune system to respond quickly to injury by secretion of ROS into an injured area while preventing damage to nearby healthy tissues that have not been injured. In this concept, a healthy conductive matrix around a site of injury, and the entire meridian system, have active roles in the healing process by limiting the spread of damage.

To appreciate this effect fully, we must look at the meridians as a system that extends throughout the body and even into every cell (the living matrix, Fig. F.2). With respect to chronic diseases, a plausible, testable and refutable hypothesis is that all chronic diseases have a single underlying cause: the stresses that produce and maintain chronic inflammation. Such stresses include environmental factors of various kinds including those that disturb physiology and those whose absence is disruptive.

A corollary to the inflammation hypothesis is that the thousands of so-called diseases that have been named may actually be an elaborate classification system of the various symptoms that can arise from a single underlying condition: inflammation. Inflammation, in turn, has a single underlying cause best described as an imbalance of electrical charge – since free radicals are generally positively charged and must be balanced by the negative charges of electrons in order to maintain health. Indirect support for the inflammation hypothesis is the abundant biomedical research on the links between chronic inflammation and virtually every chronic disease. A search of the database of the National Library of Medicine, PubMed, reveals the following numbers of peer-reviewed studies documenting relationships between inflammation and specific pathologies [24]:

- aging: 3924
- Alzheimer disease: 2145
- asthma: 12930

- atherosclerosis: 8921
- bowel disorders: 9755
- cancer: 34 871
- chronic obstructive pulmonary disease: 2626
- cirrhosis of the liver: 4708
- cystic fibrosis: 1991
- diabetes: 10 788
- meningitis: 5429
- multiple sclerosis: 3100
- osteoporosis: 823
- prostate cancer: 1015
- psoriasis: 1955
- rheumatoid arthritis: 9402.

The vital influence of nature on the proper functioning of mind and body has been known for thousands of years, and in the last century has been repeatedly confirmed by science. We know, for example, that sunlight is essential for the chemical reactions in the skin that lead to the synthesis of vitamin D, which, in turn, is vital to calcium metabolism and bone formation. Now we have learned that barefoot contact with the earth is vital to proper functioning of the immune system. Together such discoveries as these provide a scientific perspective on the ancient and mythical origins of Asian medical traditions such as acupuncture – a recognition of our place in nature: between the heavens above and the earth below [25]:

> Man proceeds from Heaven and from Earth. He is as much a part of one as of the other and incorporates within himself the principles of both.

At the beginning of this Foreword, I asked:

1. Why has modern medicine, with its powerful analytical tools, given so little attention to exploring the medicines of other cultures and other medical traditions before ours?
2. Exactly what is meant by 'healing accomplished by moving energy'?

After talking to many physicians I now believe that the main answer to the first question is that medical schools do not teach physics, biophysics and quantum mechanics (with rare exceptions, such as the recently disbanded Department of Physiology and Biophysics at Georgetown University, where the coeditor of this volume teaches). This deficit means that the average physician simply does not have the basic science that would enable a discussion of the biology of energy. When acupuncturists and other energy medicine practitioners attempt to describe the basis for their arts, the physician is often bewildered. The book you are holding in your hands would be a fine gift for such a physician and, indeed, an extremely important one for any physician, as the lack of knowledge of some basic science has had the tragic consequence of slowing the application of ancient wisdom and therapeutic techniques to modern medical theory and practice – where they are urgently needed.

With regard to the second question about healing through moving energy, we are beginning to have some sensible hypotheses to explain aspects of the nature of *qi*. As a scientist, I recognize that our scientific understandings of energetics are still limited, with the consequence that scientific understandings of *qi* remain somewhat elusive. However, I am confident that this picture will get clearer as science progresses and as health practitioners (who use *qi* every day to help their patients) learn to speak the language of physics and energetics. All of us who seek solutions to serious health issues have much to share with each other. The process is exciting and worthwhile, for not only is *qi* vital, but its understanding will be enlightening beyond our present comprehension. This book goes a long way in that important direction.

REFERENCES

[1] From a lecture, *Electronic Biology and Cancer*, presented at the Marine Biological Laboratory, Woods Hole, Massachusetts, July, 1972.

[2] Oschman JL. Energy Medicine: The scientific basis. Edinburgh: Churchill Livingstone; 2000.

[3] Szent-Györgyi A. Towards a new biochemistry. Science 1941;93(2426):609–11.

[4] Bretscher MS. A major protein which spans the human erythrocyte membrane. J Mol Biol 1971;59(2):351–7.

[5] Bretscher MS. Major human erythrocyte glycoprotein spans the cell membrane. Nat New Biol 1971;231(25):229–32.

[6] Berezney R, Coffey DS. Isolation and characterization of a framework structure from rat liver nuclei. J Cell Biol 1977;73(3):616–37.

[7] Pienta KJ, Coffey DS. Cellular harmonic information transfer through a tissue tensegrity-matrix system. Med Hypotheses 1991;34(1):88–95.

[8] Oschman JL, Oschman. Matter, energy, and the living matrix. Rolf Lines (Rolf Institute, Boulder, CO) 1993;21(3):55–64.

[9] Matsumoto K, Birch S. Hara Diagnosis: Reflections on the sea. Brookline, MA: Paradigm Publications; 1988.

[10] Langevin H. Connective tissue: a body-wide signaling network? Med Hypotheses 2006;66(6):1074–117.

[11] Finando S, Finando D. Fascia and the mechanism of acupuncture. J Bodyw Mov Ther 2011;15(2):168–76.

[12] Langevin H, Yandow J. Relationship of acupuncture points and meridians to connective tissue planes. Anat Rec 2002;269(6):257–65.

[13] Rimpler M, Bräuer H. *Matrixtherapie*. Günter Albert Ulmer Verlag, Tuningen, Germany; 2004. p. 25.

[14] Lee P. Interface: Mechanisms of spirit in osteopathy. Portland, OR: Stillness Press; 2005.

[15] Ho MW, Knight DP. The acupuncture system and the liquid crystalline collagen fibers of the connective tissues. Am. J. Chin. Med. 1998;26(3–4):1–13.

[16] Ho MW. Quantum coherence and conscious experience. Kybernetes 1997;26(3):265–76.

[17] Oschman JL. Energy Medicine in Therapeutics and Human Performance. Oxford: Butterworth Heinemann; 2003.

[18] Strogatz SH. Sync: How order emerges from chaos in the universe, nature, and daily life. New York, NY: Hyperion; 2004.

[19] Oschman JL. Can electrons act as antioxidants? A review and commentary. J Altern Complement Med 2007;13(9):955–67.

[20] Amalu W. Medical Thermography case studies. Online. Available: http://www.earthinginstitute.net/studies/thermographic_histories_2004.pdf 27 Jan 2011.

[21] Online. Available: http://www.earthinginstitute.net/index.php/research 22 Jan 2011.

[22] Sokal K, Sokal P. Earthing the human body influences physiological processes. J Altern Complement Med 2011; in press.

[23] Chevalier G, Mori K. The effects of earthing on human physiology. Part II. Electrodermal measurements. Subtle Energies and Energy Medicine 2007;18(3):11–34.

[24] National Library of Medicine database, Pub Med. Online. Available: http://www.ncbi.nlm.nih.gov/sites/entrez 21 Jan 2011.

[25] Requena Y. In: Terrains and pathology in acupuncture. Volume One: Correlations with diathetic medicine. Brookline, MA: Paradigm; 1986. p. 1.

PREFACE

A few professional texts on energy medicine have been published, and have been broadly welcomed. In the main, they have focused on practice and possible scientific mechanisms, regarding the human organism as a physical body in what we think of as 'geophysical' or 'neo-Newtonian' space and time. The current book addresses what has been called 'bioenergy' through the ancient cultural concept of *qi*, focusing on the living human organism in its bioenergetic, ecological and ecocultural contexts. It thus provides a 'natural history' in the sense of observations of the living in a natural environment.

Section 1 offers a cross-cultural approach to the history of *qi*; Section 2 lays a solid foundation for the understanding of its role in Chinese medicine, and also covers research on *qi* cultivation (*qigong*). Section 3 continues the theme of scientific research on *qi*. Section 4 looks in more detail at specific therapeutic modalities based upon *qi*, and Section 5 further explores clinical applications to specific health and medical conditions where working with an awareness of *qi* has been shown to be efficacious and meaningful for both patient and practitioner. The concluding section draws together the many themes that thread their way through the book, and an online Glossary at http://www.welwynacupuncture.co.uk/files/energymedicine_glossary.pdf provides a useful resource for further reading.

The field of *qi* is a broad and rich one, and we hope this book does it justice even if, as will quickly become clear to the reader, it is not really possible to confine experience, knowledge and understanding of it within printed pages, and certainly not meaningful simply to equate *qi* with 'energy' – although terms such as 'bioenergy' provide useful parallels. In putting the book together, we have ourselves learned a great deal about both ancient and modern aspects of *qi* and the varieties of energy medicine in practice. We hope you will find reading it as rewarding.

This book, initially proposed by Marc S Micozzi, grew from a shared interest in aspects of *qi* and energy medicine complementary to what had already published in the 'geophysical' sense. David Mayor had researched the history of electricity while compiling his textbook *Electroacupuncture*, and in the process became fascinated by the many parallels between 'electricity', 'life force' and *qi* that have been drawn over the centuries. Marc S Micozzi has investigated many forms of energy medicine in the many books he has written and edited on complementary and alternative medicine (CAM). Both have practiced extensively in the field themselves, with over 50 years of combined experience between them.

David Mayor and Marc S Micozzi

April 2011

CONTRIBUTORS

Mones S Abu-Asab, PhD
Senior Research Biologist, National
Cancer Institute, Bethesda, MD, USA

Amy L Ai, PhD
Professor, School of Social Work and
Department of Family Medicine,
University of Pittsburgh, Pittsburgh,
PA, USA

Hakima Amri, PhD
Director, CAM Master of Science
degree in Physiology, Georgetown
University Medical Center,
Washington, DC, USA

Claire M Cassidy, PhD, Dipl Ac, LAc
Director, Windpath Healing Works,
Bethesda, MD, USA

Nancy N Chen, PhD
Professor of Anthropology,
University of California, Santa Cruz,
CA, USA

Gideon Enz, DMQ
Senior instructor, International
Institute of Medical *Qigong*, Pacific
Grove, CA, USA

Kevin V Ergil, MA, MS, LAc
Professor, Finger Lakes School of
Acupuncture and Oriental Medicine
of New York Chiropractic College,
Seneca Falls, NY, USA

Peter H Fraser, BAc, BA
Chief Scientific Officer, NES Health,
Alicante, Spain

Mary Lou Galantino, PT, PhD, MSCE
Professor of Physical Therapy,
Richard Stockton College of New
Jersey, Pomona, NJ, USA

John A Ives, PhD
Director, Brain, Mind, and Healing
Program, Samueli Institute,
Alexandria, VA, USA

Wayne B Jonas, MD
President and Chief Executive
Officer, Samueli Institute,
Alexandria, VA, USA

Eric Leskowitz, MD
Psychiatrist, Pain Management
Program, Spaulding Rehabilitation
Hospital, Boston, MA, USA

May Loo, MD
Assistant Clinical Professor,
Department of Pediatrics and
Department of Anesthesia,
University Medical Center, Stanford,
CA, USA

Christopher Low, PhD, CAc(Nanjing, PRC)
Joint Clinical Director, Cambridge
Complementary Health Practice,
Cambridge, UK

Carolyn McMakin, DC, MA
Clinical Director, Fibromyalgia and
Myofascial Pain Clinic, Portland,
OR, USA

David Mayor, MA, BAc
Acupuncturist, Welwyn Garden City,
Hertfordshire, Research Associate,
Department of Physiotherapy,
University of Hertfordshire, UK

Marc S Micozzi, MD, PhD
Adjunct Professor, Department
of Medicine, University of
Pennsylvania, Philadelphia, PA,
Department of Physiology and
Biophysics, Georgetown University,
Washington, DC, USA

Phil Mollon, PhD
Head of Psychology and
Psychotherapy Services, Lister
Hospital, Stevenage, Hertfordshire, UK

Laura Muscatello, DPT
Graduate student, Doctor of Physical
Therapy (DPT) Program, Richard
Stockton College of New Jersey,
Pomona, NJ, USA

Tim Newman, LicAc, DTM, CertZB
Acupuncturist, Artist and
Ambassador of Touch, Cornwall and
London, UK

James L Oschman, PhD
President, Nature's Own Research
Association Dover, NH, USA

F David Peat, PhD, Msc
Founder, Pari Center for New
Learning, Pari, Tuscany, Italy

Franklyn Sills, MA, RCST
Co-founder, Karuna Institute,
Widecombe-in-the-Moor, Devon, UK

Cyril W Smith, PhD
Honorary Senior Lecturer (Retired),
University of Salford, Greater
Manchester, UK

Darren Starwynn, Dipl Ac, OMD
Research Director, Eastwestmed,
Phoenix, AZ, USA

Patrizia Stefanini, PhD
Director, Istituto Europeo di Shiatsu,
Milan, Italy

John L Stump, DC, PhD, EdD
Founder, Integrative Medicine
Center, Fairhope, AL, USA

Gabriel Stux, MD
Director, German Acupuncture
Society, Düsseldorf, Germany

Christopher C Taylor, PhD
Independent scholar, Birmingham,
AL, USA

Alan Watkins, PhD, MBBS
Honorary Senior Lecturer in
Neuroscience, Imperial College,
London, UK

ACKNOWLEDGMENTS

Our mutual friend Richard Hammerschlag for bringing us together back in February 2007; Mary Law, Karen Morley and Claire Wilson, our trio of successive editors at Elsevier, for their support, and Catherine Jackson, development editor, Chris Wyard, copyeditor, and Beula Christopher, project manager, for all their hard work. Inta Ozols, our first editor at Churchill Livingstone (now Elsevier), who in particular connected Marc S Micozzi with talented thinkers, researchers, practitioners and writers, some of whom appear in this book 15 years later. Yuzuru Masuda, Ariel Li-Ting Tsai and Trina Ward for their linguistic skills. John Moffett of the Needham Research Institute (Cambridge) for his generosity. Above all, our contributors for their patience, and also those who helped us find them. And, of course, our wives, for their tolerance and without whom there would be no book.

In addition, David Mayor would like to thank Marc Micozzi for his editorial expertise and companionable *randori*, Angelika Strixner for introducing him to the healing work of Bob Moore, and his Five Rhythm dancing companions on Tuesday evenings for keeping him sane (even if it didn't always look like it).

Marc S Micozzi thanks David Mayor, truly a 'treasure house' of knowledge about the history and current practice, East and West, of energy in healing; and Claire Cassidy – who has been with me as a collaborator from my first text in 1995 to this most recent one – for yet another fine contribution from her unique perspective.

ABBREVIATIONS

AB design   An experimental design comparing, for example, an active intervention (A) and a control (B)

Acetyl-CoA   Acetyl coenzyme A

ACTH   Adrenocorticotropic hormone

AD   Allergy (EAV meridian)

ADHD   Attention Deficit Hyperactivity Disorder

ADP   Adenosine diphosphate

AE   Aggressive energy

A-field   Magnetic vector potential

AIDS   Acquired immune deficiency syndrome

AK   Applied Kinesiology

AMA   American Medical Association

AMI   Apparatus for measuring the function of the meridians and the corresponding Internal Organs

AMP   Adenosine monophosphate

ANS   Autonomic nervous system

AOM   Acupuncture and oriental medicine

ART   Antiretroviral therapy

ASC   Altered states of consciousness

ATP   Adenosine triphosphate

ATP-ase   Adenosine triphosphatase

B-field   Magnetic field of flux density **B**

BMI   Body mass index

BP   Blood pressure

b.p.m.   Beats per minute

c The speed of light (approx. 300 000 kilometers per second)

C   Coulomb (SI unit of charge)

CAM   Complementary and alternative medicine

CBT   Cognitive behavioral therapy

CCT   Controlled clinical trial

CD4+   T cell (lymphocyte) expressing the surface protein CD4

CD8+   Cytotoxic T cell (lymphocyte)

CDCP   Centers for Disease Control and Prevention

CDSB   *Chun-do-sun-bup*

CF   Causative factor

CFS   Chronic fatigue syndrome

Ci   Circulation/pericardium (EAV meridian)

CM   Chinese medicine

CORE   Clinical Outcomes in Routine Evaluation

CRF   Corticotropin releasing factor

CRI   Cranial rhythmic impulse

CV   Cardiovascular

DBP   Diastolic blood pressure

DHA   Docosahexanoic acid

DMILS   Distant mental influence on living systems

DNA   Deoxyribonucleic acid

DRC   Democratic Republic of Congo

e Elementary unit of charge, charge of a single electron (1.602 176 487(40) $\times$ 10^{-19} coulombs)

EAV   Electroacupuncture according to Voll

EBV   Epstein–Barr virus

ECG   Electrocardiogram

ED   Energetic driver (fields)

EDP	External diaphragm pacer
EEG	Electroencephalogram
EFT	Emotional Freedom Techniques
EI	Energetic integrator (fields)
EMDR	Eye Movement Desensitization and Reprocessing
EMG	Electromyogram
EPA	Eicosapentanoic acid
ESP	Extrasensory perception
ET	Energetic terrain (information sequences)
FatD	Fatty degeneration (EAV meridian)
FibD	Fibroid degeneration (EAV meridian)
FM	Fibromyalgia (syndrome)
FSM	Frequency specific microcurrent
G	Gauss (non-SI unit, = 100 μT); giga (= 10^{+9})
GHRH	Growth hormone releasing hormone
GSR	Galvanic skin response
h	Planck's constant (6.626 068 96(33) × 10^{-34} Joule seconds)
H^+	Hydrogen ions (protons)
HAART	Highly active antiretroviral therapy
HbA1c	Hemoglobin A1c
HDL	High-density lipoprotein
HIA	Hemagglutination inhibition assay
HIV	Human immunodeficiency virus
HPA	Hypothalamic–pituitary–adrenal axis; hypothalamo-pituitary axis
HRV	Heart rate variability
HT	Healing Touch
5-HT	5-hydroxytryptamine (serotonin)
5-HTP	5-hydroxytryptophan
Hz	Hertz (SI unit of frequency, cycles per second)
IFN-γ	Interferon gamma
IgA	Immunoglobulin A
IL	Interleukin
IP	Identified patient
J	Joule (SI unit of energy)
JAMA	*Journal of the American Medical Association*
JD	Joint degeneration (EAV meridian)
k	Kilo (= 10^{+3})
k	Boltzmann constant (1.380 650 4(24) × 10^{-23} joules per kelvin)
K	Kelvin (SI unit of thermodynamic temperature)
kT	The energy in joules corresponding to a Kelvin temperature of T
LDL	Low-density lipoprotein
Ly	Lymph (EAV meridian)
m	Meter (SI unit of length); milli (= 10^{-3})
M	Mega (= 10^{+6})
μ	Micro (= 10^{-6})
MLC	Meridian-like channel
MOS-HIV	Medical outcomes short form HIV
MRI	Magnetic resonance imaging
MS	Multiple sclerosis
n	Nano (= 10^{-9})
N	Newton (SI unit of force)
NA	New Age
NAD	Nicotinamine adenine dinucleotide
NADA	National Acupuncture Detoxification Association
NANDA	North American Nursing Diagnosis Association
NCCAM	National Center for Complementary and Alternative Medicine
ND	Nerve degeneration (EAV meridian)
NES	Nutri-Energetic Systems
NIH	National Institutes of Health
NK	Natural killer
NMIH	National Institute of Mental Health

O$_2$ pulse	Oxygen uptake per heart beat at rest	SAM	Sympathetic-adrenomedullary system
OI	Opportunistic infection	SBP	Systolic blood pressure
OM	Oriental medicine	Sk	Skin degeneration (EAV meridian)
Or	Organ degeneration (EAV meridian)	SNS	Sympathetic nervous system
P$_i$	Inorganic phosphate		
PEP	Psychoanalytic Energy Psychotherapy	SSRI	Serotonin selective reuptake inhibitor
PG	Phosphoglycerate	ST segment	Gap between S and T waves in the heart's electrical signal indicating coronary artery blockage
pH	'Potentiometric hydrogen' ion concentration (measure of acidity/alkalinity)		
PMS	Premenstrual syndrome	T	Tesla (SI unit of magnetic flux density or **B**-field, Webers per meter^2)
PNI	Psychoneuro-immunology or psycho-neuroimmunological		
PNS	Parasympathetic nervous system	TAT	Tapas Acupressure Technique
PRE	Progressive resistive exercise	TCM	Traditional Chinese medicine
PT	Physical therapy	TDO	Tryptophan 2,3-dioxygenase
PTSD	Posttraumatic stress disorder	TENS	Transcutaneous electrical nerve stimulation
P wave	Deflection in the heart's electrical signal occurring when the atria contract	TFT	Thought Field Therapy
		TMS	Traditional medical systems
QED	Quantum electrodynamics	TNF-α	Tumor necrosis factor alpha
QG	*Qigong*		
QOL	Quality of life	TNF-γ	Tumor necrosis factor gamma
QRS complex	Deflections in the heart's electrical signal occurring when the ventricles contract	TT	Therapeutic Touch
		T wave	Deflection in the heart's electrical signal on repolarization
RCT	Randomized controlled trial	URI	Upper respiratory infection
REMAP	Reed Eye-movement Acupressure Psychotherapy	U wave	A deflection in the heart's electrical signal
		VA	Peak late left ventricular filling velocity in diastole
RNA	Ribonucleic acid		
ROM	Range of movement		
ROS	Reactive oxygen species	VE	Peak early filling velocity in diastole
RR interval	Interval between two successive R wave peaks	VO$_2$	Oxygen consumption
R wave	Most prominent deflection recordable from the heart's electrical signal	Wb	Weber (SI unit of magnetic flux)
		WHO	World Health Organization
s	Second (SI unit of time)	ZB	Zero Balancing

SECTION 1
THE ETHNOMEDICINE OF ENERGY – A GLOBAL VIEW

SECTION CONTENTS

SECTION INTRODUCTION

Ethnomedical studies open the door to understanding the health beliefs and behaviors of traditional societies around the globe. In egalitarian cross-cultural comparison, the concept of a 'vital energy' in conceptualizations of health and healing is commonplace through time and place. We are now generally familiar with how the concept of *qi* animates, informs and guides Asian medical systems as shown in the chapter by Nancy Chen. Chris Taylor takes us into the heart of Africa for an example of a corresponding metaphor outside the sphere of Asian influence, while David Mayor demonstrates the deep roots of energy medicine and many of the attributes of *qi* within the European tradition itself.

When considering the ancient medical traditions of China, India, Tibet and the Middle East it is useful to recognize that all of South, East and Southeast Asia are territories that came under the influence of two of the earliest great civilizations at the dawn of history. The cultural diffusion concepts of 'Further India' and 'Greater China' are useful to consider as succeeding waves of influence emanating from the great river valleys of the Indus and the Yellow River, respectively, carrying along common discoveries and understandings of the nature of human life and health.

A second wave occurred with the flowering of Buddhism, and ultimately a third wave, that of Islam, spread ideas from the western border of North Africa to the eastern edge of Indonesia during the 700 years from 750 to 1450 CE. This third wave carried along ancient Greco-Roman (*Unani*, or Arabic for 'Greek') concepts of health and healing that it had incorporated and preserved following the Classical Era in the West. All three of these traditions place emphasis on the concept of vital energy as central to health and healing.

This concept of vital energy (*prana* in India, and *qi* in China) is still fundamental in many Asian medical traditions. The ancient Chinese ideogram for *qi* symbolized a cloudlike vapor, as when the breath is seen on a cold day. This evanescence of the very nature of *qi* has always been difficult to capture in words. In the West, for example, *qi* has been translated to imply the flow of energy, spirit, or breath that animates living beings, as 'vital energy', or 'subtle energy'. We hope that the explications in this book, with its comparisons with other global traditions, will further understanding and encourage a wider debate on the meaning of *qi* without diluting it.

In Central Africa, flows and blockages of fluid or force also influence health and wellbeing. That there are two sides to this coin is reflected not only in the dark history of Rwanda unraveled in Chapter 2, but also in many cultures where healers may be feared for the very power they are believed to wield. *Djambe*, for example, a Central and East African concept, is an energy or power that can manifest a malign nature as well as a beneficial one. This ability of energy both to help and to harm is paralleled in medicine by the placebo/nocebo dualism, and in the 'words that heal/words that harm' concept of Dr Larry Dossey (more on this aspect of energy medicine can be found in the final chapter of this book).

Qi in Asian medicine

Nancy N Chen

I

CHAPTER CONTENTS

The concept of *qi* can be found in many Asian medical traditions. In the West *qi* has been translated to refer to the flow of energy, spirit, or breath that animates living entities. Ancient Chinese ideograms depicted the term with three horizontal strokes to symbolize cloudlike vapor, as when the breath is seen on a cold day. During the Song dynasty (960–1127 CE) the term was elaborated to include four strokes (气), above the character for rice (米) and this form (氣) continues to be used in classical Chinese (Fig. 1.1). Contemporary Chinese *pinyin* has simplified the term to the top four strokes (气), but without including the character beneath for rice.

In the Chinese language, *qi* is ubiquitous, reflecting its wide usage in everyday contexts (as in Japan, see Ch. 16). It is a compound term having many meanings, and is used in words that describe a range of entities including atmosphere, environment, flavor, feeling and emotional state. Thus context is crucial to understanding the influence of this 'energy' in plural forms.

Daoist texts, some as early as 300 BCE with later transmissions on bamboo and silk, address *qi* as an immanent elemental force that shapes both the universe and individual bodies. *Qi* comes in many forms (from refined and immaterial to condensed and heavy). It can also be cultivated by the individual through breathing and special exercises. As Livia Kohn's writings on Daoism suggest, 'breathing for life' was a critical form of accessing *qi* as an energetic force [1]. Experiences of *qi* can be quite subjective but the overall view of *qi* as energy and generative force suggests that life itself is not possible without it.

Asian medicine is diverse, comprising multiple formations of knowledge and practice interwoven within a broad range of ethnomedical traditions in the region [2,3]. This chapter offers an overview of the knowledge and practice of *qi* across these diverse healing modalities and theories of the body. Within the specific context of medicine, the subjective and social experiences of *qi* come together. In Asian medical theory, *qi* takes on a particular meaning not simply as a form that stands alone, but also as an entity that flows and brings vital energy to the organs and channels (sometimes termed meridians) it traverses or inhabits [4]. The cultivation of *qi*, and significantly its movement, is critical to wellbeing.

Asian medicine is diverse with iconic texts, notable practitioners and concepts that may date back centuries, even millennia; these medical systems tend to be

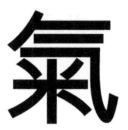

FIG 1.1   The classical Chinese character for *ki* (*qi*).

characterized as traditional or unchanging. It is crucial to realize, however, that each system of knowledge has significantly evolved, often with the intervention of state institutions. Moreover, the travel of practitioners, translated texts and pharmacopeias across Asia all contribute to multiple forms or genealogies of medical knowledge. How then to study the many different forms that come under the rubric of Asian medicine? How might it be possible to address the different historical, geographical, social, ethnolinguistic or political contexts that have shaped bodies of knowledge and medical practice? [5] A pragmatic approach could be based on textual sources and their transmission via translators. This transmission has depended in part on regional proximity and on sharing the same written language, as was the case for ancient China, Japan and Korea (where classical Chinese characters were in use until the fifteenth century CE). Another approach considers the modalities or treatment techniques that may overlap or, more often, come to define distinct characteristics of a particular system. A third comparative framework entails examining regional ethnomedical practices based on *materia medica*. In what follows, we will examine the role of *qi* through each of these lenses.

I begin by addressing how *qi* was integral for views of the body and medical practice in East Asia beginning with Chinese medicine and its later transmission to Korean and Japanese formations of medicine. These three systems refer to *qi* (*gi* or *ki*), as a form of energy that shapes all bodies. We briefly turn to the techniques and modalities incorporating *qi* that comprise these medical practices. Since other chapters in this volume address specific therapeutic modalities, my discussion will focus on the ways in which *qi* might be conceptualized in forms of energy healing. We consider notions of energy in Ayurveda, *Unani* (Greco-Islamic) and Tibetan medicines that bear resemblance to *qi* energy healing. Finally, I will address how *qigong* emerged as a social practice and global formation in the late twentieth century that greatly increased awareness of energetic forms of healing.

QI IN PREMODERN CHINESE, KOREAN AND JAPANESE MEDICINE

Chinese medicine is often referred to as traditional Chinese medicine (TCM) in Western societies, whereas in Chinese it is simply called *zhongyi* (中医, Chinese medicine). The term TCM suggests a long, storied history over several thousand years where theories and practices came to form a linear system of knowledge. In this chapter, we will identify the earlier medical theories as 'classical' or 'premodern' Chinese medicine and contemporary forms since 1950 as 'TCM'. Volker Scheid and other leading scholars of Chinese medicine note the distinction between broader traditions of Chinese medicine and the more recent formation of TCM [6]. The former is 'characterized by a diversity that encompasses every aspect of its organization and practice, from theory and diagnosis to prognosis, therapeutics, and the social organization of health care.' [7] By contrast, TCM became systematized during the 1950s in mainland China with TCM colleges, publications of medical texts, clinical and laboratory research, licensing practices and standardization of knowledge. The institutional formations of TCM as a state system transformed Chinese medicine from multiple schools of thought and practice to a streamlined body of knowledge transmitted through state-published medical texts rather than through generations of individual practitioners [8].

Classical texts in Chinese medicine date back to the second century BCE and include materials ranging from silk documents excavated from the Mawangdui Han tombs (168 BCE or earlier) to widely translated works such as the *Huangdi Neijing* (黄帝内經, *Yellow Emperor's Canon of Internal Medicine*) [9] and the *Shen Nong Bencaojing* (神農本草經, *Divine Farmer's Materia Medica*) [10] (see Fig. 1.2). The latter is less a treatise on premodern medical theory and more a compilation of plant and other material substances and their influences on the body. The earliest mention of *qi* in the Mawangdui manuscripts is in terms of vapor [11]. Vivienne Lo's analysis of the Mawangdui texts suggests that nuanced concepts of life nurturance and transformative practices were made possible with the integration of earlier notions of *yangsheng* (養生, 'nurturing generation') through breath cultivation and meditation. These 'evolving' categories preceded the more formalized notions of *qi* evident in the later manuscripts of the *Neijing* [12].

The *Huangdi Neijing* consists of two texts (the *Suwen*, 素問, or *Basic Questions*, and *Lingshu*, 靈樞, *Spiritual Pivot*) of which the *Suwen* is perhaps the most famous owing to its wide translation. The chapters consist of a dialog or series of questions between the Yellow Emperor, *Huangdi*, and his ministers. Paul Unschuld's analysis of the *Suwen* and its various translations addresses the role of *qi* as foundational to bodies. He notes that the term is often used together with, and even inseparable from, that for Blood (*xue*, 血). There is a hierarchy between these bodily substances, however, such that wherever *qi* flows so too does Blood [13,14]. Considerable discussion in the *Suwen* is devoted to the Five Organs (*zang*, 臟) – the Heart (*xin*, 心), Spleen (*pi*, 脾), Lung (*fei*, 肺), Kidney (*shen*, 腎), and Liver (*gan*, 肝) – and how each of these entities houses a different form of *qi*. This is also referred to as the Five Phases, or Five Elements (*wuxing*, 五行), and Six *Qi* (*liu qi*, 六氣). The Organs not only house but also facilitate an intimate relationship between *qi* and emotional states [15, p 161]:

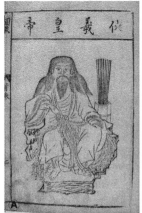
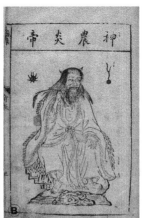
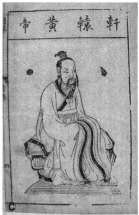

FIG 1.2   Three legendary emperors associated with the birth of Chinese medicine: (A) Fu Xi (伏羲), (B) Shen Nong (神農) and (C) Huang Di (黄帝), the Yellow Emperor. After woodcuts by the Tan dynasty artist Gan Bozong. *(With permission of the Wellcome Library, London)*

When one is angry, the qi *rises.*
When one is happy, the qi *is relaxed.*
When one is sad, then the qi *dissipates.*
When one is in fear, then the qi *moves down.*

Unschuld notes that *qi* in the *Suwen* is a multivalent term used to refer not just to vapor but also to a range of bodily states and transformations due to pathology. In other parts of the *Suwen*, he notes that 'camp' (*ying*, 營) *qi* and 'protective' (*wei*, 衛) *qi* are paired opposites, reflecting the forms of qi that are obtained from food and water and can either move within a vessel (*ying qi*) or within the skin (*wei qi*) [15, p 164]. Movement of these two forms of *qi* determined health, whereas the cessation of this movement meant pathology or death. As circulation was crucial to essential *qi*, the correlation of bodily channels and Organs to ministerial posts and functions indicated an intimate correspondence between body, cosmos and state. Nathan Sivin has also analyzed how the flow of *qi* within bodily formations informed both political formations and rightful rule, such that the greater cosmological order reflected ancient Chinese bureaucracy [16].

The original text of the *Lingshu*, the second part of the *Huangdi Neijing*, no longer exists, and translations are based on later editions from the twelfth century. The *Lingshu* (*Spiritual Pivot*) is also called the *Canon of Acupuncture* and mainly addresses the meridians (*jingluo*, 經絡) or pathways for the circulation of *qi*, and the acupuncture points (*zhenxue*, 針穴) through which *qi* enters and leaves the body. *Qi* remains a critical concept as its flow or movement within the body could be enhanced by acupuncture techniques.

Through the classical texts, it is possible to view concepts of *qi* and how these became integral to theories about the body and medical treatment. These concepts traveled widely as the transmission of medicine took place wherever exchange occurred across and beyond the Chinese empire. Both Korean and Japanese medicine utilize the concept of *gi* or *ki* based on early translations of Chinese medical texts and the introduction of medical practitioners to their courts [17].

Adoption of Chinese medical theory and *materia medica* took place sooner in Korea owing largely to its location adjacent to the Chinese empire. During the Song dynasty (970–1279), medical texts such as the *Suwen* were imported to the Koryo court [18]. Early forms of Korean medicine engaged extensively with Chinese medical theories of *yin* (陰) and *yang* (陽) (the opposite but complementary qualities of all things), meridians, acupuncture and *qi*. Later forms of Korean medicine evolved with herbal medicine indigenous to the area and with charismatic Buddhist monks who focused on healing. Eventually a hybrid system of knowledge utilizing Chinese medical concepts and local plants became the foundation of traditional Korean medicine. As with Chinese medicine, famous doctors renowned for their techniques and writings were key figures in promulgating the spread of medical beliefs and practice through texts.

During the fifth and sixth centuries, Chinese medicine was introduced to Japan through a range of travelers between the countries including court emissaries, physicians and, not least, monks. Song dynasty medical texts were a key part of this transmission of knowledge [19]. As with Korean medicine, Japanese integration of Chinese medicine incorporated basic medical principles of *ki*, *yin–yang* and notions of balance. Premodern medical texts such as the tenth-century *Ishimpo* (医心方, *Methods at the Heart of Medicine*) and a sixteenth-century eight-volume medical work by Manase Dosan, the *Keitekishu* (啓迪集, *Textbook of Internal Medicine*), utilize these theories in their discussion of diseases and their treatment [20,21]. Japanese medicine was influenced not only by Chinese medical theory but also by Buddhist and Zen practitioners, and from the late eighteenth century by Western medical knowledge introduced by the Dutch and Germans. Traditional Japanese medicine also evolved to develop specialized knowledge of acupressure (*shiatsu*), distinct techniques in acupuncture, bone manipulation and setting techniques.

Today the integrated form of Chinese medicine in Japan is referred to as *Kampo* (漢方). Like its TCM counterpart, *Kampo* has integrated evidence-based research and biomedical discourse such that *ki* in contemporary *Kampo* is described as 'a vital energy that allows the mind and body to function appropriately, which may correspond to activities of the central nervous system (CNS) and autonomic nervous system. The functioning of *ki* can be disturbed by psychosocial stressors' [22].

The transmission of Chinese medicine to other regions in Asia took multiple pathways. Besides official delegations, medicinal herb traders, spiritual pilgrims and itinerant healers contributed to the spread of Chinese medicine and its applications throughout Asia. The presence of Chinese medicine can be seen across present-day Southeast, Central and South Asia. Though diverse in practice and application, it could be argued that it is the notion of *qi* and its mutable forms that unifies these different manifestations of practice.

Today TCM is a global entity that is quite distinct from its premodern counterpart. The chief modalities that have come to characterize TCM include: acupuncture, moxibustion, herbal medicine, dietary therapy, massage and *qigong*. Notions of *qi*, its cultivation and flow are critical to each of these modalities. Moreover, the meridians or channels through which *qi* flows or can be blocked or become stagnant are key sites in considerations of pathology and therapeutic intervention. Although notions of *qi* in TCM theory and practice seem similar to those of classical or premodern forms of Chinese medicine, there has been a transition in the definition and uses of *qi* in contemporary TCM texts. In the *Suwen*, for instance, *qi* was defined as both a cosmic force and a bodily substance. The notion of *qi* in post-1949 medical texts, however, tends to reflect solely physiological dimensions and emphasizes it primarily as a bodily substance like blood and other bodily fluids. Such a transition is due in part to the medicalizing discourses of scientific Marxism where social, environmental and phenomenological meanings of the body and its forms are reconfigured into more material categories with physical properties. The body becomes less an energetic entity and is reduced to one that is more predictable and diagrammable [8].

As traders, nomads and emissaries traversed the Silk Routes, Chinese medical texts and medicinal herbs were also part of these travel circuits [21]. In what follows, I turn to other formations of Asian medical practice, namely Ayurveda, *Unani* and Tibetan forms of medicine. Chinese medicine and notions of *qi* certainly reached the Southern and Central Asian regions where these were practiced but were also part of a broader system of ideas and exchange. Nevertheless, notions of energetic healing can be found in these systems of healing. The flow of energy within a body as a source of vitality is a concept shared by nearly all Asian medical systems, although indigenous ethnomedicine based on local knowledge of plants or herbs was also critical to establishing diverse and vibrant forms of medical practice.

ASIAN MEDICAL SYSTEMS AND NOTIONS OF ENERGY

Ayurveda emerged in South Asia and is considered to have a history of nearly 5000 years. Translated as the 'knowledge or science of life', this system of healing consists of a range of practices including meditation, yoga, massage, diet and herbal medicines and tonics. Galenic medicine, and in particular its belief in humors, greatly influenced Ayurveda. Human bodies are constituted by three, rather than four, main humoral entities, or *doshas*: *pitta* (Bile), *vata* (Wind) and *kapha* (Phlegm). Another central concept is *prana*, considered to be the 'breath of life' [23], and close to the concept of *qi*. It is part of a trilogy of forces including *agni* (the spirit of light or fire) and *soma* (harmony and love). The *Upanishads*, the earliest of which date from the first millennium and are among the earliest Hindu texts, refer to *prana* as part of the physical world, providing the vital energy that sustains all living forms. The later philosophies that form the basis of yoga consider *prana* to flow through subtle channels (*nadi*, 'tubes') in the body, through which bodily fluids such as blood and semen also pass. In Ayurvedic thought, *prana* is further differentiated into five forms known as the *prana vayu* which sustain bodily processes such as circulation (*prana*), digestion (*samana*), elimination (*apana*), vocalizing sounds (*udana*) and movement (*vyana*) [24].

Like *qigong*, which is discussed in the next section and elsewhere in this volume, *pranayama* is the practice of nurturing *prana* initially through breathwork and breath control techniques. The similarities, as well as differences, between *qi* and *prana* have been much debated by scholars of Asian medicine and spiritual practices. As Joseph Alter notes about the practices of *daoyin* (導引, considered to be the precursor of most forms of *qigong*) and hatha yoga, 'To even the casual observer the similarities … are striking' [25]. However, he cautions against the quick but 'erroneous conclusion' [23, p 228] that yoga and *qigong* are the same. Instead, he suggests that these practices reflect comparable developments in notions of self-cultivation and transformation since the thirteenth century. Rather than assuming these and other vital energies to be interchangeable concepts, it is, as emphasized above, critical to address the contexts of belief and practice of the different forms of energy medicine.

Another medical system originating in the ancient world was Greek medicine, whose texts were later translated extensively by Persian scholars. Its influence can be seen today in *Unani* medicine, which, like Ayurveda, is practiced mostly in South Asia. *Unani* means 'Greek' and refers to the lineage of Greco-Islamic medical knowledge that is traceable through the treatises of Avicenna (Ibn Sina) and Galen back to Hippocrates in the fifth century BCE. During the thirteenth to seventeenth centuries, *Unani* practitioners from Persia and Central Asia gained the patronage of the Mughal court and other elites in India [26]. *Unani* overlaps significantly with Ayurvedic principles [27]. Both systems rely on notions of the humors, which shape human bodies and temperaments, and also on the concept of a vital energy that is central to life (*pneuma* in Greek). However, despite many overlaps in concepts of bodily constitution and vital energy as well as herbal formularies, *Unani* differs in several ways. An initial distinction is in their language of transmission: whereas Ayurvedic texts are mostly derived from Sanskrit and Hindu sources, *Unani* manuscripts are mainly from Arabic and Persian texts. Another distinction lies in the preparation of the remedies used for energetic healing. Ayurvedic therapies focus on detoxification and rejuvenation, with a *materia medica* derived from local plants in South Asia that includes spices and herbs. *Unani*, with its reliance on the classic Greek theory of four humors and notions of balance that can be gained from fluids, preferentially uses herbal tonics based on old *Unani* recipes for syrups (as well as powders, pills and tablets). Today these are manufactured and sold to a broad, notably youthful consumer base in urban India. Like Chinese medicine, *Unani* relies on pulse diagnosis and examination of the tongue and stool to determine the source of imbalance. Possible therapies include cupping, sweating, diuresis, bathing, massage, cauterization, purging, and use of leeches. Diet therapy tends to be used ahead of pharmaceuticals, while the last resort is surgery [28].

As with other Asian medical systems, Tibetan medicine evolved with the exchange of materials and ideas through trade and traveling practitioners. However, the extent of interregional exchange along the silk roads and the level of collaboration between foreign scholars in Tibet between the eighth and eleventh centuries appear unique. Tibetan medicine incorporated theories from multiple sources of knowledge including Ayurveda, Persian, Ancient Greek, Central Asian and Chinese medicine. Although Ayurvedic medicine greatly influenced this system, Tibetan notions of the body are more complicated, with up to 15 subcategories of humors, while also incorporating notions of *karma* and Buddhist philosophy [29]. Perhaps more than any other Asian medical system, Tibetan medicine successfully conjoined medical knowledge with the traditions of Buddhism, with its ideals of compassion and activity in the service of others [30].

Rather than singling out one form of vital energy, as in the concept of *qi*, Tibetan medicine conceptualizes the body as based on three vital *ñes-pa* similar to the Ayurvedic *doshas*: *rLung*, Wind (cold, subtle, volatile), *mKhris-pa*, Bile (hot, liquid, flowing) and *Bad-kan*, Phlegm (cool, sluggish, solid). Each has five subtypes, and in addition there are seven principal bodily constituents (saliva, blood, bone, marrow, flesh, fat and semen) [31]. Of the *ñes-pa*, the nearest to *qi* is *rLung*. Careful attention is also accorded to the breath, as every living entity is animated by the 'breath of life' [32]. Theories of causation reflect close engagement with Buddhist beliefs about physical, emotional and mental states. Initial clinical diagnosis may include pulse reading, observation, enquiry and sometimes urine analysis. The therapeutic modalities depend upon the severity of symptoms, and include golden needle treatment, moxibustion, medicinal baths, enemas, purgatives, or massage in combination with spiritual prayer, as well as Five Element color therapy, and astrological consultation. There are definite overlaps with Ayurvedic and Chinese medicine, but Tibetan medicine has evolved over the centuries to form a distinctive set of medical knowledge and views of the body. Today it faces ongoing influences and challenges from TCM and biomedicine [33,34].

GLOBAL *QI* AND SELF-CULTIVATION

During the late twentieth century, *qigong*, or the practice of breathwork and healing through cultivating one's *qi*, became an immensely popular form of exercise and healing in urban contexts, especially in China itself. Throughout major cities and towns one could always find practitioners in the early dawn in parks, on sidewalks, near public buildings, on campuses and even in streets participating in daily regimens of *qigong* exercise. Broad social awareness of this practice was reflected in mainstream state newspapers as well as popular novels.

Qigong was understood as fostering the movement of *qi* through the body either by internal visualization and meditation or through external bodily practices involving physical movement. Rather than being viewed merely as a physical substance, *qi* was embraced as a cosmological energy by practitioners and masters. Such popular views of *qi* as a healing force seemed to return to earlier, more 'traditional' notions of *qi* according to which individuals could draw upon or embody its transformative powers present in the environment and cosmos rather than merely in a body confined by everyday spaces.

Most *qigong* manuals nevertheless tend to echo traditional medical texts in the discussion of *yin–yang* and how *qi* is manifested with these dual qualities. Experiencing *qi* was a central component of practice that all *qigong* practitioners encountered and discussed on a daily basis. However, as already mentioned, *qi* is polysemous and there are multiple forms of it, such that *qi* was widely invoked to describe different forms of practice. Tracing the genealogies of *qigong* thus entails a closer examination of the concepts of *qi*.

Despite the multitude of styles and genealogies of practice, *qigong* can be distinguished into two types: external and internal. The external form, based on *waidan* (外丹) cultivation principles, tends to emphasize 'hard' *qi* and 'hard' bodies that can withstand much force and perform with superhuman powers. This martial form tends to be practiced not so much in public parks but in arenas such as streets, acrobatic troupes, or even in military compounds. The internal and meditative form, based on *neidan* (內丹) cultivation, was pursued by practitioners of all backgrounds as such forms helped to promote the circulation and transformation of *qi* as crucial steps towards enhancing vitality.

Healing in the 1980s, the initial post-Mao period prior to the formation of a massive market economy and global pharmaceutical industry later in the 1990s, emerged simultaneously as both a private act for individuals and a public performance for masters. In contrast to previous decades where socialized medicine attended to the masses with a focus on public health, the emergence of *qigong* in the 1980s was linked to the desire for self-care and individualized forms of healing and daily practice. Elderly people could attend to their complaints of rheumatism or arthritis, long-term sufferers of neurasthenia or chronic pain could seek relief, and even parents of children with congenital disorders could seek help when no other options could be found in either traditional Chinese medicine or biomedicine. *Qigong* became a practice that promised release and hope. Whether in parks or in stadiums, it became acceptable to cry openly or express fervent belief in something that was not state ideology. As some forms of *qigong* began to overlap with Daoist, Buddhist and other spiritual practices, references to *qigong* as a religion or New Age spiritualism also appeared.

During the 1990s, official state discourses about *qigong* situated it clearly apart from popular *qigong* debate. While testimonial accounts of *qigong* healing continued, there were calls to differentiate between 'real' (*zhen*, 真) and 'false' (*jia*, 假) *qigong*. This was an attempt to separate out those individuals who claimed to be masters but healed for lucrative purposes from those with 'true' abilities practicing 'more orthodox and uniform' forms. Needless to say, the state appointed bureau regulating *qigong* used scientific discourse about *qigong* (*kexue de qigong*, 科學的氣功) as a means to cleanse and discipline the ranks of 'false' masters [35].

In the past decade, medical *qigong* continues to be offered in clinical settings. More charismatic forms, however, were politicized and circumscribed through licensing.

CONCLUSION

Asian medical systems can be characterized by an extensive history of pluralism in which texts, beliefs and *materia medica* traversed mountains, steppes, plateaus, plains, deserts and seas in circuits of exchange and trade. Medical systems flourished with the integration of medical theories, translations of texts, and practitioners engaged in contributing to certain genealogies of knowledge. Despite such a plurality of texts, practices and pharmacopeias, what is shared across all these systems is the following: a sense of disease as imbalance, the image of the body as a microcosm of the broader environment, or as a reflection of cosmological order, and an emphasis on vitality and flow, often in terms of vital energy or energetic healing. These broad generalizations, taken as the main focus of comparative study, can easily be used to gloss over the multiple directions and vibrant diversity of Asian therapeutic knowledge. Scholars of Asian medical systems remind us to be careful of making direct correlations or assuming shared categories among systems [36]. Rather, we need to understand that the seemingly analogous concepts of the body, its constitution and treatment can be understood as specific to particular histories of travel, translation and transmission over the centuries.

In the face of increasingly evidence-based medicine, with its emphasis on clinical trials and an ever more tightly focused biomedical discourse, the contemporary manifestations of these Asian medical systems and therapies face new challenges of integration, or confrontation, with the globalization of medical knowledge and practice. Vitality and its expression through energetic forms such as *qi* may continue as a unifying theme in such systems of medicine as long as in their therapeutic application the body is still considered an integral part of a broader universe of order and experience, part of a greater whole that is connected by the flow of *qi* itself.

Flows and blockages in Rwandan ritual and notions of the body

Christopher C Taylor

CHAPTER CONTENTS

> ❝ The widespread concept of 'flow and blockage' is the closest to a classical African anatomy that inspires clear ideas about health and infuses numerous therapeutic practices.
>
> John M Janzen and Edward C Green [1, p 14]

INTRODUCTION

As is clear from many chapters in this book, it is now generally accepted that there are many different and culturally specific ways of thinking about the human body, its processes, pathologies and cures. Yet despite this diversity, some core metaphors recur even though the cultures in question are often distant from one another in time and/or space. One such root metaphor focuses on the idea of flows of substances or energies along bodily pathways. In the traditional medicine of China, for example, there is *qi* the orderly or disorderly movement of which is thought to underlie health and sickness. In Indian Tantric medicine, *kundalini* serves a similar role. In Rwanda (Central East Africa), there is no specifically named energy, but the flows or perturbations in flows of bodily substances – such as blood, semen, menstrual blood and breast milk – are a central preoccupation. In this chapter I concentrate on Rwandan traditional medicine and attempt to elucidate some of its principles where these flows are concerned.

I have done several stints of fieldwork in Rwanda, starting in 1983 and most recently in the spring of 2009. Although in recent years I have concentrated on issues related to the 1994 genocide, much of my earlier work there concerned local notions of the body and of healing. After my first period of fieldwork in Rwanda, I noticed that many of the case histories of patients and healers that I had collected were characterized by what I came to call 'flow/blockage disorders'. For example, the condition known as '*umu-kobwa utajya mu mihango*' where a woman of childbearing age finds herself unable to have normal menstrual periods and is thus barren, due to *ensorcellement* (see below).

Medicine in Rwanda during the 1980s was pluralistic. There was a medical school and its graduates were trained in scientific biomedicine. This was the most prestigious type of medicine and, for most disorders that could not be treated at home, it was probably the most frequently employed. Consulting a physician at one of Rwanda's hospitals did not require that the patient pay. In sharp contrast, filling a prescription at one of Rwanda's pharmacies did require payment. Since most medicines sold for prices comparable to those in Western countries, it was often difficult for Rwandans to obtain modern pharmaceuticals. This cost factor acted as something of an impetus to push Rwandans in the direction of other medical systems, such as Chinese, Indian, or Rwandan traditional medicine.

Rwandan traditional medicine, or *ubuvuzi bwa Gihanga*, employed both empirical and nonempirical treatments. Medicinal herbs were the remedies of choice in the former; ritual procedures in addition to the use of plant or animal substances were employed in the latter. Pluralism also characterized traditional medicine. Some healers concentrated on diagnosis through divination. Others were herbalists. Others employed ritual. Some used a mixture of these techniques. In addition to differences in healing techniques, healers differed over the theoretical bases of their therapies. Some healers, for example, believed that many disorders were the result of sorcery; others denied the existence of sorcery and witchcraft, maintaining that such disorders were caused by fear or by sin [2].

Both Rwandan and Chinese medical systems possess notions concerning flows and blockages. In the Chinese case there is *qi*. It is difficult to define exactly what *qi* is. At times it appears to resemble a bodily fluid. At other times *qi* is more like an energy flowing along circuits in the body and influencing the flows of Blood and other bodily fluids. There is disagreement among practitioners about *qi* and its action, but most concur that the Liver is responsible for the smooth flow of *qi* throughout the body. Problems arise when the flow of *qi* stagnates. This causes perturbations in the flows of other bodily fluids and substances and can also cause emotional disorders [3,4]. Similar to the notion of *qi*, although perhaps more unambiguously an energy rather than a substance, is the Indian Tantric idea of *kundalini*. *Kundalini* is thought to flow through the *susumna*, a central conduit along the spinal axis from a place at the base of the sacrum halfway between the genitalia and the anus to the top of the skull. The *susumna* passes through six centers or *chakras*, but energy can also deviate to right or left, through the (male) *ida* or the (female) *pingala*, respectively. The object of therapy is to rechannel energy that normally might flow through these to the central conduit. As the rechanneled *kundalini* passes upward in this way it enters each of the six *chakras*. The 'lotuses' associated with each of the *chakras* can then open. This signifies the opening of the spirit to 'knowledge' and transformation [5].

Early European and Near Eastern humoral medicine (*Unani*) are different from the above in that it is not simply the flow, obstruction, or stagnation of substances that is of concern, but rather the balance of four humors: Yellow Bile, Black Bile, Blood and Phlegm. Four reservoirs of these substances reside within the body and can affect one another: when one humor is deficient, another is in excess. The object of therapy is to regulate the flows of these humors so as to achieve their balance.

Even biomedicine has its flows and blockages. Atherosclerosis and all the maladies that follow in its wake – ranging from heart attacks and strokes to peripheral artery disease, deep vein thrombosis, pulmonary emboli and even erectile dysfunction – are said to be the result of obstructed blood flow due to plaque buildup in veins and arteries. Using empirical evidence biomedicine can demonstrate the physical existence of blockages and obstructions in blood flows. However, would experimental inquiry have been oriented in this direction had a model not already existed? It is reasonable to ask whether William Harvey's depiction of the anatomy of the circulatory system in 1616 would have occurred had it not been for traditional medicine's pre-existent conceptual imagining of flows.

Besides Rwanda there are other sub-Saharan African examples of flow/blockage symbolism. As in Rwanda these are encountered in the domains of health, fertility and ritual. One of the most striking examples concerns a group called the Komo who reside in northeastern Congo (Democratic Republic of Congo, DRC). Because this group resides not far from Rwanda, it is perhaps not surprising that their symbolism shows some similarities. In sharp contrast to Rwanda, however, their symbolism is quite explicit and conscious whereas in the former the symbolism is covert and implicit. During the Komo male initiation ritual, for example, a small reed is inserted into the urethra of the penis [6]. Elders then remove the reeds from the neophytes while they sing, 'Who obstructed the waterfall?' This ritual action signifies the transformation of infertile boys into fertile men, by the very overt action of changing a blocked penis into an open one capable of flow. Another Congolese example concerns the Sakata in north central Congo (DRC). Among the Sakata life is thought of as a 'flow of life force' [6]. When this flow is interrupted or obstructed, illness results: 'illness is like a "bubble of blood" (*kembomene ke makela*), a constipated clot of blood, blocking the healthy redistribution inside the body' [7]. (See Figs 25.1 and 25.2 for other images of flow in Africa.)

It is not my intention here to explore all the avenues of inquiry that could arise from these speculations. Instead I will concentrate on indigenous Rwandan notions of the body and of pathology. I will begin by discussing the Rwandan concept of *imaana* or supreme being and then discuss the rituals of sacred kingship that were enacted until the colonial era to catalyze the descent of *imaana* to the earth. Then I will examine material from case histories collected from Rwandan traditional medicine during the 1980s. Lastly I will show how certain specifically Rwandan notions of the body recur in the 'techniques of cruelty' employed during the 1994 genocide.

IMAANA

Before colonialism the primary embodiment of motile force in Rwandan culture was *imaana*. The term is still in use. Sometimes *imaana* refers to a supreme being. Sometimes the referent is less precise. According to d'Hertefelt and Coupez, the term refers to: 'a powerful quality, the dynamic principal of life and fecundity, which traditional Rwandans sought to appropriate by ritual techniques. In some cosmogonic tales, this same force is conceived as a conscious volitional entity, which one could term Divinity. But no religion addresses itself to this anthropomorphic hypostasis precisely because the term *imaana* does not refer primarily to a personal being whom one must honor and supplicate, but a diffuse fluid that must be captured' [8, p 460].

Imaana was thought to invest certain trees and plants, royal residences and tombs, animals and objects used in divination, and protective talismans. Diviners, ritual specialists and ancestral spirits were also believed to embody *imaana*: 'But, according to the concepts held by Rwandans, it is the king who is the supreme possessor of the fecundating fluid, *imaana*; the royal ritual is nothing else than the description of techniques which allow him to direct its effects to benefit the entire country' [8, p 460].

It is thus from the royal rituals that one can reconstruct some of the workings of *imaana* in its various guises, as these were lived in pre-1931 Rwanda. Liquids were especially favored vehicles of *imaana*. These included: water, primarily in the form of rain, but also secondarily in the form of rivers and springs, and also blood, semen, saliva, milk, honey and beer. These substances were the primary media of 'flow'. In a less direct way conceptually, but no less important, cattle were also a medium of flow. They produced precolonial Rwanda's most cherished aliment, milk, while they also mediated the transfer of human reproductive potential from one group to another by being the most important valuable in bridewealth exchange. The first Rwandan king said to have been favored by *imaana* with the possession of cattle was the legendary king, Gihanga, whose name is recalled in the term for traditional medicine, *ubuvuzi bwa Gihanga*.

The relation of kings, cattle, milk, men and *imaana* is succinctly expressed in a dynastic poem:

> *The King is not a man,*
> *O men that he has enriched with his cattle …*
> *He is a man before his designation to the throne …*
> *Ah yes! That is certain:*
> *But the one who becomes King ceases to be a man!*
> *The King, it is he* Imaana
> *And he dominates over humans …*
> *I believe that he is the* Imaana *who hears our pleas!*
> *The other* Imaana, *it's the King that knows him,*
> *As for us, we see only this Defender! …*
> *Here is the sovereign that drinks the milk milked by* Imaana
> *And we drink that which he in turn milks for us! [9]*

In this poem, we see that the beneficence of *imaana* was once conceptualized as milk. The king as the earthly avatar of *imaana* received this beneficence and channeled it downward to the rest of humanity. The Rwandan king, *umwami*, could be compared to a hollow conduit through which celestial beneficence passed. He was the kingdom's most giving or 'flowing being'. In effect, celestial beneficence could pass directly through the king's open body, and in some instances directly through his alimentary canal. A legend that is sometimes recounted in regard to the semi-mythical king Ruganzu Ndori illustrates this principle very clearly. For here fertility is restored to the earth by first passing through the *umwami*'s digestive tract.

Ruganzu Ndori was living in exile in the kingdom of Ndorwa, a neighboring kingdom to the north of Rwanda. There he had taken refuge with his paternal aunt who was married to a man from the region. In the meantime, because the Rwandan throne was occupied by an illegitimate usurper, Rwanda was experiencing numerous calamities. Crops were dying, cows were not giving milk, and women were becoming sterile. Ruganzu's aunt encouraged him to return to Rwanda to retake the throne and save his people from catastrophe. Ruganzu agreed. But, before setting forth on his voyage to Rwanda, his aunt gave him the seeds (*imbuto*) of several cultivated plants (sorghum, gourds and others) to restart Rwandan cultures. While en route to Rwanda, Ruganzu Ndori came under attack. Fearing that the *imbuto* would be captured, he swallowed the seeds with a long draught of milk. Once he regained the Rwandan throne, he defecated the milk and seed mixture upon the ground and the land became productive once again. Since that time all Rwandan kings are said to be born clutching the seeds of the original *imbuto* in their hand.

Other inferences to be drawn from this legend concern the implicit and explicit associations linking the king to the productivity of the soil, to milk, prosperity, fertility and continuity. These are supported by linguistic analysis. For example, in the nearby kingdom of Bunyoro, the king was called *Mukama*. Kinyoro (spoken in Bunyoro) and Kinyarwanda (spoken in Rwanda) have the same term, *gukama*, meaning 'to milk'. When the Bunyoro *Mukama* died, a man would ascend a ladder, pour milk onto the ground and say, 'The milk is spilt; the king has been taken away!' [10].

The terms *umwami* and *mukama* thus encompass several crucial concepts that are central to Rwandan symbolic thought: continuity, productivity, fertility, prosperity, and their metaphorization in the popular imagination as a flowing process, lactation. The verb *gukama* in Kinyarwanda and Kirundi (another Bantu language from this region) means 'to milk'. Yet it has another meaning which hints that embedded within these representations is their contrary, for *gukama* can also mean 'to dry up' [11]. In other words, one cannot 'milk' one's environment without running the risk of depleting it. The person of the *umwami* and his college of ritual specialists had to ensure that the sky's fecundating fluid fell in sufficient quantity, but without washing the kingdom away. The meteorological manifestations of excessive or insufficient 'flow' were, of course, drought and inundation, with drought more feared than inundation. The cause of either calamity, though, was the same: ritual impurity (*ishyano*). The *umwami* was a defender of the principle of 'flow' and an enemy of *ishyano*. The *umwami*'s enemies were the antithesis of 'flowing beings'; they were beings who impeded fertility. The Rwandan mythical archetype of the 'blocking being' was a small old woman (*agakeecuru*), who harbored Death in her womb. *Imaana* and the king were associated with milk and fertility, whereas Death was associated with blood and sterility, as depicted in the following legend that recounts the origin of Death: [12]

In the beginning of time, there were four brothers: Lightning, the King, Imaana and Death. One day the four were to receive their separate heritages. Lightning received his portion in the sky and in the forest. Imaana received his part upon the earth and in the sky. The King received his part on the earth, Rwanda. Death received blood. But Death was stymied in his attempts to enjoy his heritage, because each one of his brothers would protect those of his possessions that bled. In his attempts to obtain blood, Death even met with an accident and lost the sight of one eye. Dispirited and suffering from the lack of blood, Death returned to his father, the Creator, to plead his case.

The Creator (Rurema) tells Death that he shall possess whatever the others leave behind, neglect, or no longer want. Interpreting this very liberally, Death proceeds to ravage the possessions of his brothers. Finally, the three decide to join forces against Death and kill him. The King takes his bow and arrows, Imaana his heavy club, and Lightning himself. Cornering Death, the King shoots an arrow into his thigh, and when Death tries to right himself Lightning slaps him. Nevertheless, Death manages to escape into a field where an *agakeecuru* (little old woman) is gathering gourds. Death pleads with her to hide him in the fold at the front of her dress and she complies. When Lightning and Imaana arrive to see what has happened, Lightning decides to kill the old woman and thus her charge as well, but Imaana prevents him, saying that his (Imaana's) role is to oversee the multiplication of his creatures and not their demise. Besides, one day Death will have to leave his hiding place on his own and then he will be vulnerable. But Death decides that his new abode suits him well. He is protected from the rain, and he has all the blood that he wants (i.e. he has secreted himself inside the woman's uterus). Later the old woman transmits Death to all her progeny by eating with them; they in turn, take it to every corner of the earth.

In this tale we see the association between Death and beings that do not flow, because old women do not menstruate. Instead of blood or children flowing out from their bodies, the substance of fertility and its powers remain trapped within them. In this instance it nourishes Death instead of life, for Death has sought refuge in the old woman's uterus. Every woman, following the original *agakeecuru*, is born with Death already in her womb. Death, like a witch, parasitically sucks the blood of woman to sustain himself. Eventually Death destroys female fertility from within; he sucks away woman's blood and thus ultimately brings her capacity to produce new life to an end. While male fertility can endure until a man's last breath, female fertility is limited.

THE ROYAL RITUALS

In the 17 royal rituals assembled by d'Hertefelt and Coupez, the importance of liquid aliments is striking. There are dozens of references to milk (*amata*), honey (*ubuuki*) and honeyed sorghum beer (*inzoga y'inturire*), while there is only a single reference to one of the peasantry's staple foods, beans [8, p 17]. An entire ritual is devoted to another staple crop, sorghum, but even much of this grain was consumed in liquid form, either as beer (*ikigage*) or as a thick porridge-like beverage (*igikoma*). The Rwandan king performed the royal rituals with the aid of his ritual specialists (*abiiru*), his wives, and the occasional assistance of the queen mother (*umwamikazi*). Most of the rituals were faithfully enacted until the latter part of *umwami* Yuhi V Musinga's reign (he was deposed in 1931), and a few rituals were still enacted by Yuhi's Christian successors.

Of all the 17 royal rituals, which directly or indirectly concern fertility, six of them deal directly with things that flow. Two of the six, *Inzira ya Rukungugu* (The Path of Drought) and *Inzira ya Kivu* (The Path of Inundation) concern rainfall, either insufficient or excessive. *Inzira y'Inzuki* (The Path of the Bees) aims at assuring sufficient honey production, the necessary ingredient in Rwanda's most prized alcoholic beverages: honeyed sorghum beer and mead. *Inzira ya Muhekenyi* (The Path of Cattle Sickness) concerns the health of cattle and thus milk production. *Inzira y'Umuganura* (The Path of the First Fruits of Sorghum) celebrates the sorghum harvest. Probably the most important ritual, however, was *Inzira y'Ishoora* (The Path of the Watering). In this ritual, performed at the beginning of each new dynastic cycle of four kings by a 'cowherd king', all the royal cattle herds were brought to the Nyabugogo River to be watered, thus signifying the ritual revivification of the entire magicoreligious order of divine kingship.

Here I offer only one ritual example to elucidate Rwandan symbolic thought with regard to the flow of bodily, celestial and social media of exchange [8]. Bodily media include blood, semen and maternal milk. Celestial media include sunlight and rainfall. Social media include beer, cattle and women. All these things interrelate in complex ways and with varying implications, but in most domains of Rwandan symbolism they reflect similar patterns. In the origin myth of Death, for example, I discussed the relation between Death and postmenopausal women. A similar interplay of fertility/antifertility principles characterizes the royal rituals and practices related to the body. Although many of these practices have fallen, or are falling, into disuse, their underlying logic forms the ideological substrate that continues to influence much of Rwandan therapy-seeking behavior today.

In 'The Path of Inundation' [8, p 27–31] the problem of excessive celestial flow (rainfall) was ritually countered. In this instance, the king's ritualists were instructed to capture a Twa woman 'without breasts or having passed childbearing age' [8, p 28] from the forest just beyond the limits of the Rwandan kingdom. Later in the ritual her blood was shed along with other sacrificial victims: a black goat, a black bull and a sterile cow. (Black in most contexts is associated with death, sterility, bad fortune and nonproductivity.) Rwandan women without breast development (*impenebere*) and girls who had reached childbearing age without ever having menstruated (*impa*) were considered sources of ritual impurity (*ishyano*) and thus infertility to all of Rwanda. One of the king's responsibilities was to assure their elimination [8, p 286]. Usually they would be taken just beyond the limits of Rwanda and then killed; their blood as it flowed upon the earth was thought to vitiate the fertility of the foreign land, as well as bringing it other forms of misfortune. Notice that in both instances these women were 'blocked beings' (i.e. beings from whose bodies one of the two requisite fluids of female fertility, blood or maternal milk, did not flow). Because the fertility of their bodies was blocked, they were thought to threaten the productive integrity of the entire Rwandan polity. In this ritual, 'The Path of Inundation', the Twa woman's body was perceived to be deficient in at least one of the fertility fluids.

Members of the Twa ethnic group in Rwanda, comprising less than 1% of the present population, have often been considered a pariah caste by the other two ethnic groups, the Tutsi and the Hutu. One trait of the Twa particularly denigrated by the other two groups was their alleged gluttony and lack of discrimination in eating. Twa, for example, would eat mutton, an aliment spurned by both Tutsi and Hutu, because the latter valued sheep for their pacific qualities. Sheep would accompany cattle herds and were thought to exert a calming influence upon them. (This belief and the practices associated with it persist today among many Rwandans.) According to a Rwandan legend [13], the denigration of Twa was justified by the different behaviors with respect to milk of the three brothers, Gatutsi, Gahutu and Gatwa, sons of the mythical Rwandan king, Gihanga:

Gihanga gave each of the brothers a pot of milk and told him to guard it during the night. But Gatwa became thirsty and drank his pot of milk. Gahutu became drowsy and, in dozing off, spilled some of the contents of his pot. Only Gatutsi succeeded in keeping a full pot of milk until the next morning. For this reason, Gihanga decreed that Gatutsi should possess cattle and enjoy the right to rule. Gahutu would only be able to procure cattle by the work and services he performed for his brother, Gatutsi. As for Gatwa, he would never possess cattle; alternate periods of gluttony and starvation were to be his lot. It was the Tutsi, presumably, who could be trusted to keep the milk pot, which was Rwanda, filled to its brim.

According to the logic of flows, therefore, a Twa woman without breasts or not menstruating, and living in the forest beyond the borders of the Rwandan kingdom, was a 'blocked being' in both physical and social terms. She could not contribute to the reproduction of human life because of her physiological deficiency. Nor could she contribute to the prosperity of Rwanda because she lived beyond its political control and was a member of the ethnic group who, according to legend, had perturbed flows by impetuous consumption. In a situation of disordered flow (e.g. excessive rainfall) such a woman was symbolically appropriate as a sacrificial victim because her body was disordered in its flows, signified by the absence of either milk or blood.

RWANDAN SORCERY

Just as today, although not all Rwandans during the 1980s believed in sorcery, those who did frequently consulted traditional healers. What we see with sorcery spells or poisonings is that they conform to the flow/blockage logic discussed above with regard to the royal rituals. The spell termed *kumanikira amaraso* (literally 'to suspend blood') is a good example. This spell prevents a woman from being able to deliver her baby. Sometimes it prevents her from conceiving. One traditional healer explained to me that among pregnant women, the spell causes the baby to rise toward the heart instead of descending toward the birth canal. Another healer, a woman named Antoinette, told me that many pregnant women are victims of *kumanikira amaraso*, causing the baby to become turned transversally in the womb.

One method of afflicting a woman in this way is to take some of the blood and other fluid that exuded from her womb during a previous childbirth. This fluid, called *igisanza*, is placed in a packet along with other medicines and then suspended from the rafters of a house. This form of the spell prevents the woman from being able to deliver again.

Another version of this method involves taking the woman's menstrual blood (*irungu*), vaginal secretions (*amanyare*), her urine (*inkali*), or, if none of these things is available, a piece of her clothing. This item is put in a packet with medicines and (1) placed in a cave, (2) suspended from the rafters of a house, or (3) placed among rocks, where rain cannot touch it, on the summit of a high hill. In this instance, the woman's menstruation is stopped and she becomes sterile. An interesting variant of this poisoning entails putting the blood, etc. into a stream of fast-moving water. In this case, the woman's menstruation becomes hemorrhagic. This spell also causes sterility and can be life threatening. Some healers refer to this last variant as *umuvu*, whereas others consider it a form of *kumanikira*.

In effect, by suspending a woman's blood or other fluids involved in sexuality or reproduction, the woman's reproductive functions are also 'suspended'. Either she becomes unable to deliver the baby already in her womb, or menstruation stops and she becomes sterile. By suspending the woman's bodily fluids in a position between sky and earth, or in a place where rain cannot touch them, the woman's body becomes 'blocked'. When her fluids are put into a body of fast-moving water, her menses become dangerously abundant.

Healers vary in their treatment of this poisoning; nevertheless these variations possess features in common. One healer has the woman lie on her back while naked. He takes medicines and sprinkles them in a line from the woman's forehead, over the middle of her face, over her chest and abdomen, down to her genitals. The logic behind this treatment appears to be that movement must be encouraged from the top of the body to the bottom.

Antoinette uses another method. Although her treatment of *kumanikira* follows a similar line of symbolic reasoning, it engages more elements from the macrocosmic sphere in which the female body as microcosm is embedded: house, earth, sky and rain. Antoinette has the woman lie naked on her back inside her house. Someone climbs on the roof of the house, parts the thatch, and then pours an aqueous mixture of medicines through the opening onto the woman's abdomen. Another person inside the house then rubs the woman's stomach with the medicinal mixture. In this treatment the blockage within the woman's body is considered as if it were a blockage between sky and earth, and is countered by someone actually moving to the sky position (ascending to the roof of the house), and pouring fluids earthward. This time, however, the downward movement of fluids includes the woman's body in the circuit of flow from sky to earth. The cure is virtually a one-to-one homeopathic reversal of the symbolic operations accomplished in the poisoning, which removed the woman's body from the circuit of moving fluids by suspending her blood. In this cure, an analogical relation is established between the female body and the elemental forces of nature.

Another spell that is characterized by flow/blockage symbolism is the one known as *urukarango* or *umukobwa utajya mu mihango* (girl who cannot menstruate, whose menstruation has been stopped). This spell is similar to the *kumanikira amaraso* spell, and some healers consider it to be a variant of it, but according to one healer named Baudouin the procedure used to cast the spell is different.

Baudouin told me that a poisoner can inflict this spell by taking some of the girl's urine, or her menstrual blood, adding medicines (he did not know which ones) and water to it, and then cooking the mixture on a piece of broken pottery taken from a vessel which has never been used (*urujo*). The mixture is cooked until the liquid evaporates. The girl stops menstruating and becomes sterile.

Along with a number of other herbs, Baudouin usually treats this spell with the powder of a dried insect called *impanguzi*. The insect is used because its name is derived from the verb *guhaanguura*, one of whose meanings is 'to impregnate a woman, or a female, previously thought sterile' [14]. Furthermore, it lives among plants called *imvura idahita*, which means 'rain which does not cease falling'. In this instance the reasoning is that after treatment, the girl's menstruation should never fail again. In summary, a girl treated for *umukobwa utajya mu mihango* should recover her capacity to menstruate and consequently her fertility, and will so become marriageable.

TECHNIQUES OF CRUELTY – THE GENOCIDE OF 1994

Representations of the body similar to those discussed above were also apparent in the methods of cruelty employed during the genocide of 1994. One such technique was impalement. In pre- and early colonial times Rwandans impaled cattle thieves. The executioners inserted a wooden stake into the thief's anus and then pushed it through the body, causing it to exit at the neck or the mouth. The pole with its agonizing charge was then erected, stuck into the earth, and left standing for several days. Dramatically gruesome and public, this punishment carried a clear and obvious normative message intended to deter cattle thievery. In a more subtle way, the message can be interpreted symbolically. Because cattle exchanges accompany, legitimize and commemorate the most significant social transitions and relationships, most notably patron–client relations, blood brotherhood and marriage, obviating the possibility of such exchanges or subverting those that have already occurred by stealing cattle removes all tangible mnemonic evidence of the attendant social relationships. Diverting socially appropriate flows of cattle by means of thievery is a way of *gusiba inzira*, or 'blocking the path' between individuals and groups united through matrimonial alliance, blood brotherhood, or patron–client ties. It is symbolically appropriate, therefore, that people who obstruct the conduits of social exchange have the conduit that is their body obstructed with a pole or spear.

Quite obviously between the pre- and early colonial times, when Rwandan executioners impaled cattle thieves, and 1994, when genocidal murderers impaled Tutsi men and women, many things had changed. Clearly the more recent victims of the practice were not cattle thieves. Were they in some sense like cattle thieves in the minds of those committing the atrocities? My feeling is that they were, although the more recent terms used in Hutu extremist discourse to describe Tutsi only occasionally make reference to actual actions of which they might be guilty, such as theft, but instead 'Tutsi are invaders from Ethiopia', 'cockroaches', 'eaters of our sweat', or 'weight upon our back'. The Tutsi, much like the archetypal *agakeecuru* discussed above, exert their malevolent influence on the social group not so much by what they do as by inherent qualities which they supposedly embody. In that sense they approach 'blocking beings', the mythical nemeses of Rwandan tradition (*agakeecuru*, *impenebere*, or *impa*), and like these figures, they possess fearful powers. In this case they were obstructors of the cosmic unity of the nation as this unity was imagined by the Hutu extremist elite: a purified nation with a purified, reified 'Hutu culture' expunged of all elements of 'Tutsi culture' and rid of all who would resist the encompassing powers of the state. The torturers not only killed their victims, they transformed their bodies into powerful signs which resonated with a Rwandan habitus even as they improvised upon it and enlarged the original semantic domain of associated meanings to depict an entire ethnic group as enemies of the Hutu state.

Among other violence reported during the Rwandan genocide, there were frequent instances of emasculation of Tutsi males, even those too young to reproduce. Attackers also slashed off the breasts of Tutsi women. These techniques of cruelty were also employed during earlier periods of Rwandan history. Both emasculation and breast oblation manifest a preoccupation with the reproductive system and specifically with parts of the body that produce fertility fluids. In both cases, the symbolic function interdigitates with and reinforces the pragmatic function, but the symbolic function cannot simply be reduced to the pragmatic one of destroying the future capacity of a group to reproduce. The torturers were assaulting specific and diverse human subjects as well as attacking a group's capacity to reproduce. In order to convince themselves that they were ridding the polity of a categorical enemy and not just assaulting specific individuals, they had to first transform their victims' bodies into the equivalent of 'blocked beings'. A logic, *a posteriori*, was operative: reclassify through violence bodies that do not *a priori* manifest the imagined inadequacy. In other words, reconfigure specific bodies through torture so that they *become* the categorical abomination.

There were also cases of forcing adult Tutsi to commit incest with one of their children before killing them. Here the image of misdirected flows is quite clear, for incest causes blood and semen to flow backward upon one another in a closed circuit within the family rather than in an open circuit between families. Not only were the victims brutalized and dehumanized by this treatment, their bodies were transformed into icons of asociality, for incest constitutes the pre-emption of any possible alliance or exchange relationship that might have resulted from the union of one's son or daughter with the son or daughter of another family.

CONCLUSION

Representations of human health and pathology that involve notions of flow are relatively common in the world, although they differ in their specifics from one culture to another. The central African country of Rwanda possessed notions of this sort in its precolonial religious thought and in the ritual practices associated with sacred kingship. Although Rwanda has not had a sacred king since 1931 when the last 'traditional' king or *umwami* was overthrown, flow/blockage notions survive today in Rwandan traditional medicine or *ubuvuzi bwa Gihanga*. More explicit examples of these representations can be found in the neighboring Democratic Republic of Congo among the Komo and Sakata peoples. The Rwandan notions are hardly vestigial throwbacks to a bygone era. They continue to structure Rwandan thinking about the body as a physical entity subject to pathology and as a social entity involved in relationships with other human beings. Anatomical pathology and pathophysiology are characterized by perturbations in the flow of bodily fluids. But social pathology, at least as this was imagined during the genocide of 1994, has also been conceptualized as a disruption in proper flows. This was why a whole ethnic group, the Tutsi, was able to be depicted as 'blocking beings' and subjected to attack with impunity.

This metaphorical structure opposing notions of proper flows to improper flows is common because it conforms to what can be observed about the human body without the use of sophisticated technological devices. Substances enter the body and they leave the body. When a body is cut, it bleeds. When animals are slaughtered and dismembered for the purposes of consumption, flows of various sorts can be observed or readily inferred. Humans before the use of sophisticated technologies were able to make sense of human physiology by employing metaphors of the flow/blockage sort. Because the human mind seeks to make sense of the world even in those domains where its powers of observation are limited, it is no accident that where rationality and empiricism encounters limits then symbolic thought quickly takes up the slack. The flow/blockage metaphors are extended to speculation about the proper workings of social life in so far as goods, services, persons and things are constantly moving between individuals and groups. In like fashion this speculation can embrace the cosmos to explain the workings of the universe and humanity's place in it. Rwanda's representations of flow and blockage are but one permutation on what is possibly a universal system of representations.

Elemental souls and vernacular *qi*: some attributes of what moves us

David Mayor

3

> ❝ *The subject of discourse, briefly put, is the free travel and inward and outward movement of the divine* ch'i [qi]; *it is not skin, flesh, sinews and bones.*
> Neijing Ling Shu [1]

> ❝ *Streaming sensations can be felt by anyone who is not held tense by chronic contractions and who relaxes and centres the attention on immediate sensations. They are the currents of the excitement of being alive which flow within us like a silent river, and which we are not normally aware of in the urgency of our efforts to deal with the problems or difficulties that beset us.*
> David Boadella [2]

CONCEPTUALIZING *QI*

> ❝ To say that the concept of qi is the foundation stone of Chinese traditional culture (including traditional Chinese medicine) is not excessive.
>
> Liu Changlin [3]

Qi (氣) has been described as 'both a principle of unity and coherence that connects all things and a potential, an immanent life force in the world that is knowable only in the various changing aspects it assumes' [4]. Impossible to fully grasp intellectually or materially, like the *dao* (道) (see Ch. 4), it has therefore meant different things to different people and at different periods. At times it 'means the spirit or breath of life in living creatures, at other times the air or ether filling the sky and surrounding the universe, while in some contexts it denotes the basic substance of all creation' [5]. Other contemporary Western scholars have described *qi* as 'finest-matter influences' [6], 'the fine, essential matter that is the vehicle of consciousness' [7] and as itself 'neither a substance nor a spirit' [8, p 5].

As with many concepts in Chinese thought, historically its range of meanings grew by a process of accretion rather than by progressive selection [9]. *Qi* did not yet appear in the *Book of Songs* (*Shijing*, 詩經) of around 600 BCE [8], but by the time of Confucius 'blood and air' (*xueqi*, 血氣) in descriptions of the body had come to mean 'the physical vitalities' or 'physical powers' [10]. Yin Yun, who lived during the Warring States period (475–221 BCE), was the first to consider *qi* as a kind of substantial force permeating everything [11]. In the *Guanzi* (管子), based on texts from the same period, a similar position was taken; there it is described as 'the energetic fluid which vitalises the body' [12, p 101], and 'flowing between heaven and earth' [12, p 158]. In the *Classic of Mountains and Seas* (*Shanhai Jing*, 山海經) even the cosmic substance that is the eternal matter of creation was termed the 'breathing-soil' (*xi-rang*, 吸壤) [13]. *Qi* by now had the 'potential to transform' [9]. In the Mawangdui manuscripts (dateable to before 168 BCE), *qi* was not mentioned by name [14], although described as material but simultaneously volatile and pervasive (water vaporized by fire, but with the potential to liquify or even solidify as ice) [15], just as things – whether animate or inanimate – condense out of universal *qi* and dissolve back into it [9,16].

The correspondence between inner (microcosm) and outer (macrocosm) evident in the earlier *Guanzi* [9] (where 'water is the blood and breath of earth' [17]), the *Zuo Zhuan* (左轉) of around 310 BCE and the *Huainanzi* (淮南子) of around 140 BCE (where rain and wind are mentioned in the same breath as blood and *qi* [18]) is also marked in the *Neijing Suwen* (內經素問), which was compiled a little later than the *Huainanzi* (probably in the first century BCE) [7]. Here *qi* 'at the same time ... stands for everything that moves into the body, inside the body, or out of the body' [19]. In the *Suwen*, *qi* and *xue* have become distinct conceptual entities, and no longer simply the air breathed or the physical blood [10]. In contrast, by the time of Xu Shen's *Shuowen Jiezi* (說文解字/说文解字, *Explanation of Characters*) around 100 CE, the character for *qi* was analyzed as 'ascending vapour forming clouds' [8, p 10], the vapor arising from the cooking of grain, whereas originally it had signified 'to make a ritual prayer' (coming from below and rising to heaven [8, p 10]). *Qi* has thus become associated with 'movement and heat' [20] ('a kind of heat and force' [8, p 10]).

From even these brief descriptions, *qi* can be seen as having many possible associations or attributes, which are summarized in Table 3.1.

Neo-Confucianism: *qi* (氣) and *li* (理)

For the eleventh century neo-Confucian Zhang Zai (1020–1077), a proponent of the view that material reality is a process of condensing and dispersing *qi* [21], *qi* itself (both a material force and identified with the great void, *taixu*, 太虛) was governed by 'principle' (*li*, 理), in an essential unity [22] (see Ch. 11 for more details). His nephews Cheng Hao (1032–1085) and Cheng Yi (1033–1107) prioritized the permanence of *li* [21]. Later neo-Confucians differed in their views. For Zhu Xi (1130–1200), *qi* and *li* formed a duality, with *li* prior to *qi*, whereas Luo Qinshun (1465–1547) argued against the inherent transcendentalism of the Cheng brothers and Zhu and for a single unified reality of *qi*, with *li* as but one aspect of *qi*. The Japanese Ekken Kaibara (1630–1714) went further, writing on *qi* as coursing through all reality, but also that 'principle should be recognized in material force itself. For example, it is like water. The essence of water is its purity and tendency to flow downward. Water and what is pure and flows are, therefore, not two things' [22, p 143]. For Ekken, *qi* is thus 'the very lifeblood of all matter', and in one contemporary interpretation of his philosophy, 'our mutual participation in *qi* is not a claim to ownership of one another but a mutual touching of the depth of things' [22, p 66].

Table 3.1 *Traditional attributes and associations of* qi

1 Life	2 Dynamism	3 'Fire'
Life (force)*	Change	Cooking (grain)
Vitality*	Movement (between	Heat
Breath (of life)	or through)	Transformation
	Rising	
	Force	
	Power	
4 General properties	**5 'Air'**	**6 'Water'**
All-permeating*	Air	Water
Unity	Wind	Fluid*
Connection*	Vapor	
Coherence	Cloud	
Immanence*	(Ether)*	
Universality*		
Potentiality		
Consciousness* (Vehicle for)		

Asterisked terms are those shared with Mesmer's *fluidum* – see below.

In itself, *qi* may be subtly material, spirit, neither, or all these (from material condensate to volatile evanescence).

THE EXPERIENCE OF *QI* AND THE ORIGINS
OF CHINESE MEDICINE

Chinese medicine (CM) is woven together from many strands. The Mawangdui medical manuscripts, for instance, include treatises on both moxibustion and 'self-cultivation' (*yangsheng*, 養生). In the former, the *mai* (脈, vessels) are described, undifferentiated precursors to the *jingluo* (经络, channels) of acupuncture that encompass movement of both *qi* and Blood toward the *head* – but they are not blood vessel, channel or pulse but rather all of these [9]. No mention is made as yet of specific acupoints [9]. In the *yangsheng* documents, exercises are described in which *qi* is moved around the body, generally toward the *extremities*, using breath and intention [25].

The *mai*, first described in the *Zuo Zhuan* [1], were very likely developed on the basis of *subjective embodied experience* of disordered or disturbed *qi*, the 'routes of pain as it is transmitted around the body' [25], even of sensations during orgasm [26]. One of the *Maishu* (脈書) texts found at Zhangjiashan, possibly slightly earlier than those from Mawangdui, explicitly differentiates between 'blood pain' ('as if saturated') and *mai* pain ('as if flowing') [9]. Thus *qi* was often employed to describe an intensification of sensation experienced within the body – whether of heat, pain, pleasure, or passion [27]. Disorders are described in terms of pathological *qi* [7]: free flow of Blood and *qi* within the *mai* is associated with health; movement prevents stagnation [9].

The movements of *qi* in the *yangsheng* fragments were not constrained within the *mai*, but again clearly based upon inner-focused bodily experience, if then visualized in terms of the outer world, as in Figure 3.1A, which depicts the circulatory flow of *qi* up and down an interiorized Kunlun mountain (崑崙山). Later versions of such images would explicitly include treadmill waterwheels to raise the *qi* (just visible as spoked wheels in Fig. 7.2).

In the *Huangdi Neijing* (黄帝内經), or *Inner Canon of the Yellow Emperor*, and the somewhat later *Nan Jing* (八十一難經), or *Canon of 81 Difficulties* (compiled before 100 CE), the circulation of *qi* through the system of the *jingluo* became more formalized [28]. Although still of unspecified form and ambiguous course in the former [19], by the time of the *Nanjing* the *jingluo* (literally 'path' and 'network') were no longer recognizably based on the subjective experience of flow. Instead, the movements of *qi* were analyzed intellectually, albeit still in relation to the numbers of breaths taken or the time marked by a water clock [29], and in some texts *qi* was clearly more particle than flow: a small, self-contained, discrete entity taking up residence at different locations around the body, day by day [29]. Even more elaborate was the medieval *renshen* (human spirit, 人神) system, in which acupuncture and moxibustion could be performed only where the *renshen* was supposed to be located as it moved about the body in its various cycles [30]. Representations of the *jingluo* themselves became standardized (see the Figures on endpapers). It is tempting to consider the conceptual elaborations of CM as associated with its practice by the élite doctors of the imperial court [14], and the experience of flow with *yangsheng* methods that were more widely used, but this would probably be an oversimplification. The subsequent development of much of CM was based on paradigms of systematic correspondence rather than flow, on the body as conceived in thought [31] as much as (or even rather than) the *lived* body as experienced in feeling [32]. To some extent, as in Western medicine, the experience of illness had become codified in thinking about disease [33]. This is particularly true of the normative 'traditional' medicine promoted by the Chinese state since 1949. *Qi* has become a substance in the body,

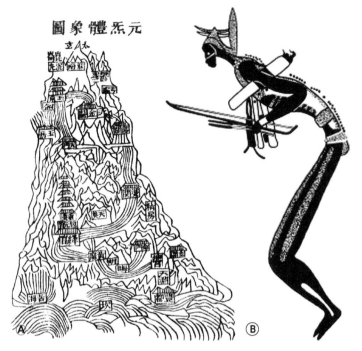

FIG 3.1 **(A) The circulatory flow of *qi* up and down an interiorized *Kunlun* mountain, showing some of the 'passes' (*guan*, 關) encountered.** *(From the fourteenth century Shang Yangzi Jindan Dayao Tu (上陽子金丹大要圖, Chart of the Great Essentials for the Golden Elixir by Master Shang), by the alchemist Chen Zhixu. (Courtesy, Needham Research Institute, Cambridge, UK.)* **(B) Rock art painting (redrawn), Harrismith, South Africa. Trance dancer of the San people in the *!kia* healing dance, showing the *kundalini*-like *n/om* as it is felt to work its way up the spine, hot and tingling.** The figure is bent over as the dancer experiences the build-up of pain in the 'stomach' before *n/om* releases in the trembling that signals transition [42]. In the symbolism of yoga [158] and of body trance, there are parallels between the sacred mountain with its waters (Fig. 3.1A), the spine and its marrow, and the world tree with its sap, which sustains life and communication between the worlds. Movements of *qi* experienced up or down the central axis of the body can be likened to climbing or descending the *axis mundi* of the mountain or tree through the levels of this tiered cosmos in shamanic trance. There may also be a homology between the 'interiority' of the body and that of the caves and shelters where much of this rock art may be found [143]. (See also Fig. 25.1.) *Reprinted with kind permission of the Rock Art Research Institute/SARADA, University of the Witwatersrand.*

no longer a cosmic force [34], or has even been redefined altogether – for example in terms of nervous system function [21] (electrical 'brain-*qi*', *naoqi*, 腦氣, according to the early Westernizing reformer Tai Sitong, 1865–1898 [35]). In the words of some knowledgeable commentators, 'traditional medical practice was saved, but the *qi* paradigm was its ransom' [23, p 52]. With the recent rise of deracinated forms of 'medical acupuncture' in the US, the use of a '*qi*-based speech code' has even been perceived as allowing more classically minded acupuncturists to 'actively construct a boundary around themselves that excluded those who might practice scientifically based acupuncture', as 'a form of resistance to … scientific integration' [36]. However, this is by no means true of all practitioners, many of whom have in fact managed to integrate aspects of the Western medical and *qi* paradigms in their work (see Ch. 20 for example).

Whatever the political overtones, it is clear that we can now add the word 'flow' and the concept of 'pathway' to the attributes of *qi* listed in Table 3.1. The contemporary Japanese philosopher Yuasa Yasuo, for example, describes it as 'a flowing energy'

Table 3.2 *Numbers of chapters in this book in which the traditional attributes and associations of qi appear*

Qi-based terms (≥ 10)		Qi-based terms (6–9)		Related terms (8)	
Flow	22	Life	9	Central axis (spine,	8
Life/vital force	20	Transformation	8	*kundalini*)	
Pathways (channels)	13	Connection	8	Dynamic	8
Breath	13	Heat	7		
Block/disruption of flow	13	Wholeness (unity)	6		
Movement	10	[Circulation]	6		

Qi-based terms in only 2–5 chapters			
Food	5	Cloud or vapor	3
Wind	5	Consciousness	3
Force	4	Universality	3
All-permeating	4	Vitality	2
Coherence 4	4	Water	2

Maximum possible score 23; Chapters 3 and 25, in which these data are discussed, are excluded.
The numbers shown for some terms are approximate only (sometimes synonyms were used rather than these exact words), and I should state that my own interest in the *qi* attribute of flow was made clear to some contributors before they wrote their chapters for this book. (See Ch. 25 for a fuller list of scored terms.)

[37], and even extracorporeally it has been described as 'the continuous psychophysical sea of stuff that constitutes the ceaseless flow of existence' [38]. Table 3.2 shows the numbers of chapters in this book in which the traditional attributes and associations of *qi* appear. It is clear that contributors to the book, despite their very different backgrounds (some unrelated to Chinese or any form of traditional East Asian medicine), have to a great extent remained true to the traditional understanding of *qi* in writing on the broader field of energy medicine.

To summarize: Life is sensation and movement. *Qi* – ungraspable in itself – is the dynamic, moving and transforming life force both within and around us, originally sensed in and then metaphorized as breath (Air), warmth (Fire), and flow (Water) in particular. Given the strong association with flow, it is unsurprising that many other ethnomedical traditions lay stress on 'the flow, transmission, and balance of life energies' [39].

AN EXCURSUS ON THE SOUL

❝ *The vaguest vegetal feeling, the reactions to physiological processes, the sense of effort and of activity, the feelings of comfort and discomfort, pleasure and pain, the sensations of touch, taste, smell, hearing, and sight, the feeling of effort in the brain (often connected with the memory-image), imagination, and thought, the emotions and the will – all these … are attached to the consciousness of self. It is, so to say, a point of insertion for all experience; its permanence is the life of the soul.*
Alfred E Crawley (1869–1924) [40]

❝ *The soul-stuff dwells in the body, proceeds from it and flows over everything that comes into contact with it.*
Gerardus van der Leeuw [41]

Most cultures have some concept akin to 'soul', although – rather like *qi* – this may be invisible and impalpable except in its effects to all but the trained shaman [42,43]. Again like *qi*, the word 'soul' is rich in associations, its meanings fluid and hard to grasp. In European languages, the term designates: (a) 'an entity conceived as the cause or vehicle of the bodily life', and (b) 'psychical activities of the individual person' [44]. Indeed, in many traditions (particularly where shamanism is practiced), souls are multiple, if usually dual, encompassing both free-soul(s) (or 'ego souls') and body-soul(s) [45,46,47], as first suggested by Wilhelm Wundt (1832-1920) in 1900 [48] and reinforced by Kruijt's observation that the 'after-death-soul' and 'life-soul' are rarely combined, at least in Indonesia [40]. In Chinese thought, for example, as early as the sixth century BCE [49] the *hun* (魂, ethereal soul), which is relatively *yang* (陽), is associated with clouds, wind and the movement of thought, rising to the realm of spirit after death, while the *po* (魄, corporeal soul), which is relatively *yin* (陰), is associated with more physical movement, at death descending into earth and lingering in the bones [50]. Wundt believed that the individual psyche (shadow, vocalized name, image, or breath-soul) was frequently symbolized by a bird, and the *embodied* soul by a snake, although the duel between solar eagle and chthonic serpent may have other meanings [51], as in the mythological history of *taiji quan* (太極拳) [52]. (In some cultures the bird becomes a butterfly or bee – all three being denizens of the air.) Others have considered the breath as an aspect of the embodied (rather than free) soul, with the body-soul defined as 'the cause or vehicle of the bodily life', or fundamentally 'the "life" of the body', closely associated with blood, breath (wind), heart and/or heat [44], as well as bone.

SEARCHING FOR THE SOUL

To determine whether the body-soul shares some attributes with *qi*, and *qi* itself in its association with the body can even be considered a type of soul, an informal and incomplete (if not exactly random) survey was conducted of the ethnographic, ethnologic and shamanic literature, on the basis of library catalogs and specialist reference lists. Some 210 useful books and papers were located, covering approximately 360 different cultures or subcultures, with mentions of around 760 souls, soul-like attributes of the individual (either named or described), or more universal forces/powers that may at times be attributes of or accessible to an individual. Partly because of the sources used, information on souls in Africa was found most frequently (246 souls, or 32.4% of the whole sample), followed by the Americas (189, or 24.9%), and Indonesia/Malaya/Papua New Guinea (I-M-PNG) (103, or 13.6%). The six other global regions each contributed less than 7% to the total.

Qi differs from the usual soul concepts – and resembles the *prana* of yoga and Ayurveda (see Chs 4 and 15) [53], and *pneuma* (πνεύμα), the cosmic breath-soul of ancient Greece – in that it combines characteristics of soul with an all-permeating universality. The latter is more usually associated with terms connoting a more general and impersonal power (if often present in all living things), such as the *mana* of many South Pacific cultures, or the force/power that arguably fills the universe for many African peoples [54,55]. However, except perhaps in some martial arts traditions, *qi* and *mana* are a world apart, and it has even been suggested that '*mana* as an invisible medium or substance or energy may be more a creation of European than of indigenous imagination' [56].

Although Ernst Arbman (1891–1958) suggested in the 1930s that the so-called 'primitive' soul concept did not differentiate between impersonal power and personal spirit, a *mana*-like force is also not characteristic of the soul as such [57]. In this sample, such an impersonal force was described in 42% of North American social groupings, 27% of Pacific cultures, 21% of Siberian peoples and 17% of South American peoples, but only 12% of those in Africa (this relatively low percentage probably resulting from the some of the sources used, which were particularly focused on the soul concept).

As described above, *qi* brings together what might be called the 'elemental' aspects of soul: Air (breath), Fire (the heat of life, combustion, distillation), and Water (flow, circulation). However, although dual or multiple souls occurred in around 60% of the 360 cultures sampled here (with the average highest number of soul types per culture in Siberia), Table 3.3 shows that there is by no means a balance of the elemental attributes of soul either globally or regionally. Other than in Europe, perhaps, the soul is predominantly aerial in nature, with the best elemental balance possibly being found in South America. It was not possible in this survey to differentiate systematically between free-soul and body-soul in their aerial aspects.

Curiously, despite the associations of soul with blood and bone often mentioned in the anthropological literature, in this sample blood-souls accounted for only 4% of all souls, and bone-souls for a mere 1.6%. About 2.8% of cultures had a belief or concept that the soul or a soul-like entity traveled around the body along some kind of pathway or conduit, or entered and left the body through a particular place on the body (the external path the soul takes to the land of the dead was not considered in this survey).

KNOTS, TIES AND DAISY CHAINS

To prevent loss of soul in this way – or even to retain the affections of the beloved – rings, anklets, armbands and different forms of knotting and weaving have all been used [59–61]. In contrast, the *un*tangling of the knots and ties that prevent

Table 3.3 *Elemental souls in different global regions: percentage of total soul numbers*			
Global region	**Air souls (%)**	**Fire souls (%)**	**Water souls (%)**
Whole world	26	5	4
Middle East	44	ID	15
I-M-PNG	35	ID	8
Asian subcontinent	33	ID	ID
Pacific	31	ID	ID
Siberia	28	ID	ID
N America	24	ID	ID
Africa	20	ID	ID
S America	19	10	10
Europe	ID	32	ID

When considering something from a different cultural milieu that is as inherently difficult to define as the 'soul', it is difficult to avoid imposing our own interpretations [58]. Many of the sources used to compile this Table are relatively old, and would not conform to modern standards of ethnologic research. Ethnographers with limited language skills – and Christian missionaries in particular – may well have misinterpreted what their informers (and their translators) were telling them.
Complete data available on request; ID = insufficient data.

a healthy flow (both internally and within the social group) is a focus of some ritual practices – in Zaire, for example [62]. Similarly, adherents of the *Shangqing* (上清, Supreme Clarity) school of Daoism used methods of internal alchemy to untie the 'knots and nodules' that form in the womb at conception and are responsible for eventual disease and death, so aiming to obtain immortality through circulation of the breath [4]. Comparable language on the 'energetic unscrambling' of knots is still used today in descriptions of *qigong* [63]. Bonds between people, links between humankind and heaven, and the connection between hunter and power animal [64], have all been described as 'threads', even in terms of a 'thread soul' [65]. More literally, Mesmer (see below) avoided knots in the ropes he used to guide the healing *fluidum* to his patients (attached together daisy-chain fashion) from specially 'mesmerized' trees [66].

> *Breath moving outwards, between the glottis and the nostrils, is, I am persuaded, the essence out of which philosophers have constructed the entity known to them as consciousness.*
>
> William James (1842–1910) [67]
>
> *Soul is only a word for something about the body.*
>
> Friedrich Nietzsche 1883 (1844–1900) [68, p 21]
>
> Goethe (1749–1832), in his poem *Gesang der Geister über den Wassern* [69], famously wrote that 'the soul of man resembles water', but this survey shows that 'soul', like *qi*, is most frequently associated with air or breath (as in William James's suggestion on the ego soul), rather than with water or flow. Again, it is far less often considered as fiery, although heat and warmth are indeed often associated with life and affection (so that cold, their opposite, may be injurious to health [70]). However, in some hot countries – Africa for example – heat is considered more dangerous [71,72,73], and the cooling properties of air [74] or water [75] may be valued as supporting life. Interestingly, the Edwardian Alfred Crawley, an early collector of souls, commented that the 'soul as a flame' is a product of what he called 'late culture' [40, p 222].
>
> **To summarize**: Both *qi* and soul are animating imponderables (not 'things'), both have strong associations with the breath, and both can be seen as mediating between different levels of experience (heaven and earth, mind and body – see Ch. 25, for example). However, despite such similarities, there are also patent differences between them, the most significant probably being that *qi* is more of a universal, and associated with flow both around and within us (sometimes along pathways or ducts) rather than being something that is in some way individualized. Thus, despite the parallels, it does not really seem possible to construct any clear general argument for one as a subtype of the other.

QI IN THE WEST: SKETCHING THE FLOW FROM HERACLITUS TO WILHELM REICH

❝ *That 'all things flow' is the first vague generalization which the unsystematized, barely analyzed, intuition of men has produced. Without doubt, if we are to go back to that ultimate, integral experience, unwrapped by the sophistications of theory, that experience whose elucidation is the final aim of philosophy, the flux of things is the one generalization around which we must weave our philosophical system.*

Alfred North Whitehead (1861–1947) [76]

❝ *There is one common flow, one common breathing, all things are in sympathy. The whole organism and each one of its parts are working in conjunction for the same purpose.*
Hippocrates (c. 460–370 BCE), *De Alimento* [77]

Qi, prana and *pneuma* are all of an air-like nature, and also have in common the property of flow: (1) each flows along ducts within the body; (2) each acts to connect body and world (or different parts of the body-mind); and (3) illness or dysfunction will occur if their flow is uneven or blocked, diverted or reversed (similar views on dynamic currents of air and fluid through undifferentiated vessels – *metw* – were held in ancient Egypt [76,78], although complicated by concern about avoiding stagnation and putrefaction in the bowels [79]). In the West, *pneuma* is closely linked to the history of vitalism, 'the doctrine that the origin and phenomenon of life are due to or produced by a vital principle, as distinct from a purely chemical or physical force' [80], a theme that winds its way throughout the history of our civilization, sometimes almost invisibly, sometimes overtly – and nowhere more so than throughout the practice of complementary and alternative medicine (CAM) [81,82].

The Greek philosopher Plato considered the *psyche* ($\psi\upsilon\chi\acute{\eta}$) to be superior to the body, or *soma* ($\sigma\omega\mu\alpha$) [83]. Aristotle considered *pneuma* as intermediary between the two [84]. In Rome, this distinction continued: the life-breath was known as *spiritus* or *anima*, the consciousness or rational soul as *animus* [85]. Fostered by St Augustine (354-430), this division between 'body-mind-soul' and 'mind-soul' became fundamental to later Western thought, paving the way for Descartes' famous dichotomy of *res extensa* and *res cogitans* (or material thing, and thinking thing). Until the Renaissance, however, Western medicine was vitalist [86], based on the teachings of Galen (129–c. 201), for whom *pneuma*-like (but still material [87]) 'animal spirits' ($\pi\nu\varepsilon\acute{\upsilon}\mu\alpha\ \phi\upsilon\sigma\iota\kappa\acute{o}\nu$, *pneuma physikon*, literally 'natural breath') occupied brain and nerves, mediating between and connecting Will and muscle [88,89]. Again, it was Descartes (among others) who was responsible for downgrading the flow of these animal spirits merely to rapidly moving particles, flame-like yet of 'a certain very fine air or wind' [90] without any inner activity of their own. In the Cartesian universe, movement itself became a mere transport of 'stuff' [91]. Correspondingly, the Galenic 'vital flame' of living matter [92], was moved from center stage and sidelined to the writings of alchemy [93] where, however, the spiritual fire retained its central importance [94,95]. Galenic flow was superseded by (or amalgamated with) other models of flow, particularly neurological [96]. Following an upsurge of interest in electricity in the mid-eighteenth century, much of the imagery and nomenclature of alchemy was transferred, virtually unchanged, into the speculations of the new electrical science; [97] now the flow or obstruction of electricity in nerves, for example, was considered by many to uphold or undermine health [98], leading in turn to the use of electrical stimulation to effect cure [99–101]. And, although the vivifying air was still considered a universal 'vital force' by the Romantic writer Novalis (1772–1801) [102], with the discovery of oxygen by Priestley and Lavoisier, and the demonstration by von Liebig that body heat derives solely from chemical processes, it lost much of its mystique. Scientific vitalism focused more on the *organizing principle* implicit in 'organism' rather than the movement or flow of life – on *li*, rather than *qi*, if you like [103]. However, although vitalism predicated on nonphysical or nonchemical agencies [104] weakened and retreated before each new scientific discovery, in the nineteenth century it migrated to an alternative medical worldview that was emerging at the time [105].

A key figure in the development of this worldview was the Viennese physician Franz Anton Mesmer (1734–1815). The invisible and intangible *fluidum* of his system of 'animal magnetism' bears many resemblances to *qi* [81] (see too Ch. 22), as shown by the asterisked items in Table 3.1 above. Significantly, right from his initial experiments, Mesmer found that the *fluidum* was associated with bodily sensations of flow, and hypothesized that a state of balance of the *fluidum* was healthy, while disease was due to unequal distribution of or 'obstacles' to flow [106]. Towards the end of his life he also described how he stoked his own internal 'invisible fire' to enhance the effect of his 'magnetic' treatments [107].

Many of Mesmer's ideas had parallels in the 'Romantic science' of the early nineteenth century (which, like alchemy, emphasized a self-investigational approach to gaining knowledge), and indeed in the Romantic movement in general [66,102,108]. Later they were seminal in the development of psychoanalysis by Sigmund Freud (1856–1939) and Josef Breuer (1842–1925), who initially proposed that disorders of the mind might result from 'a block that interferes with the normal current of feeling in such a way as to cause stagnation and overflow' [109] and used hydraulic as well as electrical language to describe their new way of working (flows, dams, charges, discharges, excitation, cathexis, currents of energy, resistance, tension) [110]. Freud – although decidedly not a Romantic – went on to develop the concept of *libido*, a term that encompassed notions of pleasure, pouring (flow) and freedom, as well as sexuality [96]. In his later writings, he redefined it as a drive towards *any* form of pleasurable bodily sensation [111] or even as the energy of all the life instincts [112]. Wilhelm Reich (1897–1957), a one-time close colleague of Freud, developed his concept of *libido* in a rather different way, concentrating on its physical expression and simultaneous psychological content [113], even interpreting the collective unconscious posited by Carl Gustav Jung (1875–1961) as a 'universal *libido*' [114]. *Libido* here became a real energy ('orgone' or 'bio-energy') discharged during emotional expression and sexual orgasm [115] and manifesting physically as static electricity [116]. Reich considered the flow of life and its block in the frozen patterns of our personal histories ('character armor') as both ultimately derived from the same *energetic* source ('orgonotic streaming') [117] (see also Ch. 25).

The flow of spirit

The 'hand', the 'burn', and the 'touch' are in substance one and the same thing.

St John of the Cross (1542–1591) [118, vol 3 p 36]

Lord! Thou art my Beloved! My desire! My flowing stream! My Sun! And I am Thy reflection!

Mechthild of Magdeburg (c. 1210–1297) [119]

The breath of the mystic turns the world.

Reshad Feild [120]

Like *qi* and 'soul', in the West the 'spirit' of God (as against the spirit of man) has been *conceived* in terms of Air, Water, and Fire (even electricity [121]). The *experience* of spirit has been described by many mystics. However, despite the obvious association between 'breath' and *spiritus*, descriptions of breath in the mystical experience appear fewer than those of fire and water. The spiritual vision of Pierre Teilhard de Chardin (1881–1955), for example, was one of the whole universe on fire with God's love [122]. By mystics such as Richard de St Victor (d. 1173) [123] and Angelus Silesius (1624–1677) [124], but particularly by the saints of the fifteenth and sixteenth centuries, God's fire was experienced as a 'consuming heat', the wound of 'a fiery spear of love', 'the living flame of love', 'the flame of sweet transformation', 'a consummating and a renewing fire') [118,125–128]. Paradoxically though, for St John of the Cross, for example, these fires of divine love were also 'seas': The 'living waters of the spirit' 'flow' and 'gush in all directions' [118, vol 3 p 57]; 'the fire and the dew' [118, vol 3 p 358] are inseparable.

Four centuries before, in a period predisposed to the 'visionary imagination' [129], Hildegard of Bingen (1098–1179) likewise experienced her visions as both 'sparkling flames' ('rutilant fire') and 'raindrops … falling from the hand of God' [130, p 8]. Another who sensed both heat and flow was the Flemish mystic Beatrice of Nazareth (1200–1268), whose experienced God's presence very much in tactile terms – his passage through her whole body, her soul pierced with the fiery sword of love, the blood of Christ's wounds flowing into her soul. As for St John, Beatrice's Beloved was a river 'which flowed in all directions' [130, p 87], and in which she wished to be dissolved, even as she burned with the fire of love while reposing in his arms.

This paradoxical conjunction of both Fire and Water appears characteristic of the mystical experience, and not just in Christianity. In his *Diwan*, for example, the Persian sufi mystic Rumi (1207–1273) wrote 'Love is a fire which would turn me into water if I were a hard stone!' [126, p 105]; St John of the Cross may well have been inspired by some of the Spanish Sufi masters. The modern mystical philosopher Franklin Merrell-Wolff (1887–1985) [131, p 37] similarly juxtaposed 'the Water of Life, the Current which is Bliss' and 'the Fire of Knowledge', as well as writing of the 'force' that he experienced as 'of fluidic character. There is something in it like breath and like water' [131, p 270]. *Debekuth*, 'cleaving unto God' in the Romantic mysticism of Hasidism, has also been described as both a 'flowing' and a 'kindling flame' [132]. In contrast, in the writings of the Indian mystic Kabir, it is the pain of separation from God that burns, while the inner experience of union with Him is a 'melting': 'his clouds of love rain on me' [133].

The conjunction of these opposites was also a central theme for Mechthild, in whose *Flowing Light of the Godhead* God is both fiery sun and gentle flowing stream, a cooling presence for her melting heart with its own burning desire for God (both of these fires very different from the raging flames of hell). She describes the overflowing stream or 'rippling tide' of love or grace as inexhaustible – although self-will may choke the channel and 'man can easily obstruct his own heart with a useless thought, so that the unresting Godhead who ever works without working, cannot flow into it' [119, p 152]. She cautions further that 'outward activity hinders the inward working of the spirit' [119, p 254] (something we need to beware of even more today, seven centuries later [131]).

For Mechthild, the pure 'burning love' of God is to be experienced 'in soul and body' [119, p 110]. 'Love melts through the soul into the senses, that the body also may have its share' [119, p 129], and the 'sweetness' that the Holy Spirit pours into her soul clearly involved bodily feelings. She writes of the sensed movement of Water, Fire and also Air, but avoids metaphors of Earth completely, as concerning the merely transient rather than divine. Her work, written in the vernacular, and outside the mainstream of medieval religious literature, derives powerfully from 'visionary description rather than theological speculation' [134].

The bodily quality of women's piety at this period, the 'experiential quality' of their mystical writing, has been contrasted with the more impersonal voice of the male church hierarchy [135, p 167]. Men whose religiosity was experiential, both embodied *and* visionary, 'often understood themselves in feminine images and learned their pious practices from women' [135, p 169]. Yet such aspects of the mystical experience were also frequently denied, or at least dissociated (see Ch. 25), and numerous (often male) Christian mystics warned against taking the spiritual experience as bodily, even declaring this 'unnatural' [136]. For example, probably partly in reaction against the popularity of Richard Rolle (c. 1300–1349), who described the 'honeyed flame' of warmth felt in the heart by the lover of God, and the 'wonderful longing flowing out in love to God', a devotion that 'even frees the body from all sorts of disease' [137], Walter Hilton (1340–1396) counseled his readers to forget the senses, emphasizing that the 'fervour and sweetness of devotion, … afire with love', being 'largely or wholly dependent on imagination rather than on knowledge', is still imperfect [127, p 318]. St John of the Cross similarly noted that perfection is attained by paying 'attention to that which is within' [118, vol 2 p 448], that the 'sensual part' of the soul should 'be stilled in the outward and inward senses' [118, vol 2 p 276], in favor of the 'rational part'. His contemporary, St Teresa of Ávila (1515–1582), notwithstanding the sensuousness of the famous sculpture of her experience of ecstasy by Gianlorenzo Bernini (1598–1680) and her own descriptions of a sweet pain 'so great, that it made me moan', of God's love as both fire and 'living water' [128, p 238], wrote that during what she called 'the rapture', 'the body is very often as if it were dead, perfectly powerless … For though the senses fail but rarely, it has happened to me occasionally to lose them wholly … But in general they are in disorder … it is as if the things heard and seen were at a great distance, far away' [128, p 144]. A century later, Marie de L'Incarnation (1599–1672), another mystic who uses imagery of both fire and flow, wrote sternly that 'nothing which falls within the scope of the senses [can adequately convey] this ecstasy and rapture of love' [138]. The erotic 'polymorphous sensuality' of the divine flood of love is put firmly in its place [139], and with Martin Luther (1483–1546), man became merely 'like a vessel or tube through which the stream of divine blessings must flow without intermission to other people' [140]. Goethe, however, although reared in the Lutheran faith, could still in his twenties write of God that 'his spirit is consuming fire, my whole heart melts' [124, p 49].

To summarize: 'Flow' in the West – of *pneuma*, animal spirits, later even electricity – was developed as a healing metaphor particularly by Mesmer, Freud and their heirs, with less emphasis on the aerial and fiery. In the experience of Western mystics, however, both fire and flow (and their conjunction) are recurrent themes.

VERNACULAR *QI* – ITS TRACES IN MODERN LITERATURE

❝ *I bless you, Father, Lord of heaven and of earth, for hiding these things from the learned and the clever and revealing them to little children.*
Jesus Christ [141]

❝ *The queen bee of all human ideas since 2000 BC has been the idea that the body, the pristine consciousness, the great sympathetic life-flow, the steady flame of the old Adam, is bad, and must be conquered.*

D H Lawrence [142, p 769]

Art is Janus-faced and may support the subjugation and rejection of the body by society observed by Reich and the English novelist D H Lawrence (1885–1930), or – like the body itself in our overrationalized and overorganized life [114,143] – may express the unconscious, disowned, 'shadow' side of society, and – again like the body [144] – may be subversive of prevailing conventional values and theories.

Mesmeric vitalism has remained a pervasive influence in literature and popular culture, consolidated in the writing of influential Romantic authors such as Shelley (1792–1822) [145], Coleridge (1772–1834) [108] and Balzac (1799–1850) [146], and later by post-Romantics such as the Austrian Gustav Meyrink (1868–1932) [147], D H Lawrence (for instance, in *Women in Love*, with its ubiquitous flows of *kundalini*-like 'fierce electric energy' [148]) and Ben Okri (whose *Infinite Riches* positively pulsates with incandescent spirits, energies and forces [149,150]). There may also be some cross-connections with the Spanish term *duende*, the magnetic fire felt from powerful performances of music, dance, or poetry, defined by Federico García Lorca (1898–1936) as a 'mysterious force that everyone feels and no philosopher has explained' [151]. Further afield, *wuxia* (武俠) martial arts fiction, which has a long history in China and is still the most widely read genre of Chinese fiction, is frequently focused on *neijin* (內勁) or *qi*-like 'internal power' [152].

To determine how pervasive the characteristics of *qi* listed above are in the modern novel – and not only in the writing of Western authors – a survey was carried out of 150 titles (novels and short story collections) by 122 authors read between 2005 and 2010 (Table 3.4). Data (phrases) were extracted according to a list of 23 keywords/concepts developed from readings on embodied language in the literature of Romanticism and the list of attributes of *qi* given above. Items were scored according to the number of titles in which they appeared (a) published since 2000, and (b) published since 1780 (Table 3.5). More specific words for feelings were analyzed for two of the keyword categories (Table 3.6). Authors of the 15 titles that scored 9 or more out of a possible 23 points are listed in Table 3.7.

Table 3.4	*Vernacular qi – material*	
Period	**Total N titles (M/F)**	**English as author's presumed first language**
1780–1899	23 (22 M/1 F)	4
1900–1949	9 (5 M/4 F)	2
1950–1989	19 (13 M/6 F)	3
1990–1999	15 (10 M/5 F)	4
2000–2009	84 (33 M/50 F; 1 M&F)	49
Totals	*150 (84 M/67 F)*	62

Table 3.5 *Vernacular qi – keywords/concepts and resulting scores*

2000–09: ≥ 30		2000–09: 20–29		2000–09: 10–19		2000–09: <10
Internal fire	63/111	Eyes	28/67	Magnetism	19/35	Block
(Other) body sensations	61/99	Blood	24/36	Spark	12/21	Bone
Flow and other fluid tropes	58/89	Air/breath/ wind	22/32			Channel/ pathway
Electricity	45/70	'Fire' between people	20/36			Life
Spine	30/44	Energy	21/34			Lightning
						Power/force

Scores indicate in how many titles these keywords/concepts appear. Left hand figure: in titles published between 2000 and 2009. Right hand figure: in titles published between 1780 and 2009.

Table 3.6 *Literary sensation – analysis of 67 words of feeling*

Most used words	Whole body sensations 59 words (88%) used	Spinal sensations 50 words (75%) used
Tingl/ing	17	3
Run or ran	12	17
Prickl/ing	8	4
Spread	8	[2]
Pain	7	4
Ris/ing	7	[1]
Shiver	6	17
Shudder	[5]	3
Snak/e	[1]	3

Numbers show in how many titles the top-scoring words occurred. Those in square brackets did not occur frequently (score highly). All terms not included scored low.

Table 3.7   *Vernacular qi – top scoring titles, by author (4 M/11 F)*

Score (max 23)	Name	Country of origin	Setting of story
14	Ben Okri	Nigeria	Nigeria
13	Kate Cole-Adams	Australia	Australia
13	Carmen Laforet	Spain	Spain
12	Syl Cheney-Coker	Sierra Leone	W Africa
12	Morag Joss	Scotland	Scotland
12	Natasha Mostert	S Africa	England
11	Sebastian Barry	Ireland	Ireland
11	Regina McBride	US	Ireland
10	Deborah Moggach	England	England
10	Holly Payne	US	Turkey
10	Andrew Sharp	Uganda	Uganda
9	Carolyn Baugh	US	Egypt
9	Faye Booth	England	England
9	Barbara Cartland	England	England
9	Francesca Marciano	Italy	Italy

Score indicates how many of the 23 keywords/concepts were used in an individual title by the author.

Note: The data in Tables 3.4–3.7 may not be altogether accurate or unbiased. Searching was conducted manually while engrossed in reading, rather than electronically and dispassionately, so some keywords were doubtless missed. Furthermore, my selection of titles was by no means random (although what leads anyone to read a particular novel may depend on many factors, which will not necessarily remain constant over several years of reading). For instance, novels in a more poetic (aural/visceral) style were preferred to the predominantly descriptive (visual) (i.e. 'fluid' rather than 'architectural' [153]), those by women to those by men (particularly once I had realized for myself – belatedly – Simone de Beauvoir's understanding that women tend to be more *yin*, attuned to their own bodies and inner processes than men, more focused on outer action, *yang*), and those by non-English/American authors as often as I could find interesting-looking covers in my local library.

Books not written in English were all read in translation, which raises the issue of whether this was true to the original language. A further difficulty – particularly with contemporary fiction – is that authors tend to be wide-ranging in their reading and very aware of other writers' language (often now learned or taught on 'creative writing' courses). It is impossible to know how much of the phraseology used, for instance, by Ben Okri (originally from Nigeria, living in London, writing in English) is based on his personal experience, how much on his early absorption of Yoruba cultural elements, how much on his impressive knowledge of European civilization (from Greek mythology to Lévi-Strauss via 'Lobsang Rampa' and the German Romantics), and how much on simple literary convention (Okri himself would no doubt dismiss the question as irrelevant).

DISCUSSION

❝ If I read a book [and] it makes my whole body so cold no fire can ever warm me, I know that is poetry. If I feel physically as if the top of my head were taken off, I know that is poetry. These are the only way I know it. Is there any other way?

Emily Dickinson (1830–1886) [154]

❝ Corporeal insides have extraordinary powers.

Maxine Sheets-Johnstone [155]

From this brief survey (Table 3.5) it is clear that the embodied experience in novels and stories, like that of the mystics, is frequently described in terms of fire (warmth) and flow, rather than breath (air, wind), which has played such an important part in conceptualizing *qi* or soul. Breath in these titles is considered less than blood, or even than the eyes ('windows to the soul'), which figure so strongly in Gothic horror and romance fiction. Sensations of electricity, magnetism and the fire between people are also described (echoing the tingling and warmth frequently reported in healing (see Ch. 25), and the 'magnetic attraction' encapsulated in the French word for a magnet, *aimant*, and the use of powdered lodestone in love potions in ancient Rome [107]).

Sixty-seven words for bodily feelings were found in the '(Other) body sensations' and 'Spine' categories. Of these, some 46% describe sensations of 'movement' (run, spread, etc.), and 19% could be construed as 'electrical' (such as prickl/ing or tingl/ing). Table 3.6 shows the most commonly used words that were found (all of these, apart from pain, being movement or electrical words). There is considerable overlap among the most frequently occurring words between sensations described in the body as a whole and spinal feelings.

Sensations in or along the spine are often used to heighten effect, but this probably has more to do with eliciting a sympathetic (ergotropic, see Ch. 25) response from readers than with *kundalini*, as sensations of cold (as in 'cold shivers') occur in this sample more than four times as often as those of heat. However, in general spinal sensations are more often described as traveling *downward* (parasympathetically? [156]) rather than upward (although perhaps less so in more recent titles), and this too is in contrast to the usual experience of *kundalini* [157,158]. Curiously, the spinal sensation was described as snakelike by three separate authors (in ancient Greece, the spinal marrow of the dead was sometimes considered to turn into a snake [159]). Apart from the possible increase in upward-moving spinal sensations since 2000, it is very noticeable that the distribution patterns of scores for major terms such as 'internal fire', 'body sensations', 'flow', 'spine' and even 'eyes' are very similar when data from most of the different periods are compared (graphical data not shown).

Looking at the top-scoring titles (Table 3.7), it is striking that over two-thirds of the authors listed are women, that most set their stories outside Anglo-Protestant culture (prominent exceptions being a post-Gothic novel by Faye Booth and one of Barbara Cartland's 'romances', a genre of watered-down Romanticism), and that at least three (Okri, Cole-Adams and Mostert) explicitly mention CAM or their own experiences with therapy or martial arts (Western *wuxia*). Other impressions gleaned from this sample are that: (a) in general, an increasing number of fiction writers now mention acupuncture, even if only in passing, and (b) a surprising number of authors who record bodily felt experiences do so using the language of synesthesia.

Of course, the language used in these books has pre-Romantic precedents as well. The fires of God's lightning-like wrath can be found in the first millennium BCE Books of Genesis and Deuteronomy, 'overflowing' in Isaiah, his anger becoming 'an overflowing shower' in Ezekiel; hearts overflow in Psalm 45, and burn in the Gospel of St Luke. 'Hot desire' is featured in *The Women of Troy* by Euripides (c. 415 BCE) [160], the hot fire of love in the heart in the plays of Plautus (c. 254–184 BCE) [159] and an 'eye of flame' in Homer [157], the late Egyptian Leyden I papyrus [74], and Virgil's *Aeneid* (c. 20 BCE) [159]. The fires of love also occur in the poetry of the troubadors [161,162] and the writings of the medieval philosopher Bernardus Silvestris (c. 1085–1178) [163]. Thus many of these metaphors are very old.

Metaphor is in fact not just the basis of poetry, but of virtually all our abstract thinking; some primary metaphors like these are so deeply embedded in (and derived from) how we experience ourselves and the world that they are virtually what Ralph Waldo Emerson (1803–1882) called 'natural symbols' [153], part of the cognitive unconscious – we are not really aware of how powerful they are. George Lakoff and Mark Johnson have plotted some of these, such as 'affection is warmth', 'vitality is a substance' (perhaps a key to some interpretations of *qi*), 'love is a physical force' (such as magnetism or electricity) [164], or 'lust is heat' [165]. Another mechanical metaphor, the basic opposition of 'blockage and movement' [166], leads on to such 'force gestalts' as 'counterforce' and 'diversion' [167], which may resonate for some readers as descriptions of pathological movements of *qi* in the channels of acupuncture. Lakoff and Johnson have also pointed out how few ways there are of conceiving life itself [168]. What they write about lifespan could in some cases equally be applied to the life force. For example, there is 'life is a path' [168], which manifests in the pathways (*jing*) of the channels (*jingluo*) in CM, or as the central metaphor of the path in the healing traditions of Fiji [169]. The importance of the village paths of the Songhay of West Africa (Mali) for the 'circulation of people, goods, and services … as vitally connected to the circulation of blood, heat, and breath in the individual body' [170, p 147] finds its echo in the writings of West African (Nigerian) authors like Ben Okri and Daniel O Fagunwa (1903–1963), or Camara Laye (1928–1980) from Guinée. In poetry itself, we have 'life is a fluid', 'life is a flame' and 'life is a fire' [165, p 52] (as in the 'vital heat' of Henry David Thoreau (1817–1862), which has itself been interpreted as *qi* [171]). However, even if derived from bodily experience, Lakoff and Johnson write about metaphors as purely conceptual entities, corporeal *concepts* (disregarding, for example, the *actual* electrical tingle that may be felt between lovers). Thus their approach has been criticized by dancer and philosopher Maxine Sheets-Johnstone for leaving out the 'embodied experience' of language [146].

So what I have tried to do here is look at use of language as embodied experience rather than just abstracted metaphors. In doing so, I have inevitably been attracted to what Daniel Stern has called 'vitality affects' [172] and Susanne K Langer (1895–1985) 'forms of feeling': the terms of 'feelings of vitality' (or aliveness) with which we become familiar even in our prenatal lives [172] and from which we have constructed our dynamic language of interiority, 'insideness' [143] or 'viscerality' [173]. This is a language of fire and breath and flow, with terms such as 'surging', 'fading away', or 'boiling up'. This is also how we feel and express our emotions. In Yuasa's words, the emotions are intimately connected with the 'splanchnic sensations of the internal organs', the undifferentiated 'dark consciousness' within [174, p 186]; to use Aristotle's example, 'anger is a surging of blood and heat around the heart' [175]. (Achilles in the *Iliad* described it as 'waxing like smoke in the breasts of men' [159, p 52].) In Jungian terms, such fiery states erupting from within often accompany a connection with the unconscious [176], the *non*-ego, in contrast to sensations from the body surface, which formed the basis of Freud's definition of the *ego* as 'a mental projection of the surface of the body' [177].

Reading a novel is not a trivial activity. 'Esthesia' means sensitivity or feeling, and the distinctive quality of art that has not been subjected to too much esthetic purification has been termed the 'intrinsic perception of sensation' [178]; in what Drew Leder calls the state of 'esthetic absorption' [173], our boundaries become porous, and in our imaginations we relive to some extent what we read, as argued by Langer for the appreciation of the artistic image [179]. For Langer, 'artistic form is congruent with the dynamic forms of our direct sensuous, mental, and emotional life' [180]. In Reichian language, the flow of images in the psyche forms a functional identity with the flow of energy within the body [114]. Just as athletes can train with visualization to improve performance [181], the act of reading a novel written with awareness of the body-self can itself develop awareness of the body in the reader, and enhance aliveness (this may be stating the obvious for those who enjoy the erotic arts [178]). I do not know whether the act of writing (or typing) has been described in terms of *qi*, but certainly Chinese calligraphy has [182], and for the painter Dao Ji (1641–1717), for example, mountains flowed like rivers and the proper way to look at them was as 'ocean waves frozen in time' [183]. The absorption required in both the act of painting and that of opening to the work of art as a feeling observer could be compared with that of *yangsheng* – tracking the movements of *qi* within both the microcosmic and macrocosmic body. The esthetic experience is one of a 'felt change of consciousness' [153, p 20], or even of liminality, 'the passage from one plane of consciousness to another' [153, p 26], and so in some ways – if we allow it to be – akin to the religious experience.

To summarize: Analyzing characteristics of *qi* in the language of the novel shows that words of fire and flow appear more frequently than do those associated with air, and that the bodily sensations described are frequently of movement, or electrical (tingling, prickling, etc.). Women are more likely to use such embodied, visceral language than men. In general the esthetic experience is essentially embodied rather than simply cerebral.

CULTURE AND COUNTER-CULTURE? WEST AND EAST

❝ I believe that, like technology, ki is something that can be useful to us in our daily lives and it should not be seen simply as a reaction against our present-day materialistic civilization.
Kaku Kouzo [184, p 10]

" The New Agers lifted up the power of nature as a healing force ... excavated the hidden vein of vitalism that had run throughout the history of biomedicine, and they challenged the biomedical focus on the anatomical body.
Linda L Barnes [185]

SOCIOCULTURAL OVERVIEW

In 1921, even before Reich published his major work, Lawrence was writing that illness may result from the blocking of flow within the body and the suppression of the sensual will. Like Reich, he believed that this attitude could also lead to psychological stunting of whole generations, not just individuals [186]. Also like Reich (and Mesmer before him), he was to some extent persecuted by the powers that be, and, again like Reich, his ideas contributed greatly to the predominantly Anglo-American 'New Age' (NA) movement of the 1970s that developed out of the 1960s counter-culture (itself partly a rebellion against postwar materialism and technocracy) [187].

It is possible to view this development as a rebellion against repression, or just part of an ongoing oscillation [72] or dynamic fluctuation of *li* and *qi* (Apollonian and Dionysian, rational and romantic [188]), or *yin* and *yang*. However, what a society considers to be its 'mainstream' views may actually be shared only by a numerical minority [189]. As Edith Turner puts it [190]: 'We now have to recognize that *this* [NA] is our "Western society", not the small enclave of rationalist scientists, however high the status and power of the enclave. This other ordinary society – its ways somewhat hidden and turned toward nature, and not appearing to be a true culture – actually predominates. This is Western society, and historically always has been.' This may appear to be an extreme view, but other respected researchers have observed that 'the consciousness of rationality' is only 'an historically situated notion constructed within a specific social context' [191], that 'popular occulture' is 'the new spiritual atmosphere in the West' [192] and that 'holistic spirituality' [193] or 'alternative spirituality' [194] (other terms for NA) is not just a passing fad, but likely to become more prevalent in the future. As one writer on the new 'centres of life' founded around 1900 has put it, 'We can best bring these things together by imagining an underground water system which, except in times of drought, always moves below the surface of high culture and professional propriety: a system that is out of our sight, and out of our sympathy much of the time, but that deserves to be studied because it is always necessary if the land is to be fertile' [195].

Interestingly, in their survey of a small Lake District town in the UK, Heelas and Woodhead found that words like *qi* and *chakra* are now more common in the general culture than traditional Christian vocabulary, that terms such as 'flow' and 'balance' are pervasive ('the great refrain, we might say, is "only connect"' [193, p 26]), and that 'energy', *qi* and *prana* have become 'functional equivalents' of spirituality [193, p 27]. Others too have observed that flow is a key holistic [196,197] or NA [187,198–200] principle – the goal being 'to remove obstructions and restore an unimpeded flow of energy' [184, p 318]; 'holism' has even been *identified* with vitalism [201]. Flow has also been invoked in discussions of US 'nature religions' [202] and definitions of NA magic as 'the art of sensing and shaping the subtle, unseen forces that flow through the world' [203, p 13].

In their analysis, Heelas and Woodhead [193] restate the difference between what the anthropologist Victor Turner termed normative 'structure' and the flow of 'communitas' [72] as one between 'life-as' (conforming to external authority) and 'subjective-life' (life-in-relation), which are deeply incompatible with each other (and with similarities to the dichotomy posited by Claire Cassidy in Chapter

13 between 'reductionist' and 'processual', or between the 'abstract, general nature of social theory' and 'the individual nature of bodily experience' described by Anne Scott [204]). Subjectivity itself, in those therapies like Chinese medicine [205] predicated on the existence of a 'subtle body' as 'open, extensive, interconnected, inherently intersubjective and processural', has been described not only as 'a response to energy, *it is* energy' [206].

ECONOMICS AND THE EDGE OF KNOWLEDGE

Today the situation for CAM modalities based on *qi* (*prana*/energy) differs from that in the counter-cultural 1960s and the early, heady days of the NA in the 1970s in that practice is very much tied in with market forces. The oppositional stance implicit in the term 'alternative medicine' has been softened to one of 'complementarity' (or even 'CAM'). 'Energy' is almost universally emphasized in folk medical systems [39], and now 'energy flow' is very much part of the Western vernacular. Even a major credit card company has used the slogan 'life flows better' with its product (although in Germany it 'runs more lightly' with it). At the same time surveys show that there is a growing nondenominational belief, throughout Europe at least, in 'some sort of spirit or life force' [207]. Given this seemingly widespread acknowledgment (if not necessarily approval) of 'flow' and 'life force', implicit in so much CAM, it is hard not to interpret the current repressive backlash against it (and against energy medicine in particular) as at least in part economically motivated, very much as in the case of the eighteenth-century rubbishing of mesmerism [107]. Capitalist economics, after all, has a great deal to do with blockage – accumulation, stagnation and retention of power and commodities (the 'spent energy' of money) – as against the relatively free flow of goodwill gift exchange and reciprocity that is found in less competitive, more 'synergistic' communities [72,169,208,209].

Attacks on CAM are also indicative of an ongoing battle against 'detraditionalization' (the shift of authority from 'without' to 'within') [210], or what may be considered by some as a wishy-washy Romantic revival [211], felt as deeply threatening to the stability of society and their own life values. They could even be symptomatic of an unwanted recognition that mainstream science is coming up against its own limitations [212,213], and that what from the centers of established science is perceived as marginal may in fact be dynamic and leading edge [214]. As Phil Mollon states in Chapter 18, 'knowledge of the energy fields, and how to work with them, has always been "forbidden"'. Such concerns may even elicit 'an enormous existential terror amongst conventional doctors' [215], who have been trained to view the body as object, mechanism, or corpse (*Körper*) [173], rather than lived body (*Leib*) [216].

DEEP ECOLOGY

❝ Our lives extend beyond our skins, in radical interdependence with the rest of the world.
Joanna Macy [217]

❝ The primary principle of magic is connection. The universe is a fluid, ever-changing energy pattern, not a collection of fixed and separate things. What affects one thing affects, in some way, all things.
Starhawk [203, p 129]

The world of the body and the body of the world have [much] in common' [170, p 141]. The associations of *qi* with life, connection and unity, and transformation (see Table 3.1), epitomized in the neo-Confucianism of Ekken Kaibara (above), link it inextricably with the deep ecology movement of Arne Naess (1912–2009)

[218], with its understanding of a flow that connects, both within communities and between culture and nature [219,220], and for some even the belief that 'all beings are ensouled' [221]. Thomas Ots's definition of *qi* as the 'bodily aware-ness of being alive' (Ch. 25), with close parallels in Yuasa's philosophy [174], has a broader parallel in the definition of 'biophilia' by Edward O Wilson as 'the innate tendency to focus on life and lifelike processes' [222], engagingly restated by Stephan Harding: 'the human organism is inherently predisposed to seeing nature as alive and full of soul … we repress this fundamental mode of percep-tion at the expense of our own health, and that of the natural world' [223]. The potentially fatal alliance between technocracy (even 'techno-addiction' [224]) and 'biophobia', explicit in the urge to reify the self [225] and control nature [226], has propelled many to take a biophiliac stance in their own lives. Some turn to the 'Gaia hypothesis' of James Lovelock [227], in which the earth's biosphere, atmo-sphere, oceans and soil form one single self-preserving system that is virtually a living organism in itself; others seek balance through the practice of *fengshui* (堪輿), or use dowsing or divining to explore the *jingluo*-like pathways taken by so-called 'earth energies' [228,229]. The biophiliac stance also often involves a turn to the softer modalities of *qi*-based medicine, perceived as working *with* rather than against nature ('a nonegoistic intention is necessary, but intention is not it. It is the allowing of an opening' [219, p 75]. This attitude of *non*-dominance has also been considered characteristic of the 'dynamic feminine' [230].

FEMINISM

There has been considerable overlap between feminism and both the counter-culture and NA ideologies. Not only did saintly medieval women experience the influx of spirit as flow [132], but generally in the literature of feminism women's bodies have been described as more 'fluid' than those of men, in many senses [231] (although the second-century theologian Origen once remarked that in general 'river is not a bad name for the body' [232], and Liebniz too compared all bodies to rivers, in a state of perpetual flux [173]). In particular, Elizabeth Grosz has written that, in the writings of men, the female body has been constructed as 'leaking, uncontrollable, seeping liquid; as formless flow; as viscosity, entrapping', whereas men's own bodies are self-contained, and they seem to want to cast out these 'liquidities' from their self-representation [233] as in some sense pathological, even to be feared [73,234]. Women's 'relational-ity' [192] and fluid permeability has been compared to 'that of ocean or air cur-rents', and again contrasted with the Cartesian (and male) vision of the reified, self-contained body [144]. This contrast between the feminine (biophiliac) 'flow of the Arche', the 'Furious Fire' of women's 'Pyrogenetic Ecstasy', and the male (necrophiliac [235]) 'State of Fixation', 'Stag-nation, and 'entrapment of gynergy', 'sapping the flow of gynergetic currents', has been powerfully described in Mary Daly's *Pure Lust* [236].

To generalize, women tend to be more aware of human energy ('biofield') phe-nomena than men [237], and more susceptible to 'transliminality' correlates of the *kundalini* experience such as hyperesthesia [238] (although *responsiveness* to orgone-acupuncture was not found to differ between men and women, unlike responsiveness to a placebo intervention (L Southgate, unpublished study, 2002); gender differences in placebo response are complex and have not yet been thor-oughly investigated [239]). Correspondingly, men are usually more skeptical than women about energy medicine [240], historically patients of mesmerists (for example) have tended to be women rather than men [241], and currently in the US this is true for CAM in general [242]. Indeed, although Western medicine as a whole tends to be deeply patriarchal in its professional structures, in most fields of CAM – as in nursing [243] – women practitioners tend to outnumber men [193,244]. Nor is it surprising that at times during its long history, despite being practiced in the past almost exclusively by men, acupuncture in China was slighted 'as the work of "women" and non-professionals' [27, p 157], or that women in China and elsewhere tend to practice internal meditative (*neidan*, 內丹) forms of *qigong* (氣功) rather than 'hard' *qigong* (*yinggong*, 硬功) [34]. Two prominent forms of *qigong* were in fact popularized by women (Liu Guizhen and Guo Lin) [245]. What is somewhat intriguing is that US women responding to a questionnaire measuring Eastern and Western thought patterns tended to be more 'Eastern thought inclined' than men [246], while Chinese ways of thinking have themselves been described as having 'feminine traits' [3].

EXPRESSION AND REPRESSION IN CHINA

❝ The sage first regulates his internal flows, and then the rivers and oceans follow in his path.

Lin Zhao'en (1517–1598) [247]

❝ The fluid presence in our bodies is our fundamental environment; we are the moving water brought to land.

Emilie Conrad [248]

Chinese-based healing practices contributed greatly to the general '*bricolage*' of NA/holistic approaches to healthcare in the West [187,199], with a predominant emphasis on meridian (channel) flow among the 'alternative' practitioners of the 1970s and early 1980s. In the late 1980s, however, a normative and more structured 'TCM' (traditional Chinese medicine) approach began its ascent to dominance. This process has parallels in Chinese history, both ancient and recent.

The demigod Gun (鯀), grandson of Huangdi, the yellow emperor, failed to restrain the great floods that threatened China by building dams. In contrast, his son Da Yu (大禹), one of the forefathers of Daoism, managed to do so by *opening* natural pathways along geographical 'lines of force' to drain the accumulated waters [4]. In the *Lingshu*, the rivers and streams of *qi* within the body were originally compared to the natural waterways of China – as with the *nadi* of yoga and the sacred rivers of India [249], the body-as-conduit and the rivers of Rwanda [250] (see Ch. 2), or the hydraulic body of the Andean Qollahuaya [251]. The same simile was used by the Roman philosopher Seneca (4 BCE–65 CE) [170]. However, once the analogy between channel and watercourse had been made [15], just as controlling and directing the flow of water was 'seen as one of the first steps to a civilized world, so channeling of *qi* into routes around the body' marked a significant stage in bringing the body under control [27, p 153]. A similar process may have occurred in the practice of yoga, whose traditional postures (*asanas*) were probably developed from more spontaneous ('natural') movements and breathing behavior [252].

Qigong, like many practices in CM, has been described as based on a 'philosophy of balance whereas biomedical science is based on the Occidental philosophy of conquest' [253]. This is certainly in keeping with a 'deep ecological' interpretation of *qi*, but given the tendency for a more formalizing approach to follow an initially freer exploration, as well as the plurality of *qigong* forms, it may be rather a romantic view, and as a generalization not altogether accurate. Similarly, taken out of context *qigong* could be considered essentially apolitical in nature, but this has clearly not been the case in China, where at times its practice has been officially encouraged, then a few years later forbidden, once more permitted (indeed flourishing during the '*qigong* fever' years of 1979–1989 [254]), and then once again restricted. Indeed the word *qigong* itself was rarely used at all before the 1930s

Elemental souls and vernacular *qi*: some attributes of what moves us

[245], receiving a government-approved standardized meaning in 1953 [255], with the first official *qigong* course after the Cultural Revolution organized only in 1982 [245].

As in the West, the Chinese body has at times unconsciously expressed what is not culturally or politically acceptable. This has certainly been the case with *qigong* [255]. With the lifting of many restrictions in China in the 1990s its more florid spontaneous forms enabled expression of much that had remained repressed under Mao (in a culture that is anyway not overly given to emotional self-expression [256]). In the words of one charismatic *qigong* master, '*qigong* releases the soul of China' [254, p 3], while another commentator has noted that *qigong* discourse became 'a symptom of repressed desires' [255], and yet another that 'a sort of Daoist body … replaced the totalitarian body' [257]. With the rise of the divisive and doctrinaire *falun gong* (法輪功) protest movement, which started in 1992, *qigong* was very definitely politicized [245] (rather as with the White Lotus rebellion of 1796 and the Boxer uprising of 1900).

Already in the 1980s, the Communist ban on *wuxia* fiction (see above) had been lifted. A few years later, even mainstream authors such as Ke Yunlu turned their attention to *qigong*. In his novel *The Great Qigong Masters* he highlights the confrontation between *qigong* and Marxist ideology, and this in turn led to real life confrontations with those such as Sima Nan, 'China's Randi', who denied the existence of *qi*, denounced what he considered the mystical fakery of some *qigong* masters, put down the effects of external *qi* to psychological suggestion and vehemently opposed the *falun gong* [255]. There were even accusations of feudal superstition and witchcraft against some prominent charismatic *qigong* teachers [254].

In response, more peaceful and meditative forms were officially promoted to counter potential political resistance [27,32], with only four classical methods permissible in the public parks [245]. The rise of 'medical *qigong*' has even been described as 'a key strategy to foster surveillance by doctors and licensed practitioners' [254, p 146]. By 2005, *yangsheng* practices were portrayed as 'dwelling in the mainstream', and included such innocuous hobbies as nature photography, disco and ballroom dancing, choral singing, chess and cards [258]. Opposition had been absorbed. In the pithy words of one feminist theoretician, 'the "civilized body" forms libidinous flows, sensations, experiences, and intensities into needs, wants, and commodified desires' [259], as is blatantly obvious in much of the health and fitness movement in the West as well [260].

CONCLUSION

A survey of concepts of the soul in 360 different cultures and subcultures indicates that some form of animating entity that is in some way akin to *qi*, if not a exactly a vital force as such, has been a globally accepted reality in almost all known cultures other than our own, both ancient and contemporary [238]. Although devalued by the custodians of our contemporary mainstream 'scientistic' worldview, an acceptance of something flowing and *qi*-like has also been an important and continuing aspect of the subterranean aquifers that keep our own culture vital, which is particularly evident in the language of embodied experience rather than that of disembodied concepts.

The balance of elemental attributes discussed and presented in tabular form in this chapter is summarized in Table 3.8 (1 to 3 = lowest to highest scores).

CAM practitioners may worry about attacks by skeptics, with their calls for evidence and cost-effectiveness. In both East and West so-called 'integrative' medicine has incorporated many techniques of CAM while rejecting their underlying vitalist philosophies [82]. In the West the New Agers and their heirs have

Table 3.8	Elemental attributes discussed in different sections of this chapter		
Term or context	Air	Water	Fire
Qi	2	3	1
Soul	3	1	1
Western thought	1	2	1
Mystical experience	1	2*	3*
The novel	1	2	3

*The conjunction of Water and Fire also appears frequently in descriptions of the mystical experience

appropriated Chinese medicine in a way that is similarly 'partial and in the image of the selector' [184, p 327]. However, the underlying stream of *qi* and its analogs has endured and, I believe, will continue to do so. As biomedical thought and practice risk becoming ever more separated from popular culture [261], the undying metaphors implicit in *qi* offer hope for a more respectful *rapprochement*.

ACKNOWLEDGMENTS

To Charles Buck and Julie Reynolds for their helpful critiques of a preliminary version of this chapter.

SECTION 2
QI IN CHINESE MEDICINE

SECTION INTRODUCTION

Here we continue to utilize the concepts of energy and flow in the analysis of *qi*, more specifically in Chinese medicine. It is striking how all of Chinese medicine, energy anatomy and pathology use functional terms relating to the overall political governance of society as metaphors for how the human body is regulated – essentially as a description of human physiology. The metaphor of a harmonious, united, smoothly functioning empire (well known, although little touched on in this book) is all the more arresting for the Western reader since biomedicine conventionally uses a very different metaphor: that of the nuts-and-bolts *machine* to describe functions of the human body. While the human body has been used as a metaphor for the political governance of a human society, for instance by Thomas Hobbes (1588–1679) in his famous treatise *Leviathan* (1651), we do not observe the reverse application in Western medicine. Leviathan was in fact the body politic made visible – a social body composed of cells of individual men, just as the human body is composed of individual cells.

Modern medicine is largely based on an understanding of the body 'from the bottom up', as essentially made up of populations of cells, these in turn comprising tissues and organs that work together as regulated by physiology, just as populations of individuals make up societies and work together under political governance. The overarching metaphors of Chinese medicine, derived from a very different way of experiencing the body, are another useful – and complementary – way of representing human functional anatomy and physiology. In contrast to the machine mode of Western medicine, as an empirical system

Chinese medicine is tremendously sophisticated and nuanced in terms of devising treatments tailored to each individual and to his or her specific conditions.

The Chinese use of metaphors in medicine that describe human physiology in terms that come from human sociopolitical organization may relate to the preoccupation of Chinese civilization with the Emperor, his Mandarins and the bureaucratic organization that provided the foundation for government administration of complex works and operations. One of the great projects of the ancient Chinese civilization, which at once created and sustained it, was the creation of canals or 'waterways' for irrigation, agriculture and transportation. Organizing the huge forced labor required for such projects had a cybernetic relationship to the development of Chinese social structures and political control. These processes and relationships were described by Karl Wittfogel (1896–1988) in his classic treatise *Oriental Despotism* (1957). The inherent relations of the contours of Chinese society – with major public 'infrastructure' projects, the political organization of the Chinese government and the Chinese pictographic language needed and used for communications – result in a rich vocabulary of metaphors useful in describing medical aspects of the human body, in particular the waterways or 'channels' (*jing*, 經) in Chinese. (The translation of *jing* or *jingluo* as 'meridians' preferred by some writers does not map so accurately to this original metaphor.)

The chapters in this section provide a new map and guide for the understanding of *qi* in Chinese medicine.

The anatomical foundations of *qi* 4

John L Stump

CHAPTER CONTENTS

❝ *Life makes shapes.*
Stanley Keleman [1]

INTRODUCTION

Most anatomy textbooks adopt the conventional Western view of the human body in emphasizing physical structures and components that interact in a very delicate and complex manner. These structures are typically mapped from the most prominent and large scale – bones, muscles, tissues and so on – down to the minutest cells and their components including genes. This structural framework forms the foundation of the archetypical theory of cause and effect that dominates Western anatomical thought.

Asian medicine is very different in that components of *process* are considered rather than just *structure*. The human body especially is seen as an energetic system in which various substances interact to generate the whole organism. The Chinese describe these basic substances, which range from the palpably physical (terrestrial) such as Blood (*xue*, 血) and Body Fluids (*jin ye*, 津液), to the more refined (celestial) such as Essence (*jing*, 精), *qi* (氣) and Spirit (*shen*, 神) [2]. What is important to remember about Eastern anatomical philosophy is that none of these was considered a separate entity. In Chinese philosophy there was and still is a continuous dynamic interaction between all things [3].

4

There is nothing more fundamental to Chinese anatomical thought than the understanding of the concept of '*qi*'. This subtle and essential energy is itself a union of cosmos (celestial) and earth (terrestrial). These two primary energies will be discussed in more detail later, but before we explore Asian medical thought more extensively, let us review some of the basic Western science that underlies our contemporary view of the physical universe.

SOME BASIC WESTERN SCIENCE

One way of understanding how Western scientific thought works is that it looks for agreement between mathematical and experimental proof of a problem [4]. This is what makes the Western scientific method so powerful. It is well suited to practical applications and has led to great discoveries, such as those in electricity (with continuing innovation in everyday audio and television technologies, for example) and in particle and submolecular physics, with developments such as radiography (X-rays), magnetic resonance imaging (MRI) and lasers.

Human knowledge progresses, and new phenomena are discovered in every scientific field, and in the anatomical world in particular. Often, these new phenomena cannot be explained fully by the theories held when they are discovered. The process of finding contemporary methods to describe unfamiliar phenomena is invariably one that expands our views, challenging current ways of thinking about the character of physical reality. This is particularly true in the case of Western anatomy, where I believe it is time for scientists to incorporate the concept of *qi* and begin utilizing a more universal concept of 'energy medicine' than heretofore.

SOME THEORETICAL CONCEPTS IN PHYSICS

Until early in the last century, much of the Western scientific worldview of physical reality was based on the physics established in the late seventeenth and eighteenth centuries by Sir Isaac Newton and his successors. They considered human anatomy as made up of solid objects, among a vast number of other solid objects in the universe, all consisting of yet smaller solid objects or particles (atoms). As science grew more sophisticated in the late nineteenth and early twentieth centuries, Newtonian physics was extended into the subatomic world, with the atoms themselves thought to be composed of solid objects – a nucleus of protons and neutrons, with electrons orbiting around the nucleus [5]. All physical reactions were seen to have a physical cause. These laws were seen as the basic laws of nature, and Newtonian concepts as comprising the ultimate anatomical (as well as atomic) theory of natural phenomena. However, in the early twentieth century, new theories were developed that went beyond the possibilities of Newtonian mechanics. With the development of powerful radio telescopes and electron microscopes, discoveries became ever more dependent on technology. Simple cells and atoms were no longer the epicenter of scientific investigation [6].

The old-world, Newtonian concepts of the human body began to change, and as science began to move out of a world of static solid form into a world of dynamic energy fields, more consideration was given to elusive and intangible aspects of the body such as emotions, consciousness and the life force itself.

For Newton, forces depended on the existence of particles. For Michael Faraday two centuries later, *fields* of force (the regions where forces operate) could have an independent existence, and in 1865 James Clerk Maxwell published his 'dynamical theory of the electromagnetic field', which unified electricity, magnetism and light for the first time under a single theoretical umbrella [7]. The concept of a universe filled with force fields that interact with each other was born [8]. In 1905

Albert Einstein developed the special theory of relativity, which demonstrated the seemingly capricious interchangeability of energy and matter [9]. Eleven years later he produced the general theory of relativity, which brought together special relativity and gravitation.

During the 1920s the explorers of the physical world moved into an extraordinary new reality within the subatomic cosmos. With the development of quantum mechanics by Einstein, Max Planck, Werner Heisenberg, Niels Bohr and others, Western science entered the age of the paradox in physics: every time a theory was established, nature seemed to respond with its antithesis, and the more scientists tried to prove their theories the stronger the paradoxes became. As the physicists penetrated deeper and deeper into the secrets of quantum matter, for example, its dual nature – as both particle and wave – became more apparent. The world of solid objects and the deterministic laws of nature were dissolving into a matrix of wavelike patterns of interconnection. Correspondingly, all particles could be created from energy, transmuted into other particles and then vanish into energy once more [10]. Yet there remained perplexing incompatibilities between the macroscopic theory of relativity and the microscopic (atomic and subatomic) world of quanta. Einstein, unconvinced that nature would prescribe totally different modes of behavior for phenomena that were simply scaled differently, and unwilling to accept that chance played such a large part in quantum mechanics, sought a theory that would reconcile such differences. This second unifying theory, the unified field theory [11], sometimes called the 'theory of everything', would reconcile the seemingly incompatible 'anatomies' of various individual fields – and in particular electromagnetism and gravitation – in a single comprehensive set of equations [12].

We are just beginning to admit these concepts as also plausible in how we understand the human body. For instance, many people are able to sense the presence of others. When two blindfolded martial arts students are put into an empty room there is a rapid *field interaction,* evident in their *randori* (sparring, 乱取り). We often use this field interaction when we feel that a person we have just met has good or bad 'vibes'. Field interaction is used daily by each of us. The consequences of Einstein's relativity theory that matter and energy are interchangeable are also relevant for the energy medicine practitioner. Mass is nothing but a form of energy [13]. Matter is simply slowed down or unobstructed energy. Our bodies are energy [14]. On a larger scale, just as the old Chinese philosophers described the *dao* and *qi* as being empty and formless yet producing all forms [13], in the new physics the whole universe can be defined as a dynamic inseparable whole.

Also relevant is the 1947 discovery of the principle of *holography* by Hungarian-born Dennis Gabor, who received a Nobel Prize for his work on electron optics in 1971 [8]. Using two laser or coherent light beams (one direct, one reflected), a two-dimensional image ('hologram') of an object can be created. Laser light can then be used again to recreate the wave pattern originally recorded, appearing now as a *three*-dimensional image. Paradoxically, from every portion of the hologram the entire image may be reconstructed. This is an instance of the *holographic paradigm*, which states that the whole is represented in each of its parts [15].

The prominent quantum physicist David Bohm wrote in his book *Wholeness and the Implicate Order* [16] that primary physical laws cannot be determined by a science that considers the universe only as comprising distinct components (see Ch. 8). His version of the holographic paradigm leads us into a new era of wholeness in science where the classical idea of dissecting the universe and humans into separate and independently existent parts no longer holds.

ASPECTS OF HUMAN ENERGY – *JING*, *QI* AND *SHEN*

Jing (精) in Chinese medicine is usually translated as Essence and, as with *qi*, is a somewhat difficult concept to grasp. It can be considered the quintessence, or the foundation, of *qi*, but should not be confused with it. Congenital *jing* forms the basis for prenatal growth and reproductive function. Fluid-like, it nurtures growth and development, and if it is weak an individual may be chronically prone to sickness and ill health throughout life. *Jing* and *qi* have somewhat of a *yin–yang* relationship: whereas *qi* is associated with movement, the slower and more methodical organic change as seen in growth is more an aspect of *jing*. Both, however, may be affected by practices such as *qigong* (see Ch. 6).

All matter, animate and inanimate, is composed of and permeated by *qi* (氣). The first known attempt to codify and explain this vital universal energy is found in the *Yi Jing* (*Book of Changes*, *I Ching*), which was traditionally compiled in the third millennium BCE and is attributed to Fu Xi (see Fig. 1.2) [8]. Here *qi* is described in terms of a polarity of *yin* (陰) and *yang* (陽), somewhat akin to the negative and positive forms of electricity described millennia later in the West by physicists, although they are inseparable: in *yang* there is always some *yin*, and in *yin* there is some *yang* – '*yin* is a becoming-*yang*; *yang* is a becoming-*yin*' [17] (Fig. 4.1). When *yin* and *yang* are balanced the living system exhibits health; when either is unbalanced a state of 'dis-ease' can manifest. Excessive *yang* may result in gross overactivity, predominant *yin* in an insufficiency of function. Another polarity is that between *li* (理) and *qi*. If *qi* corresponds to the activating force that animates matter, *li* is somewhat like matter's underlying etheric blueprint, its principle of organization [18] (see also Ch. 11). *Li* is more *yin*; *qi* is more *yang*. The earth is more *yin*; the heavens are more *yang*.

Qi may also be described in ways other than the primary terrestrial and celestial energies of the *Yi Jing*. If you imagine viewing the interior of your body, the place where you live, one of the first things you will notice is your breathing, as your lungs involuntarily pull external air in and push internal air out of the body. In Chinese medicine, this process is not just one of breathing air, but one in which *qi* enters the body as External (*kong*, 空) *qi*, and is then exhaled. The 'bioenergetics' of *qi* also involve Original or 'Prenatal' (*yuan*, 原) *qi* from the parents, Food (*gu*, 穀) *qi*, Gathering or 'Ancestral' (*zong*, 宗) *qi* from the interaction of *gu qi* with the air, and so forth (Fig. 4.2). Nutritive (*ying*, 營) *qi* flows within the blood vessels and meridians, and Protective (*wei*, 衛) *qi* outside these vessels and more superficially in the body [19].

Shen (神), or Spirit, is often also interpreted as the consciousness, emotions, thoughts and senses that make a human being unique [14]. Through practices

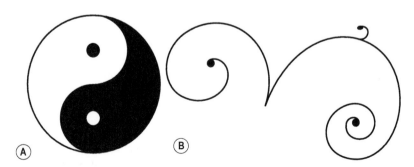

FIG 4.1　**(A) The** *taijitu* **(太极图), traditional diagram of yin and yang. (B) A contemporary image of yin and yang – opposing positron and electron spirals in a magnetic field.** *(After Lee and Bae [52].)*

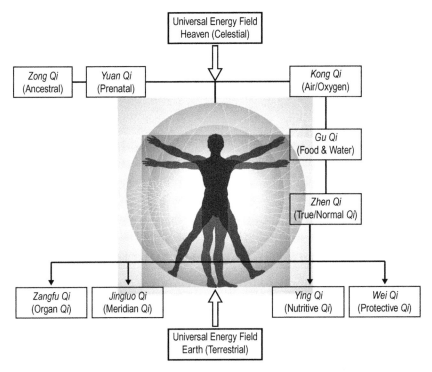

FIG 4.2   The anatomy of *qi* in Chinese medicine, as learned by the author. (In contrast, Maciocia considers zong qi as 'gathering' together gu qi and the qi from air, which he leaves unnamed, and does not differentiate between *ying qi* and *jingluo qi* [19]). (*Adapted from artist's impression, ©ag visuell/Fotolia, with permission of Fotolia.*)

such as meditation, heightened awareness of the *shen* within – and of the *shen* of others – may be developed, as in the many accounts in the world religions of experiencing or seeing light around people [8].

CONTEMPORARY ACCOUNTS OF *QI*

In an age when disease is understood in terms of microorganisms, metabolic failures and changes in DNA structure, rather than blockages in the circulation of *qi*, the modern medical model for the mechanism of acupuncture is one of cascades of biochemical and neuronal events that occur within the body. Minute amounts of peptides and other biochemicals are released, which act locally or are transported to other sites where they stimulate various biologically programmed responses.

Is there another model, however? *Qi* has been defined and described by hundreds of philosophers over several thousand years of China's history but has never been adequately scientifically explained. In the past few decades many have attempted to explain *qi* as a form of 'bioenergy' or 'subtle energy' [20]. Yoshio Manaka eloquently described what he called 'the X-signal system' (of which the acupuncture meridians are part): a primitive information system in the body whose activities are usually masked by those of the more advanced regulatory nervous system [21]. William Tiller has discussed *qi* in terms of electromagnetic energy [22]. More unconventional suggestions involve the 'innate intelligence' of D D Palmer, the founder of chiropractic [23], and a whole plethora of alternative energies such as the 'odic energy' of Karl von Reichenbach and Dean Baldwin [24]. To date none of these has been accepted by the Western scientific world, and the words of Laozi, the great Chinese philosopher, come to mind: 'The *dao* (Way, 道) that can be told is not the everlasting *dao*; the name that can be named is not the everlasting name' – meaning perhaps that, regardless of how well we try to explain *qi*, such theorizing will never be adequate [25].

Yet ideas about energy, vibration and resonance continue to exert their fascination in the world of complementary medicine, from the radionics of Albert Abrams [8] and the writings of the 'sleeping prophet' Edgar Cayce [26] to the homeopathic law of 'like curing like' and the 'energy of water' engendered by dilute doses of *materia medica* [18]. Even Candace Pert, codiscoverer with Nobel laureate Solomon Snyder of endorphins and a former section chief at the clinical neuroscience branch of the US National Institute of Mental Health (NIMH), touches on the energy of the body and *qi* when she says: 'There is Intelligence in every cell of your body. There's a form of energy that appears to leave the body when the body dies. If we call that another energy that just hasn't been discovered yet, it sounds much less frightening to me than...spirit' [27].

THE SHAPES OF *QI* – THE AURA AND THE *CHAKRAS*

The *qi* of the body is not without form (*li*). A simple way of understanding this is presented by Barbara Ann Brennan in her book *Hands of Light* [5]. She attempts to bring together the Western scientific approach and Eastern spiritual concepts in her discussion of the human 'aura', the energy field that surrounds us. In her model, there are seven energetic layers to the aura, extending within and beyond the physical body, each with its own vibration patterns [28]. These seven layers correspond to the *chakras*, or 'wheels' of energy and light, first described in the Sanskrit *Yoga Upanisads* some 3000 years ago [29] but more widely known in the West through the writings of the theosophical movement early in the last century [30], and used by many healing practitioners both past and present [31–33].

The seven major *chakras* (see Fig. 15.1) are centers where energy (*prana*) can shift between the different layers of the aura, and also where energy is exchanged between the aura of the individual and the surrounding universal energy field. They are located along the vertical axis of the body (Brennan's 'vertical power current'), and act much like electrical transformers bringing high-energy currents down to those levels we can use for our homes and businesses – in this case for the human energy body. The pathways that the energy takes within this body are termed the *nadi* ('vessels'), and there are also minor *chakras* distributed along these [28]. In the *Yoga Upanisads* some 72 000 *nadi* are mentioned.

Each *chakra* is associated with different aspects of our nervous and endocrine systems, allowing the body to utilize and distribute energy as needed (Table 4.1) [34–38].

THE ACUPUNCTURE MERIDIAN SYSTEM

Whereas the Ayurvedic system of *chakras* and *nadi* originated in India during the Vedic period, 1–2 millennia BCE [39], the acupuncture meridians (channels) widely accepted in East Asian countries – but viewed suspiciously by Western science – make up a different and probably more recent system. They, however, are similar to the *nadi* in that they form a network of communication and distribution of subtle energy within the body (and there may indeed be historical cross-connections between the two systems, with some correlations between the main *nadi* and the principal meridians – as with the *susumna*, *ida* and *pingala nadi* and the *dumai* and Bladder meridians [38]). In the meridian model, which summarizes the experience of the Chinese with disease over more than 2000 years, *qi* is taken in through the acupoints along the meridians as well as through respiration.

Table 4.1 *Neurophysiological and endocrine associations of the chakras*

Chakra name	Western name	Nerve plexus	Organs	Endocrine system	Meridian system	Biosynthesis functions	Acupoints (anterior)	Acupoints (posterior)	Ayurvedic element	Chinese element
Muladhara	Base	Pelvic plexus	Spinal column, kidneys, lower limbs	[None]	BL, KI [SI, BL, KI]	Grounding	Ren-1 *huiyin* [Ren-2 *qugu*]	Du-1 *changqiang*	Earth	Water (Earth)
Swadisthana	Sacral	Inferior mesenteric ganglion	Reproductive system, fluid balance	Gonads	SP, P [SI, BL, KI]	Centering	Ren-4 *guanyuan*, Ren-5 *shimen*, Ren-6 *qihai*	Du-4 *mingmen*	Water	Earth (Water)
Manipura	Solar plexus	Celiac plexus and celiac ganglion	Stomach, liver, gall bladder, pancreas, spleen	Pancreas	ST, LIV [ST, SP]	Bounding	Ren-12 *zhongwan* [Ren-14 *juque*]	Du-6 *jizhong*, Du-8 *jinsuo*	Fire	Wood
Anahata	Heart	Inferior cervical ganglion	Heart, blood, circulation, vagus nerve	Thymus	HT, SI [P, HT]	Bonding	Ren-17 *shanzhong*	Du-11 *shendao*	Air	Fire
Vishuddha	Throat	Superior cervical ganglia	Lungs, bronchi, vocal apparatus, alimentary canal	Thyroid and parathyroid	LU, LI [LU, P]	Sounding	Ren-22 *tiantu*, ST-9 *renying*	Du-12 *shenzhu*	Space	Metal
Ajna	Brow	Ciliary ganglion	CNS, left eye, Eustachian tube, ears, nose	Pituitary	GB [SI, BL, Du]	Facing	M-HN-3 *yintang*	Du-14 *dazhui*	None	None
Sahasrara	Crown	None	Upper brain (CNS) and right eye	Pineal	*Sanjiao*	Spacing		Du-20 *baihui*	None	None

Left portion after Cross [34], right portion after Greenwood [35], with permission. *Chakra*/Reichian segment functions in the somatic psychotherapy method of biosynthesis are also shown (see Ch. 25) [36]. Meridian variants in square brackets are after Motoyama [37,38]. Acupoint variants in square brackets are those given by Cross [34]. Slightly different acupoint correlations are given in Chapter 15.

There is not space here to describe the meridians and points and their functions in depth, but there are many other excellent books that do so [40,41]. Suffice to say that the meridians provide an essential basis for understanding the recipro-cal relation between the various diagnostic and therapeutic aspects of traditional East Asian medicine. Early on, doctors observed that pathology of the Internal Organs (*zangfu*, 臟腑) often manifests in certain external or systemic symptoms, that disease in one organ often affects another, and that many diseases follow a predictable course of development, these changes being explainable according to the meridian model [40]. Correspondingly, by stimulating distinct locations on the body surface using various methods, dis-ease in both the superficial tissues and the *zangfu* could be treated. Often these points are some distance away from the affected region of the body (the *zangfu* in particular cannot be reached directly without invasive surgery). Over time, these observations became systematized to form the basis of Chinese medicine (and then traditional East Asian medicine as a whole), with the intimate relations between the internal viscera and the periphery of the body maintained primarily by means of the meridians. Thus the system of meridians – which is comparable on one level to Einstein's unified field theory – integrates the body's separate parts and functions into one unified organism. The meridians form a web or matrix of criss-crossing pathways vertically and horizon-tally throughout the body; they run beneath the skin and link the body surface to the internal organs and all the other tissues within the body, integrating each part with the whole. This interrelationship of all parts reflects the early holistic attitude of Chinese medicine [3].

In practice, the entire framework of diagnostics, therapeutics and point selection is based upon the theory of the meridian matrix. It is this that maintains the har-mony and balance within us. From a modernist perspective, we may consider that the meridian theory reflects the limitations of understanding and scientific verifica-tion possible at the time of its development. Because of its emphasis on what might be termed 'philosophical biophysics', it is not truly appreciated or well understood in today's scientific world. However, what has clinical value continues to be used, while other parts have needed re-examination through practice and research to determine their true value in clinical application. This is especially true for those contemporary medical acupuncturists who use the meridians and points but give little clinical significance to *qi* – if even acknowledging its existence – and the other philosophical constructs of Chinese medicine [42] (Richard Niemtzow, personal communication, 2009).

THE MERIDIANS AS PATHWAYS OF *QI*

The main routes for *qi* through the body consist of 12 pairs of primary vertical (longitudinal) meridians, the *jing* (經, not to be confused with Essence) [19]. Of these, six (most on the back and sides of the body) are *yang*, and six (on the front of the body) are *yin* (see the inside cover). Each meridian is named according to whether it traverses the arm (hand) or leg (foot), is *yin* or *yang*, and by the Organ (*zang* or *fu*) with which it connects internally (Table 4.2).

In addition, there are (horizontal) connecting meridians, the *luo* (絡), which are more superficial than the *jing* [43,44]. There are also two midline 'extra' ('extraordinary' or 'ancestral') meridians: the *renmai* ('Conception' or 'Directing' Vessel, 任脈) which runs up the front of the body from the perineum to the lower lip, and the *dumai* ('Governor' or 'Governing' Vessel, 督脈), running up the back from the coccyx and over the head to the frenulum inside the upper lip. (Specific correlations of *renmai* and *dumai* points with the *chakras* may be found in Chapter 15 and Table 4.1, which also includes *chakra*–meridian correspondences suggested by John Cross [34] and Hiroshi

Table 4.2 *Derivation of the meridian names*

Name of meridian	Abbreviation	Location	Yin or yang
1. Lung	LU	Hand	*Yin*
2. Large Intestine	LI	Hand	*Yang*
3. Stomach	ST	Foot	*Yang*
4. Spleen	SP	Foot	*Yin*
5. Heart	HT	Hand	*Yin*
6. Small Intestine	SI	Hand	*Yang*
7. (Urinary) Bladder	BL	Foot	*Yang*
8. Kidney	KI	Foot	*Yin*
9. Pericardium	P	Hand	*Yin*
10. *Sanjiao*	SJ	Hand	*Yang*
11. Gall Bladder	GB	Foot	*Yang*
12. Liver	LIV	Foot	*Yin*

Motoyama [37]). Six further extra meridians have no distinct points of their own [45], including the *chongmai* (Penetrating Vessel, 衝脈), sometimes called the 'vital' meridian. This originates in the pelvic cavity and emerges at the perineum, with one branch ascending inside the vertebral column and two superficial branches that coincide with the Kidney meridian and run bilaterally up the front of the body to the throat, reuniting at the lips (Fig. 4.3) [46]. In all there are considered to be more than 70 different types of meridian, including 12 'tendinomuscular' and 12 'divergent' (or distinct) meridians, 15 *luo* [43], and other submeridians ('branches' or 'canals') supplying *qi* to the parts the *jing* cannot reach and directing it to every cell in the body [47].

The *jing* specifically connect with the upper and lower extremities, head and trunk, and internally with the *zang* (*yin*) Organs (Liver, Heart, Pericardium, Spleen, Lung, Kidney) or the *fu* (*yang*) Organs (Gall Bladder, Small Intestine, *Sanjiao* (三焦, Triple Burner/Energizer/Warmer), Stomach, Large Intestine, (Urinary) Bladder). In East Asian medicine, these Organs are *functional complexes* rather than strict anatomical structures as classified in Western anatomy.

The *renmai* is the 'sea' of the *yin* meridians, where for instance the paired *yin* meridians of the leg all meet, at points Ren-3 (*zhongji*) and Ren-4 (*guanyuan*). Its functions include regulating menstruation and nurturing the fetus. The *dumai* regulates ('governs') the *yang* meridians, which all converge at Du-14 (*dazhui*, 大椎), a *dumai* point between the lowest cervical and uppermost thoracic vertebrae. The *dumai* reflects the physiology and pathology of the brain and the spinal fluid, and their relationship with the reproduction organs. The *chongmai* is the 'sea' of all 12 principal meridians [46].

Qi itself, circulating throughout the human organism in specific directions through the meridians, is transformed, propagated, stored and distributed by the

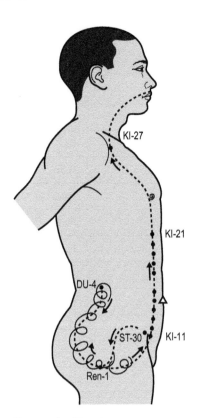

FIG 4.3 The *chongmai*, or Penetrating Vessel.

zangfu. As vital energy, *qi* also permeates every living cell and tissue. The inner circulation of *qi* in and among the Organs is often called the 'core circulation', while its circulation in the meridian pathways which lie in the peripheral or subcutaneous tissue is sometimes termed the 'peripheral circulation' [43]. Numerous internal pathways, together called the 'mediate circulation', link the core and the peripheral circulation. *The key to remember here is that qi can be manipulated only where it can be reached, and that is clearly on or near the body surface.*

MODERN THEORIES OF THE MERIDIANS

The above description of the meridians is only one of several found in the ancient Chinese classics. Further research and scientific observation is needed even to verify their existence, especially when discussing the distribution of the submeridians and subtypes of *qi* mentioned above. Although some medical acupuncturists consider the meridians to be nonexistent and simply a means for remembering acupoint locations, there are a number of speculative theories on what the meridians might actually represent anatomically. In the 1960s, for example, the Korean Kim Bonghan discovered intravascular thread-like 'ducts' that were hailed as equivalent to the meridians before being discredited during the following decade (Kim committed suicide as a result). Nevertheless, research on the Bonghan ducts and nuclei has recently revived [48]. Others have suggested that the meridians might represent the lymphatic vessels [49], or reflect patterns of division in embryogenesis [21], 'primitive lines of retraction away from noxious stimuli, or lines of reach toward favorable stimuli', 'emergent lines of shape control' [50], or some aspect of the 'connective tissue matrix' [21] or 'connective tissue planes' [51].

In some sense, these are still 'mechanistic' models of the meridians. More 'energetic' and/or vitalist models are mentioned elsewhere in this book (see for example Chs 6 and 17).

THE ACUPUNCTURE POINTS

Portals of entry on the skin, these points (*zhenxue*, 針穴, 'needle pits') correspond in some ways to the *chakras*, but additionally are places where *qi* can be manipulated and moved using acupuncture [43,52] so that *qi* imbalances, deficiencies, excesses, blockages and escapes can be restored to normal [53]. The points most used in acupuncture treatment lie on the meridians, but there are also many 'extra' surface points not on them. Traditionally, there are some 361 meridian points whose particular functions (interconnections and actions) have been known for centuries, as well as several dozen extra points whose position is well defined [43]. Most traditionally trained practitioners use these points to 'tonify' (reinforce) or 'sedate' (reduce) imbalanced *qi* flow in the meridians according to a system of diagnosis based on taking the pulse, observing the tongue and/or other indicators. They locate the points precisely by their relations to anatomical landmarks on the body surface, refined by long training in palpatory sensitivity. In addition, there are so-called *ashi* (啊是, 'ouch, that's it!') points that may be spontaneously tender or sensitive to pressure and may manifest just about anywhere on the body. The 'trigger points' used by Western doctors predominantly for pain relief are generally considered a subset of the *ashi* points, usually associated with palpable nodules in taut bands of muscle stressed by either mechanical or systemic disorders [54]. In contrast, most biomedical research has not recognized that the traditional acupoints have any commonly consistent palpable or anatomical features, although much work has been carried out on the sectional and stratified anatomy of individual points (Fig. 4.4) [55,56], there are some studies associating particular neurovascular structures with the points in general [57], and in addition the segmental innervation of the points has been mapped [58]. Charles Shang has suggested that 'singular points' originating in the process of morphogenesis during embryological development may coincide with the acupuncture points [59]. Despite such investigations, and a growing number of rigorous clinical studies which demonstrate the effectiveness of acupuncture, there remains some controversy about whether acupuncture following the traditional meridians and points method is any more effective than sham acupuncture.

The properties of each point are determined to some extent by the route and distribution of the meridian on which it lies (historically, the meridians were probably defined first [60]). For instance, the point *hegu* (LI-4, 'Joining Valley') illustrated in Figure 4.4 is the *yuan* (原, 'Source') point of the Large Intestine hand *yangming* meridian, located on the dorsum of the hand between the first and second metacarpals. Clinical indications for the point include the common cold, facial paralysis, hemiplegia, nosebleed, infantile convulsions, headache, toothache and pain in general.

Acupuncture is not the only technique that can be applied at the *zhenxue*. There is indeed no term for acupuncture on its own in China, where it is known as *zhenjiu* (針灸), or 'acumoxa', because it was originally often used with 'moxibustion', in which the herb wormwood (もぐさ, *mokusa*, in Japanese) is burnt on or over the point for stimulation. Early use of moxibustion [60] and bloodletting [61] at the points contributed to the development of acupuncture as we know it today, with some practitioners still using such adjunctive practices even more than needling.

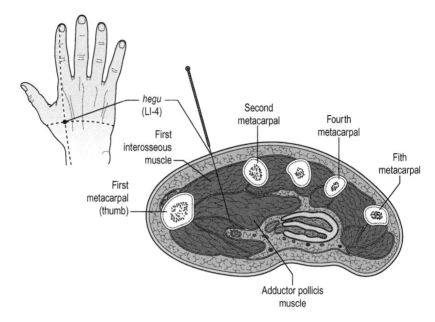

FIG 4.4   The cross-sectional anatomy of the acupuncture point *hegu*, LI-4. *(After Chen [56], with permission of Churchill Livingstone.)*

In this context, it is interesting to note that the classic text the *Huangdi Neijing* from around 70 BCE emphasized that the practitioner should let out the *qi*, but not the Blood, from the points; other texts state that Blood should be let out, but not *qi*.

CONCLUSION

This chapter gives a brief overview of some aspects of *qi* and the subtle anatomies of the Ayurvedic and Chinese medical traditions. If the nerve plexuses represent tangible aspects of the more abstract *chakras* (Table 4.1), then the meridian system and the connective tissue (neuroglial) matrix may be considered as mediating between them (Fig. 4.5), different meridians being associated with the different *chakras* [36]. This energetic anatomy provides the means whereby universal energy is 'stepped down' to a level where it can be utilized efficiently by the physical body.

Western science has successfully dissected the universe into discrete objects whose attributes it can then describe [24]. However, if we continue down this Newtonian route, will such an approach enable us to find *qi* and determine the intricacies of its workings? Questions on the complete anatomical basis for *qi* are not likely to be answered in a few short paragraphs, either by this author or even by those who have spent their lives exploring the field. Here only the surface has been scratched. To the linear, rationalist thinker who prefers material facts, attempting to describe the anatomy of something indefinable might appear implausible. To the practitioner who considers his or her art in terms of subjective experience and a multidimensional model, *qi* may lie at the core of practice. For the individual receiving treatment, healing is foremost, however it comes about.

There remain many unanswered and thought-provoking questions about the unmapped (and possibly unmappable) portions of the human (energy) body that will receive attention in the future, both from those with an interest in the gross manifestations of *qi* and from others with an interest in the more subtle consciousness of its workings. It is the author's wish that everyone's view

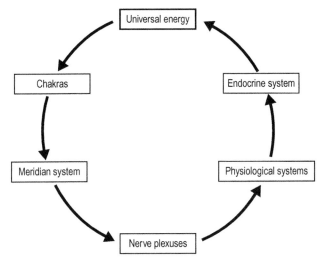

FIG 4.5 The meridian (channel) system, mediating between the *chakras* and nerve plexuses.

be allowed the same consideration, whether they approach *qi* 'mechanistically', or in the spirit of 'vitalism'. At this time in history, no scientists, physicians, or even acupuncturists can adequately explain *qi*. As practitioners, we may still work with a gross or a subtle anatomy of *qi* flow (whatever we may call it, and however we understand it). Whatever our perspective, we use what we can to help our patients alleviate their suffering.

The anatomical foundations of *qi*

Qi in China's traditional medicine: the example of *tuina*

5

Kevin V Ergil • Marc S Micozzi

CHAPTER CONTENTS

PERSPECTIVES ON THE HISTORY OF CHINA'S TRADITIONAL MEDICINE

Medicine is a human endeavor and as such is shaped by the human beings using and practicing it. Furthermore, as a human enterprise, it is embedded in and intersected by myriad other human projects. As a result, its practice sometimes has less to do with curing disease in the most simple and efficient way and a great deal more to do with economics, politics and culture. The same is true of medical research, and even the choice of how to conduct a medical procedure or what kind of healthcare to choose may have more to do with ideology, belief, habit or economics than with rationality or efficacy.

More generally, our own individual and cultural perspectives on medicine and our experiences with the medical systems familiar to us will fashion our ideas regarding what is normal or typical in the practice of medicine. We may have stereotypical expectations of other traditional systems, for example imagining Chinese herbal medicine as a gentle therapy using nontoxic ingredients, preferring to overlook its use of substances that are highly toxic or obtained from threatened species of animals or plants. Or we may have an opposite view: that only Western biomedicine is safe and reliable.

Medical systems are thus rooted in their respective cultures, in turn molding our understanding of how minds and bodies function, and the disease conditions we fall prey to. For example, neurasthenia *(shen jing shuai ruo,* 神经衰弱, a vague fatigue once thought to be caused by psychological factors) is an important syndrome in traditional Chinese medicine and Chinese psychiatry, despite the fact that this diagnosis has fallen into disrepute among Western psychiatrists and it is no longer classified as a disease entity in diagnostic manuals. Neurasthenia was an exceptionally popular diagnosis in the nineteenth century during periods of extensive medical exchange between the United States and China and Japan. The diagnosis continued to be clinically important in China into the 1990s because it corresponded well with certain traditional medical models and responded well to cultural and political concerns about mental illness [1]. Americans and Europeans who encounter neurasthenia within the corpus of Chinese medicine sometimes find it an unusual or obscure concept despite its relevance for Chinese medical practice and the resemblance it bears to the equally mystifying chronic fatigue syndrome described in Western medicine (see Ch. 23). Considerations such as these are important when we try to understand the concept of *qi* in Chinese medicine.

ENCOUNTERING *QI*

When encountering an unfamiliar idea, it is often difficult for us to grasp unless we can relate it to something with which we are already familiar. One example is the use of the word 'energy' to express the idea of *qi*. An extension of this is the common practice of describing the therapeutic method of draining pathogenic factors from channels as 'sedation'. Neither energy nor sedation has much to do with the concepts that underlie *qi* and draining; however, these terms are more familiar to us and make Chinese medicine feel more accessible. Unfortunately, this practice can obscure the breadth of meaning of these terms [2].

We try to make sense of the world from our position in it, historically as well as culturally. Within our basically monotheistic culture we tend to view history as progressing, as if by design, to a specific end, rather than in terms of cultural pluralism. Events of the past viewed from the perspective of the present offer tempting opportunities for reinterpretation in relation to current experience. For example, in the context of perspectives on disease causation, the Ming dynasty physician Wu You Ke's statements that 'pestilential *qi*' (*li qi*, 疠氣) could cause epidemic disease, and his concept of 'one disease, one *qi*' (N Wiseman, unpublished work, 1993), have led contemporary sources in China to suggest that such an insight, coming as it did before the invention of the microscope, is quite remarkable [3]. The implication that Wu You Ke's observation was a precursor of germ theory is attractive to Chinese practitioners who are trying to find a place for traditional practices in an increasingly biomedicalized world. In fact, the concept of miscellaneous *qi* (*za qi*, 杂氣) or pestilential *qi* has been used extensively in adapting traditional theory to the management of human immunodeficiency virus (HIV) infection. However, as Wiseman points out, this concept was never explored in relation to the causation of disease by microscopic organisms, nor was it ever conceived as such.

In contrast to the historical progression of Western medicine, with its comparatively recent attempts to pare away inconsistencies within the system and its cultural commitment to a unitary model, the breadth of traditional Chinese medical thought has always been sustained by an intellectual climate that retained all possible ideas for use and exploration. A given philosopher or clinician might reject an idea, but the idea itself would remain available for future use.

Taking the example of Wu You Ke (1592–1672) once more, he was the leading exponent of the 'offensive precipitation sect' (*gong xia pai*, 攻下派) of physicians, whose tenets included a distinctive set of ideas concerning the management of epidemic disease and a wholehearted rejection of many established principles in Chinese medicine [4]. He was subsequently viewed first as a contributor to Chinese medical thought, then as a proponent of a divergent and uninformed theory, and finally as the intellectual antecedent of Koch, the discoverer of the tuberculosis bacillus. At no point were his ideas discarded.

Interestingly enough in modern China, where the sheer volume of information and the nation's healthcare needs make it necessary to teach a standard curriculum to thousands of students each year, this tolerance for varying clinical perspectives continues to some extent. For instance, there are herbal physicians known as 'Minor Bupleurum Decoction' (*xiao chai hu tang*, 小柴胡汤) doctors because their prescriptions are *organized* around one formula from the *Treatise on Cold Damage (Shang Han Lun*, 傷寒論), an early text on diagnosis and herbal therapy written during the Han dynasty (206 BCE–220 CE). In contrast, some herbal physicians reject traditional formulas entirely and use contemporary perspectives on the Chinese pharmacopeia to organize their prescriptions. There are acupuncturists whose clinical focus is dedicated almost entirely to six acupuncture points and who use computed tomography scans to plan clinical interventions. At the same time, two floors down in the same hospital, physicians base their selection of acupuncture points on obscure and complex aspects of traditional calendrics and systems such as the 'Eight Techniques of the Magic Turtle' (*ling gui ba fa*, 灵龟八法). Chinese medicine is thus a broad and varied tradition with many manifestations and philosophies, and an extensive history. As with most medical traditions, this history can itself be approached from several perspectives.

One such perspective is the ancient mythology of Chinese medicine, which attributes the birth of medicine to the three legendary and semimythical emperors Fu Xi, the *Ox Tamer* (伏羲, circa 2953 BCE), Shen Nong, the *Divine Husbandman* (神農, 2838–2698 BCE), and Huang Di, the *Yellow Emperor* (黄帝, 2698–2598 BCE) (see Fig. 1.2). Fu Xi (associated with the West) taught people how to domesticate animals and breed silkworms, and divined the *Ba Gua* (八卦), the eight symbols that became the basis for the *Yi Jing* (易經) or *Book of Changes*. Shen Nong (associated with the South and with Fire) is considered the founder of agriculture and herbal medicine, having learned the therapeutic properties of herbs and substances by tasting them. Later authors attributed their work to him to indicate the antiquity and importance of their texts. The *Divine Husbandman's Classic of the Materia Medica (Shen Nong Ben Cao Jing*, 神農本草經) is a case in point. Probably written in the Han dynasty (around 200 BCE), it was later reconstructed by Tao Hongjing (456–536 CE). Huang Di, the third mythical emperor (associated with the Center), was responsible for the principles of Chinese medicine, and acupuncture in particular, as set out in the *Huangdi Neijing* (黄帝内經) or *Yellow Emperor's Inner Classic*, which is of uncertain date but was very likely compiled in the first century BCE [5] (see too Chs 1, 3 and 4).

Another perspective is offered by the careful study of available ancient texts and records. These records indicate, for example, that there is no reference to acupuncture as a therapeutic method in any Chinese text before 90 BCE [6], and that the oldest existing texts to discuss medical practices that faintly resemble current Chinese medicine date from the end of the third century BCE [6].

Finally, there are interpretations of archeological evidence and textual materials that seek to establish the ancient character of certain Chinese medical practices. One somewhat extravagant interpretation, for example, is the common assertion that the stone 'needles' excavated in various parts of China are remnants of ancient acupuncture [7, 8]. This assertion is based on references in texts from later periods to the ancient surgical application of sharp stones and on morphologic similarities between the excavated stones and the metal needles that were used later. A link between them is by no means proven.

QI AND THE ESSENTIAL SUBSTANCES OF THE BODY

Apart from the ideas of *yin* and *yang* and the Five Phases ('Elements'), there is no concept more crucial to Chinese medicine than *qi* – the idea that the body is pervaded by subtle material and mobile influences that cause most physiological functions and maintain the health and vitality of the individual. This idea is not common to biomedical thinking about the body. *Qi* is often translated as 'energy', but this translation conceals *qi*'s distinctly material attributes. Furthermore, although energy is defined as the capacity of a system to do work, the character of *qi* extends considerably further.

As described elsewhere in this volume, the Chinese character for *qi* is traditionally composed of two radicals (ideographs), with that for breath or rising vapor positioned above the radical for rice (See Chs 1, 16). *Qi* is thus linked with the concept of 'vapors arising from food' [6]. Over time this concept broadened but never lost its distinctively material aspect. Unschuld favors the use of the phrase 'finest matter influences' or simply 'influences' to translate the term [6], while more recently Sivin has used 'the fine, essential matter that is the vehicle of consciousness' [9]. Thus Wiseman points out that some phenomena labeled as *qi* do not fit conventional definitions of substance or matter, further confusing the issue [3]. Because of this confusion, many authors prefer to leave the term *qi* untranslated.

The idea of *qi* is extremely broad, encompassing almost every variety of natural phenomena. The body contains many different types of *qi*. In general, the features that distinguish each type derive from its source, location, and function. There is considerable room for debate in this area, and exploration of a wide range of materials suggests a variety of different ideas about categories of *qi*. In general, *qi* has the functions of activation (including transportation and raising), warming, defense, transformation and containment (Table 5.1).

Qi is sometimes compared with wind captured in a sail; we cannot observe the wind directly, but we can infer its presence as it fills the sail. In a similar fashion, the movements of the body and the movement of substances within the body are all signs of the action of *qi*. Thus *qi* is important to many aspects of Chinese medicine. *Qigong* (氣功) for instance is a general term for the many systems of meditation, exercise and therapeutics that are rooted in the concept of mobilizing and regulating the movement of *qi* in the body, or *qi* cultivation (see Ch. 6). Acupuncture can be used to influence organ and channel *qi* (see Ch. 4), and in fact one characteristic feature of much acupuncture treatment is the sensation of 'obtaining the *qi*' or *deqi* (得氣).

In relation to *qi*, blood (*xue*, 血) and body fluids (*jin ye*, 津液) constitute the *yin* aspects of the body (see too Ch. 20). Blood, which nourishes the body, is understood to have a slightly broader range of actions in Chinese medicine than it does in biomedicine. *Qi* and blood are closely linked: *qi* generates blood and moves it,

Table 5.1 *Some types of qi and their functions*

Type (Chinese)	Type (English)	Function
Ying qi (營氣)	Nutritive or Construction qi	Supports and nourishes the body
Wei qi (衛氣)	Defense qi	Protects and warms the body
Jing qi (經氣)	Channel qi	Flows in the channels (felt during acupuncture)
Zang qi (臟氣)	Organ qi	Flows in the organs (physiological function of organs)
Zong qi (宗氣)	Ancestral or Gathering qi	Promotes respiration and circulation

while blood nourishes *qi* [10]. This relationship is expressed in the Chinese saying, '*Qi* is the commander of blood and blood is the mother of *qi*.' It has been suggested that *qi* and blood are linked in the same manner as a person and his or her shadow.

Fluids (*jin ye*) are a general category of substances that serve to moisten and lubricate the body, and may be thin or viscous. 'Liquid' (*jin*) is thin and responsible for moistening the surface areas of the body including the skin, eyes and mouth. 'Humor' (*ye*) is thick and related to the body's organs; one of its functions is the lubrication of the joints.

TUINA (CHINESE MASSAGE)

Tuina (推拿), literally 'pushing and grasping', is a comprehensive system of massage, manual acupuncture point stimulation, and manipulation (Fig. 5.1). It has been practiced for at least as long as moxibustion (see Ch. 4), if not longer, and so, as with all aspects of Chinese medicine, regional styles and family lineages of practice abound. However, the first Chinese massage training course was not created until 1956 in Shanghai [11], and the formal curriculum available in Chinese programs, although extensive, is probably not a complete expression of the range of possibilities. Today, *tuina* can serve as a minor component of a traditional medical education or an area of extensive clinical specialization.

A distinct aspect of *tuina* is the extensive training of the hands necessary to accomplish focused and forceful movements in clinical practice. Techniques such as pushing, rolling, kneading, rubbing and grasping are practiced repetitively until they become second nature. Until their hands develop the necessary strength and dexterity, students practice on a small bag of rice.

Tuina is applied routinely to patients with orthopedic and neurological conditions, but also to patients with conditions that may not generally be thought of as susceptible to treatment through manipulation, such as asthma, dysmenorrhea and chronic gastritis. It can be used as an adjunct to acupuncture to increase the range of motion of a joint, or instead of acupuncture when needles are uncomfortable or inappropriate, as in pediatric applications.

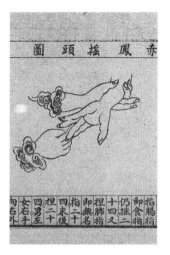

FIG 5.1 **'Red phoenix shaking its head'.** From the Qing period *Xiao'er tuina guangyi* (小兒推拿廣義, *Overview of Pediatric Tuina Massage*) by Xiong Yingxiong. *(With permission of the Wellcome Library, London.)*

TUINA AND *QI* CULTIVATION

Although Daoist and Buddhist practices of *qi* cultivation (*qigong*) are aimed ultimately at spiritual realization, given the fundamental importance of *qi* to health and wellbeing it is not surprising that one important aspect of the practice of Chinese medicine is the systematic cultivation of *qi*. This is relevant to *tuina* in three specific areas. The first is to allow the practitioner to cultivate the demeanor and stamina to enable him or her to perform the strenuous activities of *tuina*, to sustain the constant demands of clinical practice and to quiet the mind to facilitate diagnostic perception. The second involves cultivating the practitioner's ability to safely transmit *qi* to the patient. Practitioners may direct *qi* to the patient either through needles or directly through their hands. This activity may be the main focus of treatment or an adjunctive aspect, in which case the *qi* paradigm is expanded to include direct interaction between the patient's *qi* and that of the clinician, as in *daoyin* (導引, conduction or guiding and pulling, described in Ch. 10). Finally, patients may be taught to do specific *qigong* practices that are useful for their illnesses. As in the martial arts traditions of China, the intention of *qigong* practice is to increase the quantity, smooth movement and volitional control of *qi*, in this context thus strengthening the body of both practitioner and patient.

Qi cultivation makes extensive use of the principles of China's traditional medicine, and its history is intertwined with that of famous physicians as far back as antiquity, pointing to an early recognition of the importance of exercise to health. In Master Lü's *Spring and Autumn Annals* (*Lüshi Chunqiu*, 呂氏 春秋), a famous aphorism relates the importance of movement to the maintenance of health and function: 'Flowing water will never turn stale, the hinge of the door will never be eaten by worms. They never rest in their activity: that's why.' [12] This describes the role of dance and movement in correcting the movement of *qi* and *yin* within the body and benefiting the muscles [13].

Descriptions of *qi* cultivation practices and exercises are attributed to the early Daoist masters. Zhuangzi, writing in the fourth century BCE, reveals the role of breathing and physical exercise in promoting longevity, yet disparaging the sage intent on merely extending his life [14]: 'To pant, to puff, to hail, to sip, to spit out the old breath and draw in the new, practicing bear hangings and bird-stretches, longevity his only concern.' [15]

Among the texts recovered from tomb three at the Mawangdui site in Hunan province (datable to 168 BCE or before), as well as the earliest known manuscripts on moxibustion are a series of illustrated guides to the practice of *daoyin* that provide guidance to the physical postures and therapeutic properties of this form of *qi* cultivation [14]. The famous physician of the second century CE, Hua Tuo, is credited with the creation of a series of 'exercises of the five animals', the *wuqinxi* (五禽戲). Based on the movements of the tiger, the deer, the bear, the monkey and the bird, these exercises were to be practiced to ward off disease. Zhang Zhongjing, another renowned second-century physician, in his *Golden Cabinet Prescriptions* (*Jingui Yaolue*, 金櫃要略) recommended *daoyin* together with the *tuina* of the breath (exhalation and inhalation) to treat disease. From the 1950s on, in line with Mao Zedong's well-known 1958 dictate that 'Chinese medicine is a great treasure house! We must make all efforts to uncover it' [16], *qigong* training programs were implemented and sanatoria were built, specializing in the therapeutic application of *qigong* to the treatment of disease.

Examples of *qigong* exercises used in the practice of *tuina*

Most discussions of *qi* cultivation address relaxation of the body, regulation or control of breathing, and calming of the mind. *Qi* cultivation generally is performed in a relaxed standing, sitting or lying posture. Once the correct position is achieved, the practitioner begins to regulate breathing in concert with specific mental and physical exercises.

For example, one form of *qigong* involves visualizing the internal and superficial pathways of the channels and imagining the movement of the *qi* along these channels in concert with the breath. As the practice develops, the practitioner begins to experience the sensation of *qi* traveling along the channel pathways. Traditionally, it is believed that the mind guides the *qi* to a specific area of the body and that the *qi* then guides the blood there as well, improving circulation in the area. From this point of view, this particular exercise trains the *qi* and blood to move freely along the channel pathways, leading to good health.

Another exercise involves the use of breath, visualization, and simple physical exercises to benefit the *qi* of the lungs, and is recommended for bronchitis, emphysema and bronchial asthma. It begins by assuming a relaxed posture, whether sitting, lying, or standing, breathing naturally and allowing the mind to become calm. The upper and lower teeth are then clicked together by closing the mouth gently 36 times. As saliva is produced it is retained in the mouth, swirled with the tongue, and then swallowed in three parts while the person imagines that it is flowing into the middle of the chest (corresponding to the acupuncture point Ren-17, *danzhong*, 膻中, or 'Chest Center') and then to an area about three fingerbreadths below the navel (the lower *dantian*, 丹田, or 'Cinnabar Field', associated with point Ren-6, *qihai*, 氣海, 'Sea of *Qi*'). The individual now imagines that he or she is sitting in front of a reservoir of white *qi* that enters the mouth on inhalation and is transmitted through the body on exhalation, first to the lungs, then to the lower *dantian*, and finally out to the skin and body hair (white is the color associated with the lungs, which control the skin and body hair). This process of visualization is repeated 18 times [17].

This practice uses the relationship between the mind and *qi* to strengthen the function of the lungs and to pattern the region of *danzhong* where the Lung and respiration *qi* (肺氣) is stored. The lower *dantian* is considered important in the production and storage of the body's *qi* in general.

Further information on *qigong* can be found in Chapter 6.

Qi cultivation in qigong and taiji quan

6

Gideon Enz

CHAPTER CONTENTS

The quest to understand and enhance the energies of life has been an essential part of all human cultures since the dawning of time. And, since time immemorial, human beings have studied the ebb and flow of vitality in nature (soil, plants and animals) to deepen their understanding of the patterns and polarities that govern themselves and their lives. Over millennia of observation, systems of governance, science, art and medicine have been explored, tried and perfected. Among the cultures of the world, a great volume of historical records documenting the methodology, experimentation and accumulated knowledge on these subjects lies within the shadows of the Himalaya or Kunlun mountains (崑崙山).

THE ORIGINS OF QIGONG

The cultures of China, Tibet and India have preserved countless streams of endogenous research in music, medicine, martial arts and spirituality. For thousands of years, these streams have interacted with, developed from, or poured wholly into other streams, thus providing a vast and unmatched wealth of information and experiential data on the processes and principles behind the mystery of human experience.

From the prehistoric methods passed down to the *wu yi* (巫醫), or shamans, who simultaneously functioned as doctors, priests, psychologists and sorcerers, the Chinese techniques for cultivating vitality and wellbeing have centered

73

around the mastery of *qi* or life-force energy. This 5000-year-old exploration of *qi* has led to the evolution of thousands of varieties of *qigong*. However different they appear, all systems of *qigong* share a common foundation.

THE MEANING OF *QIGONG*

The word *qigong* is a combination of two characters: *qi* (氣) and *gong* (功). *Qi* translates most simply as 'energy' (but see Chs 5 and 8) and refers specifically to the life energy that animates the tissues of the human body, while the word *gong* is usually translated as mastery. To properly understand *qi*, however, we must also understand the concepts of *jing* and *shen*. The ancient Chinese conceived of *jing*, *qi* and *shen* as forming the triad of substances that make up a human being [1], sometimes known as the Three Treasures (*sanbao*, 三寶).

Jing (精), which is usually translated as 'Essence', is the most obvious of the three and refers to the basic material from which tissues are made. As such, *jing* is often confused with the sexual essence (sperm or ovum). However, *jing* refers to a wide range of substances, and to the overall *yin* of the body. In newborn babies, for example, the *jing* circulates throughout the infant's body, governing the growth and formation of specific tissues. It is the predominance of *jing* that gives babies their characteristic flexibility and resilience. During the process of puberty, *jing*, having already completed its job of forming the overall matrix of the body, descends and condenses into the sexual organs. During the rest of a person's adult life, whenever the *jing* is not expressed sexually, it circulates throughout the rest of the body strengthening and nourishing the tissues.

Qi (氣), as mentioned above, is the life energy of the body. The production of *qi* is derived from a sort of internal combustion of physical substances, in which *jing* plays a central role. Food, drink and air also play an essential role in the production of *qi* (see too Chs 4 and 20). When a person's food, drink and air are from natural sources and taken in moderation, and the person's *jing* is abundant, there is an abundance of high-quality fuel for the production of *qi*. When *qi* is abundant, a person will feel healthy and vital, always having sufficient energy available to do whatever is required. When *qi* is deficient, the person will feel drained, tired or exhausted and even the simplest of tasks will seem nearly impossible. Children display so much energy and vitality because their *jing* is circulating throughout their system and transforming into *qi* everywhere in their body. Different emotions also affect the flow of *qi* within the body [2]. Grief, for example, causes the body's *qi* to become 'thick and sticky' [3, p 441] (Fig. 6.1), whereas anger heats up the *qi* and directs it away from the body (Fig. 6.2). Similarly, a feeling of peace and 'everything in its place' occurs when the *qi* is spread evenly and coherently throughout the body.

Shen (神) is even more subtle than *qi*, and is usually translated as 'Spirit' or 'Mind'. The term *shen* denotes the overall character of a person and is used to refer to thoughts, emotions and general awareness. Positive states of thought and emotion such as love, peace, trust, honor and faith are all manifestations of a healthy *shen*. States of thought and emotion such as anger, anxiety, obsession, sadness and fear will be quickly processed by a person with a healthy *shen*; if a person's *shen* is unhealthy, he or she may hold on to any of these negative emotional states for a prolonged period of time, eventually damaging their *qi* and *jing*. It is said that when the eyes are bright the *shen* is strong; when the eyes are dull, the *shen* is deficient. The brightness in the eyes of babies reflects the purity and strength of their *shen*. However, the sparkle of *shen* in the eyes is also apparent in people who are in love, in pregnant women and in those who are just about to die. In all of these individuals, *jing*, *qi* and *shen* are transforming into each other at a rate far above average.

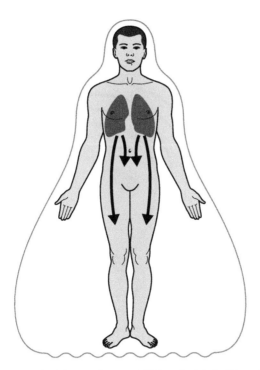

FIG 6.1   Grief causes the body's *qi* to become 'thick and sticky'. *(Adapted from Johnson, [3, p 442] with permission.)*

So, the term *qi* in *qigong* refers to the life-force energy that is the bridge between a person's physical body and the intangible qualities of his or her character. *Qi* then is something like the biological equivalent of Einstein's '*E*' in his most famous formula [4]. This formula, the first to define mass–energy equivalence clearly in physics, reads 'energy = mass × (the speed of light)^2, or simply:

$$E = mc^2$$

In the above equation, 'c^2' is the conversion factor required to convert from units of mass to units of energy. In *qigong*, a similar formula can be applied:

$$\text{abundant } qi = \text{physical substance (properly converted)}^2$$

The real challenge comes with the 'properly converted' part of the above equation. How can we train our physical substance so that our life-force energy multiplies itself to the point where it becomes a tangible and usable force? This is where *gong* comes in.

The same *gong* as in *gong fu* (or *kung fu*), the term *gong* (功) refers to mastery gained through consistent practice. However, consistent practice alone is not enough. To develop *gong*, the student must practice using a proper method. The saying 'practice makes perfect' is not exactly correct; it would be better stated as 'practice makes habit'. If the practice is incorrect or incomplete, so is the 'skill' it develops [5]. Over the past 5000 years of Chinese culture, many variations of 'proper method' have been embarked upon, explored, then either cast aside, absorbed into other traditions, or refined. The successful results of these experiments, as well as the signs of success and what to avoid, have been passed down in secret from master to student, with each generation attempting to build upon the experience of their teachers. Some of these lines of teaching survive into the present day, while many more have been lost in the vast river of Chinese history.

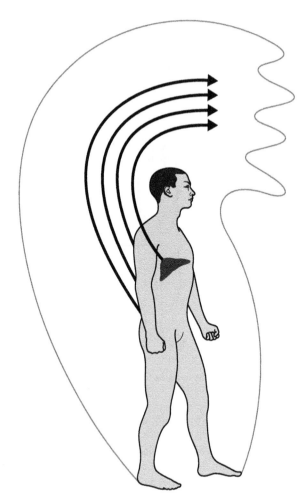

FIG 6.2 **Anger heats up the *qi* and directs it away from the body.** *(Adapted from Johnson, [3, p 437] with permission.)*

LEVELS OF TRAINING

Given the wide variety of styles and training methods in practice today, it would be impossible (and unnecessary) for any one person to learn them all. Generally speaking, there are three levels of teaching, each level revealing substantially more about training methods than the previous one:

- techniques given to the common people (students)
- techniques given to disciples
- techniques passed down from a master to his/her successor.

In classical Chinese society, students were given the least attention. They were taught various external forms (such as a *taiji* form or specific *qigong* exercises) and given instruction in morality and philosophy, but they were not actually taught how to refine and use the exercises on their own; nor were they instructed in how to discover their own personal morality and philosophy.

Before being taught anything deeper, students would generally be required to 'take a firm foothold in daily life' [6] and then ask again and again to be taken on as disciples; they would be repeatedly turned down. Eventually, however, most tenacious students would be selected, after which they would be put to work cooking, cleaning and running errands for several years to test their character and commitment. Any character defaults were to be ironed out through the rigorous workload that the student would carry out night and day. After a period of months or years, such a student would be taught a basic technique, such as the 'immortal embracing the post' or 'holding the balloon' posture (*cheng bao zhuang*, 撐抱樁) [7], which he would practice whenever possible. Over time, the student would gradually be introduced to key concepts such as breathing into the belly and pressing back the *mingmen* (命門) or Gate of Vitality, which is located in the lumbar region behind the navel. Similar techniques would be learned and mastered along the way to becoming a disciple. Once accepted, a disciple would then be taught the purpose and function of the various exercises he had previously learned, as well as how and when to apply each exercise.

THE IMPORTANCE OF THE LOWER *DANTIAN*

In all systems of *taiji* and *qigong*, the cultivation of the lower *dantian* is paramount, as this is viewed as the center of the body. The lower *dantian* 'is the body's center of gravity as well as the energy center. The *dantian* stores *qi* and drives it throughout the body. By concentrating on this point one learns to harvest, cultivate and nourish qi energy' [8, p 101]. The term *dantian* (丹田) translates as 'elixir field', referring to the function of a *dantian* as an area in which one substance is transformed into another [9]. For example, the lower *dantian* (abdominal region) is the primary region where *jing* is transformed into *qi* [10] (Fig. 6.3). The middle *dantian* (heart

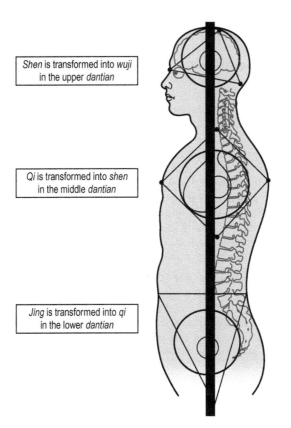

Shen is transformed into *wuji* in the upper *dantian*

Qi is transformed into *shen* in the middle *dantian*

Jing is transformed into *qi* in the lower *dantian*

FIG 6.3   The three *dantians*. *(Adapted from Johnson, [10, p 207] with permission.)*

center) governs the transformation of *qi* into *shen*; the upper *dantian* (head center) governs the transformation of *shen* back into *wuji* (無極, infinite space) [11].

Because the lower *dantian* is the main fueling station for *qi*, cultivation of *qi* always begins with gathering energy in the lower *dantian* by focusing on exercises that gently increase the heat in the abdominal center over a period of weeks or months. This heat eventually causes an accumulation of extra *jing* in the body that then transforms into *qi*. As this infusion of *qi* builds up in the body, the disciple experiences greater and greater levels of health and vitality.

However, before beginning the practice of energizing the lower *dantian*, practitioners are required to undergo some manner of purification. For example, the disciple would be taught that the first level of training in any system involves an exercise that cleanses and prepares the body, breath and mind [3]. Often this included exercises such as 'pulling down the heavens' (*yin xia tian*, 引下天) (which brings energy and awareness from the head to the feet), meridian brushing (which cleanses the acupuncture meridians along the arms, legs and torso), or a simple set of exercises that warm up each of the body's joints. Once he was proficient in these exercises and the school's basic and intermediate levels of forms, the disciple would begin *qi* cultivation in earnest.

This process begins with increasing the amount and quality of *jing* by refining the health and structure of the body through the use of medicinal foods and herbs and practicing personalized exercises tailored to the disciple's strengths and weaknesses. The disciple would then combine visualizations (*shen gong*, 神功) with the exercises in order to speed up the process of filling the lower *dantian*. An example of the above combination of posture, breath and imagination is as follows:

- **Posture:** Stand with the feet shoulder-width apart, holding the arms and hands to form a large circle at the height of the navel. The hands should be 4 to 6 inches (10–15 cm) apart, and the palms should face the area immediately below the navel.
- **Breath:** Breathe deeply into the abdominal area. With each inhale, feel and slightly exaggerate the expansion of the abdomen. With each exhale, feel and slightly exaggerate the contraction of the abdomen back in against the spine. Make each breath as long and full as possible while still breathing comfortably.
- **Imagination:** With each inhalation imagine a vibrant gold color flowing in through the nostrils and down the front of the body to the navel. With each exhalation, imagine and feel the golden energy penetrating into the body and spiraling into a smaller and smaller ball of bright hot energy suspended just in front of the spine and just behind and below the navel.
- **Guidelines for practice:** Continue to practice the above exercise for a minimum of 100 days, with a minimum of 100 breaths per practice session. In order to ensure both quality and quantity of *jing*, it is important to avoid consuming overstimulating food or drink (such as alcohol, coffee and overly spiced or fried foods) and to remain celibate while engaging in this practice.

Here it is worth noting that not all disciples – nor all teachers – were celibate monks. Therefore the methods of practice for celibate monks differed slightly from the methods used by householders. Monks were taught how to remain celibate by taking herbs that eliminated the sex drive and by engaging in practices that drove any remaining sexual energy upwards. Householders were taught techniques that allowed them to retain or even increase their *jing* while still enjoying the pleasures of married life.

Traditionally, the process of filling the lower *dantian* was continued until a sensation of intense heat or burning pain was felt at the bottom of the spine, at which point the disciple was taught the beginnings of the 'small heavenly cycle' (*xiao zhou tian*, 小周天) [3, p 99–100]. In the small heavenly cycle, and then later in the 'large heavenly cycle' (*da zhou tian*, 大周天), the *qi* developed in the lower *dantian* was gradually distributed throughout the body along the eight extraordinary channels or meridians (*qi jing ba mai*, 奇經八脈). These practices linked the lower *dantian* to the torso and then linked the torso to the limbs.

Once this stage had been completed, different practices would be undertaken depending on the goals of the student and the nature of the *qigong* system being taught. In medical *qigong* (see below), one uses the energy thus developed for the purpose of healing others, utilizing medical *qigong* treatment either as a stand-alone procedure or in conjunction with other modalities such as acupuncture or herbology. Practitioners of spiritual *qigong* continue the process of *qi* cultivation, circulation and transformation until they reach the level of 'immortality'. For practitioners of martial *qigong*, this extra energy is used to protect oneself and overcome an opponent.

QI AND *TAIJI QUAN*

The martial art of *taiji quan* (太極痊), pronounced 'taaee chee chwaan', is more commonly known outside of China than is *qigong*. In recent times, *taiji quan* (often called *taiji* or *tai chi*) has been taught primarily as a health-promoting exercise practice. However, *taiji quan*, which literally translates as 'supreme ultimate fist', was traditionally taught as a powerful martial art – only in the past 50 years has 'real *taiji* fighting been ignored' [12]. Though the first secret to the art of *taiji* lies in its slow gentle movements, some systems of *taiji* still incorporate fast aerobic movements as well as in-depth training in the martial applications of each movement within a given exercise set.

All Chinese martial arts, *taiji* included, are normally referred to by the term *gong fu* (or *kung fu*). As mentioned above, *gong* (功) translates as 'mastery developed by consistent training using correct method', while the character *fu* (夫) means 'man'. The term *gong fu* can thus be used to describe mastery in any area of life. *Taiji*'s nearest relatives are the two other internal martial arts of *bagua* (八卦, 'eight trigrams') and *xingyi* (形意, 'form/intention'). All three share the same theoretical principles as well as many fighting and training techniques.

In the practice of *taiji*, one learns to develop a powerful structure based on a gentle integration of the entire body in each posture. This is referred to in classic literature on *taiji* with instructions such as: 'The whole body should be linked together through every joint; do not show any interruptions.' [13] Because this is very difficult to learn and extremely powerful once mastered, few people are actually taken through the entire spectrum of *taiji* training. Instead, as mentioned earlier, people are taught *taiji* for health.

Even though *taiji* is at its essence a martial art, the health benefits it provides are numerous. Because the slow controlled stepping inherent in *taiji* develops strong thighs, flexible hips and steady balance, simplified versions of *taiji* are popularly used as exercise routines for seniors. The meditative motions emphasize relaxation and the path of least resistance [14], a feature that ranks *taiji* high among the stress-relieving practices sought out by today's overworked 'type A' personality. Additional health benefits are derived from precisely coordinating deep abdominal breathing with the expanding and contracting movements of a *taiji* form. However, all of the above characteristics and benefits of *taiji* are also common elements of nearly all types of *qigong* practice. To understand some of the distinctions between *taiji* and *qigong*, it is necessary to briefly overview the history of Chinese *gong fu* and the Buddhist revival brought about by the Indian sage Bodhidharma.

BODHIDHARMA, *GONG FU* AND *TAIJI QUAN*

Born a prince in Southern India around 500 CE, Bodhidharma was the acknowledged founder of the Chan (禪, later to become Zen in Japan) tradition of Buddhism and the individual responsible for turning the Shaolin monastery into a martial arts mecca, a position it maintained for the next 1500 years. After being invited from India as an envoy of Buddhism some time in the early sixth century, Bodhidharma made the difficult journey to China where he became known as Damo. During a decade of teaching and practice in China, he reinvigorated the meditative traditions of Buddhism and introduced physical exercises into the daily practice routines of the Shaolin monastery. These physical training methods integrated Indian martial arts and temple dances with Chinese medicine and Buddhism, eventually leading to the creation of Shaolin *gong fu*. Bodhidharma also emphasized the *qigong* practices of 'tendon changing' (*yi jin jing*, 易筋經) and 'marrow washing' (*xisui*, 洗髓).

A few hundred years later, a Daoist ascetic named Zhang (or Zheng) Sanfeng is said to have combined elements of Shaolin *gong fu* into a system of slow movements based on the principles he observed in nature. For this creative combination of infinite softness and devastating martial power, Zhang Sanfeng became known as 'the originator of the internal martial arts' [8, p 29], the most notable of which is the art of *taiji quan*. In this new martial art, all the movements were practiced slowly in order to emphasize the gradual development of internal structure and the accumulation of *qi* in the lower *dantian*. Since *taiji* places importance on training and utilizing *qi* rather than training structure alone, years of practice enabled *taiji* practitioners to develop near-mystical fighting abilities.

All of the apparently gentle postures that make up a *taiji* form are actually fighting movements designed to cause maximum damage to an opponent with a minimum of effort. Since each movement is coordinated with deep abdominal breathing and the integration of opposing muscle groups, anyone practicing *taiji* correctly will improve their health and increase their sense of vitality. However, these benefits have traditionally been secondary, the primary goal of *taiji* practice being to enhance one's martial skill.

The methods of *taiji* training can be incredibly effective, and for this reason many of the turnkey concepts and principles have either been kept secret or deliberately misinterpreted to the public. This ensured that the master and his own family always had power and ability beyond anything that was available to students or to the public.

QI CULTIVATION IN *TAIJI QUAN*

Once the basics of a *taiji* form have been mastered, a disciple then begins the long task of learning to emit and control *qi*. At this point a system of basic *qigong* exercises is practiced, such as the filling the lower *dantian* technique previously outlined, until the practitioner has an abundance of *qi* flowing throughout the body and is able to direct it at will. Once the practitioner gains control of his or her own *qi* in the solo *taiji* form, he or she then learns to manipulate the *qi* of an opponent in predesigned sets of martial applications performed with a partner.

QI CULTIVATION IN *QIGONG*

Qigong in essence refers to any practice that leads to the mastery of *qi*. For this reason, there are literally thousands of different styles and systems of *qigong* in practice today. However, there are a number of easily identifiable characteristics and concepts that can always be found in any quality system of *qigong*. These concepts boil down to three simple ideas: purifying, nourishing and harmonizing.

- **Purifying:** The first and most important step in any *qigong* practice is cleansing or purification. This includes exercises that cleanse the physical body (fascia, internal organs, etc.), those that cleanse the energy body (meridians, *chakras*, etc.), and those that cleanse the spiritual body (chronically held patterns of thought or emotion). The primary concept in purification exercises is one of identifying areas of toxic energy within the body and moving those energies out of the body.
- **Nourishing:** Beyond mere nourishment through food and drink, in *qigong* the term 'nourish' refers to the process of adding or increasing energy in the body. As with purifying, the process of nourishing can be performed physically, energetically and spiritually. Nourishing practice essentially involves identifying areas within the body that are energetically depleted or deficient and then gathering energy from outside the body and adding it into those areas.
- **Harmonizing:** This refers to the overall action of balancing and integrating different energies within the body. Though harmonizing techniques can be designed to target physical, energetic or spiritual levels, most *qigong* harmonizing practices involve an integration of all three aspects. The essence of a *qigong* harmonizing exercise involves a set of complementary actions that balance inside/outside, up/down, right/left and front/back.

THE THREE SCHOOLS OF *QIGONG*

Before going any deeper into general *qigong* training methods, it is important to understand that differences among the various exercises practiced by different *qigong* systems are not necessarily a matter of correct or incorrect methods, or even of what is taught to the public and what is hidden, but rather are defined by three distinct purposes or goals. These differing goals divide *qigong* practice into three primary branches or schools of *qigong*: medical *qigong*, martial *qigong* and spiritual *qigong* [10]. All three branches share the same basic characteristics and utilize common principles but apply them in different ways. This difference can sometimes seem more pronounced than it is. In actuality all three branches of *qigong* rely heavily on the foundation of medical *qigong*. Here, the term 'branch' is used to refer to the overarching goal and function of a *qigong* practice. Throughout history, masters of *qigong* have endeavored to master all three branches, and to be a successful practitioner of *qigong* it is necessary to be proficient in at least two.

MEDICAL *QIGONG*

In medical *qigong*, a practitioner seeks to correct imbalances at the physical, energetic and spiritual levels of a patient in order to help the latter achieve optimum health. Medical *qigong* is actually one of the original components of Chinese medicine; due to its shamanic roots, many people claim that medical *qigong* is the oldest and most effective branch of Chinese medicine. Until recent times, a doctor of Chinese medicine was schooled in acupuncture (*zhen bian*, 枕邊), herbology (*zhong-yao xue*, 中藥學), massage (*tuina*, 推拿) and *qi* manipulation (*qigong*, 氣功), along with miscellaneous techniques such as moxibustion (*jiu*, 灸), scraping (*guasha*, 刮痧), cupping (*baguan*, 拔罐) and bloodletting (*fang xue*, 放血). Only with contemporary attempts to 'modernize' Chinese medicine has medical *qigong* been taken out of the curriculum for acupuncture students. The practice of medical *qigong* involves techniques ranging from simple *qi* massage for relieving pain, to combined sound and *qi* projection for dissolving tumors and cysts, to complex soul retrieval techniques for reviving patients who are comatose or incapacitated. Since medical *qigong* specializes in techniques that maintain and increase health, it provides the practical basis for both martial *qigong* and spiritual *qigong* training.

MARTIAL *QIGONG*

In martial *qigong*, practitioners seek to use the techniques of *qigong* to increase their own strength, enhance their own perception and manipulate the *jing*, *qi* and *shen* of their opponent. In this form of *qigong*, defensive techniques such as 'iron shirt' (*tieshan*, 鐵衫) are practiced in order to make the body resistant to an opponent's blows. On the offensive, specific *qigong* techniques (e.g. *dim mak*, 點脈) are mastered in order to paralyze or even kill an opponent by the proper use of certain acupuncture points. In essence, many of the martial *qigong* techniques are simply medical *qigong* techniques applied in reverse. Additionally, a martial artist needs to learn the techniques of *qigong* that relate to traumatology in order to heal both his/her own and others' injuries.

SPIRITUAL *QIGONG*

In spiritual *qigong*, practitioners seek to purify, increase and expand their *qi* and *shen*. Its techniques emphasize confronting and transforming oneself in order to enter fully into deeper spiritual states of union and transcendence [15]. Through transcending one's attachments to society and one's own personal history, a practitioner of spiritual *qigong* endeavors to realize the underlying unity of all things – referred to as *nirvana* in Buddhist traditions or as 'realizing the *dao*' in Daoist traditions. Different from mere philosophy, spiritual *qigong* practice allows an individual to see beyond his or her own limitations and reach experientially into realms and states of being well beyond the 'reality' of ordinary persons.

Most Daoist spiritual *qigong* systems, for example, stress that the goal of *qigong* cultivation is 'immortality' – a concept that seems to the Western ear to ring of delusional fantasy, and something more in the realm of myth and fairytale than a state that can actually be achieved by any human being. But, as often happens when the practices of one culture are introduced into a foreign culture, the difficulty is primarily in the translation.

Though much literature and tradition emphasize the longevity-producing effects of proper *qigong* and *gong fu* training, the concept of immortality in the Chinese tradition does not simply refer to having a physical body that lasts forever. When Daoists talk of immortality they are often referring to the end product of a long series of internal practices that result in the ability to fully gather one's consciousness and identity and launch it away from the physical human form at will. This is referred to as 'having a body outside the body', or 'release from the matrix' [1, p 58] and it is similar to the Western understanding of astral projection, in which one is able to enter a sleeplike (hypnagogic) state and project one's spirit out of the physical body. This understanding of a human being's innate capacity to leave the body at will is not unique to China. In the Indian and Tibetan traditions the ability to project one's awareness and identity out of one's body has been a closely guarded secret for millennia, while research on astral projection has been conducted in the Western world for well over a hundred years.

The difference between astral projection and the Chinese 'immortality' is that in astral projection one is still very much tied to the physical body, whereas once one has completed the processes of internal alchemy that are prerequisites for immortality, one is no longer bound to return to one's physical form.

COMPARISON OF *QIGONG* AND *TAIJI*

Having overviewed both *taiji* and *qigong* it is easy for us to see the similarities in appearance, style and function between the two. While newcomers may see no real difference between the two, purists may argue that *taiji* and *qigong* are entirely different systems that share only a few common training techniques and principles. In reality the truth is somewhere in between, as there are no training systems that exist independently of those who practice them. Historically, *qigong* has provided a base for the practice and development of *taiji* and of all the internal martial arts. However, as we have seen, *taiji* is primarily a fighting system, whereas *qigong* is broader in its applications. With its emphasis on breathing, movement and structure, *taiji* provides general health benefits and has been the subject of numerous studies both in China and in the Western hemisphere. In contrast, *qigong* can be tailored to suit individual goals and needs, and it has been used successfully to accomplish everything from healing chronic disease states (such as cancer and diabetes) to achieving enlightenment and immortality. When compared side by side, although *taiji* provides numerous important benefits, *qigong* proves to be the more flexible of the two disciplines. Both systems rely on the same underlying principles, and both ultimately provide vehicles for personal self-expression.

Qi cultivation in qigong and taiji quan

Qigong theory and research

Amy L Ai

7

CHAPTER CONTENTS

INTRODUCTION

This chapter summarizes the most important research on *qigong* (QG) over the past decade. Despite public interest in QG and the theories behind it, whether QG practice can 'cure' medically diagnosed diseases remains an underinvestigated subject by Western standards [1]. One reason is that this mindful practice focuses on promoting health-related wellbeing rather than on curing diseases according to modern diagnoses. *Qigong* is the phonetic juxtaposition of two Chinese characters: *Qi* (氣), meaning 'flow of air' in a more literal sense or 'vital energy' in a more symbolic sense, and *gong* (功), meaning 'perseverant practice' [2]. Integrating different perspectives, QG can be seen as an energy-based practice and mind–body therapy involving deep breathing and meditation together with movement (internal or external) that may benefit health [3]. QG can be classified into two systems: *internal* QG: self-practice to harmonize healthy *qi* flow, and *external* QG: the manipulation of *qi* by a master with healing power (see Ch. 6).

The concept of 'vital energy' in living beings is shared by many Western and non-Western healing traditions, as well as by shamanic traditions globally [3]. *Qi*, in Chinese thought, is uniquely characterized by: (1) a concern for

85

holistic health in terms of multilevel energy patterns, (2) circulation within the pathways of the meridian system, and (3) an underlying rationale that the activities of this energy are fundamental to both humans and the universe. *Qi* refers not only to the essence of all material objects, but also to their dynamic interactions in terms of the rhythmic alternation of two forces termed *yin* (陰) and *yang* (陽), which may be seen as similar to positive and negative electric charges. This energy-centered worldview can be at odds with clinical research based on Western materialistic science, which is ultimately traceable to Aristotle's view of the world as a systematic structure and Democritus' concept of the atom as the basic unit of natural substances [4]. To appreciate the essence of QG, it is necessary to understand the basics of its guiding philosophy, Daoism (Taoism), which has shaped the ontology and epistemology underlying QG as well as many other forms of traditional Chinese medicine (CM). This chapter therefore focuses first on Daoism before discussing current scientific investigation of internal and external QG.

DAOIST DIALECTIC VIEW OF THE WORLD AND HUMANS

Dao (道), or *tao*, refers to the way, or the universal order, to be followed in life and in nature [2]. *Dao* is the ultimate, indefinable principle underlying all energetic movements, all processes in the universe. The principles basic to QG, such as concentration, emptiness of desire, quiescence, flexibility and infant-like breath, were first described in the influential *Daodejing* (*Tao Te Ching*, 道德經), attributed to Laozi (Lao Tsu). Ancient Daoists sought to achieve a conscious awareness and philosophical understanding of universal principles, or the manner and development of change in cosmological processes. In keeping with its image as an invisible yet perceivable 'flow of air', the word *qi* was used as a vivid metaphor to illustrate the ever-altering energy patterns in the universe. Capra [5] suggests that the Daoist ontology resembles that of quantum physics. Both traditions propose that all forms of substance are nothing but the materialization of energy, a theme that frequently recurs within this book. Both view the dynamic patterns of energy as primary in nature, whereas the substantive aspects are secondary.

ONTOLOGICAL DIFFERENCES UNDERLYING WESTERN AND EASTERN MEDICINE

Fundamental differences between Eastern and Western medicine are deeply rooted in their culture-based worldviews. The Daoist energy-centered outlook underlying QG differs remarkably, both ontologically and epistemologically, from the operative philosophy of science that supports western medicine, with its origins in Aristotelian empirical materialism [4]. Biomedicine, as the offspring of this outlook, focuses primarily on the material structure of the body, as broken down into systems, organs, tissues, cells, chromosomes, genes and molecules. This view led to the great achievement in allopathic medicine of universal diagnosis and disease-specific treatment. Ontologically, however, Daoism is more interested in the interactive phenomena that occur at multiple levels in nature and their ever-changing energy patterns [2]. Thus CM and QG do not follow the Cartesian dualism of mind and matter (*res cogitans/res extensa*). Rather, they consider all energy patterns as organized at symptomatic, psychobehavioral, environmental and cosmological levels in one coherent system. Concurrently, the activation of *qi* as health-related energy is seen as the primary principle underlying health in QG practice.

Laozi used *nonbeing* ('non-existence', *wu*, 無, referring to the *formless and timeless dao*), and *being* ('existence', *you*, 有, referring to *everything with a certain space-time form in the universe*), to summarize the energetic and substantive aspects of all things. According to the *Daodejing*: 'The Tao is abstract … Without form or image, without existence, the form of the formless, is beyond defining, cannot be described, and is beyond our understanding. It cannot be called by any name [Ch.14] … All things are born of being; *being is born of non-being* [Ch. 40] … All living things are formed by being, and shaped by their environment, growing if nourished well by virtue; the being from nonbeing' [Ch. 51] (emphasis added) [6]. In other words, an invisible energetic force as the origin of the world existed before all material substances emerged, whereas the visible materialistic aspects of the world are transitory phenomena in a cosmos sense. However, Daoist *nonbeing* tends to differ substantively from the Buddhist *nothingness* or *emptiness*. The former concerns the nature of ultimate reality itself, conceptualizing the origin of the universe or all objective being as energetic *nonbeing*, implying a void field filled with the dynamic movement of *qi*. The latter, however, usually involves subjective reflection on that ultimate reality, offering a cognitive solution as detachment to human suffering through emptying the mind.

DAOIST DIALECTICAL EPISTEMOLOGY UNDERLYING ENERGY-CENTERED *QIGONG*

Daoist dialectical epistemology is also fundamentally different from the laws of *formal logic* underlying Western science, traceable back to ancient Greece. Central to this are the three laws of *identity, noncontradiction* and *the excluded middle* [7]. The first law claims that everything must be identical with itself, the second insists that no statement can be both true and false, and the third declares that *A* is either *B* or *non-B*. For example, in *The Republic* Plato emphasized the incompatibility between opposite concepts such as beauty and ugliness, justice and injustice, good and bad, and all such paired terms (forms) [8]. Accordingly, at least until recently, the order of the world from the Western perspective tended to follow a path of *certainty, specification* and *a linear logic that links cause to effect*. For example, if *A* leads to *B* and *B* leads to *C*, then *A* also leads to *C*. Formal logic defines relative truths concerning contingent reality within structures so rendering natural laws comprehensible within specified domains, particularly those of science.

In contrast, Eastern tradition values intuitive thinking above rational thinking [5]. Daoist knowing tends not to employ *formal* logical thinking, empirical observation and linear deductive reasoning but rather dialectical thinking, intuitive imagery and cyclical patterning. Central to Daoist dialectical epistemology are three different but interrelated principles: *change, contradiction* and *holism* [7]. The first principle claims that reality is *in constant flux*, the second states that reality is full of paradoxes and the third declares that all things are interdependent and interactive. According to the *Daodejing*: 'When living by the Tao, awareness of self is not required, for in this way of life the self exists and is also non-existent, being conceived of not as existentiality nor as non-existent' [Ch. 7] [6]. Formally, this passage states that both *B* (existence) and *non-B* (non-existence) are true. From the Daoist perspective, the order of the world, including that of humans, tends to follow a path of *uncertainty, mutuality* and a *circling logic that links the individual part to the whole*. This last principle (holism) is the essence of dialectical thinking and the consequence of the first two. Thus truth is often presented in a fluid sense in relation to its context, or to opposite but related aspects, rather than as something isolated and absolute. As stated in the *Daodejing*: 'We cannot know the Tao itself nor see its qualities directly, but only see by differentiation, that which it manifests. Thus that which is seen as beautiful is beautiful compared with that which is seen as lacking beauty' [Ch. 2] [6].

THE THREE BASIC PRINCIPLES

In accordance with the last principle, *holism*, Daoists believe that all things in the world are interrelated and affect every other thing in mutually interactive and cyclical ways. Parts become meaningful only in relation to the whole context. Daoist dialectics did not lead to classic, Newtonian science or modern medicine, but it can help us to comprehend the dynamic energetic totality in QG, and perhaps modern physics. In keeping with the second principle, *contradiction*, the polarized *yin–yang* aspects of all paradoxical relations define each other, as in being and nonbeing, energy and substance, spirit and matter, or mind and body. The S-curve dividing line between the *yin–yang* halves of the *taijitu* symbol (太極圖) (see Figs. 4.1A and 7.1) implies a constant cyclical movement of opposing pairs that are at the same time interdependent, mutually controlling (creating and consuming) and interpenetrating. Each may influence and transform into the other in certain ways, as in the ever-changing relationship between health and illness. From this relativist perspective, the metaphors of *qi* and the *yin–yang* relation aptly describe the energetic and functional relationships within and between humans and the universe.

Finally, in correspondence with the first principle, *change*, Daoism uniquely focuses on the constant movements of the *nonbeing* aspect of nature rather than on its *being* aspects, such as its visible (e.g. physical landscape) or invisible properties (e.g. the concept of *spirit* in many cultures). The universal principle of all change is presented by a single word, *dao* – law inherent (immanent) in nature rather than law determined by a (transcendent) creator. This law of nature is not perceived as a fixed order but as a continuous *flow* in the constant movement of both *nonbeing* and *being* aspects within a hierarchical or even a nonhierarchical system. As stated in the *Daodejing*: 'When the consistency of the Tao is known, the mind is receptive to its states of change [Ch. 16] ... Man's laws should follow natural laws, just as nature gives rise to physical laws, whilst following from universal law, which follows the Tao' [Ch. 25] [6]. The law of the universe, not of human logic, is what Daoism intends us to comprehend philosophically, to appreciate esthetically, or to worship spiritually [9].

THE *YI JING* (易經): A CODING SYSTEM FOR UNIVERSAL CHANGES

Daoism uniquely employs mathematics to predict changing patterns in nature and humans. Unlike in science, however, even the mathematical patterns of such principles are displayed in symbolic ways. This approach derives from the pre-Daoist *Yi Jing* (*I Ching*) or *Book of Changes*, which is traditionally dated to the third millenium BCE, and has profoundly influenced East Asian traditions including QG. This book is entirely devoted to the basic ordering principles of change in the dynamic energy patterns of the universe (including human health), and has been used to calculate such predictable changing patterns since ancient times. Its 64 hexagrams register all the possible combinations of *yin* and *yang* in six lines, as shown in Figure 7.1. This dichotomized coding system resembles, but emerged thousands of years before, the binary zero–one language of computer science. Capra has also seen close similarities between the system of the *Yi Jing* and Heisenberg's S-matrix theory, forerunner of string theory in quantum physics, not least because 'in both systems, the emphasis is on the process rather than object' [5, p 281].

Although Legalism and Neo-Confucianism probably played significant roles in the development of acupuncture [10], throughout Chinese history Daoism has been the most influential intellectual tradition underlying the development of QG. In keeping with Daoist ontology, QG in theory is a function- and

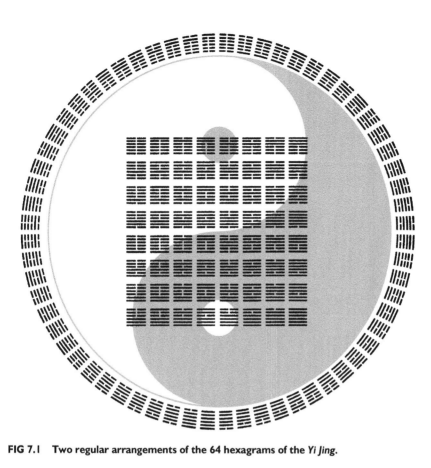

FIG 7.1 Two regular arrangements of the 64 hexagrams of the *Yi Jing*.

health-centered rather than a structure- and disease-oriented system. Each person is considered to be an energetic cosmos in miniature. QG theory is literally a systematic elaboration on the changing patterns of *qi* with respect to the interconnectedness of body, mind and spirit, as well as their interactions with the energetic environment (i.e. nature, society and cosmos). One's energy movement manifests the same pattern as that of the universe. Thus, in one traditional Daoist diagram of 'the regeneration of the primary vitalities' in internal alchemy (Fig. 7.2), not only are the physical body parts represented, but also the *renmai* and *dumai* meridians, some acupuncture points and major energy centers, along with images of the changing moon (in accordance with the 24 fortnightly periods of the traditional Chinese lunar calendar) and other symbols, to indicate that the changing *qi* patterns within humans correspond to those of the seasons and other cosmic movements.

HEALTH: A HOLISTIC BALANCE IN EVER-CHANGING *QI* PROCESSES

Consistent with Daoist epistemology, in QG human phenomena are viewed as a complex hierarchical web of *qi*, rather than as merely isolated physical matters. Health is maintained only when the overall internal and external energetic (*qi*) contexts of each individual are taken into account and is perceived in terms of its constant *changes*, *contradictions* and *holism*. According to the principle of *holism*, illness conditions are often individually assessed and addressed using multiple

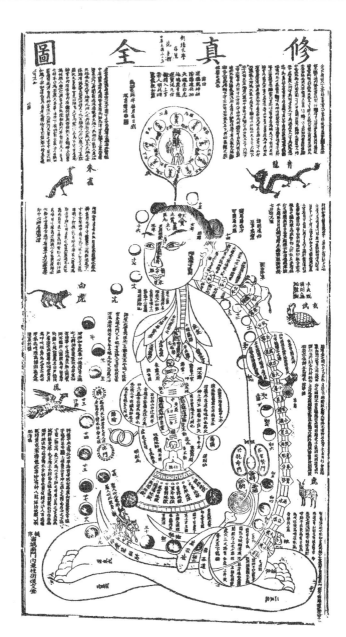

FIG 7.2 **'Regeneration of the primary vitalities' in Daoist internal alchemy, representing elements of the physical and subtle bodies together with the macrocosmic circulation of qi.** From a Chengdu woodblock print, 1922. *(Courtesy, Needham Research Institute, Cambridge, UK.)*

principles concerning one's (or the patient's) whole energy system rather than a standardized diagnosis and assessment for structural abnormality. Because of *contradiction,* health is not viewed as a state of opposition to or absence of disease but rather as an uncertain process of constantly balancing normal and abnormal *qi* patterns. Because of *change,* health and illness can be transformed into each other, depending on interaction between the stage of the ailment and the individual's health practice.

This Daoist essence is reflected in the Chinese character for CM, *Zhongyi*. *Yi* (醫) means 'medicine', while *zhong* (中) refers to 'middle'. Yet *zhong* also means the internally balanced 'golden mean'. *Zhongyi* therefore does not mean the 'Medicine of the Middle Kingdom' (Chinese medicine), but actually refers to 'Medicine for Inner Balance' [11]. Guided by these principles, QG is essentially a method of mind–body practice and spiritual cultivation, with an emphasis on breathing technique for holistic health. As indicated in the *Daodejing* [6] [Ch. 10], by breathing as a sleeping babe, one can maintain harmony and achieve enlightenment. As with early Hippocratic medicine [12], the approach of QG is 'psychosomatic', with mental activities guiding the *qi* flow through constant meditative exercise, and so spontaneously affecting physical health. Clearly, the principles involved can make the application of empirical research methods to QG highly challenging, because their goal is to investigate definable and specified objects through objective and replicable observations. Accordingly, contemporary clinical research does not aim to address questions on the essence of *qi* in QG but to ascertain the measurable outcomes of QG practice.

STUDIES ON INTERNAL *QIGONG*

As recently noted by this author [3], clinical studies conducted up to the 1980s dealt primarily with internal QG and were by Chinese researchers. Most were descriptive in nature, and very few were reported in peer-reviewed journals in English. These investigations especially involved cardiovascular diseases and function, as well as some other chronic conditions. Despite claiming a wide range of measurable outcomes, these reports mostly fell short of accepted standards for sound design in clinical research, especially for randomized controlled trials (RCTs). Information on some good studies can be found in the above review [3]. Over the past decade, however, a growing number of RCTs on QG have been conducted worldwide, including in China. New studies have also offered more solid evidence on its health benefits and underlying mechanisms. The following sections review the efficacy studies of QG published in English after 1997, including over a dozen RCTs and three additional systematic reviews (meta-analyses).

META-ANALYSES ON QG EFFECTS

Ng and Tsang [13] conducted the first review, focusing on the health benefits of QG and its underlying psychophysiological mechanisms. They identified some 24 RCTs conducted between 1997 and 2006, involving a total of 750+ subjects with a mean age (±) of 52.5 years (among the 26 reports, 4 publications appeared to have been generated from two samples in Korea). Some articles were published in Chinese. Of these RCTs, 12 used a comparable control group (e.g. conventional therapy or attention placebo), while the rest used a no-treatment control group. In the selected programs the participants received instruction from a QG master or followed audiovisual training materials. All studies used individual and/or group-based QG practice as the main intervention, although in some QG was integrated with other interventions (e.g. mindfulness). The authors concluded that QG had some clinical effects in reducing blood pressure, total cholesterol level and depressive symptoms and posited that the explanatory pathways or underlying mechanisms were related to *stress reduction* via the QG regulation of neuroendocrine and immune functions.

In the second review, Rogers et al [14] selected 36 reports of research on QG and *taiji* (太極), conducted between 1993 and 2007 with a total of 3700 participants (aged 55 or older). Identified categories of study outcomes included fall and balance, physical function, cardiovascular diseases, and psychological and additional disease-specific responses. The reviewers concluded that QG and *taiji* interventions may help improve physical function, reduce blood pressure, decrease fall risk, and mitigate depression and anxiety. Major trials identified in my own literature search and in Ng and Tsang's review [13], including a few overlapping studies, are summarized in the following sections. To be conservative this chapter discusses only the four trials from Rogers et al's review (2009) that clearly identified QG as the primary intervention.

HYPERTENSION, METABOLIC SYNDROME AND CARDIAC FUNCTION

Consistent with Chinese researchers before 1997 [3], both Ng and Tsang [13] and Rogers et al [14] found support for the view that QG may lower both systolic and diastolic blood pressure (SBP and DBP). Lee and various colleagues in Korea randomly assigned study participants to one of two groups: a *shuxin pingxue gong* (舒心平血功, 'calming the heart and stabilizing blood circulation') QG group, or a waiting-list, no-treatment control group [15–18]. After 10 weeks of QG practice (30 minutes per session, twice per week), the QG group showed a significant decrease in both SBP and DBP compared with the control group ($P < 0.001$). For the QG group, the average reduction in both SBP and DBP appeared to be more than 10 mmHg as judged from a data figure, but actual values were not reported. However, Cheung et al [19] did not find a significant difference between the practice of *Guolin* QG for 60 minutes in the morning and 15 minutes in the evening for 16 weeks and conventional exercise in the treatment of mild hypertension, although blood pressure was significantly reduced in both groups. (*Guolin* QG is a moving form of QG, developed by teacher Guo Lin to treat her own cancer, and mostly used for cancer patients.) In Australia, Liu et al [20] used a pretest–posttest design to assess the effect of QG (three times per week for 12 weeks) on blood pressure among inpatients. SBP decreased by 11.64 mmHg on average (mean) and DBP decreased by 9.73 mmHg ($P < 0.001$). Because there was no adequate control, however, such numbers may serve only as references for others' trials. All these studies had a small sample size.

Further, most hypertension trials also documented the impact of QG on the physical and/or hematological indicators of metabolic syndrome. Lee et al [15] showed significantly reduced levels of total cholesterol, triglycerides and apolipoprotein A-I in their QG-exercise group, compared with no treatment. Cheung et al [19] reported a similar significant reduction in triglyceride level, body mass index (BMI) and waist circumference in both the QG group and the regular-exercise control. Liu et al [20], however, did not find changes in triglyceride level, cholesterol or fasting blood glucose level, but a significant improvement was seen in insulin resistance, hemoglobin A1c (HbA1c) level, BMI and waist circumference. In addition, Liu et al [21] in China compared a 3-month regimen of Eight Brocade QG (*ba duan jin*, 八段錦) with a control regimen of walking and attention in patients with hyperlipidemia. Significant improvement was found in levels of total cholesterol, high- and low-density lipoprotein cholesterol profile and triglycerides in the QG group but not in the controls.

In Japan, Iwao et al [22] found no difference in the effect of QG walking and conventional walking (30 minutes after lunch) on plasma glucose levels in 10 patients with diabetes mellitus associated complications. Participants in both walking groups showed significantly lower plasma glucose levels, compared with those who did not practice postlunch walking. Yet the group on conventional walking had significantly higher pulse rates than in the QG-walking group or the control, suggesting a calming effect of QG walking. Concerning glucose metabolism, Tsujiuchi et al [23] observed the significantly reduced levels of HbA1c and C peptide among type-2 diabetic patients who practiced QG over 4 months, especially in patients with higher preintervention levels of HbA1c levels. The results were compared with those who employed dietary advice and exercise treatment as the control to test the effect of QG.

A few studies investigated cardiac function in participants with or without cardiac disease. In Italy, Pippa et al [24] compared QG training with waiting-list controls in older patients with chronic atrial fibrillation. Results on the 6-minute walking test were improved in the QG group but declined in the control group, although no significant changes were found in ejection fraction, BMI or lipid levels. In Sweden, Stenlund et al [25] studied 109 older patients with coronary artery disease (aged 77.5±). After 3 months, the QG group demonstrated considerable improvements in their self-estimated physical activity and performance on a one-legged stance test and coordination and box-climbing tests, compared with the usual-care control group. In China, Du et al [26] (using 69 patients, aged 60.6±) and Wang et al [27] (using 220 patients, aged 50-70) employed an echocardiogram to test the effect of *yi jin jing* (易筋經, 'muscle/tendon changing') QG (five times per week for 6 months) on cardiac function indices, compared with a no-treatment control. Both studies reported significant improvements in stroke volume, peak early transmitral filling velocity (V_E), and peak late transmitral filling velocity (V_A) across time and between groups.

OTHER CHRONIC CONDITIONS, AGE-RELATED FUNCTIONS AND STRESS BIOMARKERS

Xu [28] in China randomly assigned older patients with chronic obstructive pulmonary disease to practice respiration QG (20 minutes twice per day) and self-massage or to receive external diaphragm pacer (EDP) therapy. After 20 days, both groups exhibited improvement in lung function (forced vital capacity, forced expiratory volume in 1 second, peak expiratory flow rate), blood gas values (arterial partial pressure of oxygen and carbon dioxide, arterial oxygen saturation), and descending and ascending excursion of the diaphragm. Yet QG was superior to EDP in enhancing lung functioning. Mannerkorpi and Arndorw [29] in Sweden found that, compared with a no-treatment control, practicing dynamic QG for 3 months improved movement harmony in patients with fibromyalgia. However, no improvement was seen in fibromyalgia symptoms or physical function. They also reported an adverse event related to the practice of standing QG. Astin et al [30] in the United States indicated comparable improvement (e.g. reduced pain and disability scores on the Fibromyalgia Impact Questionnaire) in patients with fibromyalgia who practiced mindfulness meditation and Phoenix QG, compared with an exercise control. Likewise, Tsang et al [31] in Hong Kong showed the similar effect of both Eight Brocade QG and conventional rehabilitation activities (i.e. physical and occupational therapies) in improving physical health, ability to perform activities of daily living, and social function in 50 adults (aged 74.7±) with chronic disabilities. These findings, along with others trials [19,22], suggest that QG can be an alternative to regular exercise for management of certain chronic conditions for older patients.

Concerning physical status, Tsai et al [32] in Hong Kong compared *yi jin jing* QG with a no-treatment control in 71 women (aged 45 to 55). After 8 weeks of practice, the QG group showed significant improvement in muscular endurance, body fat, waist-to-hip ratio and BMI. Wenneberg et al [33] in Sweden explored the benefit of QG in 31 patients (aged 51.4±) with muscular dystrophy. After 30 months of practice, the QG group reported better perceived health (Medical

Outcome Study Short Form Health Survey) and coping skills (Ways of Coping Questionnaire) but not physical ability (Berg Balance Scale), compared with the no-treatment control. In the United States, Yang et al [34] examined the effect of QG and *taiji* on falling and balance in 49 healthy adults aged over 65. The QG group demonstrated significantly better scores than the waiting-list control on Sensory Organization Test vestibular ratios and on quiet stance Base of Support measures, but not on visual ratios of the Sensory Organization Test or on feet-opening angle. German researchers Schmitz-Hübsch et al [35] compared the effects of integrated Crane and Eight Brocade QG on Parkinson's disease with a no-treatment control (56 patients, aged 63.8±). More patients in the QG group than in the control showed improvement in motor symptoms (Unified Parkinson's Disease Rating Scale, motor part) at 3- and 6-month follow-ups, but not at the 12-month follow-up. These results indicate the need for a long-term commitment to practicing QG.

Perceived stress can interact with many age-related health conditions, and a number of RCTs investigating the benefits of QG have assessed neuroendocrine, immune and other biomarkers associated with both stress and chronic diseases (see too Ch. 21). Chen et al [36] in China found a significant reduction in interleukin 6 (IL-6) levels and maintenance of bone mineral density in those who practiced Eight Brocade QG for 12 weeks (87 women, aged 45.2±). In contrast, the usual lifestyle controls showed a significant reduction in bone mineral density. Testing 29 naive subjects, Manzaneque et al [37] in Spain showed significantly decreased numbers of total leukocytes and eosinophils, decreased number and percentage of monocytes and lower complement C3 concentrations following QG training (30 minutes of daily practice for 1 month) compared with controls. Lee et al [38] in Korea compared *Chun-do-sun-bup* (CDSB) QG with similar movements but without the breathing exercise and the associated mental technique in 60 subjects (aged 36±). After a 2-hour practice, levels of peripheral blood leukocytes and lymphocytes increased among CDSB participants, but not among controls. In another sample (18 individuals, aged 26.5±), Lee's group found that NK cell cytotoxicity, but not NK cell numbers, significantly increased in the CDSB group but not in the no-treatment control [39]. They also reported a significant decrease in plasma levels of norepinephrine and epinephrine [38] and a decrease in urinary levels of norepinephrine, epinephrine and the latter's metabolite metanephrine [17] in a group of hypertensive patients practicing QG. Finally, Yang et al [40], studying 50 older adults (aged 77.2±) with a history of flu immunization and sedentary lifestyle, reported higher immune function in a group practicing QG (hemagglutination inhibition assay (HIA) increase 109%) than in waiting-list no-treatment controls (HIA increase about 10%). Results from these RCTs indicate that QG may have certain effects on modulating immune functions and on the sympathetic nervous system.

MENTAL HEALTH AND ADDICTION

Some previously mentioned post-1997 research also assessed certain aspects of mental health and psychological conditions. Astin et al [30] found that QG practice reduced depression (Beck Depression Inventory) in patients with fibromyalgia. Lee's group reported increased levels of general and exercise self-efficacy [16] and decreased levels of stress [18] in hypertensive patients. Tsang et al [41] examined Eight Brocade QG in 72 older adults (aged over 65) with a history of depression and chronic illness; the QG group experienced significantly decreased depression (Geriatric Depression Scale) and increased wellbeing, perceived benefits and self-efficacy compared with controls (newspaper reading). Zhang et al [42] reported the benefit of *Yi jin jing* QG in older adults in improving both cognitive performance (e.g. reaction time, digit memory) after 6 months of practice and psychological health (e.g. depression, obsession and anxiety, using the Symptoms Checklist 90) after 1 year of practice, compared with no-treatment controls (124 versus 214 subjects, aged 61±; it is unclear, however, whether these two samples overlapped).

Finally, in a study of detoxification treatment (60 subjects, aged 32.4±), Li et al [43] found that a *Pangu* QG group showed negative urine test results (for morphine) by day 5, whereas the usual-care controls had negative results only by day 9 (*Pangu*, 盤古, was the creator of the world in Chinese mythology, responsible for separating *yin* from *yang*, Earth from Heaven). The QG group also experienced more rapid reduction of withdrawal symptoms (e.g. hallucinations, behavioral deviation, nausea, vomiting) and had significantly lower anxiety scores (Hamilton Anxiety Scale).

STUDIES ON EXTERNAL *QIGONG*

Surging public interest in mind–body medicine prompted several RCTs funded by the US National Institutes of Health (NIH) on the role of external QG in the treatment of medically diagnosed conditions. Conforming to a higher standard of research design, such investigation has involved interdisciplinary collaboration and multiple standardized assessments of physical and mental health outcomes [1,44,45]. This initiative has involved considerable methodological challenges, especially regarding possible 'placebo' effects (see Ai et al [1]).

The first NIH-funded study involved multiple-session assessments of 26 patients (aged 18 to 65) with treatment-resistant late-stage complex regional pain syndrome type I with six 40-minute sessions of either QG or placebo treatment (sham QG) over 3 weeks (22 patients) [45]. Comprehensive evaluation was performed at baseline and at 6- and 10-month follow-up (Symptoms Checklist 90, Sickness Impact Profile, Beck Depression Inventory and Cognitive–Somatic Anxiety Questionnaire); 82% of QG patients reported less pain by the end of the first session, compared with 45% of control patients. By the last session, 91% of QG patients reported analgesia compared with 36% of control patients. The results demonstrate that external QG led to transient pain reduction and long-term reduction of anxiety in the experimental group, even in such a small sample. This report suggests that by using a sound design it may be possible to provide valid scientific evidence of QG effects.

A second NIH/NCCAM-funded, large-sample trial randomly assigned 400 in-hospital rehabilitation patients following open-heart surgery to three groups receiving: (1) no treatment, (2) sham QG from trained actors, or (3) real QG from a QG master (see Ai et al [1]). The study design combined the methodology of an RCT in clinical medicine with that of a multiwave survey to achieve multiple interrelated objectives. The RCT part had three layered goals to examine: (a) the efficacy of QG, (b) underlying mechanisms, and (c) the placebo effect. Researchers, patients, surgeons and evaluating research assistants and physicians were all blinded to the intervention assignment. The efficacy of QG was assessed by measures of wound healing, pain relief, use of pain medication and length of hospitalization. To test for placebo effect, patients were questioned on whether they believed they had received the effective (real) treatment. Various assessments were made at 2 weeks before hospitalization, 2 days before surgery, during 4 postoperative days in hospital, and at 1 month, 6 months and 3 years after surgery.

Unfortunately, the principal investigator and designer of this trial left the University of Michigan Integrative Medicine Program immediately after the NIH funding became available. The trial data were collected, cleaned and analyzed, but results were not delivered for publication by the subsequent investigator.

A personal contact indicated only a placebo effect. Several factors may help explain this finding: (a) no QG effect in this difficult condition, (b) insufficient 'dosage' due to only three to four in-hospital treatments of QG intervention, limited by the duration of postoperative hospitalization, and (c) the limited healing power of the QG practitioners tested in this trial. Students of the QG master participated in the RCT, but not the master himself who had practiced QG for over 60 years. Whereas the author once witnessed this master healing the lower leg of an elderly hypertensive and diabetic man within only 3 weeks (the leg had been broken in eight places), none of the students had this healing power after less than 10 years of QG healing practice. One of these healers was later tested by a biophysics professor and researcher in the University of California system; after multiple biophysical assessments he indicated that the tested level of this particular healer was only at what he could call 'B+'.

The third NIH-funded trial randomly assigned 112 patients with knee osteoarthritis (aged >50) to receive either genuine QG from one of two QG masters or sham QG from one sham master for five to six sessions over 3 weeks [44]. Of the 106 patients who completed the trial, those in both QG groups reported significant reduction in pain scores (Western Ontario and MacMaster University Osteoarthritis Index). Results from the two healers were then analyzed separately, and compared with those in the sham control. Patients treated by healer 2 reported greater reduction in pain (mean improvement -25.7 ± 6.6 vs. -13.1 ± 3.0; $P < 0.01$) and more improvement in functionality (-28.1 ± 9.7 vs. -13.2 ± 3.4; $P < 0.01$), as well as a reduction in negative mood, but not in anxiety or depression. Patients treated by healer 1 experienced improvement similar to those in the control. These results persisted at 3-month follow-up for all groups. Mixed-effect models confirmed these findings when controling for possible confounders (e.g. gender, BMI, belief in CAM therapies, and duration of osteoarthritis pain). Consistent with the third possibility raised for the second NIH-funded RCT, this study suggests that the master-dependent efficacy of external QG requires further investigation into the healing-power level of different practitioners.

Jang and Lee [46] in Korea assigned 36 college students with premenstrual syndrome (PMS) to receive either real QG treatment or a sham QG placebo eight times during the two consecutive menstrual cycles following 2 months of screening. With subjects completing a treatment diary, significant improvements were reported by the QG group (e.g. negative feeling, pain, water retention and total PMS symptoms) compared with controls.

Information on laboratory studies of external *qigong* can be found in Chs 9, 10 and 12.

CONCLUSION

The long-term efficacy and effectiveness of QG can be established only with sound research and evidence-based practice. Current research gives initial support for some efficacy of QG, especially regarding age-related chronic conditions and associated wellbeing. New RCTs have also offered a balanced view of QG, including its limitations in treating certain heritable and highly debilitating diseases for which there is as yet no definitive pharmaceutical cure. However, with only a small number of well-designed trials and small samples in most studies, research gaps remain. Future investigation should improve several aspects of methodology: (a) using creative sham QG as a control [38], (b) examining the match of effective forms of QG with given chronic conditions [29], (c) testing adequate confounding factors, (d) investigating underlying mechanisms and the interplay between QG and personality traits, and (e) using innovative biophysical methods to assess the level of healing power and inter-healer consistency or treatment reliability.

At the end of their research article, Ai et al [1] described the implications of the new investigation of QG for clinical sciences as follows:

Inquiry into controversial issues surrounding QG does not arise only from the need to improve the quality of research design in energy healing trials. It is also a call for continuing innovation of research methodology to address the unique challenge of evaluating the complicated frameworks of CAM modalities. Through close cooperation ... the blossoming of research on energy healing may eventually enrich methodologies used in clinical research on other types of health care.

ACKNOWLEDGMENTS

The author has been supported by National Institute on Aging training grant T32-AG0017, National Institute on Aging grant R03-AGO-15686-01, National Center for Complementary and Alternative Medicine grant P50-AT00011, a grant from the John Templeton Foundation, and the John Hartford Faculty Scholars Program.

SECTION 3
THEORY AND EXPERIMENT IN *QI* RESEARCH

SECTION CONTENTS

SECTION INTRODUCTION

During the twentieth century, Romanticism had its revenge on the Enlightenment world of the Great Machine, as developments in quantum theory and special and general relativity changed forever the available metaphorical base of the language used in discussions about energy and matter [1]. In 1906 a Nobel Prize was awarded to British physicist J J Thompson (1856–1940) for his discovery in 1897 that electrons are particles, rather than waves or atoms. A generation later, his son George P Thompson (1892–1975) shared a Nobel Prize for his discovery that electrons *can* also be considered as waves.

To explain experimental findings that did not fit with classical (Newtonian) theory, Niels Bohr (1885–1962) developed a model of the atom in which electrons take instantaneous, discontinuous 'quantum' jumps from one atomic orbit to another, with no intervening time and no travel through space – an impossible act for a Newtonian particle. A decade later, Werner Heisenberg (1901–1976) showed in his famous Uncertainty Principle that the position and momentum of an individual subatomic particle cannot both be known precisely at the same time, again something unthinkable in classical physics with its solid material particles. Finally, it was found that electrons can regularly tunnel through a solid barrier that, classically, would be impenetrable.

On the basis of these findings, the basic principles of quantum mechanics (often known as the Copenhagen interpretation) modify a materialist worldview: (1) no solid matter; (2) no strict causality, as precise predictions for individual subatomic particles become impossible and there is no way to trace strict causal relations among individual particle; (3) no locality, as quantum

mechanical equations indicate that two particles, once they have interacted, are instantaneously connected even across astronomical distances (this property defies the strictly local connections allowed in classic materialism);
(4) no reductionism, because if apparently separate particles are actually connected nonlocally then a reductionist view based on isolated particles is untenable.

Although the Copenhagen interpretation could not be tested experimentally for decades, by the 1980s a number of actual research results consistently contradicted the theories of materialism (often called local realism) and consistently confirmed the predictions of quantum mechanics. These results do not invalidate materialism altogether. In the everyday world of 'large' objects, the mechanistic causation of Newtonian physics is approximately correct. This is why much of Western medicine continues to rely on it, without incorporating these many clues and observations about the nature of reality from fundamental physics into its perspectives on health and healing. Western society has advanced into the twenty-first century using modern cutting edge technologies still guided by nineteenth-century theories of materialist physics (and also typological biology).

In quantum field theory, first developed in the 1920s, the probability wave for a particle is described as a fluctuation in an underlying, nonmaterial field (a force field or matter field). In more recent 'superunified' theories, all the force and matter fields that make up the universe have been described as modes of vibration of one underlying, unified field: a 'superfield' or 'superstring field'. All the order and intelligence of the laws of nature arise from this one fundamental, nonmaterial field – as does all matter. Not only are particles really just waves, but those waves ultimately are made of an underlying field, as ocean waves are 'made of' ocean water. Returning to the metaphor of water, and waterways or channels, theory and research on *qi* as well as observations from contemporary practices of energy medicine may be seen in this new light.

In this section, systems theory and contemporary physiology also offer fresh interpretations of *qi*.

The language of *qi*, quantum physics and the superimplicate body

8

F David Peat

CHAPTER CONTENTS

LANGUAGE AND REALITY

This discussion of *qi* opens not with an exploration of the new visions brought about by quantum physics, nor with an exploration of energy in the body, nor with an examination of Oriental philosophy, but rather with a discussion of language because there is a very deep and subtle relation between the language a society speaks, its perception of the world around it, and thus our understanding of that world and the various concepts we create. In other words, the way we act towards the world and to others is profoundly tied to the language we speak.

For linguists this reality is embodied in the ethnolinguistic Whorf–Sapir hypothesis [1] on the relation between language and worldview – which is accepted in some quarters, but still controversial in others. One can also appeal to a far more ancient authority: that of Confucius himself who, when asked for advice during the troubled times in which he lived is attributed with replying, 'first purify the language'. The problem was interpreted by Laozi in his much-discussed saying [2] that 'the *dao* that can be told is not the eternal *dao*. The name that can be named is not the eternal name' (*dao ke dao fei chang dao. Ming ke ming fei chang ming*; 道可道, 非常道. 名可名, 非常名) [3].

Of course there have been later attempts to 'purify the language'. Leibniz tried, in vain, to create a 'philosophical language' in which all terms would be unambiguously defined [4]. In the twentieth century Bertrand Russell attempted something similar with his Logical Atomism [5]. After all, if matter could be broken down into its most primitive elements – atoms – why not break down philosophical arguments into atoms of clear and unambiguous meaning? As it turned out, the sorts of things that could be stated by Russell ended up being rather trivial and obvious, such as 'water boils at 100 degrees centigrade'.

Wittgenstein followed Russell with an even braver attempt to build a wall around the garden of language [6]. Within that garden, statements could be made clearly and arguments resolved with precision. But not everything was contained within that garden. Indeed Wittgenstein argued that the wilder land outside the garden was the province of poets and dramatists – the world of Keats, Goethe or Shakespeare. Nevertheless, for many philosophers it continued to remain the province of the 'great philosophical questions'.

But later Wittgenstein was to admit that his whole approach had been oversimplified, that language just cannot be made to work in this way [7]. It is a highly creative human endeavor that cannot be bound by a simple set of rules. Wittgenstein's own way out was to suggest that many of 'the great questions' of philosophy were no more than pseudoproblems. He compared the philosopher to a person trapped in a room. The chimney is too narrow for escape, as is the window. And so the philosopher frantically looks for a way out without ever realizing that the door has been open all the time.

So philosophy has already made strenuous efforts to resolve this issue of language and reality, but what about physics? After Werner Heisenberg had discovered quantum mechanics in 1925, he and Niels Bohr began to ask about the nature of what could be called 'quantum reality'. For Heisenberg the reality lay in the mathematics itself. However, Bohr pointed out that when physicists gather around a blackboard to discuss these equations they are always talking to each other. They are using language – German, Danish, English or French for example – and these languages always contain a number of subtly hidden assumptions about the nature of space, time, matter and energy. In other words, as soon as we begin to talk about the quantum world and the nature of quantum reality we find ourselves importing assumptions from our large-scale world. Bohr's conclusion was that 'we are suspended in language such that we do not know what is up and what is down' [8].

Bohr's observation is the crux of the matter and applies, I believe, as much to the world of atoms and electrons as it does to the world of *qi*. We may go so far, but then language, the very tool we use to communicate with each other, steps in and produces its own distortions derived from the large-scale, everyday world.

But there may be an atom of hope. The physicist David Bohm, of whom we shall learn more later in this chapter, pointed out that those European languages we speak are strongly structured around 'subject, verb, object', and so 'the cat chases the mouse'. We begin with two well-defined objects in space and time and connect them with a verb, an action word. In fact this sort of structure is a mirror for the Newtonian world of classical physics in which we have well-defined objects in space and time that interact via forces and fields.

Is there any way out of this dilemma, this linguistic grip of the Newtonian world? Bohm himself experimented with the development of an alternative, strongly verb-based, language he termed the Rheomode (or flowing mode) (David Bohm, personal communication, 1970s) [9]. Although he did not have much practical success with this approach he did end up meeting speakers of the Algonquian family of languages (which includes Blackfoot, Ojibwe, MicMac, Cree, among others). Their languages are very strongly verb based and, not surprisingly, their worldview is one of eternal flux and change. It is a world in which a person's name changes throughout their life and in which objects do not have a permanent basis. Indeed it is a world close to that revealed through quantum theory and far from that of Newtonian physics. Moreover it may well be a world in which it would be much easier to speak of *qi* [10].

METAPHOR AND CONFUSION

There is yet another area in which language can give rise to confusion. This occurs because there are many words in common use that also appear in specialized areas of physics. We have, for example: 'energy', 'force', 'potential', 'field', 'local', 'work' and so on.

A person may be a great force for good in the community, but we also have the phrase 'the weak nuclear force'. Does the word 'force' have the same meaning in both contexts? A particular person may have great potential as an artist but does that word 'potential' have the same meaning as in the phrase 'the vector potential'? We may organize a football game in a field but surely that use of the term field must be very different from that of 'the electromagnetic field' – a place not normally used for football!

Generally we do not really have problems when we use these terms – after all, their meanings are generally established by the context in which they are used – and there is a clear distinction when a word is used about a person, or about an experiment in the laboratory. But there is one area in which confusion does arise and in particular where one should be cautious in speaking or writing about qi as energy. That is when some people, maybe with the best of motives in mind, attempt to make a particular subject 'scientific' by importing terms from the world of physics; for example, by using a word such as 'field' or 'energy' that is in common use, but 'dressing it up' as it were to make it appear more 'scientific'. It is quite common in everyday usage to speak of a 'field of influence', and by that the speaker generally wishes to convey a rather vague and intuitive feeling experienced when they enter a particular building or encounter a powerful person. However, psychiatry has now begun to speak of the 'field' between patient and therapist, with the intention of suggesting that this is in some way related to the fields found in physics which all have very rigorous definitions and usages. In this way it is subtly suggested that the interaction between patient and therapist has been placed on a firmer and more 'scientific' basic.

We all know what 'local' means, but in physics the term 'nonlocality' is also used. This term is used to describe the correlated behavior of two quantum systems but in a way that does not involve any force or exchange of signals. If the correlation takes place via a signal or force then it is termed 'local'; nonlocality by contrast, while appearing counterintuitive, is firmly based on quantum physics. However, it is but a short step to make something like telepathy more 'scientific' by suggesting that this is a 'nonlocal effect' similar to the 'quantum entanglement' of two quantum systems.

Yet another term increasingly in use is 'subtle energy'. This would suggest, amongst other things, that subtle effects may indeed occur within the body that are not amenable to normal methods of measurement. We shall speculate on such subtle effects later in this chapter, but it should be made clear at this point that no rigorous scientific connection has yet been made between possible subtle effects in the physical body and the brave new world of the quantum (for a contrary view, see Ch. 9).

All this discussion is by no means intended to shut a door on debate or the creative development of new ideas and insights, but more to act as a word of caution, so to speak, and to suggest that confusions can occur such that we must always be alert to the use of language and the mixing of common and scientific terms within the same conversation.

HISTORY AND DEVELOPMENT

Let us now take a step backward and look at some of those language terms in the world of Newtonian physics. Classical physics in essence viewed the cosmos as a giant mechanism – the Newtonian clockwork. Hence, when used in physics, words such as force, energy, potential and so on all had a strongly mechanistic connotation.

But then came quantum theory and with it such notions as the uncertainty principle, the role of the observer, quantum wholeness and absolute chance. Faced with these new concepts the dominant worldview of Newtonian mechanism began to lose its power, although one shadow remained and that was with the concept of force and potential.

If an electron passes a charged body it experiences an electrical potential. The closer it approaches the charge the larger is this potential. And the larger the potential, the greater is its effect on the electron. Thus while we have thrown away certainty, a world independent of any observer, and a world built out of 'independent elements of reality' we have still retained the mechanistic notion of pushes and pulls. The electron is attracted or repelled by a particular potential and the amount of that push or pull depends upon the size of the potential. So, deep within the new quantum theory, physics has retained the notion of a mechanical effect on the motion of physical bodies.

THE QUANTUM POTENTIAL

In addition to his concerns about language David Bohm had always been unhappy with the conventional version of quantum theory. Back in the 1950s he had attempted an alternative approach, generally known as 'hidden variables' but, with one or two exceptions, this approach was not taken seriously by the scientific community. Then in the early 1970s he revisited his approach in a radically new way. In addition to the conventional (and, as we have seen, mechanistic) potential whose effects depend on its size, he proposed what he termed the 'quantum potential'. Unlike a conventional potential the effect of this quantum potential does not depend on its size but on its 'form' or shape [11].

What is this quantum potential? It could be said to be an expression of the nature of the experimental apparatus encountered by the electron. Or to put it another way, it is an expression of the particular physical disposition of this apparatus. In other words, encoded within the complex shape or pattern of the quantum potential is information about the physical environment a particular electron encounters.

To make this clear David Bohm used to say that the quantum potential is 'IN-FORM-ATION'.

What is more the electron is able to 'read' or decode the information within the quantum potential. In other words, the electron is no longer some tiny feature-less particle but has considerable internal complexity. In David Bohm's terms the electron has 'proto-mind'. So mind was not something that evolved at a particular point in history or at a particular level of an organism's complexity. Proto-mind was present from the beginning and cannot be fragmented away from matter itself.

It is now clear that this 'information', within the quantum potential, is not something passive, like words printed on this page or binary digits on a computer's hard drive, but has an activity of its own. It is 'active information'.

Think of the following analogy. A ship approaches a harbor in dense fog. By means of radar the ship detects an image of the harbor indicating that one of the docks is free. The radar signal uses very little energy when compared with the energy used to drive the ship through the water. However, even while this energy is weak it is packed with information. Via the ship's computer the radar signal is then able to direct the ship's motion through the water and toward the empty dock.

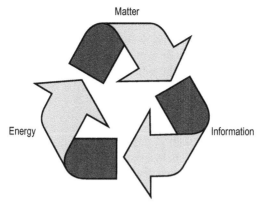

FIG 8.1   The triad of energy–matter–information.

Thus what could be termed a very subtle but information-packed energy has directed the gross energy of the ship.

Thus we have a triangle (Fig. 8.1), in which:

- information acts on energy to direct and modify its effects
- energy acts on matter to move matter or to transform it (solid to liquid, liquid to gas, for example)
- in turn, information 'reads' the particular orientation of matter
- and so on.

All this suggests that a new form of movement is possible, one that does not take place in response to a mechanical force. Likewise a new form of transformation is possible, one that takes place in response to what could perhaps be called, with some validity, 'subtle energy'. And by 'subtle energy' we mean an energy effect arising out of 'form' or 'information'.

ACTIVE INFORMATION IN THE BODY

Clearly the term 'subtle energy' could also be applied to a person's physical body. At one level the body's processes are responding to electrochemical processes such as a flow of hormones. Yet another more subtle level may also be present. Here I can only speculate since I do not have an in-depth knowledge of the traditions of *qi*, although it would be true to say that within the 'inscape' of my own body I am aware of sensations and movements that it may be possible to interpret within the verb-based language of *qi* [12].

It is certainly true to say that the body already operates with an impressive system of active information, in some aspects even more complex than that of the brain. Here I refer to the immune system, which is constantly gathering information from the environment and protecting the body from intrusion. Other systems of active information are also almost certainly present in the body, other proto-mind collectives perhaps.

THE IMPLICATE BODY

Up to now we have dealt only in part with Bohm's new approach to quantum theory. Indeed the physicist wished to go further, not simply to propose a new approach in physics but a radically new order he termed the 'Implicate Order'. In

The language of *qi*, quantum physics and the superimplicate body terms of active information we had understood the electron as a rather complex particle capable of reading what is encoded in the form of the quantum potential. However, at that level the electron is nevertheless an object well defined in space and time but one whose path is determined by the quantum potential – in other words, by active information. In this sense we are still partly within the Newtonian world of objects defined in space and in time, albeit with the addition of something new – an activity of information. We are, as Bohm had pointed out, still following the subject–verb–object convention and not in the world of flux and transformation of the Blackfoot language. Bohm termed this conventional world the 'Explicate Order', an order of objects well defined in space and time and, on the large scale, interacting via forces and fields. But according to Bohm this is no more than a surface manifestation of the much deeper Implicate Order.

The Implicate Order could loosely be compared to an *enfolded* order. One analogy is between the image on a photograph and that on a holograph. In a conventional photograph of a person each spot on the person corresponds to a spot on the photograph. If two regions are very close together on the person they will be close together on the photograph. If they are far apart on the person they will be far apart on the photograph. Both are expressions of the Explicate Order [11].

Now take a holograph. In this, laser light is reflected from a point on the person and distributed across the whole holographic plate. Thus the image of the person could be said to be enfolded across the whole of the plate: two areas that are distant on a person will be enfolded together at every point on the plate. Further, every part of the hologram contains information about the whole subject. No longer do we have objects well defined in space but objects that are distributed together within the Implicate Order. This now makes sense of nonlocality or quantum entanglement since two objects far apart in the Explicate Order remain correlated or co-related because within the Implicate Order they are enfolded one within the other.

While within the Explicate Order an object could be said to have a path or trajectory in space, we now have the explanation that this object is in a constant process of unfolding and enfolding out of a deeper order to manifest itself in an Explicate Space. In his thinking Bohm always stressed the importance of flux and movement and coined the term 'holomovement' to refer to 'the movement of the whole'. According to such thinking the physical body would not be some fixed object well defined in space and time, with its Cartesian split from the realm of mind. Rather it is the manifestation of a process of constants unfolding and enfolding out of a domain in which what we call mind and what we call matter are as inseparable as the two poles of a magnet. In Bohm's words, 'the deeper reality is something beyond either mind or matter, both of which are only aspects that serve as terms for analysis' [13].

We could perhaps go further, from the individual body-mind to society itself. After all, if we believe that the world is an organic, living thing, flexible and ever changing, this status should indeed be reflected in the social world that surrounds us. Yet the institutions we have created to deal with this fluid world are all too often rigid and insensitive, and do not behave in the same way as sentient beings. Similarly our attempts at intervention in society and the environment can at times be inappropriate. It is for this reason that this author has explored the notion of a new and more creative form of 'gentle action' [14].

THE SUPERIMPLICATE ORDER

So far we have only reached the first level of Bohm's new order. By way of an analogy the Explicate Order could be compared to the spaceships displayed on the screen of a video game. They are well defined and move on fixed paths. They are, however, not a primary reality in themselves but the manifestation of an underlying program held in the videogame's computer. This program moves through its iterations, sending data to the screen where it appears as spaceships. In this sense the computer and its program could be compared to the Implicate Order.

But there is a third factor to the video game, the player who watches the movements on the screen and then moves the joystick in an appropriate matter. By observing the manifestations of the Implicate Order, in its Explicate form on the screen, the player is then able to make transformations to the computer program and change the motions of the spaceships. In other words as the Implicate Order manifests itself in the Explicate it allows for a new order, the Superimplicate, which has the capacity of modifying the Implicate. As Bohm often remarked 'creativity has been added to the picture' [15].

Thus, by allowing its own manifestation via the Explicate Order, the Implicate begins to 'know itself' and thereby brings about its own creative transformation. Just as we earlier had the triad of matter–energy–active information, we now have the triad of Explicate–Implicate–Superimplicate Orders.

THE SUPERIMPLICATE BODY

We have long known that the human body is plastic in nature rather than being a fixed, rigid structure. After all, cells are born and die, continually replacing themselves throughout the life of the body. Neural networks are constantly being created in the brain while others atrophy and die. But now we reach another level of insight: that the physical body is an expression of an Explicate Order and beyond this lies the Implicate Order. In other words, the elements of the body are in constant flux, unfolding and enfolding out of a deeper ground. Moreover, their manifestation in space and time is observed and guided by a Superimplicate Order. In other words, the integrity of the body's various processes is maintained by what could perhaps be called a 'watchful activity of information'. It is here, I believe, that the insights of modern physics, at least in David Bohm's reformulation, can find a marriage to the ancient Chinese notion of *qi*, as further discussed in this book.

Qi and the frequencies of bioelectricity

Cyril W Smith

9

CHAPTER CONTENTS

INTRODUCTION

To avoid having to find metaphors or even definitions for something that has been recognized in Chinese medicine (CM) for millennia, the present starting point will be a concept of '*qi*' as some part of the 'being alive' experience of human existence. Frequencies are measures along a time span as illustrated in Figure 9.1.

Over the past 30 years, my research has taken me into the ways that living systems make use of frequencies and fields. Frequencies as an aspect of bioelectricity include time variations of electric fields, magnetic fields and radiation but also of mechanical vibrations through piezoelectricity. The lowest frequency that can be of significance to a living system must be that corresponding to its lifetime. Higher frequencies relevant to living systems range from circadian rhythms through heart and brain waves, muscle activity, acoustic frequencies and onwards to the frequencies of heat and light (visible and ultraviolet) characteristic of chemical reactions (e.g. combustion)

109

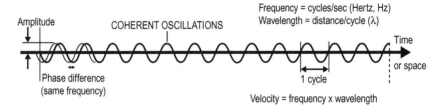

FIG 9.1 **Frequency and its units of measurement.** For a regular variation in any quantity its frequency is the number of complete cycles completed in unit time. This is usually taken as one second and one cycle per second is termed one Hertz (Hz). Multiples and submultiples are often used, e.g. 1 MegaHertz (MHz) = 10^6 Hz, 1 GigaHertz (GHz) = 10^9 Hz, 1 milliHertz (mHz) = 10^{-3} Hz.

and luminescence. The fundamental link between frequency and chemical structure is the basis of chemical analysis by spectroscopy.

FREQUENCIES AND PHYSICS

This section covers the physics of how living systems make use of frequencies and introduces the frequencies of fields, quantum effects and the memory of water for frequencies. If this is not of interest, the reader can go straight to section three, which introduces acupuncture meridians and endogenous frequencies and leads to the measurement and interpretation of frequencies associated with *qi*.

COHERENCE AND LONG-RANGE ORDER

The importance of frequency in biological systems was recognized by Herbert Fröhlich. In the 1930s, when told that the cell membrane potential was only a fraction of a volt but across an extremely thin cell wall, he realized that this represented an electric field of enormous strength that should resonate at around 100 GHz (10^{11} Hz). Such a field would be strong enough to align molecules over the distances involved in assembling biomolecules. By 1967, he had applied the theory of coherent modes of oscillation in nonlinear systems and long-range phase correlations to biological order and showed that the excitation of organs to their correct frequency could be achieved by energy from metabolic sources. The subsequent development of his ideas and the work of his worldwide circle of collaborators he edited into his two 'Green Books': *Coherent Excitations in Biological Systems* [1] and *Biological Coherence and Response to External Stimuli* [2].

I was privileged to collaborate with Fröhlich from 1973 until his death in January 1991. During this period, I and my students provided experimental support for his theoretical work [3]. From 1982, I became involved in the diagnosis and treatment of patients suffering from electrical hypersensitivity [4], extending the Miller technique of provocation–neutralization for this purpose. I found that frequencies that neutralize a patient's symptoms can be imprinted into water and used for therapy.

COHERENCE DOMAINS IN WATER

In 1995, Giuliano Preparata with Emilio del Giudice and coworkers showed through quantum electrodynamics (QED) theory that phase coherence is a fundamental property of water, arising from the exchange of radiation at the natural resonances of the water molecule [5]. This coherence is in the *unexcited* (ground) energy state of water – therefore, unlike the coherence of a laser, it needs no energy supply. Fröhlich's theory needed metabolic energy to elicit coherence.

COHERENCE AND FRACTALITY OF FREQUENCY

The distance over which order persists within a coherent system is termed the 'coherence length'. In a coherent system this feature becomes a constant parameter, making the velocity with which the coherence propagates proportional to the frequency being propagated. This makes frequency a quantity with no absolute scale of magnitude, as any velocity that the system can support will have a corresponding and proportionate frequency. It is this that enables chemical and biological frequency effects to interact and to be influenced by frequencies from manmade electronic equipment. That is, frequency has become a *fractal* quantity (see the Glossary for definitions of this and other technical terms).

FREQUENCIES AND FIELDS

In mathematics, a field is a region of space containing objects, rather like the 'field of view' seen with a camera or binoculars. In physics, a *field* is a region in which a force acts, for example the gravitational field. The 'classical electromagnetic field' is the basis of electronics and radio; it describes physical states of a system for which the phase is well defined but the large number of particles (quanta) involved is undefined. In contrast, a 'quantum field' has a fundamental uncertainty determined mathematically by the Heisenberg Uncertainty Relation:

$$\Delta\Phi. \; \Delta N \geq \hbar / 2$$

in which the uncertainty in the phase is $\Delta\Phi$, the uncertainty in number of coherent particles involved is ΔN and $\hbar$ is Planck's constant (6.63×10^{-34} J.s) divided by 2π. Within a water coherence domain, the more the uncertainty is taken up by fluctuation in the number of particles the more perfect is the phase coherence of the field [3].

Electric charge is associated with matter (electrons, atoms and molecules): unlike charges attract, like charges repel; in contrast, *unlike* currents repel, and *like* currents attract. A *moving* charge generates a magnetic **B**-field (the bold underline indicates a vector or directed quantity). An *accelerated* charge radiates energy as an electromagnetic wave at the frequency of its acceleration. A magnetic field (**B**-field) can exist only in closed loops. A mathematical consequence is that a further field called the 'magnetic vector potential' (**A**-field) must exist. If an **A**-field oscillates, it generates an alternating electric field in space of magnitude proportional to the frequency [6].

All this is going on in three dimensions. A current of water flowing down a drain provides a convenient image: the closed loop of vortex around the current is analogous to the **B**-field, while the vortex being sucked into the waste pipe is analogous to the vector potential (**A**-field) along the current or flow path (Fig. 9.2).

Electric and magnetic fields and energies are not continuously variable, however; they come in *quanta* just as matter comes in atoms. One quantum of electromagnetic radiation equals Planck's constant h multiplied by the frequency v. One quantum of magnetic flux is $h/2e = 2.07 \times 10^{-15}$ Wb (Webers) where e is the charge of the electron. If two coherence domains are weakly coupled together, this constant can describe the voltage/frequency relations (≈ 500 MHz/μV) between them through the Josephson effect [7].

If living systems have phase coherence extending over the distances of biological structures then they can behave as large-scale quantum systems in which

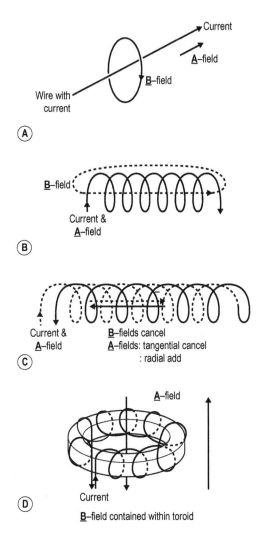

FIG 9.2 **Coils and fields.** (A) A vortex of water flow is analogous to the magnetic **B**-field generated by a flow of electric charge through a wire. The **B**-field circles the wire (in a right-hand corkscrew around the current), while the **A**-field is in the direction of the current. (B) For a simple coil (solenoid), the **B**-field is uniform within the solenoid and loops around the outside, while the **A**-field is in the direction of the current. (C) A caduceus coil consists of two solenoid windings in opposite directions, so that the **B**-fields cancel. The *tangential* **A**-field components also cancel, but the *radial* **A**-field components add, and are present both within and outside the caduceus coil. (D) For a toroid (ring), the **B**-field is contained within the torus, while the **A**-field loops around it. *(Adapted from Smith & Best [4], with the authors' permission.)*

a domain of coherence behaves like an enormous single atom. Mathematically, any such system can be described by a wave equation having amplitude, phase and frequency. The **A**-field affects the phase of this wave function, and it is in the **A**-field that frequency information in biological systems resides [8]. Marcer and Schemp [9] created a mathematical model representing the brain and conscious-ness in terms of a holographic image coded in the phase of a coherent quantum field. Since an **A**-field can affect the phase of a wave function, it must alter the body's holographic image of itself.

WATER MEMORY FOR FREQUENCIES

Samuel Hahnemann, the founder of homeopathy, prepared his remedies (*potencies*) by *potentization*, a process called *succussion* that involved taking a vial containing a dilution of the original material (the 'mother tincture') in water and banging it on the cover of a leather-bound book. The combination of succussion with serial dilutions changes the pattern of frequencies imprinted, and these remain in the water even after all the original chemicals have been diluted away [10] (see Ch. 12).

Not only can a frequency be imprinted into water by succussion, it can also be imprinted by a strong **B**-field. The **B**-field component merely has a potentizing or formatting role; its frequency does not matter so long as it is below that of the **A**-field frequency being imprinted [8]. Frequency may also be imprinted by a train of seven unidirectional voltage pulses, by certain frequencies (e.g. 7.8 Hz, which is readily available from the heart *chakra*), or by chemically induced effects.

An **A**-field is produced in the space around a toroidal coil. The **B**-field is contained *within* the toroid so there is no risk of its potentizing effect imprinting a tube of water when being used to measure frequencies. In that process the specimen is positioned near to but *outside* the toroid-exciting coil (Fig. 9.2D). The same set-up is used when imprinting a signal frequency passed through the coil, but in this case the tube is concurrently succussed by banging the base of the tube on the wooden bench.

However, a frequency imprint in water (or a homeopathic potency) is permanently *erased* if the geomagnetic field is shielded, for example by placing the water briefly inside a steel box and putting the lid on. Erasure occurs if the **B**-field is reduced to less than 380 nT as then the magnetic energy in the volume of a coherence domain becomes less than the thermal energy (kT), which can break up the order that gives rise to the memory. This shows that a coherence domain in water must have a diameter of exactly 53 μm.

In addition to the North–South magnetic **B**-field of the Earth, there is an **A**-field component in an East–West direction that biases the alternating field from the toroid. If an imprint is made on the North side of the toroid it stimulates biological activity, whereas if the imprint is made on the South side it depresses such activity – presumably generating *yang* and *yin* phases respectively.

In 1983, we showed [11,12] that living systems can respond to magnetic resonance conditions at geomagnetic field strengths. This allowed later speculation that a frequency might be retained in a water coherence domain if the magnetic resonance of its protons could be synchronized to an applied frequency. The protons would then generate their own internal magnetic field to satisfy proton resonance conditions exactly [3]. This condition becomes independent of frequency if a very specific number of protons satisfy this condition. Such a memory would be stable unless the coherence were broken up by removing the geomagnetic field – as happens in *erasure* (described above). The physics involved in the instrumentation of measuring frequencies in water memory has been described [6].

The measured bandwidth of a water imprint is of the order of parts per million. This is consistent with statistical fluctuations in the number of protons involved and is confirmed by an observed increase in pH on imprinting frequencies into water, which returns to its original value on *erasure*. An increase in pH implies that fewer protons are available [13]. Although it is sufficient for most purposes to make frequency measurements to four significant figures, it is necessary to emphasize the precision with which nature uses frequency (see the comments to Table 9.6 below).

ACUPUNCTURE MERIDIANS, ENDOGENOUS FREQUENCIES AND MEASUREMENTS

In 1982, Dr Jean Monro asked me for help with the problems experienced by chemically sensitive patients who had become hypersensitive to their electromagnetic environment [4]. The symptoms provoked in them by chemicals to which they had acquired a hypersensitivity were identical to those triggered by specific frequencies in their environment. It quickly became clear that it was frequency that mattered and that this was patient specific. When we had extremely electrically sensitive patients who could not even tolerate an oscillator switched on when they were anywhere in the building, I had them imprint their body frequencies into water and I developed a dowsing technique [14] that covers the frequencies necessary for clinical purposes. The dowsing response involves a phase comparison between the left and right side Heart and Pericardium meridians. If either of them are joined by a wire the response is lost. I have worked on instrumentation for this measurement and could confirm that the frequency measured by dowsing was the same as that measured electronically, although it has taken me 25 years to understand the physics involved [6].

These patients were sensitive to the $\underline{A}$-field produced by an alternating current in a toroidal coil, and the frequencies to which they were sensitive ranged from milliHertz to TeraHertz. It took some time to realize that we were seeing reactions at the endogenous frequencies of the acupuncture meridians and *chakras*.

When an acupuncture point is needled, acupressure applied or a target organ stressed, its endogenous frequency spreads throughout the body. This can be measured by imprinting it into a vial of water held in the fist and succussed on wood. These frequency imprints identify stressed meridians and a therapeutic frequency imprint (potency) can then be made. However, the therapy will not be permanent if frequency signatures from chemical toxicity remain.

The autonomic nervous system (ANS) is usually the first to become compromised. Between stable states of health and disease, there may exist a region in which a patient is in a state of mathematical chaos [15]. The various complementary and alternative medicines can operate within chaos and restore a patient to a state of stable health. The nature of chaos means that it is not possible to do repeatable 'double-blinded' trials, since a chaotic system started from similar initial conditions never reaches the same endpoint each time.

QI AND THE ACUPUNCTURE MERIDIANS

In Chinese and some other medical systems, *qi* or its equivalent is considered as a 'vital force' or 'energy' that flows along meridians, freely in health but becoming disturbed in illness. These acupuncture meridians probably originate at the presomite stage of embryo development, when layers of cells, ectoderm, endoderm and mesoderm are in close contact. Then it only needs the frequencies of adjoining cells to become phase coherent and for this coherence to be retained as the organism develops to provide channels or meridians of coherent frequencies linking target organs to the acupuncture points [16].

FREQUENCIES AND MERIDIANS

Once it was realized that endogenous frequencies exist for the acupuncture meridians and *chakras*, it was not difficult to map them out. Table 9.1 lists nominal values measured for these endogenous frequencies (note that there are two fractally related frequency bands – high and low – for each acupuncture meridian). The remainder

Table 9.1 *Acupuncture points and chakras with nominal values for endogenous frequencies*

Location	Target organs	Point measured	Low-band frequency	High-band frequency
Acupuncture points (body in anatomical position)				
Hands				
Thumb:				
Outside	Lymphatic tissue Lungs	Ly-1	6.0×10^{-2}	$2.95 \times 10^{+6}$
Inside	Lungs	LU-1	4.8×10^{-1}	$2.40 \times 10^{+7}$
Index finger:				
Outside	Large intestine	LI-1	5.5×10^{-2}	$2.70 \times 10^{+6}$
Inside	Nerve degeneration	ND-1	5.5×10^{-4}	$2.70 \times 10^{+4}$
3rd finger:				
Outside	Pericardium/ Circulation	P-9	5.0×10^{-2}	$2.46 \times 10^{+6}$
Inside	Allergy	AD-1	2.0×10^{0}	$9.84 \times 10^{+7}$
4th finger:				
Outside	Organ degeneration	Or-1	7.8×10^{-2}	$3.85 \times 10^{+6}$
Inside	*sanjiao* (Triple Burner)	SJ-1	$6.0 \times 10^{+3}$	$\approx 3.00 \times 10^{+11}$
Little finger:				
Outside	Heart	HT-9	7.8×10^{0}	$3.84 \times 10^{+8}$
Inside	Small Intestine	SI-1	2.5×10^{-2}	$1.23 \times 10^{+6}$
Feet				
Big toe:				
Inside	Spleen/pancreas	SP-1	5.5×10^{-2}	$2.70 \times 10^{+6}$
Outside	Liver	LIV-1	4.8×10^{0}	$2.36 \times 10^{+8}$
2nd toe:				
Inside	Joint degeneration	JD-1	3.0×10^{-1}	$1.48 \times 10^{+7}$
Outside	Stomach	ST-45/left	4.4×10^{-1}	$2.20 \times 10^{+6}$
	Stomach	ST-45/right	4.4×10^{-2}	$2.20 \times 10^{+7}$
	Stomach	ST-45/balanced	2.1×10^{-1}	$8.1 \times 10^{+6}$
3rd toe:				
Inside	Fibroid degeneration	FibD-1	$8.0 \times 10^{+2}$	$\approx 4.00 \times 10^{+10}$
Outside	Skin degeneration	Sk-1	3.5×10^{-3}	$1.72 \times 10^{+5}$
4th toe:				
Inside	Fatty degeneration	FatD-1	7.4×10^{-1}	$3.60 \times 10^{+7}$
Outside	Gall Bladder	GB-44	5.0×10^{-2}	$2.46 \times 10^{+6}$
Little toe:				
Inside	Kidney	KI-1	9.5×10^{-4}	$4.70 \times 10^{+4}$
Outside	Bladder	BL-67	5.5×10^{0}	$2.70 \times 10^{+8}$

Qi and the frequencies of bioelectricity

(Continued)

Table 9.1 *Acupuncture points and chakras with nominal values for endogenous frequencies—cont'd*

Location	Target organs	Point measured	Low-band frequency	High-band frequency
Further Points				
Posterior	*dumai* (Governing Vessel)	Du-14	4.3×10^{0}	$1.49 \times 10^{+8}$
Anterior	*renmai* (Conception Vessel)	Ren-24	$1.4 \times 10^{+1}$	$7.30 \times 10^{+8}$
Middle finger	Pericardium*	P-9*	2.5×10^{-1}	$1.30 \times 10^{+7}$
	Anmian I & II		$3.0 \times 10^{+3}$	$\approx 10^{11}$
Chakras				
Crown	*sahasrara*		2.5×10^{-1}	$1.2 \times 10^{+7}$
Forehead	*ajna*		3.0×10^{0}	$1.5 \times 10^{+8}$
Thyroid	*vishudda*		$8.1 \times 10^{+1}$	$3.9 \times 10^{+9}$
Heart	*anahata*		7.8×10^{0}	$3.8 \times 10^{+8}$
Umbilical	*manipura*		$2.3 \times 10^{+1}$	$1.1 \times 10^{+9}$
Pubic	*svadhisthana*		$8.1 \times 10^{+1}$	$3.9 \times 10^{+9}$
Coccyx	*maladhara*		$8.1 \times 10^{+1}$	$3.9 \times 10^{+9}$

Included in the writer's presentations at the International Annual Symposia on 'Man and His Environment in Health and Disease' in Dallas, Texas, 2000, 2005, 2007.

of this chapter describes findings that demonstrate possible relationships between *qi* or 'energy' flow and the endogenous frequencies of the acupuncture meridians.

COMMENTS ON TABLE 9.1

1. The *jing*-Well acupuncture endpoints [17] are located at either corner of a nail bed. Reinhold Voll, creator of the EAV (Electroacupuncture according to Voll) system [18], listed connections between specific acupuncture points and the ANS. For example, ND-1a is the summation point for the entire ANS, ST-10a the summation point for the parasympathetic division and GB-20 for the sympathetic division.
2. There are additional frequencies at points that link with the ANS (sympathetic $\approx 0.003\,\mathrm{Hz}$, parasympathetic $\approx 0.3\,\mathrm{Hz}$).
3. At a *luo* point, frequencies of both connecting meridians are found.
4. For the *sanjiao* (Triple Burner) meridian a total of 31 frequencies from imprints made by 22 patients had a mean equal to $6.018\,\mathrm{kHz}$ (SD $\pm 0.20\%$). For the Heart meridian and a total of 53 frequencies from imprints made by 38 patients, the mean was $7.788\,\mathrm{Hz}$ (SD $\pm 0.92\%$).

   The fractal ratio of the two frequency bands detected is $49.19 \pm 0.08 \times 10^{+6}$ (SD $\pm 0.15\%$).

FREQUENCY SYNCHRONIZATION OF ACUPUNCTURE MERIDIANS

There is a band of applied frequencies within which any meridian will depart from its endogenous value and become synchronized to that frequency. It may change by ± 30% before the meridian frequency jumps back to its endogenous value. The *dumai* meridian (Governing Vessel) is unique in that it can synchronize itself to almost any environmental frequency, selecting only that with the strongest signal.

A subject was exposed to the high-band frequency of the Heart meridian by sitting in front of a microwave oscillator for 3 minutes (microwave power density was estimated as of the order of mW/m^2). After this, the frequencies at HE-9 were immediately imprinted into water and measured. The frequency measurements took about 5 minutes following exposure and by this time the acupuncture point frequency had reverted to the unexposed value. At 260 MHz and at 500 MHz there was no synchronization. From 270 MHz to 480 MHz the endogenous frequency at HT-9 had become synchronized. The corresponding low-band frequencies had shifted in proportion to 5.245 Hz and 9.657 Hz respectively. Similarly, if a practitioner's *qi* activity results in the emission of frequencies, these should be able to entrain a subject's acupuncture meridians and *chakras*.

FREQUENCY CHANGING BY INTENTION

It is possible to change the frequency of a meridian and what is imprinted into water by intention, thereby linking frequency and *qi*. Some healers consider their 'energy' is emitted from the pad of the middle finger, where the acupuncture point P-9* (EAV Pericardium-9*) is positioned by some teachers (see Table 9.1). Experiment showed it was possible to change the frequency at the P-9* acupuncture point by *intention* from 0.2012 Hz to 7.575 Hz. A healer might do this in response to what is sensed as a need for the patient. The endogenous frequency of the Heart meridian (7.8 Hz) is generally regarded as therapeutic and covers not only the function of the heart and circulation but also consciousness, the function of the brain and mental activity. The heart *chakra* can effect potentization (see above). However, the present investigation did not cover consciousness and intention effects in general [19,20].

FREQUENCIES AND *QI*

Frequency itself is unlikely to be a complete description of *qi*, although it may be at least a measurable correlate. Sometimes when tracing the endogenous frequency along a meridian one arrives at a blockage to frequency, and so presumably to *qi*. It may be that the proximal side of an operation scar has the normal frequency of the target organ, but the distal side shows no frequency at all, or some entirely different frequency. Imprinting the correct frequency here may restore normality to frequency and *qi* along the entire meridian.

Classical Chinese acupuncture describes 12 meridians and groups these into three sets of paths along which *qi* is supposed to flow, namely: LU–LI–ST–SP, HT–SI–BL–KI and P–SJ–GB–LIV. In each path, the *yin* and *yang* Organ frequencies can be combined for calculation purposes according to their geometric means. When tubes of water are imprinted with two mean *yin* and two mean *yang* frequencies respectively (e.g. LU + LI and ST + SP) and then placed close together, all four frequencies disappear (become undetectable). If one attempts to imprint all four frequencies into a single tube of water, three will imprint normally but then at succussion to imprint the fourth frequency there is erasure of *all* frequencies [21]. This may be an example of 'nilpotency' [22]. So long as the four meridians indicate a healthy condition, these combinations of frequencies will be zero, giving living systems a very refined error detection mechanism.

QI IN ACTION

This section describes measurements made in cooperation with *qigong* expert Birinder Tember. It includes measurements made during his *qi* demonstrations. Glass tubes of water were imprinted either by succussion with the tube held in the fist, or imprinted by intention from a distance of about 1 meter using the well-known *baduan jin* (八段锦) or 'Eight Pieces of Silken Brocade' *qigong* routine – of which Birinder practices a form developed by Grandmaster Peng Qing, his own teacher's grandfather, acknowledged as one of China's greatest *Shaolin* grandmasters (L J Wen, Personal communication to BT, 1993).

FREQUENCY MEASUREMENTS OF *QI* IMPRINTS INTO WATER

The following Tables and Comments list measurable properties of *qi*. These are expressed in terms of frequencies related to acupuncture meridians (use Table 9.2 to aid interpretation; in these Tables ↑ is used to denote a frequency stimulating biological activity and ↓ to denote a frequency depressing biological activity).

Table 9.2 Initial trial measurements of qi frequencies imprinted by Birinder Tember (27 June 2009)						
Imprint	**Tube**	**Measured frequencies (Hz)**				
		↑	↓	↑	↓	↑
After 5 min standard relaxation	1	1.012×10^{-3}	5.422×10^{-2}	7.515×10^{0}	$6.002 \times 10^{+3}$	$1.233 \times 10^{+6}$
Note: tubes 2–6 were all stimulatory		↑	↑	↑	↑	
Spiraling energy	2			7.522×10^{0}		
Meditative imprint	3		5.003×10^{-2}			
Mudra (hand positions)	4			7.802×10^{0}		
Mantra-based imprint	5	1.413×10^{-3}	3.312×10^{-1}	7.213×10^{0}	$6.002 \times 10^{+3}$	
Balancing Spleen and Stomach (self-treatment)	6			7.213×10^{0}		
↑ = stimulatory; ↓ = depressive.						

COMMENTS ON TABLE 9.2

Tube 1 was imprinted by succussion, held in the hand after a 5-minute period of relaxation exercises. It shows Birinder's initial condition and his meridians then under stress. These frequencies follow the usual pattern – alternately stimulatory (*yang*) and depressive (*yin*) of biological activity. Table 9.1 identifies meridians and *chakras* from their frequencies. Here, the frequencies associated with the Kidney, Large Intestine and/or Spleen, *sanjiao* and Small Intestine meridians appear, although they should not normally appear in the *whole* body field. In contrast, the Heart meridian *is* normally present, but here its frequency is off the normal 7.8 Hz.

Tubes **2 to 6** were imprinted by 'directed *qi*'; there was no physical contact with the tubes. These imprints differ from Tube 1 showing that the exercises and mental concentration of the *qi* routine can overcome personal characteristics. These frequencies were *all stimulatory*, which is a feature of imprints made by healers.

Tube 2 had a frequency of 7.522×10^0 Hz, which is nearer to the 7.515×10^0 Hz of Tube 1 than to the nominal Heart meridian frequency 7.8 Hz. This may be due to incomplete relaxation.

Tube 3 had the frequency 5.003×10^{-2} Hz. This would stimulate the Gall Bladder and Pericardium (Voll's 'Circulation') meridians.

Tube 4 had the frequency 7.802×10^0 Hz – precisely the Heart meridian value.

Tube 5 had frequencies that would stimulate the Kidney, Joint degeneration meridian and Parasympathetic ANS, Heart and *sanjiao* meridians.

Tube 6 was imprinted after Birinder had used a *qi* self-treatment to balance his Spleen and Stomach meridians, which he knew were stressed. Only the Heart meridian frequency remained, still off the normal endogenous value.

Table 9.3	Trial measurement of qi therapy applied to a 'Fire type' subject by Birinder Tember (27 June 2009)			
		Measured frequencies (Hz)		
	Tube	↑	↓	↑
Baseline control	7	2.131×10^{-3}	3.114×10^{-1}	7.803×10^0
Subject after CF treatment	8			7.803×10^0
↑ = stimulatory frequency (Hz); ↓ = depressive frequency (Hz).				

COMMENTS ON TABLE 9.3

The 'Causative factor' (CF) is a principle used within a branch of Five Element acupuncture developed by J R Worsley, which categorizes individuals into five constitutional or 'CF' types according to the five 'Elements' of antiquity: Fire, Earth, Metal, Water and Wood [23]. These can be related to the endogenous frequencies of the classical acupuncture meridians [21].

Tube 7 was a control imprint made by succussion. Stress on the sympathetic nervous system is characterized by the appearance of the frequency $\approx 3 \times 10^{-3}$ Hz, and on the parasympathetic nervous system by $\approx 3 \times 10^{-1}$ Hz. The Heart meridian appears at 7.8 Hz as wanting stimulation, as to be expected in a 'Fire type' CF.

Tube 8 was imprinted by succussion after CF treatment and shows only the Heart meridian.

	Tube	↑	↓	↑	↓	↑
Table 9.4 Frequencies (Hz) from 'Healing sounds qigong' imprinted by Birinder Tember (22 July 2009 at 14.30)						
Initial test – imprint with no sound	I	1.001×10^{-2}	4.313×10^{-1}	7.802×10^{0}		
'He' sound corresponds to Heart	2	7.802×10^{0}				
'Ho' sound corresponds to Heart	3	$6.005 \times 10^{+3}$				
'Hu' sound corresponds to Spleen	4	$6.005 \times 10^{+3}$				
'Fu' sound corresponds to Spleen	5	7.805×10^{0}				
'Xu' sound corresponds to Liver	6	2.004×10^{-1}	7.802×10^{0}	$6.005 \times 10^{+3}$		
'Xu' sound corresponds to Liver	7	3.003×10^{-1}	7.801×10^{0}	$6.001 \times 10^{+3}$		
'Hey' sound corresponds to Triple Burner (sanjiao)	8	2.005×10^{-2}	3.002×10^{-1}	7.803×10^{0}	$8.001 \times 10^{+2}$	$6.001 \times 10^{+3}$
'Chui' sound corresponds to Kidneys	9	7.801×10^{0}				
'Aum' for stimulating/ awakening the kundilani	10	1.002×10^{-2}	7.802×10^{0}	$6.002 \times 10^{+3}$		

↑ = stimulatory frequency (Hz); ↓ = depressive frequency (Hz).

COMMENTS BY BT AND CWS ON TABLE 9.4

Tube 1: Initial test, no sound. Tube succussed on wood six times. The frequency 1.001×10^{-2} Hz is not near that of any meridian. 4.313×10^{-1} Hz is that of the left-side Stomach meridian. 7.802×10^{0} is the Heart meridian frequency.

Tube 2: The 'He' sound corresponds to Heart, and gives the Heart meridian frequency 7.802×10^{0} Hz.

Tubes 3 and 4: These sounds have imprinted $6.005 \times 10^{+3}$ Hz, the *sanjiao* frequency, rather than the Heart or Spleen frequencies.

Tube 5: This sound has imprinted 7.805×10^0 Hz (Heart rather than Spleen).

Tube 6: 2.004×10^{-1} Hz is the frequency of balanced Stomach meridians. The other frequencies are those of the Heart and *sanjiao* respectively. The Liver frequency is not present.

Tube 7: 3.003×10^{-1} Hz is the frequency of Joint degeneration and the parasympathetic ANS. The other frequencies are those of the Heart and *sanjiao* respectively. The Liver frequency is not present.

Tube 8: These sounds have correctly imprinted the *sanjiao* frequency $6.001 \times 10^{+3}$ Hz. Of the other frequencies, 2.005×10^{-2} Hz is near the Small Intestine frequency, 3.002×10^{-1} Hz is that of the Joint degeneration and parasympathetic ANS. 7.803×10^0 Hz is the Heart frequency, and $8.001 \times 10^{+2}$ Hz is the Fibroid degeneration frequency, which is uncommon.

Tube 9. This sound has imprinted 7.801×10^0 Hz (Heart, not Kidney).

Tube 10. This sound has imprinted 1.002×10^{-2} Hz (also present in the initial test), also Heart 7.802×10^0 Hz and *sanjiao* $6.002 \times 10^{+3}$ Hz.

Table 9.5	Baduan jin *posture imprints by Birinder Tember (25 July 2009 at 20.00)*		
Baduan jin **posture**	↑	↓	↑
Posture 1 (pressing the sky)	5.001×10^{-1}	7.801×10^0	$6.001 \times 10^{+3}$
Posture 2 (shoot eagle with bow)	3.336×10^{-2}	3.336×10^{-1}	3.336×10^0
Posture 3 (pressing heaven and earth)	3.617×10^{-1}	7.801×10^0	$6.001 \times 10^{+3}$
Posture 4 (looking backwards)	7.804×10^0		
Posture 5 (shake head, wag tail)	2.232×10^{-2}	3.126×10^{-1}	7.801×10^0
Posture 6 (tapping heaven and earth)	2.413×10^{-2}	3.034×10^{-1}	7.801×10^0
Posture 7 (punching with angry eyes)	5.747×10^{-3}	3.133×10^{-2}	7.801×10^0
Posture 8 (swimming dragon)	2.013×10^{-1}	7.801×10^0	$6.001 \times 10^{+3}$
BT relax (3 breaths, hold 2 breaths)	7.801×10^0		
BT relax again (3 breaths, hold 2 breaths)	7.801×10^0		
↑ = stimulatory frequency (Hz); ↓ = depressive frequency (Hz).			

COMMENTS FROM BT AND CWS ON TABLE 9.5

Birinder imprinted each tube by cupping it between both hands following each of the eight postures of *baduan jin* and the two relaxations. Two names are listed below for each posture, together with their basic benefits.

Posture 1 'Pressing the sky' or 'Holding the gates of heaven': This exercise relates to the *sanjiao* meridian and aids fluid transportation of Blood and *qi* within the body. 5.001×10^{-1} Hz stimulates the Lung meridian, 7.801×10^0 depresses the Heart meridian, and $6.001 \times 10^{+3}$ Hz stimulates the *sanjiao* meridian.

Posture 2 'Bending the bow' or 'Shoot the eagle with the bow': The emphasis here is in the upper *jiao* (chest region). Contraction and expansion of the chest cavity and arm muscles facilitate intake of oxygen and the flow of Blood and *qi*, so quickening regeneration of cells and muscle fibers. Tiredness

9

Qi and the frequencies of bioelectricity

121

will give way to a feeling of liveliness. The results are unusual in that the three frequencies are exactly decades apart.

3.336×10^{-1} Hz is depressing the activity of the parasympathetic ANS. The other two frequencies do not correspond closely with any meridian. This decade pattern is occasionally seen in patient imprints and occurs in the signatures of chemicals such as somatropin. 3.336×10^{0} Hz may stimulate the *dumai* meridian.

Posture 3 'Pressing upwards and downwards' or 'Separate heaven and earth': This helps the function of the Stomach and Spleen, which in CM have the role of transportation and transformation of digested food, producing food *qi* (*gu qi*, 穀氣). It thereby helps improve digestion and absorption of nutrients by the body. The frequency 3.617×10^{-1} Hz might be a combination of stimulation for the parasympathetic ANS and the left-side Stomach meridian. 7.801×10^{0} Hz is depressing the activity of the Heart meridian, while $6.001 \times 10^{+3}$ Hz is stimulating the *sanjiao* meridian.

Posture 4 'Looking backwards' or 'Looking behind': This is excellent for the spine, loosens neck muscles and calms the nerves. It is also said to assist in overcoming exhaustion of the *zangfu* (Internal Organs) and injuries caused by imbalance (excess or deficiency) of the seven emotions Joy, Sympathy, Grief, Fear, Anger, Hatred and Desire. The only frequency here is 7.804×10^{0} Hz, stimulating the Heart meridian.

Posture 5 'Looking around and up' or 'Shake head and wag tail': This settles the emotional state and affects the Heart meridian primarily. It removes excess Heat from the Heart (a condition in CM with symptoms such as 'feeling disturbed', 'a constant uneasiness', 'insomnia', 'constant thirst' and 'a dry sensation on the tongue, especially on the tip and a redder than normal color'). 2.232×10^{-2} Hz is stimulating the Small Intestine meridian, 3.126×10^{-1} Hz is depressing the parasympathetic activity of the ANS, and 7.801×10^{0} Hz is stimulating the Heart meridian.

Posture 6 'Bouncing on the toes' or 'Tapping the earth with the heels': This regulates *qi* throughout the body. It also helps relieve worry and anxiety to some extent. 2.413×10^{-2} Hz is probably stimulating the Small Intestine meridian, but is further from the nominal value than in Posture 5 so other factors may be involved. 3.034×10^{-1} is depressing the activity of the parasympathetic ANS, while 7.801×10^{0} Hz stimulates the Heart meridian (as for Posture 5).

Posture 7 'Punching with angry eyes' or 'Punching with glaring eyes and fist': This exercise helps store the *qi* in the lower *dantian* when in the horse stance. If done isometrically (not recommended if you suffer from hypertension), it increases both muscular strength and stamina. Widening the eyes helps release stagnation of *qi* from within the meridians (which is especially good for the Liver meridian). This further helps release locked-in emotion, easing frustration and inappropriate anger (a great exercise for many women with premenstrual syndrome). 5.747×10^{-3} Hz is not specific for any meridian but may stimulate the sympathetic ANS; 3.133×10^{-2} Hz may depress the activity of the Small Intestine and the right-side Stomach meridians; 7.801×10^{0} Hz stimulates the Heart meridian.

Posture 8 'Swimming dragon' or 'Gathering qi': This harmonizes the middle *jiao* and regulates the pancreas (so can help reduce blood sugar). 2.013×10^{-1} Hz stimulates balanced Stomach meridians, the Pericardium meridian and the crown (*sahasrara*) *chakra*; 7.801×10^{0} Hz stimulates the Heart meridian and $6.001 \times 10^{+3}$ stimulates the *sanjiao* meridian.

Tubes 9 and 10 were imprinted successively after each of two relaxation periods following the above exercises. Both show the Heart meridian at its normal value.

Table 9.6 *Birinder Tember energized these tubes of water using different qigong and yogic breathing patterns as stated (21 August 2009 at 16.30)*

Qigong patterns	Tube	↑	↓	↑
Initial test: tube tapped on wood 6 times	1	7.801×10^0		
Baduan jin	2	7.801×10^0		
'Collect the moon's reflection from the sea bed'	3	7.801×10^0		
'Steel thumbs of Lohan'	4	6.313×10^{-2}	5.113×10^{-1}	7.801×10^0
Sound qigong – 'Hu' corresponding to the Spleen	5	7.801×10^0		
Mantra	6	3.615×10^{-2}	4.123×10^{-1}	7.801×10^0
Indian yogic breathing exercises				
Bastrika	7	7.801×10^0		
Anulom vilom	8	7.801×10^0		
Kapalbhati	9	3.151×10^{-2}	6.413×10^{-1}	7.801×10^0
'Brahmri'	10	6.227×10^{-2}	6.902×10^{-1}	7.801×10^0

↑ = stimulatory frequency (Hz); ↓ = depressive frequency (Hz).

COMMENTS BY BT AND CWS ON TABLE 9.6

In Table 9.5, Tubes 1–8 each showed three frequencies and all but one included that for the Heart meridian. Here, all imprints included the Heart meridian 7.801 Hz frequency precisely.

Tube 1 Initial test: Tube of water succussed on wood six times – Heart meridian imprinted.

Tube 2 *Baduan jin*: After performing the entire routine of eight postures, Birinder then energized Tube 2 (in Table 9.5 this was done posture by posture). Here only the Heart meridian was imprinted, at a frequency identical to that of Tube 1.

Tube 3 'Collect the moon's reflection from the sea bed': Results are identical to those for Tubes 1 and 2.

Tube 4 'Steel thumbs of Lohan': A Buddhist meditation exercise holding a specific posture with thumbs pressed into the Kidney back-*shu* points (BL-23). 6.313×10^{-2} Hz is nearest to the Liver and Bladder meridian frequencies.

Tube 5 'Sound *qigong*': This was the sound *'Hu'* corresponding to the Spleen. However, this imprinted the Heart meridian frequency (in Table 9.4, this was for the '*Fu*' rather than the '*Hu*' sound). There was no response to 5.500×10^{-2} Hz from the oscillator (the nominal frequency of the Spleen meridian), but there was a response to an imprint copied from an actual Spleen meridian.

Tube 6 Mantra: This was a different *mantra* to that used in Table 9.2, hence the differing frequencies.

Tube 7 Bastrika: Heart meridian imprinted.

Tube 8 Anulom vilom: Heart meridian imprinted.

Tube 9 Kapalbhati: The frequencies 3.151×10^{-2} Hz and 6.413×10^{-1} Hz are not close to any meridian, 7.801×10^{0} Hz is the Heart meridian.

Tube 10 Brahmri: 6.227×10^{-2} Hz is near the Lymphatic meridian frequency, 6.902×10^{-1} Hz near that for the Fatty degeneration meridian, 7.801×10^{0} Hz is the Heart meridian frequency.

The depressive frequencies in Tubes 4, 6, 9, 10 might arise from intention-directed changes in Birinder's Pericardium meridian frequency. In Tubes 4, 6 and 9 only, the Heart meridian also had an acoustic resonance at the same frequency. This is characteristic of an imprint made from the Heart Chakra point. It can only be erased by exposure to the 1.42 GHz molecular hydrogen frequency.

All imprints in Table 9.6 contained 7.801 Hz. Tube 1 was held in Birinder's hand and succussed on wood to imprint his 'whole body field' as a control. This gave as is usual the normal value for the Heart meridian. (The actual resonance was between 7.801 040 Hz and 7.800 720 Hz, representing a highly coherent bandwidth of 41 p.p.m.) When these tubes were measured singly at 7.801 Hz using an oscillator connected to a toroid coil, each gave the same stimulatory response. Hence, one might assume that all tubes were identical in so far as 7.801 Hz was concerned and measuring them in pairs should make no difference to the result.

However, when they were excited in pairs with 7.801 Hz, some responded only to a toroid field, and others only to a caduceus field (see Fig. 9.2C). When placed in pairs next to a tube imprinted from a heart *chakra* at 7.801 Hz, all gave a stimulatory response. When placed in pairs in a caduceus coil, there was zero response in each case. Any four or eight of these 10 tubes measured together in a toroidal field also gave zero response. A possible conclusion is that one is dealing here with macroscopic quantum systems and must therefore expect to find such integer intervals.

The greatest distance over which any pair of tubes would interact was 6.4 meters, implying that this is the coherence length for ambient air. This would seem to be consistent with an entertaining YouTube demonstration of a *qi*-master in Beijing projecting his energy [24].

These results indicate that there is something more to *qi* projection than resonances between *qi* imprints and oscillator frequencies even though the latter are at least a measurable parameter.

THE ENVIRONMENT AND *QI*

To effect a potentization or imprinting there must be some boundary to the medium used. It is not possible to potentize sea or air in general. However, a sealed plastic bag containing ambient air can be potentized, although this does require the air to be humid. If some silica gel is put into the bag, no potentization is possible.

Accordingly, an experiment was carried out in which three tubes of water were set up in front of Birinder. The centre tube was inside a plastic bag containing sachets of silica gel as desiccant. *Qi* was directed towards them. The two outer tubes acquired an imprint of 7.801 Hz. The tube in the dry atmosphere received no imprint that could be stimulated *electrically*, implying that this projection and imprinting of *qi* requires air of normal humidity. However, it did acquire an acoustic resonance at 7.801 Hz.

CONCLUSION

The results in the above tables show that frequency is something that can be measured in respect of *qi* activity, thereby assigning numbers to it. Frequencies can be imprinted into water by *qi* projection, succussion or self-*qi*-treatment.

The stated intention of a particular *qi* procedure does not always result in the imprinting of a frequency as measured electrically corresponding to the endogenous frequency of the acupuncture meridian intended as the target. There is a clear difference between measurements comparing a frequency generated by an electrical oscillator and the same frequency copied from an actual acupuncture point. This may be due to differences in the field configurations or to some other field as yet unidentified. The comparison by dowsing techniques of pairs of tubes imprinted by different *qi* procedures with each other and against a set of tubes imprinted from acupuncture meridians should provide a useful measurement tool. The transmission of *qi* and the potentization of water vapor in a contained space warrants further investigation.

ACKNOWLEDGMENTS

Thanks are due to David Mayor for challenging me to write this chapter on *qi* and frequencies and for his encouragement and support during the process, and to Birinder Tember for his demonstrations of *qi* in practice and for providing me with something to measure.

Systems theory: tracking and mapping healing with *qi*

10

Christopher Low

CHAPTER CONTENTS

INTRODUCTION

The core theme of this chapter can be put as a direct question:

Is there a way of thinking about qi which will enable us to bridge the gaps between the measurable truths of modern biomedical science, the embodied experience of 'energy', and metaphysical description?

For the past three decades there has been expanding public awareness of the potential safety, economy and perceived therapeutic efficacy of healing practices that purport to generate, strengthen and regulate *qi*. Predictably, this interest has created a need to understand the bodily phenomena associated with *qi* and the reputed health benefits in concrete, rather than metaphysical, terms. From a Western perspective this means asking 'how' and 'why' *qi* has the effects on the mind and body that are claimed for it and observed and experienced by many.

Alongside this development there are growing doubts within both complementary and alternative medicine (CAM) and orthodox biomedicine in relation to the current over-reliance on the prevailing scientific model as an investigative paradigm for the appraisal of health and disease. Fundamental questions remain about the nature and quantification of phenomena occurring within the therapeutic dyad of practitioner and patient. Some of these phenomena are widespread and include nonspecific (placebo) effects [1,2], nonlocal healing [3,4] and the therapeutic agency itself. Importantly, the last of these can be viewed as a discrete property of the healing encounter, distinct from the matrix of pharmacological and physiological effects in which it may be embedded.

In concrete terms, how can *qi* simultaneously be described as, for example, a force with measurable magnetic properties [5] and also as a metaphor for mediation and interconnectedness [6,7], an intangible notion that is arguably bigger than the human mind can fully grasp? The phenomenon of *qi*, a Chinese term often loosely translated as 'energy', can be viewed from a dualist philosophical standpoint as the mediating principle between the polar opposites of *yin* and *yang*. In the human body this mediation is expressed as physiological process, structural change and substance generation (e.g. blood and body secretions). What is interesting about *qi* in relation to health and healing is that it does not presuppose a split between mind and body. In fact mind and body are seen as a 'whole', which leads to a worldview and a type of medicine that considers all bodily phenomena, including thinking and felt experience, as a continuum of denser or more rarefied aspects of *qi*. Moreover, *qi* may be considered as a metaphor with extended possibilities for linking image with bodily and mental processes. Given the Daoist origins of much Chinese medical philosophy, with its ancient roots in animism and the natural world, the concept of *qi* is clearly manifold and all-encompassing, and cannot simply be 'trimmed to fit' the requirements of modern scientific method.

DEFINITION OF INTERNAL AND EXTERNAL *QI*

One distinctive and remarkable feature of *qi* is that it can be experienced directly both within and outside the body (i.e. intrinsically and extrinsically). This property is at the core of extant health promotion practices such as *daoyin* (導引) healing, *qigong* (氣功) and later *taiji quan* (太極痊). For example, using certain simple techniques within Daoist health promotion practices it becomes possible for individuals to sense the *qi* of another person [8,9] in addition to observing and experiencing their own responses to the interaction within the dyad. When applied systematically for the purpose of health promotion, this cultivation of *qi* is known as *qigong* – literally '*qi* work'. The precursor and generic core of *qigong*, however, is the much older practice known as *daoyin*, meaning 'guiding and pulling [of *qi*]' [10–12] described below.

Internal *qigong* (Box 10.1) refers primarily to self-applied health promotion practices for the purpose of mobilizing, regulating, enhancing and transforming one's own *qi* [13]. Essentially, internal *qigong* utilizes internal aspects of *qi*. In practice, this refers to qualitatively different forms of *qi* following the *jingluo* (經絡) or meridian circulation, the *qi* associated with the 12 *zangfu* (臟腑) organs within the trunk, and the 'Three Treasures' (*san bao*, 三宝) or resources of *qi*, known individually as *jing* (Essence, 精), *zhen qi* (True *qi*, 真氣) and *shen* (Spirit, 神).

BOX 10.1 Practitioner experience of internal and external *qi* through the practice of internal and external *qigong*

Internal *qigong*
- Health promotion practices applied to oneself
- One person is affected by the process, i.e. 'self-healing' is considered to occur
- e.g. *qigong*, *taiji quan*, *xingi quan*, etc.

External *qigong*
- 'Therapy'/'healing' given to another person or group
- All participants are affected by the interaction, with the healer facilitating 'healing' in the others
- e.g. *daoyin* healing, external *qigong*, *buqi*, variants of acupressure using *daoyin* principles rather than physical pressure

---

In contrast, external *qigong* refers to the mobilization of an external *qi* field by the practitioner to effect healing in the environment (proximally or at some distance away) [8]. In this way, healing can be given either to a single recipient or to a whole group within what we could loosely call the 'healing space'. External *qigong* utilizes external aspects of *qi*, including the field that is apparently generated and transmitted from healer to patient. Although the situation is more complex in practice, because of other interaction effects, we can say that external *qigong* has a number of distinctive features irrespective of the specific skills of individual *qigong* masters or healers and their particular lineages (Box 10.1).

Within this basic division, there is a wide range of therapeutic modalities that utilize *qi*: from the ancient practice of *buqi* ('spreading qi', 布氣), to more recent practices such as *qigong* massage. Essentially these are hybrid forms of *qigong* where the 'healing space' is shared between practitioner and patient and both internal and external *qi* may be used. It must be emphasized that laying on of hands with actual physical contact is not strictly necessary for *qigong* healing. In fact, *qigong* with touch is a hybrid healing modality, and in itself sets up complex interactions within the therapeutic setting that research may find difficult to unravel.

Finally, artificial '*qi*' devices exist that have been designed to replicate an energy field, usually a correlate of *qi* (e.g. electromagnetic radiation) and probably not the 'real thing'. This is an ill-defined area of enquiry since the range of devices is varied and the potential research parameters ambiguous.

WHAT PART DOES INTENTION PLAY IN HEALING WITH *QI*?

Qi does not just 'sit there', but has to be generated, mobilized and given direction and form. In the Daoist healing and medical traditions, *qi* can effectively be 'made to happen' in three ways according to three different kinds of intention blended into one integrated act of volition. These three activities comprise the generic core of healing practices using *qi*:

- **Visualization:** Thought with specific imagery generates the *qi*.
- **Breathing:** Breath gives power to what has been imaged.
- **Form:** Sequencing of movement, together with specific bodily postures, moves, directs and issues the *qi*.

These three aspects of intention are known as mental, breathing and postural *daoyin* in Chinese therapeutics and together can be considered to represent the therapeutic agency within the various Chinese internal and external healing modalities. The concept of *daoyin* predates that of *qigong* by at least 1500 years [10], and can therefore be considered a precursor of the healing and health-promoting modalities developed in China since ancient times.

Daoyin, the '*way of quiding and pulling*', was originally applied to health promotion practices designed to stimulate and regulate the flow of *qi* throughout the *jingluo* or meridian system – a Daoist medical concept which was well established by the Western Han Dynasty (c. 200 BCE). Deeply embedded in the Chinese medicine tradition for millennia [10–12], *daoyin* is considered a significant and innocuous health promotion practice in its own right. Moreover, *daoyin* is still considered an important part of Chinese medicine in the present day [8].

EXPERIENCING *QI*

Arguably the two most distinctive properties of *qi* in the healing context are the fact that it can be *felt* and also that it *moves*. In other words, *qi* has an impact on both consciousness and the physiological dynamics of the body.

With the latter, interactions may be experienced in many individuals as a 'felt sense' that can vary in intensity from the extremely subtle to strong physical sensations [14]. Such responses to *qi* can include involuntary movements and tingling of the body, limbs and extremities, for example. Other sensations may be subtler and include perceptions of light inside the body, increased sensitivity to and appreciation of sound, a feeling of lightness and shifts in perceptions of body image.

NEW RESEARCH PERSPECTIVES

The last four decades have seen the development of chaos theory and the emergence of the new science of complexity. In the fields of physiology and therapeutics, for example, it may be possible to describe the structural and functional organization of the body – indeed health itself – in terms of a complex system with definable properties [15–18]. In recent years it has become possible, using computer software, to map fluctuations in robust markers such as heart beat intervals over extended periods of time. Far from being arbitrary, this dynamic behavior can be shown to contain hidden rhythmic order embedded within it. For example, different research groups have established that the rhythmic order of heart rate degrades to a more random condition in certain heart pathologies such as angina and congestive heart disease [17,19] and also, importantly, with healthy aging [20,21]. These findings suggest that complex rhythms are vital in maintaining the plasticity of our adaptive responses. This development has the potential to bring new insights to current perceptions of *qi*.

Here data are presented from recent original research [22] that appears to demonstrate that *qi* may itself be the therapeutic agency effecting cure. In this study, non-contact *daoyin* healing was adopted to investigate the aspects of qi outlined above (i.e. mental, postural and breath *daoyin*). These three approaches can be blended by the practitioner in many different ways – so making *daoyin* healing a useful model for researching *qi*. Using this approach, and new complexity measures for analyzing heart rate variability, this research reveals exciting new possibilities for mapping subtle physiological impacts, for example tracking the impacts of *qi* on the neuroregulation of heart beats during, and following, a healing session with *daoyin* healing using data from the electrocardiograms (ECGs) of both practitioner and recipient.

The fractal measure known as 'Alpha' can now be used to quantify the persistent patterns, or time structures, embedded in long sequences of heart beat intervals. As a robust measure, Alpha (generally split into Alpha-1 and Alpha-2) has been shown [20,23,24] to characterize the 'landscape' of complex heart beat fluctuations (heart rate variability, HRV) in a meaningful way by quantifying its 'ruggedness' (for these and other technical terms see the Glossary). Alpha-1 and Alpha-2 can be understood to represent the short- and long-term 'memory', respectively, of the neural networks that regulate the heart rate when the body is at rest. These correlations break down to a more random pattern in certain diseases and in healthy aging [25,26], leading to the suggestion that such quantitative measures of rhythm fluctuation might be useful in predicting certain disease states [27,28]. Figure 10.1 shows, for example, how HRV changes with healthy aging. Both traces exhibit a property known as self-similarity, but it is clear that complexity of variation is lost in the lower graph.

The question arises whether this ordering and pattern of heart beat intervals is sensitive to the emergence of *qi* in the 'healing space' and could consequently be used to track and map the healing process. (See also Ch. 24.)

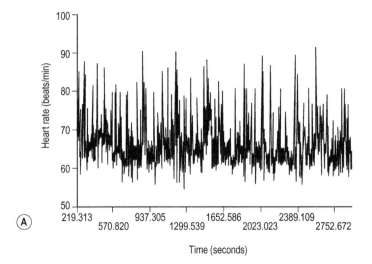

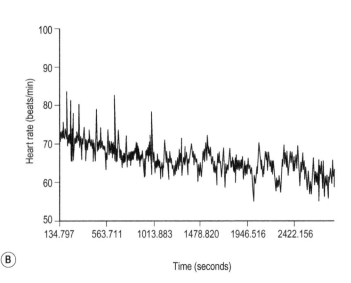

FIG 10.1 Two graphs of heart rate variability, in a young and an elderly person, showing loss of complexity with normal aging: (A) Male, 22.5 years; (B) female, 80.6 years.

EXPLORING THE CHAOS CONNECTION TO *QI*

A randomized baseline and placebo-controlled study was conducted to investigate the behavior of external *qi* reputed to be associated with *daoyin*. A total of 27 individuals ranging in age from 22 to 81 years were screened, of whom 25 met the entry criteria and were recruited. Participants attended for three sessions within 8 days. Continuous ECG recordings were collected for 45 minutes throughout each of the three sessions: baseline (BL), an intervention session – split into a mid-portion where *daoyin* and sham interventions of 5 minutes each were given in a randomized order – and a final 24-hour follow-up (FU) (Table 10.1). In each session the ECG recording was divided up into three equal time blocks for analysis, so that they could be compared. The raw ECG signal was delivered via a bipolar lead,

Table 10.1 *Experimental design of daoyin study: intervention session (2nd visit)*				
Pre-Intervention	**Intervention**			**Post-Intervention**
15 min.	5 min.	[5 min.]	5 min.	15 min.

Session lasted 45 minutes divided into three 15-minute segments – intervention, pre- and post-intervention. The middle segment consisted of two 5-minute interventions (*daoyin* and sham, in randomized order), separated by a 5-minute interval. Baseline and follow-up sessions (i.e. first and third visits) also lasted 45 minutes, the 'intervention' segment being replaced with a clear 15-minute interval.

recording RR inter-beat intervals in normal sinus rhythm from participants lying flat and in a relaxed wakeful state throughout the collection period (the 'R' wave is the most prominent feature of the normal ECG). Baseline recordings were made 1–7 days before the intervention session in all cases. Entry to the intervention session was conditional upon there being a normal ECG at baseline. Follow-up recordings were collected 24 hours after the intervention session. *Daoyin* and sham interventions were single blinded with a block randomized AB design [29], the ordering of interventions being independently assigned by a statistician. The assigned *daoyin* and sham interventions were performed in the middle 15-minute segment of the intervention session and were separated by an interval of 5 minutes (Table. 10.1). All ECG data collected were checked and analyzed by an independent observer to internationally accepted standards [30] before the heart beat data were analyzed statistically.

Interventions were performed for exactly 5 minutes by the researcher standing at a distance of 2 meters from the subject. Subjects lay supine on a treatment couch without physical contact with the researcher throughout. The researcher adopted a simple standing *daoyin* posture combined with horizontal hand movements, with arms parallel and extended forward and approximately 30 cycles of movement during the intervention. The 'sham' movements outwardly appeared identical but differed in that they lacked focused mental activity or attention to breathing by the researcher.

RESULTS OF STUDY WITH *DAOYIN* HEALING

Heart rate and fluctuation measures from baseline, intervention and follow-up sessions were obtained from 24 participants. Results revealed no significant differences in mean RR interval between first and last 15-minute segments of the baseline and follow-up sessions, whereas for the intervention session the mean RR interval varied slightly between study phases. The bar chart in Figure 10.2 shows how heart beat intervals changed during the Intervention. The 'Active' bar shows that, on average, intervals increased in the middle 15-minute portion of the session. As this segment contained the two 5-minute intervention periods, this result indicated the combined effect of the randomized interventions. The increased interval translates as a reduction in heart rate – a response normally associated with relaxation. This effect has also been broken down into separate bars for the *daoyin* and sham interventions. Interestingly, there was no significant difference between these, suggesting that, in this experiment, the presence of the practitioner was more important than the interventions themselves!

Whereas conventional linear measures, such as 'mean RR interval', inadequately describe HRV, nonlinear fractal analysis is able to reveal additional information embedded within the ECG, including changes in the subtle rhythmic order of heart beats as a consequence of the interventions described above. The fractal

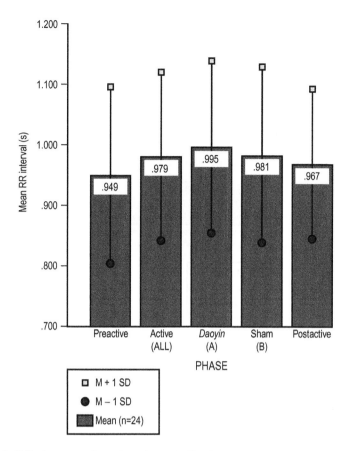

FIG 10.2 Shifts in average heart beat intervals ['RR intervals'] during different phases of the intervention session with *daoyin* and sham healing (*n* = 24). M = mean; SD = standard deviation. The difference between the preactive and *daoyin* phases was highly significant ($P < 0.001$), as was the difference between the preactive and sham phases ($P = 0.005$) and between the preactive and entire active phases ($P = 0.001$) containing 15 minutes of data, *including* both interventions. Differences between preactive and postactive phases and between *daoyin* and sham interventions were, however, not significant.

measures Alpha-1 and Alpha-2 for each of the study phases in the intervention session are shown in Figure 10.3A and B. Variation of these measures for the whole sample across the study phases is clearly apparent, with significant differences in Alpha-1 between the preactive and *daoyin* phases ($P = 0.050$) as well as between the preactive and postactive phases ($P = 0.011$). In contrast, there were no significant differences between the preactive phase and other study phases for Alpha-2.

The behavior of continuous series of heart beat fluctuations may be visualized for single subjects, using data from complete sessions. Plotting beat-to-beat behavior of the heart beat shows up distinctive fractal attractors for discrete time periods during the intervention session (Fig. 10.4). The salient feature of these attractors appears to be their ability to map the emergence of a more even distribution of points in the 'swarm' by the postactive phase compared with marked differences between the clustering evident in previous phases. The clinical utility and esthetic appeal of this method are compelling, and could greatly assist in making holistic appraisals of the transition states and subtle interactions that appear to be involved in the healing process.

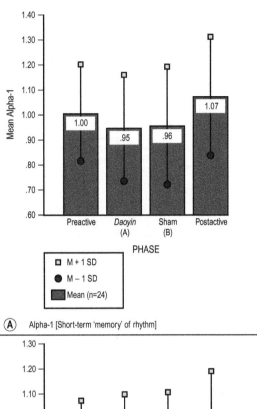

(A) Alpha-1 [Short-term 'memory' of rhythm]

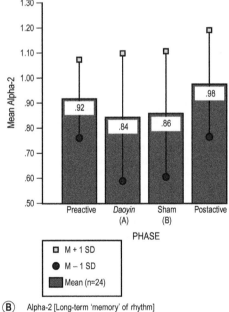

(B) Alpha-2 [Long-term 'memory' of rhythm]

FIG 10.3 Shifts in rhythmic order during different phases of the intervention session with *daoyin* and sham healing. An Alpha value of 1.0 indicates the presence of persistent fractal patterns associated with a dynamic and healthy physiological state. M = mean; SD = standard deviation. **(A)** Short-term 'memory'. There were significant differences in Alpha-1 between the preactive and *daoyin* phases ($P = 0.050$) as well as between the preactive and postactive phases ($P = 0.011$). **(B)** Long-term 'memory'. Both *daoyin* and sham phases were significantly different with respect to the postactive phase ($P = 0.018$ and 0.036, respectively). Note that, whilst the Alpha values fell during both interventions, the final Alpha value in the postactive phase is increased with respect to the preactive phase; this is associated with a more dynamic fractal pattern in the heart beat variation.

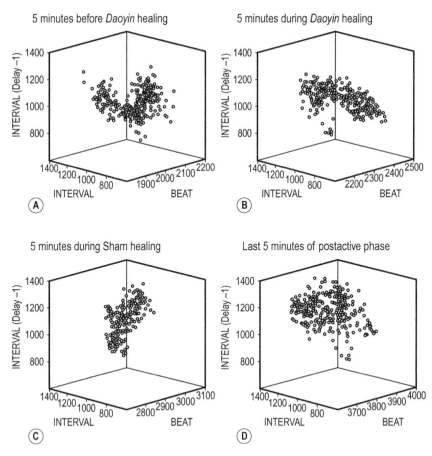

FIG 10.4 Three-dimensional phase space plots indicating behavior of heart beat fluctuations during discrete 5-minute phases of external *qi* healing (*daoyin* before sham) in a single study participant. 'Swarms' of points, or fractal attractors, are realised by plotting how each RR interval in the series [INTERVAL] varies over time [BEAT] in relation to the interval that precedes it [INTERVAL (Delay -1)]. (A) Preactive – 5 minutes immediately prior to *daoyin* intervention; (B) 5 minutes during *daoyin* intervention; (C) 5 minutes during sham intervention; (D) last 5 minutes of postactive phase. *Note:* There was a 5-minute pause between the *daoyin* and sham interventions (see Table 10.1).

This study therefore provides new information about the effects of subtle therapeutic impacts on the complex neuroautonomic output that regulates normal cardiac rhythm in healthy individuals. Both interventions appear to produce physiological impacts on the rhythmic patterns of heart beat fluctuations embedded in the ECG, since these were detectable during both *daoyin* and sham phases. Moreover, these investigations showed that neither the time domain measure (the RR interval) nor the fractal measures (Alpha-1 and Alpha-2) could detect any meaningful differences between the *daoyin* and sham interventions. This interesting finding suggests that, within the therapeutic dyad, the researcher's proximity and presence during both interventions produced a measurable effect, whereas purported healing effects attributable to *daoyin* did not.

COMPLEXITY, CHAOS AND *QI*

The study above sought to map one of the key outputs of a complex system – the patient–practitioner dyad – during the application of a non-contact form of *daoyin* healing. Are we justified in ascribing therapeutic agency to this procedure? Observed changes in the linear RR measure in the present study suggested that the effects of both *daoyin* and sham interventions were transient and confined at most to the active phase itself. However, the nonlinear response, according to the Alpha-1 and Alpha-2 measures, appeared to be indicative of a more persistent effect. This impact could now be characterized in terms of altered correlation properties, the correlations reflecting changes in the self-organizing character of the heart beat fluctuations. This presents us with the counterintuitive notion that a healing intervention can evoke, for the duration of the procedure, a temporary degradation to a more chaotic state of the self-organizing behavior of the neural networks regulating the heart rhythm. Moreover, after this shift there appears to be a reinstatement to a more ordered condition than existed previously.

We have associated *qi* with altering physiological functions in potentially profound ways. In the new science of complexity such impacts on the whole organism are interpretable as shifts in self-organization, which can include abrupt, apparently unpredictable, *nonlinear* behavior indicative of transitions from order to chaos and vice versa. As we have seen, these insights have brought about new ways of tracking and mapping processes that remain 'hidden' to conventional, *linear* methods of analysis. Indeed, 'subtle energy' may be considered as an aspect of self-organizing behavior arising out of the complexity of the living state. For several decades theoretical biologists [31,32], through observations on the processes of evolution and change in living organisms, have referred to this property as autopoiesis – literally 'self-creation' – and the implications have been extensively studied on a cellular level. Might this also be an aspect of *qi*? This idea, together with the physiological adaptive responses and both ancient and modern ideas of connectedness (i.e. Daoist philosophy and systems theory), yields a holistic paradigm that is based on broader biological themes rather than narrower medical ones. Such a perspective offers the potential of bringing deeper insights into the purpose and mechanisms of self-healing, itself a key component of health restoration and health maintenance.

Taking all of the above into consideration, there are several features that appear to characterize the healing 'encounter':

1. The independence of the recipient's system is challenged by healing.
2. A paradox arises: the healer provides the recipient with another system, making possible a combined field of interaction and an extended range of responses, putting both participants in a position of *inter*dependence during the initial exchange ('meeting') phase of their therapeutic encounter.
3. In this encounter an exchange of information occurs that can have physiological potency. The subtle physiological impacts that arise can be detected, tracked and mapped as witness to this process.
4. Within this encounter the recipient 'cherry picks' information created by the combined information field generated by healer and recipient. This new input empowers the recipient to recreate a newly independent state.
5. Healing, through this relationship of encounter and information exchange, therefore eventually creates or reinstates a condition of wholeness, wellbeing and health on all levels.

This presents us with the unusual insight of 'subtle energy as information exchange' (see Ch. 12), which is suggestive of a pragmatic systemic response on the part of the body to ensure optimum creativity and, ultimately, survival of the individual.

However, clinical experience demonstrates such a 'healing space' is far more complex, and often conditions are far from ideal. For example, we could envisage the above scenario in the physiological domain, affecting the somatic level. What is less clear is the impact on mental, intuitive and spiritual levels of being. For example, which, and how much, of these aspects of consciousness are shared – either with the healer in the therapeutic dyad, or collectively? Another factor concerns the operation of the therapeutic agency as a discrete aspect of healing and the extremely wide spectrum of treatment modalities that may be associated with it. By its very nature, this agency will contribute more to the subtler treatment modalities, particularly those involving no physical contact. Moreover, 'misreading' real events occurring within the healing encounter could account for them being labeled as the 'nonspecific' effects frequently associated with a treatment modality. This circumstance could also help explain why subtle treatment interventions relating to *qi*, such as *daoyin* healing, *qigong* massage and *buqi*, may perhaps be equated with nonspecific effects in a dismissive way that belies their intrinsic therapeutic potency.

COMPLEXITY, CHAOS AND HEALTH

In the prevailing worldview, core assumptions are made in therapeutics about the 'way we are made' and about our relations to the external world which mitigate against a holistic approach to problem solving. The new perspectives brought by chaos and complexity theory to the life sciences, in particular, have already delivered insights into previously inaccessible areas of scientific enquiry. For example:

- There are ubiquitous aspects of complex nonlinear processes that occur throughout the natural world. As an instance, a power law relationship appears to exist between the size of naturally occurring forest fires and their frequency [33].
- These processes are seen to occur on all scales of magnitude [18,34].
- This ubiquity and scale invariance suggests that simple rules underlie complex biological systems. For example, quarter-power scaling may predict the essential features of transport systems, from blood vessels and bronchial trees in mammals to plant vascular systems [35] The Fibonacci number series and the 'golden mean' explain the embodied proportion and structural organization in many living things, from the human body to sunflowers, and are another well-known example.
- Simple rules provide explanations of transitional states from order to chaos and vice versa, such as bifurcations – abrupt shifts in behavior which bear no linear relationship to the parameters governing the complex system where they occur [36–38].
- There is a concept of criticality ('the edge of chaos') in complex systems operating far from equilibrium [16,34,39].
- Dynamic far-from-equilibrium behavior appears to be the norm rather than the exception in the complex living system [40–42].

Implicit in these notions of agency, potency, chaos and order are many and diverse possibilities for health and healing. Treatment interventions of one kind or another will have varying degrees of success assisting in the restoration, maintenance and promotion of health in the event of injury or disease. If this process is basically helping the body help itself (self-healing), then it is clear that a *subtle* intervention is just as likely to be effective as a *radical* one – a common principle in many holistic practices of CAM.

Clearly a means of detecting, observing and mapping the 'agency' that enables the body to restore, maintain and promote health would assist in understanding ambiguities inherent in the therapeutic encounter. Moreover, orthodox medicine is effectively in the same position as CAM when it comes to characterizing and quantifying therapeutic potency in terms of a more protean health-promoting impact on the body as distinct from pharmacological effects, which tend to be described in terms of linearly deterministic processes.

In the science of complexity the healthy state can be seen as a dynamic interplay between form and function, with each part of the organism capable of relating to and influencing the whole, mediated in turn by the form, function and constituents of its component cells. Within this maelstrom of activity, it has become possible to delineate the ubiquitous mathematical 'design principles' upon which the structural and functional integrity of the human body depend. For instance, West et al have derived a general model describing how essential materials are transported through space-filling networks of branching tubes [35]. This work was significant for two reasons. First, it appears to indicate that allometric scaling relations are ubiquitous among organisms. Second, the model predicts the structural and functional properties of vertebrate cardiovascular and respiratory systems and other distribution networks. Both findings were found to rest on fractal properties of structural and functional elements. Of particular interest is the fact that the fractal concept also applies to the functional domain. For example, a fractal process may yield an output signal with a complex time structure that is neither periodic nor random, but with the property of scale invariance or self-similarity. These ideas are important in as much as fractal structure and function seem to characterize the healthy living state on different scales of magnitude. A subsequent study by West's group [18] asserts that these fractal-like networks endow life with an additional fourth spatial dimension that appears to apply to all organisms and is independent of the detailed processes expressed conventionally in linear reductionist terms.

CONCLUSION

The concept of *qi* as something both tangible and intangible – that is, at one and the same time actual, subtle and metaphorical – contributes to its potential as a therapeutic phenomenon with considerable explanatory power. *Daoyin* and the healing modalities derived from it have survived through millennia and appear to confer therapeutic benefits. These facts suggest that within the Daoist healing and medical traditions a successful synthesis of human talents and faculties could be employed to understand human health, in addition to the application of problem-solving strategies when health has failed. This corresponding union of left and right brain activity, of systematic thought with mindfulness and feeling, is arguably the greatest legacy of Daoist healing in modern times, yet presents researchers with considerable methodological difficulties. As these challenges are understood and overcome, a discourse about *qi* within the therapeutic domain appears to be converging around several key themes, notably: mind–body interaction, the role of *qi* as a factor in health restoration and health maintenance, the therapeutic mechanisms of so-called 'nonspecific' (placebo) effects, and nonlocal interactions in space and time attributable to a '*qi* field'.

Qi can therefore be seen as a linking phenomenon in an interconnected view of both the body and its environment, and can help explain many of the phenomena seen in therapeutics and within patient–practitioner relationships. This connectivity can take several forms. For example, the use of *qi* as a metaphor is linked with its imaginal components and they themselves may be capable of creating nonlocal, affective responses and sensations [43–45] when practitioner and recipient

10

are separated by considerable distances. Similarly, a 'felt sense', experienced both inside and beyond the physical envelope of the body, provides a more tangible manifestation of *qi*.

Qi transcends boundaries, not just in mind and body, but in the transpersonal domain as well. Hence, in contrast with modern biomedicine with its overpowering emphasis on symptom control and physiological manipulation, the *qi* healing modalities described above appear to offer a broader range of therapeutic possibilities. Their manifold effects are consistent with a systems-oriented view of the body that is open to fluctuations in the body's internal and external environments. From these, the body can orchestrate a healing response – sometimes in spite of the effects of constraint-oriented forms of concurrent therapy such as medication.

This chapter has presented a new approach to the quantitative study of therapeutic agency as distinct from the specific active components of the treatment accompanying it. A method is described for the mapping of subtle therapeutic impacts to quantifiable changes in the fractal variation of heart beat intervals using a non-contact healing variant of *daoyin* as an experimental model. The results from this study appear to show that resting heart beat rhythms are a sensitive yet robust tool for mapping real-world encounters between practitioners and their patients. These results suggest further research possibilities:

1. The variant of *daoyin* healing employed, being independent of verbal and physical contact, could provide an effective and holistic model with which to demonstrate and characterize therapeutic agency as a discrete phenomenon that has clinical value in its own right.
2. Opportunities may be created for observing the genesis, physiological impact and importance of therapeutic agency within the patient–practitioner relationship. The present study delineates a method that may be adapted for either single (patient) or concurrent (patient and practitioner) ECG recordings, and so may be helpful in this regard.
3. The availability and clinical utility of previously 'hidden' information derived from normal resting ECGs could be extended to the fields of complementary medicine and health promotion, outside the current focus on such ECG data as a diagnostic and prognostic indicator in heart disease and aging.
4. Insights of systems theory, in particular those from the new science of complexity, could enable more effective combinations of allopathic and holistic systems of therapeutics for integrative medicine.

There are clearly many possible interpretations of the findings of this study. Arguably, the most interesting conjecture concerns the existence of nonlocalized physiology as a new generic category of human function, with potentials for biological control, health maintenance and therapeutic interactions not confined within the envelope of the human body.

side running titleSystems theory: tracking and mapping healing with *qi*

page number139

The physiology of *qi*

Hakima Amri • Mones S Abu-Asab

> **“** *Respiration is a slow combustion of carbon and hydrogen, similar in every way to that which takes place in a lamp or lighted candle and, in that respect, breathing animals are active combustible bodies that are burning....*
>
> Antoine-Laurent de Lavoisier 1790 [1]

INTRODUCTION: THE UNDERSTANDINGS OF *QI*

There is a lot of mystery surrounding the nature of *qi* (氣) and its connection to the energy of living organisms. This confusion is reflected in the many meanings and contexts of *qi* that have been written over hundreds of years. Partially responsible for this is the focus of Chinese medicine (CM) on function rather than anatomical models; this has left room for a wide interpretation of *qi*. Some define *qi* as the spirit or breath that gives life to living creatures, the air, or the material filling the universe; it may also denote the basic building blocks of all life forms [2]. *Qi* is associated with wind (*feng*, 風) in Chinese mythology [3], and there are a few modern cultural uses of the term [4]. So, how could a concept be that amorphous and poorly defined and still be useful in medicine? Could all these definitions be correct? After all, they are based on the experience and perception of thousands of people for hundreds of years (see Chs 1 and 3). If so, how are they connected? Is there a conceptual framework that can tie them together? And, what are the modern biological explanations that will make sense in both Western medicine and CM? In other words, is there a similar concept in Western medicine that is congruent with CM's *qi*?

Concepts within traditional medical systems (TMS) are mostly based on introspection, observation, induction and deduction, and rarely on experimental data. Besides *qi*, there are other major shared deductive concepts that make up the principles of TMS. For example, they share the concepts of 'elements' and 'temperaments', neither of which are based on atomic physics; the 'humors' too are not based on biochemical analysis of body fluids. However, these concepts form the theoretical frameworks that guided medical practices for thousands of years and helped explain biological and medical phenomena without the need for sophisticated equipment. As we are going to see later in this chapter, some of these concepts are plausible assessments and congruent with our current scientific paradigm.

The confusion over the nature of *qi* has not only been festering for a long time within CM and modern translations of CM; it is also pervasive in other TMS (see Chs 1–3). The literal meaning of *qi* is 'breath', which is exactly equivalent to 'spirit' in English. *Unani* medicine (the Greco-Arabic traditional medical system) has an identical concept/term to *qi* called *pneuma* [πνεύμα] and *rouh* [ح و ر], which also means spirit [5], and Ayurvedic medicine has *prana* [6]. So it appears that the concept of *qi* is universal, and whether these Old World systems arrived at it independently or copied it from one another is still an open question.

In this chapter, we will put forward our own understanding of *qi* by interpreting CM and other TMS within the conceptual framework of modern biology. Our aim here is to find the scientific basis and explanations that connect the *qi* concept with biological and medical sciences. To achieve this goal, we will draw on the similarities between *qi* and the fundamentals of modern biology. It is imperative to reconcile the concepts of CM and other TMS with our current medical knowledge and paradigms as long as their concepts are congruent with modern science. Failure to do so will keep TMS in the realm of voodoo medicine, and hinders the integration of TMS and allopathic medicine.

A BRIEF HISTORY OF *QI*

Although the initial pictograph of *qi* referred to heat waves rising from a hot surface, it later evolved to signify exhaled breath seen on a cold day, and remains to the present day associated with breath [4,7]. The ancient Chinese understood that *qi* is the basic ingredient of all things, including the universe, as well as metaphysical concepts [8]. However, the dominant version is that *qi* is the vital air in the atmosphere, which is essential to sustain life, assimilate nutrients and produce the sound of the voice (as noted in *The Six Junctures and Manifestation of the Viscera*, Chapter 9 of the *Neijing Suwen*), and that the quality of air can be diminished by polluting elements [4].

There are a few salient features of *qi* in Chinese medicine [7]; among these is that *qi* is naturally associated with air and wind. *Qi* is the very source of life entering the human body through breathing and circulates throughout the body. Furthermore, it is responsible for the functioning of organs, its imbalance causing malfunctioning of organs and disease. Medical treatment therefore usually aims to get rid of stagnant *qi* or to strengthen normal *qi*.

Culturally nowadays *qi* refers to air in different contexts – even that within tires; however, it may also refer to the overall metabolic health and vitality of a person, or of the body organs [4].

QI IN HEALTH AND DISEASE

Despite having different meanings, the term *qi* is invoked in a healthcare context by many CM practitioners. Whether it has culturally evolved to have a number of different meanings is irrelevant to the practitioner, since *qi* can have different meanings for different practitioners and remains useful for medical purposes through the techniques that can influence it. The consensus is that, for a human body and all of its organs to remain healthy, a stable level of *qi* is needed throughout the body and its organs; any disruption of the *qi* supply or its distribution will cause first a temporary illness that may turn into a degenerative and chronic disease if it persists for a long time.

Most clinical applications in TMS center on manipulating *qi* to its optimal levels within the body or a specific organ to end a pathological condition and to re-establish the healthy status. Manipulations can be done with one or a combination of modalities that include needle acupuncture, herbs, diet, massage (e.g. *tuina*, *shiatsu*) and breathing exercises (*qigong*). The last modality has external and internal forms; the external involves the use of the mind, the hands or a ritual object, without necessarily touching the body; the internal involves exercises by the individual aimed at balancing their own *qi* (e.g. *taiji quan*).

The Western notion of disease begins with the appearance of symptoms; however, pathogenesis begins much earlier, at the cellular level according to allopathic physicians. In all TMS, though, it is assumed that disease begins with a disruption in flow of energy, such as *qi*, through the body (e.g. in the meridian and body organ system of CM). Therefore, TMS treatments aim at restoring the flow of energy or *qi* to normal. Practitioners working on *qi* manipulation claim that such treatment can be effective against a wide spectrum of illnesses; these include allergies, hypertension, general weakness, chronic pain, cancer, insomnia, rheumatism, stress, etc.

MODERN UNDERSTANDING OF TRADITIONAL MEDICAL SYSTEMS

According to the World Health Organization (WHO) [9], TMS are the sum of the facts, skills and practices based on beliefs and experiences indigenous to respective cultures that are employed to maintain health as well as prevent, diagnose and treat physical and mental illness; however, the theories and modalities of TMS have not yet been reconciled with modern scientific knowledge. TMS are therefore pragmatically oriented paradigms that are less focused on understanding the mechanisms of action in modern scientific terms. Nevertheless, within the context of the global evolution of knowledge, the twenty-first century seems like the most appropriate time for TMS and the latest technological advancements to interact, and this may lead us into a new era of medical systems.

The biggest challenge that TMS face in our times is the academic and Western mainstream acceptance of their principles and practices. Although lack of scientific evidence for TMS modalities is often cited for marginalizing them, it is rather the conceptual misunderstandings of TMS that constitutes the main reason for holding back their integration within mainstream Western allopathic medicine. If a TMS modality works and patients benefit from it, then we should pursue and understand its mechanisms of action and connect the modality to modern medicine.

In China, CM is not only culturally accepted and practiced, but it is an important part of the mainstream medicine of the Chinese people as well. CM and allopathic medicine are practiced side by side in many Chinese hospitals. The persistence of CM in its native land and its spread to the West are attributed to its medical and cost effectiveness.

QI AND *LI*: THE CONCEPT AND THE PRINCIPLE

We are relying on the neo-Confucian synthesis in most of our CM concepts and their meanings to understand the reasoning behind *qi*. According to the great neo-Confucian philosopher Zhang Zai (1020–1077), human nature is the result of the interaction between primordial life and *qi* (air, breath) [10] – this idea is analogous to and totally compatible with our current evolutionary understanding that the interaction between primitive anaerobic life forms and oxygen was responsible for the appearance of the sophisticated eukaryotic forms of life that eventually gave rise to human species. Zhang's idea represents an evolutionary thinking that is akin to Darwin's theory of evolution, and the later synthesis of organic molecular evolution. Zhang went on to add that the effects of *qi* were controlled by the physical phenomena of *tian qi* (天氣) – the universal rules that *qi* follows. Accordingly, because *qi* shaped human nature, it was also responsible for the evolution of the human mind. Zhang's ideas mirrored similar ones in Greek and Arabo-Islamic philosophies and indicated that, given the limited molecular-based scientific knowledge of their times, the world philosophers of different cultures were able to put forth interesting hypotheses for the evolution of life on earth. The ultimate goal of the neo-Confucian philosophers was to show that natural principles apply to both human beings and the universe, that both can be connected together by the same principles and concepts, and that both have the same nature. Therefore, the neo-Confucian CM concepts such as *qi* and the elements were put forth as the connections between human and nature (i.e. the universe), and the principle (*li*, 理) to explain how these connections work [10].

In CM, from a neo-Confucian perspective, the *qi* has a complement – the *li* – and both operate in mutual dependence [8]. *Li*, like *qi*, is a term that has suffered modern misusage. The neo-Confucian school recognized that everything is made out of *qi* and *li* – where *li* is the pattern or principle that determines the nature of things and *qi* is the existence in different forms: rising and falling, moving and still, etc. *Li* can be thought of as the mold that holds the *qi* and gives it a function; in a modern sense, we can also think of *li* as the physical rules that govern energy production and distribution. There are metaphorical explanations of *li* in CM. For example, if *li* is a cup, then the *qi* is the water in the cup; the *qi* can be replaced many times, and the cup used over many times. However, CM interprets the different types of *li* (let us assume that *li* is an anatomical organ here) to be different manifestations of several types of *qi*; that is, it attributes the different functions of the body organs to different types of *qi*. It is similar to *Unani* medicine in this respect, where the specific function of an organ is attributed not to its unique cellular differentiation but rather to the type of *qi/pneuma/rouh*/spirit that it takes in from the air. This notion is incorrect in all TMS since we now know that there is only one type of *qi* (homologous to oxygen) and several types of *li* (the number of differentiated tissue types within the body). As you will see later in the chapter, this concept of *qi* and *li* will apply well to our physiological interpretation of *qi* within the modern scientific paradigm.

HEALTH AT THE CELLULAR LEVEL: THE *YIN* AND *YANG* OF ENERGY PRODUCTION

From the different types of energy that energy therapists claim to be using or affecting within the body, we need to clearly find out which energy therapies affect the processes of cellular energetics. Within the conventional biological paradigm, there is a well-resolved view of cellular metabolism especially its energetics. In this section we will briefly summarize the parts that are relevant to our understanding of *qi* and *li*.

According to the modern cellular theory, the cell is the unit of life and the functional unit of the body [11]. The human body is made up of billions of cells, the vast majority of which are differentiated into organs and specialize in specific functions. Only a tiny fraction of the cells, termed 'stem cells', are not fully differentiated but are located within the organs and give rise to the cells that will undergo a full differentiation [12].

The term 'differentiation' is important here, because it also defines the health state of the cell: a well-differentiated cell should be able to carry out the functions it is supposed to do, whereas a cell that undergoes a loss of some aspects of the differentiation process is an unhealthy cell. Loss of cellular differentiation may occur when the cell lacks sufficient energy to carry out its functions (Fig. 11.1). If the cell is able to regain its normal energy supply then it will recover from its temporary illness. However, a chronic and irreversible loss of energy could unravel the cellular differentiation and lead to a degenerative disease initiated within the organ. In cancer, mutations in the DNA accompanied by disruption of energy supply within affected cells may produce malignant tumors [13].

The main intracellular energy storage and carrier molecule is called adenosine triphosphate (ATP) [1]. All the intracellular metabolic processes require ATP including biosynthetic reactions, motility and cell division. It also produces the heat necessary to maintain homeostasis. The basic chemical structure of ATP is that of a nucleotide, similar to the basic building blocks of deoxyribonucleic acid (DNA) (Fig. 11.2) [14]. ATP is synthesized in the mitochondria from inorganic phosphate (symbol P_i and chemical formula PO_4^{3-}) and adenosine diphosphate (ADP) or adenosine monophosphate (AMP).

When ATP is used in a metabolic process it loses one phosphate group and is converted back to its precursors:

$$ATP \rightarrow ADP + P_i + energy$$

or:

$$ATP \rightarrow AMP + PP_i + energy$$

It is estimated that the human body turns over its own weight of ATP every day [15].

ATP is produced by cellular respiration, a process that starts in the cytoplasm of the cell and is completed in the mitochondria (the plural of 'mitochondrion'); these are tiny organelles where almost all energy is produced. There are between 300 and 400 mitochondria in each cell depending on the organ.

The physiology of qi

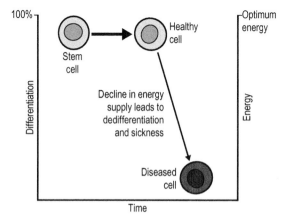

FIG 11.1 Relationship between energy supply and cellular differentiation. Optimal energy is needed for a fully functioning cell; a decline in energy supply will lead to dedifferentiation and sickness (© Mones Abu-Asab).

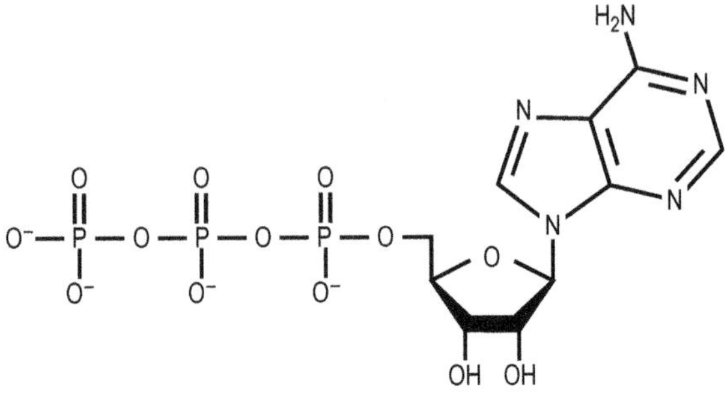

FIG 11.2 ATP structure.

Respiration is a multistage process that takes place within each cell of the body to produce the energy needed by the cell. There are three main stages of respiration: glycolysis, the Krebs cycle and oxidative phosphorylation. Glycolysis is the breakdown of glucose, a six-carbon molecule that is the basic building block of complex sugars like starch, to two three-carbon molecules called phosphoglycerate (PG). In a healthy cell PG is converted to pyruvate. Glycolysis can be simply summarized as follows:

one molecule of glucose → two of phosphoglycerate → two of pyruvate.

The next stages of cellular respiration take place inside the mitochondria. There, pyruvate is oxidized to acetyl-CoA (acetyl coenzyme A). This is the step that precedes the Krebs cycle (also called the citric acid cycle or tricarboxylic acid cycle), in which acetyl-CoA fuses with oxaloacetate to form citrate; then a series of oxidative reactions catalyzed by enzymes results in the release of carbon dioxide and a net release of water, as well as reduction of two other molecules, NAD (nicotinamide adenine dinucleotide) and ubiquinone (coenzyme Q), to be used later for ATP generation within the electron transport chain by a process termed 'oxidative phosphorylation' (Fig. 11.3) [14].

The importance of the Krebs cycle cannot be overemphasized. Besides being the engine of the energy production that is needed for cellular differentiation, recent published reports have implicated problems within the Krebs cycle, such as mutations of enzymes, in a large number of diseases including cancer as well as metabolic and storage disorders [13,16]. One defective enzyme leads to the accumulation of its substrate molecule and the destruction of the mitochondria, and in turn to the death of the cell or malignancy. Additionally, mitochondria can induce the death of the cell by a process termed 'programmed cell death' or apoptosis, an evolutionarily conserved mechanism in the vast majority of living organisms [17].

ATP is the universal currency of energy in all living organisms; they all need to produce ATP by oxidative phosphorylation. The process starts by transferring electrons from electron donor molecules to electron acceptors such as oxygen [14]. These donors and acceptors are protein complexes on the inner membrane of the mitochondria (Fig. 11.4). The energy release from such transfer of electrons is used to pump the hydrogen protons (H+) from the inner to the intermembrane space of the mitochondria (between the inner and outer membranes, see Fig. 11.4), thus creating a concentration potential across the membranes resulting in chemiosmosis. A large enzyme unit called ATP synthase utilizes the potential energy of chemiosmosis, and through allowing the

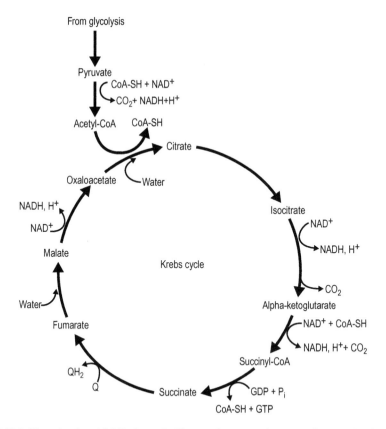

FIG 11.3 The mitochondrial Krebs cycle. The transformation of pyruvate (from the breakdown of glucose) to carbon dioxide, water, NADH.H$^+$ (reduced NAD) and QH$_2$ (reduced coenzyme Q). The last two products go through the electron transport chain to produce ATP. (GDP = guanosine diphosphate; GTP = guanosine triphosphate, another energy-storage and carrier molecule; P$_i$ = inorganic phosphate © Mones Abu-Asab).

hydrogen protons to return to the mitochondrial matrix (see Glossary) it produces ATP by adding one molecule of P$_i$ to ADP. Two of the returning protons unite with oxygen, which has already taken their electrons from the electron donors to form a molecule of water.

Oxidative phosphorylation is where the oxygen is utilized in energy production. Without oxygen the hydrogen protons will accumulate in the intermembrane space, and electrons will fill the electron transport chain leading to the degradation of the system [1]. This is the *yin* (陰) and *yang* (陽) of cellular energetics; a proper balance of the requisite supplies and well-functioning mitochondria are essential for the health of the cells and the whole body. Disorders within oxidative phosphorylation produce reactive oxygen species such as superoxide and hydrogen peroxide, which lead to propagation of free radicals that damage mitochondria and cells and contribute to disease and aging. Also the enzymes of oxidative phosphorylation are affected by many drugs and poisons that inhibit their activities [16].

Oxygen is the molecule that drives the respiration metabolism to its conclusion. The appearance of sufficient quantities of oxygen in the earth's atmosphere allowed the evolution of land organisms from their marine ancestors, and diversity

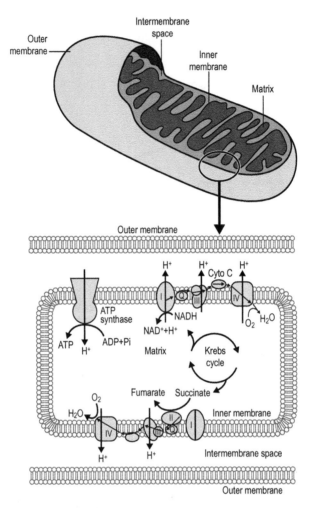

FIG 11.4 A whole mitochondrion (top) and a section through its outer and inner membranes (bottom). Components of the electron transport chain are located on the inner membrane where the process of oxidative phosphorylation (i.e. ATP production) takes place (© Mones Abu-Asab).

of life forms. In humans, the oxygen taken in by inhaling air diffuses into the lung tissue, and reaches the capillaries where it binds to the hemoglobin molecules packed into the red blood cells. Oxygenated blood travels to the heart where it is pumped to all body parts, diffuses out of capillaries and enters the cells to be used in oxidative phosphorylation.

A MODERN SYNTHESIS OF *QI* AND *LI*

The authors firmly think that TMS, based on lengthy accumulations of experience in health, pathology and healing as well as valid conceptual frameworks, represent a valuable body of knowledge that can and should be interpreted in the light of the current dominant biological paradigm. There are two factors that influence our approach to a modern synthesis of *qi*; one is to explore the homology of similar concepts to *qi* in other TMS and determine their conceptual congruence and their compatibility with modern interpretations, and the other is to match the *qi* concept to our modern knowledge of physiology. Correspondence between the two factors will strengthen our reasoning and interpretation.

Our experience in reinterpreting *Unani* medical concepts tells us that the process can be done [5]; however, one should not shy from pointing out conflicts and the invalidity of some ancient concepts when incompatibilities arise. For example, physicians and philosophers of TMS did not recognize tissue differentiation as a criterion that is responsible for organs' special functions; rather they attributed organ specialization to the different types of spirits (*pneuma, rouh*) or *qi* that either entered the body from air or were generated by the heart – as in *Unani* for example. As we understand it now, there is only one type of spirit and *qi*, and that is oxygen [4,5].

The spirits (including *qi*) as they have been used by TMS, and also philosophically and culturally, blurred the difference between the energetics of the body and the theological and mystical spirits. However, if we are to reach meaningful explanations, we need to distinguish vernacular uses and interpretations from science-based understanding of TMS. The fact that oxygen was not known till the eighteenth century led many to assume that it was a mysterious vital force in the air that was necessary for life [18]; that was despite the attempts of some, like Avicenna hundreds of years before, to point out clearly that the 'spirits were purely physical objects' [19]. In a biological sense, the spirits are strictly physical and signify oxygen, tissue differentiation and cellular energetics [5].

Kuriyama [3] pointed out the striking similarity between the ancient concepts of *qi*, *pneuma* and *prana* among different TMS – Chinese, Greco-Arabic (*Unani*) and Indian – arguing that these three concepts are identical and share a similar timeline of conceptual evolution. Kendall [4, p 141] matched the *qi* energy concepts with our current knowledge of respiration physiology; he equated *qi* with oxygen and described respiration as the 'true or genuine function' (*zhenqi*, 真氣) that is responsible for energy production and all vital functions of the body. Kuriyama did not comment on the *Unani* concept of *ignis* that is always associated with *pneuma*; it signifies the heat or energy produced in the tissue. In a modern sense, *pneuma* and *ignis* are equivalent to blood oxygenation and mitochondria-generated heat and chemical energy as ATP.

Our novel analysis shows, in a biological context where *qi* and *li* are necessary to life, we have arrived at the understanding that the CM concept of *qi* is basically homologous to the element oxygen, and that the principle *li* fits within tissue differentiation and its cellular respiration, including mitochondrial function in the Krebs cycle and oxidative phosphorylation. Therefore, we propose that the *yin* and *yang* of respiration is an interplay between the *qi* (oxygen) as the *yang*, and glucose supply from mostly starch and sugary foods, and fat, as the *yin*; furthermore, the respiration apparatus of the cell is the *li* (Fig. 11.5).

The goal of all therapeutic intervention is to return the body or one of its organs to its usual healthy homeostatic condition, which includes primarily a narrow range of body temperature [20]. Humans are endothermic creatures maintaining a constant body temperature that is needed for the optimal function of their cellular metabolism. Respiration, through its three segments mentioned above, is the source of our energy and heat that maintains homeostasis and therefore a healthy status. Consequently, therapies of all types and forms have to preserve and enhance cellular respiration since it is the basis of a healthy body.

Therapies and interventions that affect mitochondrial respiration are numerous; these processes seem very vulnerable to a wide range of chemicals and appear to be the Achilles' heel in many pathologies, both acquired and inherited [16]. Thus, it is not surprising that many therapies may affect or claim to affect respiration and

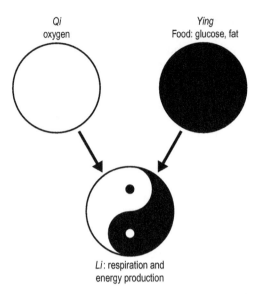

FIG 11.5 The yin and yang of cellular energy is an interplay between the supplies of two components: qi, or oxygen from air (yang) and ying, mainly glucose from starchy and sugary foods (yin). *(After Toshihiko Hanawa [7]).*

particularly ATP production. The health benefit of ginseng (*Panax ginseng*), a well-known *qi*-invigorating herb, is attributed to its positive effects on ATP production and its related compounds in the mitochondria [21]. Other purified and whole herbal products have been shown to affect cellular energetics. *Yang*-invigorating herbal extracts were found to enhance ATP generation, whereas *yin*-nourishing herbs did not or decreased it [20]. Cisplatin inhibition of adenosine triphosphatase (ATP-ase), the enzyme responsible for the release of energy from ATP, was alleviated by the Chinese herbal compound *jian pi yi qi li shui tang* (健脾益氣利水湯, decoction to strengthen the Spleen, benefit *qi* and regulate water) [22]. Others have measured ATP up-regulation due to the in vitro application of electric current in skin tissue [23].

As we have demonstrated here, our understanding of the *qi* concept and *li* principle can be elucidated and enhanced by coupling them with the current biological paradigm, and finding the homologies that bring out logical explanations of the principles and practices of TMS. However, at this stage the connections we have made are still partially hypothetical. They will become plausible only when basic and clinical research fully explains the molecular workings of the cell and verifies the modes of action of the modalities and treatments of TMS.

SECTION 4

QI AND ENERGY MODALITIES IN CONTEMPORARY PRACTICE

SECTION INTRODUCTION

This section explores different varieties of treatment predicated on an understanding that *qi* (or its equivalent) is somehow central to practice, and not merely a matter of philosophy or belief. The first chapter, by John A Ives and Wayne B Jonas, leading on from the preceding section on research, examines 'bioenergy' and describes both laboratory and clinical research that goes some way to support arguments for its existence. They follow this with a discussion of possible mechanisms giving rise to bioenergy effects, ranging from the 'biofield' hypothesis, through the thickets of the placebo effect, and back to possible quantum mechanisms. The next two chapters, by Claire M Cassidy and Tim Newman, are more about the *experience* of *qi* as something that *flows* and whose effects can be felt, not just something intangible or merely conceptual. Building on this experience, Gabriel Stux outlines the approach he has developed to combine different subtle modalities that emphasize the *awareness* of energy flow by both patient and practitioner.

This theme of awareness and self-development is interwoven by Patrizia Stefanini with an interpretation of the acupuncture (*shiatsu*) meridians in biophysical and macroquantum terms. Following this, Darren Starwynn explores the world of microcurrents (both within the body and applied), and how they are related to *qi* and affect it. He provides a clear account of some of the cost-effective microcurrent and microlight methods he has developed. Phil Mollon describes the methods of energy psychology, working with what he calls the 'mind–body information fields', which allow the practitioner to cross the Cartesian divide and work with both mind and body aspects of the whole person in a very practical and literally 'hands-on' way.

This section closes with Franklin Sills taking the reader on a journey through the many levels, fields, flows and tides of the hands-on approach to the life energy represented by craniosacral therapy, once again focusing on awareness of the interior world in the creation of the healing relationship.

Energy and medicine

John A Ives • Wayne B Jonas

CHAPTER CONTENTS

ENERGY MEDICINE AND BIOENERGY

Energy medicines – such as *qigong*, *reiki* and Therapeutic Touch – are thought to involve putative forms of energy. However, the 'energy' in so-called 'energy medicine' is not of the same nature as the electromagnetic energy of conventional science. First and foremost, it is not directly measurable. Secondly, it does not appear to fall off in power with distance (according to the inverse square law, for example). Finally, it is not blocked by barriers that block conventional energy. This distinction in 'energies' is important because often these two very different concepts are used interchangeably and confusion results. Yet both types of 'energy medicine' have been placed in this category by the US National Center for Complementary and Alternative Medicine (NCCAM).

Here we make a clear distinction between the two uses of the term 'energy', but summarize research primarily on what might be termed 'bioenergy'. Western allopathic medicine is skeptical about many aspects of energy medicine, mostly because it is based on philosophy, historical use and/or tradition but without much modern scientific empirical evidence. Lack of an accepted mechanistic explanation for the 'energy' (or energies) in energy medicine also presents a fairly large hurdle to acceptance. In general, it is thought to involve some kind of interaction between the *energy field* of the patient and the energy field or the *intention* of the healer. However, in addition to questions about the efficacy of energy medicine modalities, there have not been any unequivocal demonstrations that either known or heretofore unknown forms of energy are emitted by the healer or involved in the interaction between healer and patient. We will return to the idea of *intention* and interaction with forms of energy when we discuss the *quantum enigma*.

Although recent literature on forms of bioenergy (*qi*, *ki* or *prana*) and their biomedical application has significantly increased, the form of energy involved in energy medicine remains largely mysterious, and there is no universal agreement as to what it might be. Despite this, phrases such as 'subtle energy', '*qi* energy' or *prana* are often used. However, there are some recent attempts in the English language literature to characterize the energy [1], although these studies have not been replicated by other groups. To date, probably the most complete, criteria-based, systematic review of this area is a book by Jonas and Crawford [2]. Benor [3] has compiled an additional comprehensive survey.

In addition, over the past 30 years there has been considerable work done on measurement of external *qi* as physical energy. The majority of publications in this field are in Chinese and therefore not easily accessible to the Western scientific community. The few English language references dealing with bioenergy include a book by Lu [4]. A more complete review by Zha is included in the 2001 Proceedings of the Samueli Institute Meeting in Hawaii [5]. A thorough review of previous work on physical measurements of external *qi* is outside the scope of this chapter and the previous references are included as those most accessible, at least to readers in the US. It appears from these documents that previous experiments had neither been conducted in a rigorously controlled way nor utilized instruments that were current state of the art. At best the documented experiments reveal very low levels of physical energy associated with external *qi* emission by *qigong* practitioners/healers [6].

Finally, any putative bioenergy involved in energy medicine must be internally consistent and allow for consilience (unity of knowledge) with the known energies of accepted physics, chemistry and biology. An appropriate cybernetic or systems analytic approach consistent with conventional descriptions of electromagnetic energies but which also usefully describes bioenergy transfer is shown in Figure 12.1. This abstract model is based on the concepts of: (1) an information source, (2) a medium for carrying the signal and (3) some form of receiver. Here the underlying physical basis for transferring information is intentionally hidden in order to allow discussion of the transfer of bioinformation without deciding *a priori* what the physical mechanism is for that transfer to occur [6].

The input and output coupling in this model depends on properties of the source and the transfer medium, and likewise for the sink. 'Perception' is used, rather than simply 'reception', to imply an active process that uses some form of perceptual intelligence in processing the information based on its content.

We can define a bioenergy system as one that comprises:
- a source that generates energy and modulates it in some manner such that it conveys information
- a coupling mechanism connecting the bioenergy source to a transfer medium
- a transfer medium through which the bioenergy flows
- a coupling mechanism connecting the transfer medium to the bioenergy 'sink'
- a terminal sink that includes a mechanism for the perception of information.

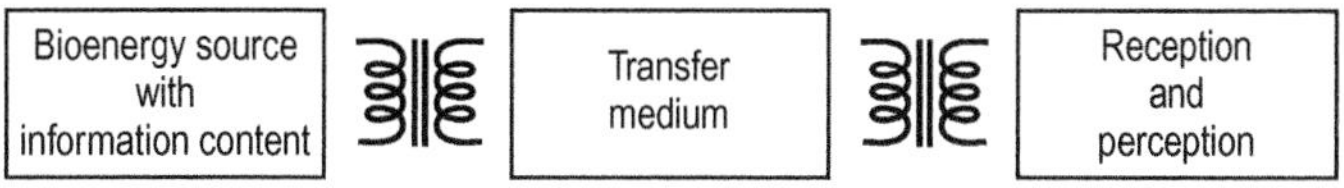

| Bioenergy source with information content | | Transfer medium | | Reception and perception |

FIG 12.1 Block diagram of bioenergy transport mechanism components.

The means by which information is transmitted and interacts with the system, in the sense that physicists understand it, is not clear. Feedback loops in biosystems are examples of information transfer. In most, if not all, cases the physical means by which the feedback is provided to the system is either understood or is assumed to involve interactions among actual physical objects. However, in the case of bioenergetic explanations of the placebo, for example, it is not always self-evident how the information is transmitted even though, *de facto*, it appears to be.

Thus, in studies on placebo, information alone is capable of significantly influencing a biological system and its response to pain. Similarly, although we have some understanding of the biological consequences of energy medicine [7], the means involved – the 'energy' – remains unknown. For example, *qigong* has been demonstrated to have antidepressive effects in patients but although the psychological mechanisms underlying these have been described their neurobiological mechanism remains unclear [8]. The same may be said of hypnosis where the clinical effects are now widely accepted (thanks in part to statistical profiling) but the neurobiological mechanism has remained unclear since the time of Mesmer, whose own understanding of his results in terms of a universal energetic *fluidum* was disparaged by the scientific community of his time [9] (see Ch. 22). Further research is clearly needed to elucidate the biology of energy medicine and consolidate its scientific base.

STANDARDS AND QUALITY IN ENERGY MEDICINE RESEARCH

Although it is facile to recommend that complementary and alternative medicine (CAM) be held to the same standards as conventional medical science, the complexity and intricacies of CAM, as reported in the US White House Commission on CAM, remain understated [10]. This is particularly true for energy medicine.

A search of the literature attests to the fact that studies are conducted in nearly all the CAM disciplines that lend themselves to the hypothesis-driven paradigm. Essentially, CAM scientific research follows the same standards used for conventional research (i.e. use of statistically significant number of subjects, specimens or replicates, introducing internal and experimental controls, defining response specificity and reproducibility). The last is perhaps the most challenging criterion. In several cases, experiments show positive results but when repeated, sometimes in the same laboratory, do not work despite rigorous attempts to maintain identical experimental conditions.

This challenge is illustrated in the work published by Yount and colleagues [11]. The group investigated the effect of 20 minutes of *qigong* on the healthy growth of cultured human brain cells. A rigorous experimental design of randomization, blinding and controls was followed. Although both a pilot study that included eight independent experiments and a formal study that included 28 independent experiments showed positive effects, the replication study of over 60 independent experiments showed no difference between the sham and treated cells (there are several possible explanations for this negative result). This study represents an excellent example of basic science research on energy medicine being held to the highest standard of experimental methodology.

However, this level of rigor is rarely achieved in energy laboratory research. For example, we reviewed the basic and clinical research in the area of distant mental influence on living systems (DMILS) and energy medicine. The quality of research was quite mixed: whereas a few simple research models met all quality criteria, such as in mental influence on random number generators or electrodermal activity, much basic research on DMILS, *qigong*, prayer and other techniques was poor [2]. In setting up these evaluations, we established some of the necessary criteria required for all such laboratory research [12,13].

In basic science research, formulating the testable hypothesis is sometimes not the major issue; it is setting up and testing the practice itself. In the example of Yount et al [11], who followed the most rigorous methodological and experimental designs, the practice under investigation was not a simple treatment with defined doses of a pharmaceutical compound or the antagonist of a specific receptor. Instead it was an unknown amount of energy of unknown characteristics emanating from the hands of a number of *qigong* practitioners, with variable skills.

Mind–body-based therapies are often not considered energy medicine, especially when applied to one's self, although they are for the purposes of this book. Thus, when the goal is to produce a change in an outside entity through meditation, for example, then we claim this is a form of energy medicine. As such, it is very challenging to explore in a laboratory setting. Although there are several studies showing the effects of meditation on cell growth [14], differentiation [15], water pH and temperature change, as well as on the development time of fruit fly larvae [16], we believe that in these studies the necessary level of methodological rigor has not been met. Independent replication has been especially problematic. In contrast, some CAM applications, such as dietary supplements, homeopathy and phytotherapy (herbs or herbal extract such as those used in Ayurveda or Chinese medicine) are relatively easy to translate to the laboratory setting. This is because such practices and their products of use are essentially similar in many respects to conventional interventions using pharmaceutical compounds, allowing dose and time-course experiments to be designed. However, most also involve individualized prescribing according to very specific principles, and if these are not followed correctly then poorly structured studies may give meaningless or falsely negative results, as in one on homeopathy for muscle soreness after long-distance running [17]. By contrast, a more methodologically sound trial of homeopathy for fibromyalgia generated positive results for this notoriously refractory condition. Interestingly, a subgroup of excellent responders was identified, not only by clinical response, but also by using a novel form of electroencephalography (EEG) screening (alpha concordance measurement) to identify likely positive responders to homeopathy [18]. We will return to homeopathy as a form of energy medicine later in this chapter.

THE EXAMPLE OF HEALING AT A DISTANCE

Let us now look at a set of studies that we performed to examine the effects of a healer employing distance healing on cells in culture. The healer explained that he uses intention to focus his mind and channel 'Divine love through his heart' to perform healing. This and similar energy medicine practices are often called 'distant healing' because the practitioners do not place their hands on the patient or subject. They believe that distance is not a factor in their healing although most, in fact, do their work within a foot or so of their patients. In this study the healer usually placed his hands within inches of the person on whom he was working. As an aside, he also performed diagnoses by positioning his hands near to but without touching the person. We will return to the issue of distance later in the description of our findings. His approach is typical of the so called 'laying on of hands' practiced in many cultures and accepted and associated traditionally with healing in Western medicine as well as the Judeo-Christian tradition

The explanation often given for any benefit seen from energy medicine of this kind is that it is due to a strong placebo effect resulting from belief and expectation generated during the encounter [19]. We intended to minimize this effect by using cells grown in laboratory culture. The healer came to our laboratories one morning each week throughout much of two sequential winters. We wanted to understand how he 'communicated' with cells in the laboratory and influenced them with his 'intention' in a positive and healthful way. The study would not involve diagnosis or even a human subject. Working with cultured cells in a laboratory setting we increased our power over the experimental and control parameters by comparing the effects of the healer to no treatment, sham treatments, and treatments using different doses, time periods and other various environmentally controlled conditions including the effects of expectation with blinding.

We asked the healer to alter the calcium flux in such a way as to increase the concentration of calcium ions inside the cells. We would measure any change in cellular calcium using a scintillation counter before and after the 'treatments'. A demonstration of significant effect would be powerful evidence that something, some form of energy presumably, flowed from the healer to the cells and changed their biochemistry in a targeted, intentional and specific way.

In our studies we used Jurkat cells, an immortalized line of T lymphocytes, derived from human immune system T cells. They were established as an immortalized line in the late 1970s and are available for purchase and easy to grow and maintain in the laboratory. They are a favorite choice for cellular immunobiologists interested in understanding cellular mechanisms of the immune system and have been used extensively to study mechanisms of action for HIV and anticancer agents.

The experimental setup was quite simple. Jurkat cells were grown in tissue culture dishes to near confluence, and on the day of the experiment the cells were suspended in a balanced salt solution, 'loaded' with calcium sensitive dye (fura-2) then placed inside a square cuvette. In the presence of calcium, the dye fluoresces and so the cells emitted light, the amount of which was proportional to the quantity of free calcium ions inside the cell. Measured spectrofluorometrically, this technique provides an accurate and objective measure of free calcium inside the cells.

The healer was asked to increase the internal concentration of calcium ions inside the cell. He told us that he would need 15 minutes of relative quiet while he placed his hands near the cuvette of cells and concentrated on his intention (Fig. 12.2). The experiments were repeated in six independent trials conducted on different days. Internal cellular calcium concentrations were significantly increased by 30% ± 5% ($P < 0.05$, Student t-test) compared with controls run in parallel. Varying the distance from the healer's hands to the cuvette between 3 and 30 inches (7 and 75 cm) did not seem to affect the outcome [20].

Three independent attempts were made by the healer to affect calcium concentration in this system from approximately 10 miles away. He tried first with internal visualization, then with a photograph of the cells to focus his attention and finally with a video camera displaying a 'live' version of the cells. None of these tests produced any noticeable change in the calcium concentration. Anecdotally, we ran a few noncontrolled tests in which his hands were kept behind his back rather than toward the cuvette of cells. This relative position seemed to interfere with his ability to affect calcium concentration. This was in spite of the fact that we documented a 'linger effect' in which cells placed on the table where he had focused his intention, but after he had left the laboratory, showed an increase in calcium concentration similar to the cells that had been directly subject to his

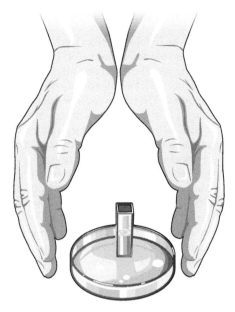

FIG 12.2 Use of non-contact bioenergy healing to increase the concentration of calcium ions in cells derived from the human immune system.

intention. This linger effect disappeared over time: fresh (untreated) cells placed on the table at intervals after he left still exhibited fluorescence, but fluorescence from cells placed there 24 hours later were no different than from controls.

Finally, we attempted to block the healer's 'energy' or intention by placing a grounded copper Faraday cage around the cuvette containing cells. Thus the healer, while still within 30 inches of the cells, had to keep his hands outside of the wire enclosure surrounding the cells. There was no significant difference in effect on the internal calcium concentration. It was still raised by the healer's 15-minute 'treatment'. This suggests that, whatever the energy is, it is not blocked by a Faraday cage in the way an electric field would be. (For other studies on non-contact 'energy' or *qi* transmission see Chs 9 and 10.)

THERAPEUTIC TOUCH, HEALING TOUCH AND ENERGY THERAPIES

Reiki, Healing Touch (HT), *qigong* and Therapeutic Touch (TT) are all 'energy therapies' that use gentle hand techniques that are thought to help repattern the patient's energy field and accelerate healing of the body, mind and spirit. They are all based on the belief that human beings are fields of energy that are in constant interaction with other fields of energy from others and the environment. The goal of energy therapies is to use the energetic interaction between the practitioner and the patient in a purposeful manner to restore harmony to the patient's energy system. Western allopathic approaches focus on diseases and their underlying mechanisms; cure is the be-all and end-all. In contrast, most energy therapies are based on a holistic philosophy placing the patient within the context of their life and an understanding of the dynamic interconnectedness with themselves and their environment [21]. They are about healing rather than cure [22].

The most common contemporary touch therapies used in US nursing practice are TT, HT and *reiki*. The first two were developed by nurses whereas *reiki* was developed in the 1920s in Japan and, although not targeted for nursing, is being used today by many in hospital settings [22–24]. Controversy has accompanied the use of these therapies even after their inclusion in the practice of the North American Nursing Diagnosis Association (NANDA). The controversy has not prevented their increasing popularity within the profession for the purposes of promoting health by reducing symptoms and ameliorating treatment side effects. Practitioners use TT and HT to improve health and healing by addressing a patient's 'Disturbed Energy Field: disruption in the flow of energy surrounding a person's being that results in a disharmony of the body, mind, and/or spirit' [25]. Like many other energy therapies, TT is designed not to treat specific diseases but instead to balance the energy field of the patient or, through a boosting of energy, improve the patient's energy. It was developed by Dolores Krieger, PhD, RN in the 1970s. She borrowed from and mixed together ancient shamanic traditions and techniques she learned from well-known healers of her time. Like acupuncture, *qigong* and *yoga*, HT is based upon the idea that illness and poor health represent an imbalance of the personal bioenergetic forces and fields that exist around and through an individual's body. Rebalancing (or boosting) these energies is done through a clear intention to support and harmonize the subject with his or her innate energy balance. These practices therefore typically begin with the practitioner performing some form of ritual that clears and focuses the intention to bring harmony and balance to the person who is in need (for further information see Ch. 22).

There has been sufficient research on TT published in peer-reviewed journals to perform a meta-analysis of the combined results from separate studies. Two meta-analyses have determined that there is a moderately positive effect on psychological and physiological variables hypothesized to be influenced by TT, primarily anxiety and pain [26,27]. A systematic review of the healing touch (TT or HT) research published in 2000 included 19 randomized controlled trials (RCTs) involving 1122 patients [28]. The authors found 11 studies (58%) that reported statistically significant treatment effects. Another systematic review of the literature on wound healing and TT found only four studies that met the authors' criteria for quality. Of these, two showed statistically significant effects while the other two found no effect from TT. The evidence is therefore insufficient to conclude that TT works for wound healing [29].

TT and HT seem to work well for anxiety, improving muscle relaxation, aiding in stress reduction, relaxation and a sense of wellbeing, promoting wound healing, and reducing pain. In addition, no serious side effects have been associated with these healing modalities [22]. One review of touch therapies looked at studies with outcomes such as pain, mood, anxiety, relaxation, functional status, health status, wellbeing, wound healing, blood pressure and immune function. The authors found the studies were of mixed quality, providing a variable degree of evidence in support of the effectiveness of touch therapies on these outcomes [30].

Reiki was originally intended as a self-practice, and today has become the most widely known of the hands-on energy therapies while perhaps the least substantiated, in part due to the apparent ease of training – typically attendance at a weekend workshop grants the practitioner Level 1 mastery. No graduate-level training or clinical experience is required, as it is not intended to be restricted to healthcare professionals [31]. However, it is often used by practitioners to help their clients enhance their wellness, to help cope with symptoms such as pain or fatigue, or to support their medical care, sometimes in the case of chronic illness or at the end of life. *Reiki* was developed in the 1920s by Mikao Usui in Japan as a spiritual practice (*reiki*, 霊気, may be translated as 'spiritual *ki*'). With Usui's help, one of his master students Chujiro Hayashi extracted the healing practices from the larger body of practices. Hayashi began to teach these practices and opened a clinic to treat patients. The practice itself is extremely passive. Practitioners lay their hands gently on the patient or hold them just above the patient's body without moving their hands except to place them over another area. The *reiki* practitioner does not attempt to adjust the patient's energy field or actively project energy into the patient's body. Also, unlike other forms of energy medicine but more like meditation, *reiki* does not involve an assessment of the patient's energy field or an active attempt to reorganize or adjust the patient's energy field. Instead *reiki* practitioners believe that healing energy arises from the practitioner's hand as a response to the patient's needs. It is in this way customized to the patient's needs and condition.

In one study, 23 *reiki*-naïve healthy volunteers participated in standardized 30-minute *reiki* sessions. They often reported experiencing a 'liminal state of awareness' characterized by novel and paradoxical sensations, which were often symbolic in nature. The experiences covered the gamut from disorientation in space and time to altered experience of self and the environment, as well as relationships with people, especially the *reiki* master. In another study, quantitative measures of anxiety and objective measures of systolic blood pressure and salivary IgA were altered significantly by the *reiki* experience; anxiety and systolic blood pressure were lowered while immunoglobulin A (IgA) was increased. Skin temperature, electromyographic readings and salivary cortisol were all lowered, but not significantly. Taken together it is apparent that in this study *reiki* induced states of lowered stress and anxiety and should be considered salutogenic in nature. The authors conclude that the liminal state and paradoxical experiences are related to the ritual and holistic nature of this healing practice [32]. A review of *reiki* research published in 2003 concluded that, as with TT, the most tightly controlled studies demonstrated subjective improvements rather than organic changes [33].

A 2008 Cochrane systematic review of touch therapies for pain relief included HT, TT and *reiki* [34]. The authors evaluated the effectiveness of these therapies for relieving both acute and chronic pain. They also looked for any adverse effects from these therapies. RCTs and controlled clinical trials (CCTs) for treatment of pain that included a sham placebo or 'no treatment' control arm met the criteria for inclusion. Twenty-four studies (16 TT, 5 HT and 3 *reiki* studies) were found that met these criteria. A small but significant average effect on pain relief was seen (0.83 units on a scale of 0 to 10). The greatest effect was seen in the *reiki* studies and appeared to involve the more experienced practitioners but the authors concluded that the data were inconclusive as to which is more important, experience or the modality of therapy. In spite of the paucity of studies, the authors concluded that the evidence supports the use of touch therapies for pain relief. These therapies also decreased use of analgesics in two studies. No statistically significant placebo effect was seen, and no adverse effects from these therapies were reported. The authors pointed out the need for higher-quality studies, especially in HT and *reiki* [34].

LIGHT, HEALING AND BIOPHOTONS

To understand more about the role of light in biology and human health we have examined the spontaneous emission of ultraweak photons, often called biophotons, in humans [35]. Although these photons are in the visible range (470–570 nm) they are too low level to be seen in normal background light. We thus developed a very efficient photomultiplier and ran our experiments in a completely light-tight environment. We theorize that reactive oxygen species (ROS) are the principle source of the photons as these are very reactive molecules and take part in reactions which involve interactions of high enough energy to result in spontaneous photon emission. Measuring human photon emission (biophotons) may therefore be a noninvasive method for measuring oxidative state, general health, chronic disease and healing.

We also found that biophotons were emitted in a generally symmetrical pattern from the human body. This was not true for individuals with chronic diseases such as diabetes and arthritis. Furthermore, we demonstrated reproducible emission patterns in meditating individuals and a different pattern in sleeping individuals. We believe this approach holds promise for a real-time, continuous and noninvasive method for monitoring health, wellness, healing and chronic disease, and perhaps even states of consciousness.

An important focus for future research is on whether energy medicine modalities exploit these biophotonic emissions. It is not hard to imagine the ability for some or perhaps all of us to detect these emissions. If this is possible, it is a small step to imagine that healers 'learn' to detect these biophotons and their correlations with health or the lack of it. Finally, is it possible that healers interact with their clients' biophotons and use this system not only to gain information and knowledge but, in fact, to transmit biological information and instructions to clients through these interactions? Is it possible that healers emit biophotons in patterns such that patients' biosystems and biophotons will respond and interact with them? At this point, these are all untested hypotheses. Only by researching these questions further will we learn the answers (see too Chs 16 and 17).

THE QUANTUM ENIGMA

❝I cannot seriously believe in [quantum physics] because ... physics should represent a reality in time and space, free from spooky actions at a distance.
Albert Einstein [36]

❝The universe begins to look more like a great thought than a great machine.
Sir James Jeans [37]

We feel that the incorporation of quantum physics into the discussion on energy medicine provides a possible explanation for some of the empirical observations, anomalies and hallmarks of these therapies. In addition to helping to explain the role of consciousness in healing, and energy medicine in particular, quantum mechanics and physics may explain some of the anomalous observations that have been made in aspects of energy medicine such as *distant healing*.

Most forms of energy obey an *inverse square law*. That is, the effect or force drops as an inverse square of the distance from its source. In contrast, quantum effects do not show this drop-off with distance. Furthermore, all other energies exert their influence either at or below the speed of light whereas quantum effects, like many phenomena in energy medicine, seem to happen immediately without an appreciable time delay. Thus, two of the anomalous aspects of energy medicine, *independence of time and of distance,* are also observed in quantum effects [38]. In this way we may go some way toward explaining the exchange at a distance of healing information, or 'subtle energy', between healer and patient [39].

We are not alone in making this connection. Cyril Smith (see Ch. 9) has also postulated that the body functions as a macroscopic quantum system [40]. This idea may also be applicable in the related field of energy medicine. In a 2003 guest editorial, Smith went further and suggested on the basis of his experimental data that the acupuncture meridian system is made up of quantum domains and networks [41]. Jahn and Dunne have even proposed that consciousness and intention are connected through quantum mechanical means to our body's healing potentials [42].

However, there are serious problems with this hypothesis (see also Ch. 8). Specifically, quantum effects have been demonstrated only on an extremely small scale and are thought by most physicists to be inapplicable in domains larger than those defined by Planck's constant (i.e. than photons and electrons), only traditional Newtonian mechanics being considered applicable to the domains we experience in everyday life. Smith's proposal is that there is a hierarchical series of networks and domains in which quantum effects are transmitted to molecules through their electrons, with molecules transferring this information to cells, and so on, until the intact organism is involved and influenced by quantum effects.

HOMEOPATHY AS ENERGY MEDICINE: A POSSIBLE ROLE FOR QUANTUM ENTANGLEMENT

Homeopathy is defined as yet another form of energy medicine by the US National Institutes of Health (NIH) [43]. This may make sense as standard pharmacology is surely *not* at work in what are called 'high-potency' remedies – those in which the original active substance is diluted to such an extent that there is no possibility that any atoms of the original constituents are present. Dilutions of 30 000, 100 000 or even a millionfold are quite common in this type of homeopathy. Quantum theory is currently in vogue and, perhaps partly because of its mysterious nature, is sometimes invoked to explain all aspects of energy medicine including homeopathy. This is usually not done in a rigorous way and often by novices to the world of quantum mechanics.

However, Harald Walach and his colleagues have addressed this gap in a formal, mathematical way and in 2002 published a paper in *Foundations of Physics* in which they describe how quantum mechanics and quantum theory could be applied to macroenvironments and to nonphysical activities such as intention and thoughts. Their theory, called 'weak quantum theory and generalized entanglement', demonstrates that, mathematically at least, transfer of information between consciousnesses in a nonphysical way is possible [44]. Walach has also produced experimental data to support this hypothesis, although it needs independent replication.

Walach has gone on to present a case for the application of weak quantum theory and generalized entanglement to homeopathy [45]. He contends that the remedies are entangled with both the system and the condition (symptoms) and that even when the original substance has been diluted out of the solution the entanglement remains. Furthermore, he proposes that this explains both the efficacy of homeopathy when it works and the difficulty conventional researchers have in demonstrating this efficacy in clinical trials. Milgrom has also developed formal models for mapping how quantum mechanics could be used to explain the effects of homeopathy and has made suggestions for testing these models in clinical settings [46–48].

Because entanglement is not fully understood, may not operate inside normal time and space boundaries, and is certainly complex and counterintuitive, conventional, linear, cause–effect experiments may not properly test the system as it actually exists, i.e. *entangled*. Certainly physicists have demonstrated how counterintuitive and mysterious this property can be, and how difficult it is to demonstrate even when you know what you are looking for and specifically set up sophisticated experiments to do so. Standard biomedical research methods and study designs, including RCTs, would not demonstrate entanglement. Walach believes that weak *quantum effects and entanglement underlie much of CAM practice and especially energy medicine* [49]. If true, this could at least partially explain the difficulty of attempting to demonstrate the efficacy of energy medicine using conventional experimental approaches, while simultaneously providing an explanation for the empirical effects that are clinically observed but without apparent causal connections. For example, two salient characteristics of energy medicine are the apparent lack of dissipation of 'subtle energy' effects with distance and our inability to block effects with conventional energy barriers [28]. This same pair of phenomena is observed in quantum entanglement. Thinking in this way and designing tests to support or refute the weak quantum theory and entanglement hypothesis represent important directions for future research.

SOME CONCLUSIONS ON MECHANISM

We are not so bold as to suggest that we know *the* mechanism for energy medicine. On the contrary, we contend that there is legitimate debate over whether there even is such a thing as 'subtle energy'. Our goal in this chapter was to present some of the discussion that is occurring in the field and the literature around energy medicine. There are at least three theories as to the underlying mechanisms giving rise to the effects of energy medicine: (1) the *conventional energy* explanation and the *biofield* hypothesis, (2) *placebo* effects and (3) *quantum entanglement*. We have focused primarily in this chapter on the quantum mechanics approach, not because we feel that it is the most correct one, but because it is the most novel and perhaps least understood of the theories, and it also best fits the best data collected so far in all forms of energy medicine.

THE BIOFIELD HYPOTHESIS

The idea of a 'vital force' is often used to explain therapeutic practices in the West such as mesmerism, magnetic healing and faith healing (see also Ch. 22). It has been a core aspect of traditional healing practices for millennia (in the form of *qi* or *prana*) and has also been part of discussions in Western science at least since 1907 when Henri Bergson proposed it as an explanation of why organic molecules could not be synthesized at the time [50]. This thinking held that electricity – the physics and engineering wonder of the time – was somehow connected with this vital force [9].

The modern expression of this idea is often called the 'biofield hypothesis'. As Rubik pointed out: 'The biofield is a useful construct consistent with bioelectromagnetics and the physics of nonlinear, dynamical, nonequilibrium living systems' [51]. For our present discussion the important aspect of the biofield hypothesis is its dependence on classical electromagnetic fields and forces. (See Rubik's paper for a more thorough description of this concept and discussion.) Although some aspects of energy medicine may be explained with the biofield, there are at least two aspects of some forms of energy medicine that it does not adequately explain. One is the apparent independence of distance. The other is the apparent instantaneous change of state that can occur. Neither of these can be explained by classical mechanisms.

THE PLACEBO EFFECT

Another mechanism that might also explain the effects from energy medicine is the *placebo* effect. That is, whatever is going on is the result of patients convincing themselves that they are healing or being healed – they feel less pain, they have fewer complaints and so forth – but that 'nothing' 'really' happened between healer and patient. However, this explanation is not really any more satisfactory and also does not fit some of the best data (for instance, in the field of homeopathy) [52]. The placebo effect itself is not understood or well defined and thus still begs the question of mechanism. Secondly, if patients actually experience healing and/or feeling better, then something 'really' is happening *consciously* and we are back to our first point of still not knowing the underlying mechanism while in fact having authentic healing. Thus, we find invoking the placebo effect to be equivalent to confessing that something really is happening with the patient but we do not know how, nor whether it is coming from within or from without. In addition, the known mechanisms of placebo such as belief, expectancy and conditioning do not account for some of the best-replicated data on the direct effects of intention in living and nonliving systems and blinded, distant effects [2].

QUANTUM MECHANISMS

It is possible that the most fundamental aspects of energy medicine as well as the above-mentioned anomalies, which are not explained by either the biofield hypothesis or the placebo effect, have their explanation and source in quantum physics. We acknowledge that others disagree outright with this idea [53], whereas still others feel that, although this is not the whole explanation, some aspects of quantum physics may be relevant and play a role in energy medicine [54]. If it is true that energy medicine is often working through nonclassical and quantum forms of energy, it is now possible to visualize a future where energy medicine uses a *combination* of classical and quantum energy fields and forces to target and regulate endogenous processes and fields within the body in order to affect healing and salutogenesis. If energy medicine and distant healing are fundamentally forms of information transfer then quantum mechanics may provide the explanation and means for this process.

In addition to explaining the transfer of healing energy between people, quantum mechanics may underlie the natural self-healing process itself. Rein has proposed that this flow of information within the body is necessary for health and that when it is impeded ill-health and disease result [55]. In this thinking, energy medicine is also the flow of information through quantum effects between healer and patient. In an analogous fashion, salutogenesis and health can be seen as the free flow and transfer of information within the body and the interchange of information with the environment to augment this flow. Thus, we feel that the fields of information and quantum models will be important areas of focus for future research and practice. Indeed, if testable theoretical models can be developed that explain data from both conventional and putative forms of energy medicine, a new paradigm of understanding in science and healthcare may emerge that is as important and revolutionary as were our biochemical models in the twentieth century.

What does it mean to practice an energy medicine?

Claire M Cassidy

CHAPTER CONTENTS

INTRODUCTION

An essential characteristic of *qi* is that it flows . . . it moves . . . it responds to, even forms, its own environment. That *qi flows* creates demands that guide Oriental medicine (OM) practice, in North America and Europe, in ways that make it distinctly different from biomedicine. In part 1 of this chapter I support this assertion by asking readers to listen in on acupuncture practitioners as they explain their medicine. In part 2, I offer a social science grounding for my argument.

CONTEXT OF ACUPUNCTURE PRACTICE IN NORTH AMERICA

The medicine I practice is called 'acupuncture' in the United States – though my scope of practice is wider than acupuncture *per se*. Acupuncture is one modality of five within the world medicine called Oriental or East Asian medicine. Oriental medicine originated in China, spread to Korea and Japan and all over East Asia, then to the wider world. Like any world medicine it is highly variable, offering many styles of practice. Additionally wherever it goes it takes on cultural tonality from its new home.

The issue of cultural tonality matters because, generally speaking, no single label can honor the whole medicine, yet each label captures some relevant characteristic. In North America, acupuncture has been called a *hands-on* medicine, *holistic, patient-centered, integrative* and an *energy* medicine. From a social science point of view, it utilizes a processual or relational *medical model*. Remembering that *qi* is not 'just' energy, what matters is that in OM the 'way in' to the suffering body is through studying the movement and character of *qi*, or what I have previously called the 'energetic body' [1]. From that point, Oriental medicine expands to 'embrace the entire breadth of the energy–matter continuum' [2].

In practical terms, from the 1960s, people began to seek holistic patient-centered care that purported to treat the 'whole body, mind, and spirit'. Buoyed by positive news reports, interest in acupuncture rose, and professional training schools began opening their doors by the mid 1970s, purposefully framing acupuncture care as holistic. Today the practice of AOM – acupuncture and Oriental medicine – is widely established and highly professionalized in the United States and its user image is one of offering effective energy-based, hands-on, holistic, patient-centered care.

THE PRACTITIONER'S VOICE

Saying that AOM is an energy medicine because of its focus on *qi* flow is theoretically interesting, but more important is to find out whether it is actually practiced that way; that is, is its practice dynamic, emergent, active, or is it formulaic? If so – if theory is actualized in practice – we can move on to ask what significance this might have for topics such as patient wellness and for the relevance of 'traditional' clinical research designs such as the randomized controlled trial (RCT) to the assessment of acupuncture.

Practitioners quoted (using their initials) in part 1 of this chapter are participants in my ongoing Acuperceptions Project. This qualitative study uses semistructured interviews with practicing acupuncturists to explore how these clinicians view their work. Eleven provide perspectives in this chapter.

With the exception of myself, the practitioners quoted are not clinical researchers or social scientists; they are exclusively practitioners of acupuncture medicine. They vary by age, sex, residence, place of training, styles of acupuncture practiced and years in practice. They typically do not know each other. Yet despite this variability in person and experience they offer remarkably similar images of acupuncture care, and – as I think you will see – these images well fit the concept of an energy medicine.

Qualitative research focuses on *meaning* issues; it is not statistical in character or intent. My interview data are analyzed to identify shared *themes* so as to reveal the *perceptual universe of the respondents* – in this case acupuncturists. In this chapter, practitioner *voice* emerges in the form of quotations; each such quotation illustrates a particular issue, and should be interpreted as a *data point* drawn from a larger sample – *not* as 'anecdote'.

Table 13.1 *Participants in the Acuperceptions Project*			
Practitioner code	**Sex**	**US state**	**Years in practice at time of interview**
CB	M	DE	3.5
OD	F	NC	9
JE	F	MD	6
MF	F	WI	5
EF	M	MD	24
NH	F	CO	26
MM	F	NC	6
YN	M	NJ	9
FR	F	CO	6
HR	M	MD	21
MU	F	MD	12

13.1 EXPERIENCING *QI*

WHAT IS *QI*? THEORIES OF PRACTICE

YN: Qi is energy and structure.

Qi for practitioners of AOM is an ever-present substance that is more or less material, more or less ethereal. Imbuing all things in the universe, taking appropriate forms, its fundamental nature is to *flow*, and it is dynamic, changing expression continually. In the body it takes different forms in different areas, as also in abnormality. Most of the time it cannot be seen, but it can be felt, and its behavior can be followed. Thus *yang qi* is more like Fire, having little substance, but dry and warm and tending to rise. The upper half of the body is relatively *yang*, as is the back. *Yin qi* is more like Water, heavier, flowing downwards, tending to be cool. The lower half of the body is more *yin*, as is the anterior. Good health comprises a balance of Fire and Water, cool and warm, dry and wet. In good health, *qi* flows smoothly to every part of the body, taking its proper form. Thus *qi* in the chest is more like breath, but *qi* in the gut is more like chyme. We may say that health is a condition of *transparency* with regard to *qi* – it does its work and we, emanations of *qi*, get on with our lives often without giving it much thought, like breathing.

Complaints, symptoms and signs arise when there is *maldistribution*, or abnormal *character* of *qi*. Maldistribution can be caused by mechanical barriers to movement, such as scars, by malfunction of the Organs and emotions, by external invasions or by trauma. It creates areas of excess, stagnation, sharp pain, usually accompanied elsewhere by areas of deficiency, weakness or numbness. Abnormal character can show up as *qi* being too Hot or too Dry, too Damp or too Cold or too 'sticky' (Phlegm). Examples of these ideas applied to real patients are given below (and see standard texts such as Helms [3] or MacPherson and Kaptchuk [4]).

How is healthy *qi* sourced in the treatment room? Two models offer complementary explanations. Good *qi* flow reappears when acupuncture care creates balance within and between the regions in excess and those in deficiency *in the patient*; or the practitioner can *subtract qi from* or *add qi to* the patient's system by accessing the apparently inexhaustible supply of the universe. These two models are rarely segregated. For even as the practitioner works with the energy of the patient guiding excess to regions of deficiency, so also is the person of the practitioner transmitting energy. Thus – presumably, and especially if the practitioner is acting with awareness – externally sourced energy can be inserted (or removed) with every needle.

> *EF:* After 23 years of practice, I don't think it's possible to deliver acupuncture without transmitting energy.

A practitioner could use his or her own *qi* to treat, but that is not wise because the sum of one's personal energy is limited.

> *OD:* I am always working with energy, but you burn yourself out if you are using your own energy. You must channel it from other sources. [What other sources?] Heaven, Earth . . . the Universe is filled with energy and we are working to get energy aligned and balanced instead of in chaos, or being stagnant and stuck.

SENSING *QI*

Diagnosis – sensing the distribution and character of *qi* – is done by assessing *color, smell* and *taste, touching* (palpation and 'pulsing', or taking the pulse) plus *listening* to the patient's story and emotional tone. Different practitioners are drawn to different tools. Some are especially sensitive to the movement of the breath, others to the tongue, the pulse, the hands, or to 'listening' with their whole being:

> *YN:* I'm an average pulse taker. I'll use the tongue for reinforcement. But honestly, my forte is really . . . listening with everything that I have and . . . hearing the gap in what one is saying and what one is living. . . . I live for that role, because it's where the juice is. It's where the *qi* is. Right? *Qi* is energy and structure.

Another practitioner uses her hands but:

> *MU:* My hands feel as if they are turning into ears. I would like . . . when touching with intention, to hear what's inside of where the hands are. And sometimes . . . I just have to wait . . . [and then] I'll touch some part, whether it's a pulse, a foot, whatever, . . . and there'll be a little 'aha!' that will tell me where to go. . . . If a place feels cool, depressed, as if there's nothing there under it that's vital, that area might send me to . . . warm the belly, or something like that. If a place feels hot and dry, it might send me to the inside of the knee, to . . . put moisture somewhere. [Points around the knee and elbow are 'sea' points useful for increasing moisture in the body.]

> In my case, I consider my hands my most important tool. I use them both to diagnose and to assess the effectiveness of treatment. I remember the moment my hands awoke. I had been an intern for some weeks, still raw and anxious. One day I stepped out of my cubicle in search of a teacher, when suddenly I felt my hands tingle, light up, change gears. I stopped in the midst of the passing white-coated crowd, staring at my palms. They

were the same shape, the same color, patterned with the same lines as before . . . but now they were . . . *alive to acupuncture.*

Since then I've felt my hands grow in knowledge, the nourishing blood vessels expand, the individual fingers develop specific skills. In taking pulses one always uses the same three fingers on each wrist. Thus one finger becomes wise to sensing *Lung qi* activity, while its neighbor learns to sense *Spleen qi* activity, and so on, six fingers in all. Again, the lateral side of the tip of the left index finger becomes exquisitely sensitive to finding acupoints, even those very tiny or located some distance from the standard 'map' position. My hands *know* things that my brain cannot compute – putting one's hands on a patient provides data that one cannot get in any other way.

Another practitioner who relies on his hands links his assessment to the underlying task of managing balance for the patient:

> *EF:* For me, the pulses always were my best way in, you know, I could have a conversation with people, I could listen to color sound odor emotion, but the place where I really got down to business and made the treatment choice is when I was taking pulses . . . I saw myself as an artist, . . . sort of plucking the right strings that created the harmonious music.

There is also the crucial moment when one meets the patient. That moment can be richly used to assess the patient's *qi*.

> *MF:* After doing this for a while it's pretty easy to pick up on the kind of energy that a person has, just what's happening in their body, and what needs to happen in the relationship. It's kind of an intuitive thing, and yet there are so many markers for it. You know, you can look at their body type, their facial expression, you listen to their voice, what they're wearing . . . just how they're taking care of themselves, how they sit, . . . whether they're comfortable or if they fidget a lot.

OD, a nurse-acupuncturist, comments:

> I shake their hand. Just shaking their hand gives me a lot of ideas. Is it edematous? What are the fingernails like? How is their voice, how were they sitting in the waiting room – eyes closed? Magazine? Are they weak? If they are in pain I look to see how they walk, how they get out of the chair, how they hold themselves to sit.

SENSING THE NEEDLE AND THE ACUPOINT

In training, one learns to insert needles and locate the acupoint. Modern acupuncture needles are thin, flexible, solid (filiform) stainless needles with handles, finely honed, and today often coated to make them slide in more easily. They are sterile and used only once before disposal. Acupoints are located all over the body, organized into 'channels' or 'meridians' with names like Stomach channel or Heart channel. The points along each channel are used to treat the named functional Organ, but their use is much broader, and guided in a complex way. Thus Stomach points can also hone the immune system, treat shoulder or ankle pain, and support other channels and Organs, besides treating the stomach and digestive system.

For our purposes, what's most important about the acupoints is simply finding them. They have been 'mapped', but the map location is often not the active location, and it is the task of the practitioner to find the active point. Detection of acupoints can be done with sensitive fingertips, but there are other methods, including inviting the patient to participate in their care by commenting if the point is active: 'Yes, that's it. I feel it!'

The theory of acupuncture states that the needle must be inserted so that the *practitioner feels the qi*. This is called 'getting *deqi*'. The patient may also feel the *qi* but practice styles vary as to whether they consider this important. In my experience, I know I've hit the point when I sense my needle going into something more softly solid, more mildly resistant, than the surrounding tissue. I know I've missed the point if there's no resistance. But if the patient – or the point – is very deficient, resistance is unlikely to show up. In that case I might determine that I had 'hit the point' because the deficient pulse changes. In fact, one can accurately select points by pulsing with one hand, while touching points along the meridian with the other. When point palpation changes the pulse picture, *that* is the point to needle . . . and after needling, one checks the pulse again to make sure the desired change has occurred. *Qi* moves fast – change can be expected within seconds to minutes.

Other practitioners report:

> CB: I don't move on to the next point until I know I've gotten the *qi* at that point, and really, when you get right down to it, once you get the *qi* at the point, you did the right manipulation with the needle, it's done its job, you can take the needle out. [What do you feel?] Kind of – kind of – like a pressure, or a light feedback in the needle.

> HR: When I feel like my hands are touching energy it gives me like, a chill up and down my spine. And with needles I get the same thing, [even though] one is a needle and one is an extension of my finger. I can actually ignite an acupuncture point with my finger; I don't need a needle to do it. I know from touching something that I can feel that energy move and because of that chill up and down my spine. Or if I'm using a needle, I feel something from the needle go into my fingers, like a little charge.

There are also relations among touch, needling and effectiveness that most practitioners sense, but HR expressed well as he was talking about patients who are afraid of needles:

> If . . . the client feels comfortable with your touch, then it really makes the insertion of the needle very near and dear. If someone is tense and really uptight about receiving a needle, then guess what? Even when you put a needle in, it might not do anything. Because they are blocking it.

CLINICAL CARE

ESTABLISHING A RELATIONSHIP

Acupuncturists typically emphasize the importance of establishing a relationship with the patient. It is a hands-on practice – practitioners must spend a relatively long time with a patient to talk, examine, and insert needles. In addition, US acupuncture care is also (almost always) an *intentionally* patient-centered practice, and this feature arises organically from the focus on the flow of *qi*.

How important is this relationship? Simply consider the last quotation. If, in fact, patients can 'block' the effectiveness of acupuncture by fearing needles or by disliking the practitioner's touch, then treatment success depends partly upon the practitioner's ability to create a safe environment and warm relationship from the outset. Practitioners do this in different ways. Some try to create distinctly 'healing' treatment settings; others rely more on their interpersonal skills and healing intentionality. Practitioners also 'train' patients. Because acupuncture care is not normative in the US, the need for such training applies to each new patient, and practitioners develop their own methods for drawing patients into becoming active participants in the treatment dyad.

But there is another level of implication here. It is that – in this medicine – the acupuncturist and acupuncture treatment are not *doing something to* another body-person, but rather, enabling that body-person to *engage itself in functioning in the best possible way.* This understanding emerges repeatedly during interviews, but MU provides a particularly clear summary:

> [Acupuncture is] this ancient process of using needles . . . to affect the vitality of another human being in a way that helps that person become more in a homeostatic state, or more who they're meant to be. Basically all that an acupuncturist is trying to do is help the person show up in the best possible wellbeing. And sometimes that means living with their pain. It may be that what they're carrying can't really be gotten away, but can be lifted, or heartened, or made more bearable. . . . What I would like to do best is to be so present to someone when they come in that I get out of the way, and . . . understand that they are already whole, and that all I am doing is providing a space for them finding their own wholeness.

This perspective is clearly an energy-centered view of the body, with the practitioner transformed from hierarchic authority to partner enabling positive self-change [5]. This shift in practitioner function is another reason why practitioners focus on *the patient* and their *energetic relationship to healing the patient,* often noting that they are themselves altered by the act of delivering medical care. They work to be aware of the flow of energy within themselves, inside the patient, and between themselves and the patient, often reporting following various daily meditative practices so as to clarify their own energy before seeing patients.

In sum, 'establishing relationship' in acupuncture care has (at least) two aspects. The first is the familiar one about establishing a relationship so that treatment can be offered, which is characteristic of most medical care. The second is specifically characteristic of an energy medicine – and has to do with recognizing how energy flows among practitioner, patient and the universe, and in encouraging a healing flow.

DIAGNOSING THE PATIENT, DELIVERING TREATMENT

As noted, AOM offers several methods of diagnosis, and each patient visit includes hands-on assessment varying with style. In a typical session, after receiving the patient's report, the practitioner begins the physical examination with a biomechanical assessment (if needed), and moves on to body palpation, pulse palpation and tongue examination, usually with the patient lying on a treatment table (examination details may be found in standard texts [3,6-8]). Using my practice as an exemplar, which reflects techniques drawn from both Chinese and Japanese styles, I start with abdominal palpation (brushing, pressing, probing), seeking temperature and texture changes, each of which offers a diagnostic clue. Next I take the pulses.

Taking the pulses in AOM is different in intention and technique from taking pulses in biomedicine. AOM takes three pulses at each radial position, on each wrist. Each position represents a different *yin* Organ at the middle level, and a different *yang* Organ at the superficial level. Counting 3 levels (superficial, middle, deep) and 6 positions, there are 18 locations to assess to find out how much *qi* is expressed, and whether it is abnormal in character. Some positions may be deficient – feeling empty, slow, weak. Others may thump against the fingertips.

Pulses can flow evenly, hang static or beat irregularly. I once felt something like a sail billowing in the wind – this occurred in a hyperthyroid patient.

Two examples ground this discussion of touch assessment.

1. A man complained of pain behind the knees. His abdomen remained rock-hard as I palpated and he felt nothing. His pulse picture was excess in Urinary Bladder (an energy channel comprising points that can be associated with back-of-knee pain), and deficient in Heart. Palpation on his back revealed soft, yielding flesh, and as I ran my fingers down his spine, I seemingly 'fell off a cliff' at T4–T5. He had no pain until I palpated his buttocks and sacrum to seek sources for knee pain. But why the 'cliff'? Checking again to be sure I was not imagining it, I heard him murmur: 'I was abused.' Pieces fell into place: armored in front, vulnerable and deficient in back in the region over Heart and Heart Protector [Pericardium]. Partial treatment plan: reduce knee pain, tonify Heart *qi* and Spirit.

2. An elderly woman said she'd had bronchitis but was well now since she'd been taking antibiotics. My full body assessment revealed that all reflexes relating to immune system and Lung were active, her Lung pulses were in excess, and she had swelling in the lymph nodes in her neck. Hmmm – *not energetically well!* – even if antibiotics had changed the mucous from green to clear. I proceeded to treat the Lung.

Once diagnosis is initially completed, it is time to select points and insert needles. Diagnosis can lead to naming one or more patterns of disharmony that in turn suggest appropriate needling strategies. One could proceed in strict protocol fashion – classical point patterns to treat a wide range of complaints are listed in textbooks [6,7]. Experienced practitioners – at least those intent on tending the issue of energy – may use a protocol approach but continually assess its effectiveness, modifying the intervention if pulses do not normalize, sore reflex points disappear, patient pain ameliorate or range of motion improve. In fact, treating a patient is (potentially) a very active process in which the practitioner is continually checking back to ensure that the choice of points is making a difference.

Another way to say this is to say that, *in AOM, diagnosis and treatment are not separate and sequential activities, but linked in an active feedback loop.* This is, in fact, one of the most powerful and distinctive aspects of AOM: it enables the practitioner to determine whether a treatment is *being effective, even as treatment is happening.*

In some styles of practice, the patient is regularly brought into the treatment equation, and not treated as a passive recipient. One such style is that taught by Kiiko Matsumoto (with David Euler, and Stephen Birch). For example, if the patient reports discomfort in the left lower abdominal quadrant, one interprets this as stagnation of Blood and *qi* there, or *oketsu* [8]. This is treated with LIV-4 on the inside of the left malleolus and LU-5 on the inside of the left elbow. However, the best way to treat *oketsu* is to *engage the patient in determining the best position for the needle* at LIV-4. Thus, the practitioner puts one hand on the site of the *oketsu* and asks the patient to pay attention to the pain, then puts a finger on LIV-4, moving it to several positions until the patient says 'That helps [the abdominal pain]'. Now the needle is inserted at the position and angle that *the patient* has signaled as effective. Needles are left in for up to 20 minutes while other treatment tasks are carried out. Meanwhile, the patient *knows* that the treatment is being effective because pain in reflex regions is steadily diminishing. This is *energy medicine in action* – the points chosen are distant, and guided not only by theory (the relationship of Liver and Lung to stagnation) but also by practice – the actual and prompt relief of symptoms, which both practitioner and patient can judge independently.

By the end of a particular acupuncture session, the practitioner looks for normalization of the pulse picture, normalization of the reflex point picture, and patient-reported changes such as relief of pain or other symptoms and improved movement, energy and/or mood. Also, since acupuncture is ordinarily delivered in a series of visits, at subsequent visits the practitioner will look for improvement in pulse and reflex signs at the *outset* of treatment – a way of assessing how well the previous treatments have been integrated into the patient's body-being. The patient should also be reporting symptomatic improvements: less reflux, better bowel movements, less coughing, fewer headaches, improved stamina, steadier mood, less pain, improved range of motion, better sleep, relief of grief and so on, depending on the patient's initial complaints.

Practitioners in the Acuperceptions study offer more insight on the link between diagnosis and treatment, and how energy-based treatment and patient-centered care are actualized.

> OD: When I start to palpate I try several points before they lie down and ask them to say if there is pain. . . . I ask them to tell me if the point feels funny, tight, etc. I use the abdomen, then neck . . . I talk with the patient and say what I'm doing; they get an idea of how [my AOM diagnosis] relates to the biomedical diagnosis and how Chinese medicine is different. . . . I'm checking [reflex points] every few needles.

> MF: I do it differently for different people. My goal is to meet people where they're at. Some are sensitive, so I keep needles at the surface. Some people have difficulty accessing their energy, and they're really strong, so for them *qi* is hard to obtain. For them I needle deeply, vigorously, with very strong stimulation, and that means grasping hard with my fingers and manipulating back and forth, using my *qi* to do that. And what I've found is that when I meet them where their energy is at, the treatment is just right for them.

To close this section, EF describes a nonprotocol approach:

> What I discovered was that by asking the patient's body which points to use and in what sequence – you know, 'Now I've done this, what's next?' – I could eliminate pain while the patient was on the table . . . and this also works for emotional issues. By asking the patient's body, you can always get the right answer.

FEEDBACK LOOPS AND ASSESSING TREATMENT EFFECTIVENESS

As presented so far, delivering acupuncture care demands that the practitioner pay close attention to how energy moves in the patient. Not everyone practices that way – one could deliver protocol care as a technician and without seeking immediate feedback from the body. In my experience, however, most practitioners are acutely aware of the interactive nature of acupuncture care. As they check back repeatedly during care delivery to see whether the pulse picture has improved, the sore spots recovered, the range of motion enlarged, or the swelling diminished, they create a series of feedback loops between the needle and the body, their intention and their choice of acupoint, the intervention and the patient's experience. Thus they measure continuously whether an acupoint stimulation has been effective. Prompt feedback also serves to enhance practitioner confidence in the quality of their perception and intervention. Assessing rapid feedback is not unique to acupuncture; it is characteristic of hands-on practice, but it is not characteristic of pharmaceutical or herbal practice.

In the Acuperceptions study, practitioners who described patient care distinguished between the relative ease of treating musculoskeletal pain and the longer-term tasks associated with treating chronic conditions and emotional complaints. I have limited the quotations to two mainly about pain relief because they best illustrate the issue of feedback.

EF: With physical situations, conditions, in many cases it's possible to get the pain to zero. So I may ask [the body] 'is there another point needed?' and . . . I may get a 'no' answer. And then I'll turn to the patient and say 'Is there any pain left?' – 'Yes.' – 'So how much?' 'Well, maybe 10%.' ' Well, is that pain placed any differently than I was working before?' 'Yes, it's medial.'. . . or something. So then, because I've now eliminated the pain behind the knee, then I go and search for the points that will eliminate [the new pain]. [In] more emotional kinds of things, . . . I'm more likely to ask the patient what they notice within themselves, what has changed emotionally, and . . . sometimes it changes on the table and sometimes it doesn't. And when it doesn't change on the table, what I'm looking to do is to determine when to stop treatment. When I'm happy with pulse balance, I stop. When doing the Kiiko method, the way you know to stop is when the reflexes are normal.

MF: If I'm working with pain, I want a response right away. So this morning I was working with shoulder pain. I went to the shoulder, then put two needles in lower opposite leg, move the shoulder and there was a little change but not much . . . so I put another needle down in the leg, and go up and move the shoulder again. I went back down to the leg, put another needle in, went back to the shoulder and the pain was gone. So I said 'OK, I got what I wanted here.' Then I put one needle in her hand on the affected arm, as a guide. As a guide for the energy to move up from leg and down arm to [her] hand. I would call that success, in the moment. And several things can happen. The pain can not come back at all, and that's just great. It doesn't typically happen that way – usually you need 2–3 more treatments and then the pain might come back but it won't come back to the same degree. And I expect people with acute pain to be in for three treatments and then for the pain to be gone, and that's what I tell them. But people who've had longer pain, I tell them it's going to take longer, but . . . I still expect some pain decrease on the table, and if I don't get any, I'm not happy. So that's how I'm thinking about pain: I want to be judging what I do in the moment.

BRIEF CASE STUDIES

Case studies demonstrate theory and practice in action, and offer a living flavor of the treatment process. Each case below illustrates a point of theory, a practice technique and/or a problem of practice.

CASE STUDIES

1. MM reports a case in which correct diagnosis was paramount:

   I had a case that surprised me. It was a patient with asthma. She was born with it and now she was age 32. Whether a case is easy or hard depends on diagnosis and if the right thing is done at the beginning. The diagnosis must be correct. The treatment protocol is easy and fast if you've got the diagnosis right. In this case she had asthma and allergies and was constipated. Most asthma is a result of coldness in the lungs – but this person had Lung Heat – this was a surprise. If she overdresses in winter she gets asthma and it's worse in summer. She used to go around in shorts in the middle of winter. I found a protocol in the *Shang Han Lun* [220 CE [9]], and found her LU-10 was painful, which confirmed my diagnosis. [LU-10 is a Fire point.] I treated her with Metal-Water [protocol to cool Fire]. She tried herbs for 6 days, and Lung Fire cleared. It was winter – she bundled up; no asthma. I was totally amazed by this. After I treated her for asthma, I spent the last 5 minutes – touch up – on the constipation issue . . . . Afterwards, she never had constipation. Then she tried to eat fiber, and she got constipated. (laughs) So I did the points again.

2. Sometimes a single judiciously chosen acupoint can make a major body-wide difference, as in this case. Du-2 (GV-2) is a point on the sacrococcyx. In this position it affects the craniosacral movement, and can indirectly affect the whole body. It is specifically helpful for Lung issues [10], and Lung includes the entire respiratory system and the skin.

OD: This was the fourth treatment of a woman with allergies and asthma . . . . One note [from the other acupuncturist] said this woman had spina bifida . . . so I thought about GV-2 and sinuses. I asked her 'Do you mind if I touch a spot near your [tailbone]?' She said 'No.' She also had neck/shoulder/low back pain. As soon as I did GV-2 her neck and nose opened instantly and I was [delighted]. She said she felt 100% when she left.

3. Different styles of acupuncture practice offer somewhat different perspectives on care, and different protocols. Here is a case in which a change of protocol made a difference.

MM: One more interesting case, a guy with high blood pressure. Kiiko [Matsumoto style] points didn't work. I looked at Master Tung's points – he is very protocol-based . . . But he had a very specific point for high blood pressure, which I tried. [The patient's] BP was 162. I added the point, and did a 5-minute check – it was 148. At 1 hour it was 138. By night it was 128. That was dramatic. It stayed down several days and then [it went up and] he took BP medicine. I treated again – this was recent – he was at 130/80, so already low. I tried the point and in 10 minutes it was down to 120, and he wanted to go to sleep, like turning a light switch off.

4. Scars are common and sometimes mechanically constrict the flow of qi. From my experience:

(1) A woman complained of icy feet and sore swelling in a knee where she had recently had surgery. I treated her twice with needles and electroacupuncture (electrical leads to needles to magnify the needling effect). After the first session her knee was neither swollen, sore, nor too warm; after the second *her husband* joyfully announced that her feet were warm and he could slumber without fear of a toe touching him in the night. Interpretation: *Yang qi* was not reaching her feet, and the recent surgery created a second barrier to the free flow of *qi*. Acupuncture care removed the barriers.

(2) A man received a soccer wound in his teen years that developed as a depressed purple scar adherent to the tibia above the medial malleolus. Now nearing 40 he complained of foot pain and inability to play. The foot was mottled and swollen, what AOM calls *Blood stasis* – clearly *qi* (and blood and lymph) could not flow past this scar. I used distant needles, and cupping (creating a vacuum) over the scar. After about six treatments, the scar had lifted off the bone, allowing liquids and nervous sensation to flow beneath. Mottling and swelling in the foot disappeared. Three years later he proudly displayed the scar, soft and normal in color, and reported that he was still playing soccer.

(3) A woman complained of chronic cystitis with pain and inability to have intercourse. She had a 'smile' scar on her lower abdomen, souvenir of multiple

Caesarian deliveries, the last 10 years previously. Ten years! – but the scar lying over her bladder, vagina and uterus had not healed. I used a Japanese technique involving triple ion-pumping cords (a diode forces one-way flow of bioelectrical charges). After two treatments she dropped out of care, leaving me wondering if I'd been helpful to her. Six months later she phoned for an appointment, and when I asked how she was, sounded startled – 'Oh, that's all gone! I'm well. I still use a special diet, but what you did, did the job!'

5. As noted earlier in this chapter, the absolute amount of *qi* in one's body can vary – it can be *lost by overuse* or the passage of a lifetime, or it *can be added to* by accident, evil intention or curative intention. We are not surprised when the elderly become frail, meaning that their supply of *qi* is seriously diminished. But it can also happen to youthful people who work too hard. One former patient who worked in war zones desperately wanted to become pregnant. Every time I saw her on home leave she arrived exhausted in body, mind and spirit. Able to use only my *words* as 'needles', since she was soon off again, I wrote out a system for energetic rejuvenation to permit pregnancy, and accompanied the letter with a serious warning about the state of her *qi*/health. This time she changed her behaviors and 6 months later, back home, announced that she was pregnant.

6. AOM also recognizes that illness can enter from the outside, an invader, 'evil *qi*'. The commonest expression of this is a 'cold' or infection – invasion by Wind – but one can also be invaded by another's emotions. MM, explaining how she became curious about AOM, tells a story about herself suffering the effects of Wind and Cold invasion when a sophomore in college:

When you wash your hair, [Chinese medicine practitioners] say, don't go out in the wind with wet hair. It didn't make any sense to me. I went out to run and there was a huge wind storm on the track and I got a huge migraine headache, with vomiting.

This form of evil *qi* can often be pushed out of the body using 'Wind' points on the upper back.

Emotions that 'invade' or 'attack' can enter a vulnerable energetic system from the inside or the outside, and make one's behavior unpredictable. Worsley [11] provides specific protocols for dealing with 'aggressive energy' (AE) cases such as the next two. YN reports:

[There is] this one new client . . . um . . . who is quick to anger, you know, temper on the job. And I've been treating him for about 6 weeks now, and his fellow coworkers in construction will come up to him and ask him if he's okay . . . because he hasn't been the hot head, alright? And that was after AE.

In a case in my experience, a woman said that she could not stop shaking 3 days after a guest in her home harshly accused her of prejudicial behavior. I used the Worsley protocol to chase the invading *qi* out of her body. It 'worked' in that the patient stopped shaking and allowed the event to take an ordinary place in her psyche as a 'rotten event . . . and one can learn from rotten events'.

In both forms of invasion, follow-up treatments would focus on improving the ability of the body to resist invasion. In 'Western' terms we might speak of strengthening the immune system, or improving emotional resilience.

7. A clinical suggestion is also, potentially, an invader – something that many acupuncture practitioners well know. Here the acupuncturist suspected

that her failure to help partly stemmed from another practitioner's suggestion that the patient (unfortunately) had integrated into his being. The patient had sciatica – generally relatively easy to treat with acupuncture – but he did not respond to her care.

> MF: The interesting piece was that he'd gone to a chiropractor before he saw me, and [the chiropractor] told him that he wouldn't treat him, that this wasn't treatable by anybody and if it got better while he was seeing somebody, it was just that it resolved on its own. I said 'I have never heard any practitioner say that!' But I did question whether there was that [suggestion] sitting in his mind, a kind of a block. I didn't question it with him, but at the same time I put in an extra needle to settle the mind, because I thought, if I settle the mind I might get a piece here that I might not have gotten otherwise. But that didn't change things either. So the whole thing was that he left in pain, and I don't know if he got any relief at all.

8. In an energy medicine, the entire body is considered as a whole even when a complaint appears to be more or less confined to one functional region. For example: A woman complained of chronic diarrhea, with no other symptoms except fatigue. Palpating her body, I found she was distinctly cold over the middle of her abdomen, and on the inside of both lower legs. The middle abdomen includes a major point called Ren-12 (or CV-12) that signals digestive abnormality. The inside of the lower leg contains the point called SP-6, a major point that treats three Organs at once, Spleen (in charge of digestion), Liver (in charge of the smooth flow of *qi*), and Kidney (in charge of Water). I also found that her medial shins were lined with rubbery lumps, none painful, not edematous. AOM considers such lumps to be signs of accumulated sticky Damp *qi*, called Phlegm. Adding the pulse picture, this pattern pointed me toward a diagnosis of *Deficient Spleen qi with Damp*. I chose to treat with needles to move *qi*, and moxa (warming herbs) to warm and dry the Damp and Cold. At the third treatment, the patient reported normalizing stools and better energy. Her shins were smooth to the touch. I mentioned this to her, and she exclaimed, 'Yeah, isn't it neat? But I didn't think it was part of the treatment!' True: lumpy legs would probably not be a sign to a gastroenterologist treating chronic diarrhea, but in an energy medicine, concern with correcting the character and flow of *qi* applies to the whole body. Remember the logic: energy channels in her legs are part of her Spleen function, and her Spleen represents her digestive system . . . *so too do her legs.*

9. In this last case, the practitioner was interested in the larger issues of care, or how the patient 'transforms' so that in future she may be healthier and more connected to life. This is an example of how a holistic practitioner 'embeds' physical care in a larger framework that includes the patient's entire life.

> FR: I have a patient who came in with blisters all over her hand and severe eczema and couldn't touch anything, was in pain every day. So first transformative is if that goes away, they get the quality of their life back, but also transformative is realizing and recognizing why that might be happening and making those changes in the lifestyle and becoming happy in their life because they feel better. In that case, she had an allergy to dairy, even though she had all the tests done that said she didn't, and we came to assess that she did, based on helping her recognize her behavior and her lifestyle and when things were happening and testing it out a couple of times, having it come back. And then there's some restrictions in life which people have a hard time accepting, saying 'I'm going to do that anyway because it's something that I've always enjoyed', so putting those limitations could be difficult for them, but then coming to a place of acceptance and then having that quality of life . . . .

What does it mean to practice an energy medicine?

CONCLUSION TO PART I

Based on what the sampled practitioners revealed, we can now propose what an 'energy medicine' looks like *from within*. In brief, it involves:

- whole body-person focus
- patients viewed as responsive and participatory, not passive
- practitioners skilled at sensing *qi*
- diagnosis and treatment linked in a feedback loop
- a healing or transformative goal.

13.2 THINKING ABOUT *QI* AND ACUPUNCTURE

In part 1 we were concerned with *feeling qi*; in part 2 we *think about qi*. It is good to remember that our ultimate task is pragmatic – we want to know if the way AOM practitioners are behaving has general implications for the understanding and delivery of healthcare, and how it is applicable to the design of quality clinical research.

We found in part 1 that selected practitioners of AOM explain themselves using terms like 'energy' and/or by reporting behaviors that one might expect to emerge from utilizing a medical model that emphasizes flow and fluidity. We continue by trying to answer three questions: How representative are these practitioners? Is there a larger context for their style of medical care – that is, for the energy medicine model? Can we usefully generalize from practitioner behaviors to the larger scene that includes public health outreach and clinical trials design?

HOW REPRESENTATIVE ARE THE QUOTED PRACTITIONERS?

Studies of patient response to AOM show them to be, with few exceptions, highly satisfied with their care. They are pleased by relief of symptoms, but more than that: they report appreciating other benefits, which can be recognized to derive from delivering a medicine that utilizes the characteristics summarized above.

Cassidy [12,13], Gould and Macpherson [14], MacPherson et al [15] and Mulkins and Verhoef [16] all report, in somewhat different language, that acupuncture patients attribute 'feeling better' not only to the specific effects of acupuncture care, but also to features such as the close therapeutic relationship, individualization of care, care focused on the 'whole person' or on 'overall wellbeing', and on the transformative nature of the intervention. Price et al [17] found that the practitioner's ability to be empathetic – or successfully create a trusting safe relationship – was highly important to the success of outcome in both the short and long-term (for more reading on patients and the patient–practitioner relationship in professional acupuncture care, plus methodological discussions, see Cassidy and Thomas [18] and Paterson and Schnyer [19]). Paterson and Britten [20,21] followed patients from the outset of treatment for several months and reported that patients sought holism when reporting on the therapeutic relationship, new understandings of themselves and even the acupuncturist's diagnostic and needling skills. These studies were done with patients of professional acupuncturists. Interestingly, a study in Germany of patients of biomedical doctors providing acupuncture did not find that care was 'holistic' from the point of view of patients [22]. Thus an acupuncture needle can be an instrument of non-holistic therapy when delivered by hands (and minds) guided by a reductionist philosophy (see below).

Kaufman and Salkeld [23], working with professional acupuncturists to find out how they viewed their work with hospice patients, found that they expected a broader outcome than relief of symptoms – particularly an improved ability to deal proactively with end-of-life issues. Ethnographic data on practitioners reported by Emad [24] offer close parallels to the depth-interview data reported in part 1. Ryan [25] interviewed practitioners to find out how they made clinical decisions and concluded that, while they drew on 'traditional', 'experiential' and 'reflexive' sources of knowledge, they did not typically consult research data partly because most did not seem relevant to clinical practice.

In sum, limited data on the practices of professional acupuncturists and their patients in the USA, Canada and the UK suggest that the 'holistic' or 'energy-framed' model of acupuncture care is normative.

A METAPARADIGMATIC CONTEXT FOR AOM AS AN 'ENERGY MEDICINE'

Social scientists and historians of medicine, who have long tried to analyze health-care systems, recognize that medical practices tend to assort into two groups:

— those that emphasize the person and the movement of life
— those that emphasize order and disorder.

These two major models can be framed into the yet larger context of society-wide perceptual preferences, or *metaparadigms.*

Metaparadigms have been discussed by a wide range of thinkers [26]. Each is known by multiple names. Thus, the position that emphasizes persons and movement has been called *processual, relational, ecological, feminist, holistic, integrative* and, with regard to medical models, *physiological* or *process-oriented.* The metaparadigm that emphasizes order and disorder – still dominant in Euro-American societies – is termed *hierarchical, reductionistic, paternalistic, Newtonian,* or, in medical contexts, *reductionist* or *ontological.*

Table 13.2 summarizes some medically relevant differences, discussed in terms of AOM. Readers should remember, however, that lists are artificial, and real people, real systems, ordinarily do not rigidly conform to such premises. Nevertheless, because so much of metaparadigm is out of consciousness, the assumptive *tendencies* are likely to show up repeatedly, and be resistant to change.

A useful mnemonic for thinking about these two spans on an intellectual continuum is to speak of verbs and nouns. Focused on movement (e.g. metabolism), *processual models* are more like verbs. Focused on states of being (e.g. cells, tissues, diseases), *reductionist models* are more like nouns. Of course, sentences have *both* verbs and nouns, and though medical models can be reasonably segregated into movement-oriented types and state-of-being types, all deliver medical care.

As one would expect of a model also called relational, *processual medical models* emphasize the whole body-person – that is, the integration of parts and the interaction and interrelationships of this body-person with its human and natural environment. Each person creates a distinctive network of relations with his/her surroundings, which, if it supports a productive life, can be described as 'balanced'. But 'balance' is not fixed; it is constantly moving, presumably around someone's own center of 'best function'. Thus it is dynamic,

What does it mean to practice an energy medicine?

and change is normal at different ages and in different settings, and even at different times of day. In bioscience it is common to call this point of physiological balance *'homeostasis'*. Since the focus here is on the fact that it *moves*, a better term is *homeodynamis*: a point of balanced flowing movement, not an achieved state.

Continuing the logic, disorder emerges from disturbances in the network of interactions – that is, interior or exterior abnormal relationships, or *imbalance*. Meanwhile, there are so many potentially intervening factors that it is accepted that people vary, and interventions to return the body-person to balance must account for the whole person in his or her environment. Also, because people vary, intervention must be *individualized* – that is, the practitioner must figure out how imbalance is showing up in this *particular* body-person. A corollary of the need for individualization is that it is difficult to find predetermined protocols that will work for everyone. Instead, the practitioner must immerse him/herself in diagnosis, offer an intervention, check to see if improvement is occurring, repeat a diagnostic process if necessary, and treat again until her repeated assessment indicates that the patient has achieved an acceptable degree of homeodynamis. This integration of diagnosis and treatment demands fluidity from the practitioner; in short, the concept of movement does not apply simply to the response of the individual body-person, but also to the diagnostic and treatment process, and to the behavior of the practitioner.

Again, it is assumed that when an intervention is offered the whole body-person will respond. Even if the complaint appears to affect primarily one part or system, the whole body is out of balance, and treatment will draw the whole body back into balance. No part is truly separate. In this case not only will complaints of which the patient is aware ameliorate but, potentially, treatment will have far-reaching effects up to and including transformation or change, and learning from change, that allows the patient to live thereafter with more comfort and productivity.

The focus on balance is also played out in the preference for forming more equal partnerships with patients, offering 'patient-centered' care. One can form such 'equilateral' relationships partly *because* patients respond. In the case of AOM specifically (for the 'energy' model applies to a wide range of medical systems), the *qi* of patients can be accessed, can be guided, and patients will respond physically, emotionally, energetically: their symptoms will ameliorate, their *spirit* will improve, they will be able to take better charge of their lives. Note that, although this characteristic could be merely an intellectual command from a medical model, in fact real patients report such responses and, furthermore, say that they enjoy receiving healthcare that assumes responsiveness as against simple compliance.

A metaparadigm is an identifiable philosophical model preferred society-wide during an extended period of time such as several centuries; such preference is revealed by common usage and shared understanding. An important component of metaparadigm is that many of its premises and much of the resulting logic remain *out of the awareness of users*, who simply feel and act as if these ideas were 'normal' and 'self-evident' (as in 'We hold these truths to be self-evident'). Challenges arrive – people discover that their 'truths' are assumptions not necessarily shared or 'proven'– when they meet novel ideas. Today we live at a time when the long-dominant *Newtonian* [reductionist] metaparadigm is making less cultural sense, while the *relational* [processual], which was formerly almost unseen by North Americans, is making more cultural sense.

This shift affects medical care, for every medical system partakes in metaparadigm, and its own professional paradigm reflects its preferred allegiance. Several terms are used more or less interchangeably to refer to professional paradigms, including 'medical model', 'explanatory model' and 'reality model'. The latter reminds us that the model underlying a medical practice *makes sense* and *creates medical reality* for those practicing that medicine. People must remember this when observing medical actions different from their own or the 'conventional'. That 'other' way of practicing medicine is typically not the product of foolishness or ignorance, but the result of working from a different intellectual starting point: a different set of underlying assumptions.

Yet another expression of the focus on movement shows up during diagnosis and treatment. Diagnoses are unlikely to involve assigning labels like biomedical disease labels ('you have X') because the expression of the body *right now* will change with treatment, and may or may not show up similarly next week. Instead in AOM 'patterns of disharmony' are identified, usually several per patient, and these are named to describe what is currently happening with energy in this body. For example, one might have a patient complaining of severe headache whose diagnosis is *Rising Liver Fire*. Once this is treated – by reducing Fire excess – the patient's headache should disappear, *as will the diagnostic label*. So what will this patient express next time he/she comes in? Some practitioners enjoy the mystery that this feature of a processual medical model presents; the patient's condition varies from week to week, thus diagnosis must be made anew at each visit.

This could seem like a burden to a reductionist thinker who might prefer to have a 'clear label', but to a practitioner focused on movement it is ordinary and doing diagnosis at each visit is also ordinary. At the same time, it is well known

Table 13.2 *Two major metaparadigms described in medical terms*

Processual	Reductionist
Focus on movement, flow, verbs	Focus on states of being, nouns
Whole body-person focus	Physical body focus
Imbalance	Disease
People vary; individualize care; minimize interventive protocols	Diseases vary; people similar; interventive protocols normative
Diagnosis and treatment integrated	Diagnosis precedes treatment
Whole person responds	'Placebo effect' problematic
Transformative	Curative

that people tend to malfunction in somewhat predictable ways in terms of their constitution. Thus a person who complains of a Liver issue may have difficulty ensuring the smooth flow of *qi*. Next time this person who *had* Liver Fire comes for care, one might again expect to find a Liver issue, perhaps *Liver qi stagnation*.

APPLYING THE ENERGY MODEL TO CLINICAL RESEARCH

The premises undergirding the processual medical model are sufficiently different from those of the reductionistic medical model that they produce serious difficulties for clinical researchers, nearly all of whom are primarily enculturated to the reductionist medical model, for which their research is designed and for which it is suited. For example, the famous random-assignment placebo-controlled protocol-based clinical trials design was developed for the assessment of pharmaceuticals, and is based on the assumptions listed in the second column of Table 13.2. *Attempts to apply it directly to the study of acupuncture medicine yield difficult-to-interpret results* of uncertain relevance to actual clinical practice. A full discussion is too large for this chapter, so I shall flag just a few issues to keep our 'thinking' fresh and moving.

> "The reason for practicing acupuncture, and for researching it, is to improve the quality of patients' lives . . . . However, when it comes to research, the patients' perspective and subjective experience is often removed . . . When this happens . . . research cannot answer the question of whether and how acupuncture addresses people's health needs and improves their lives" [19].
>
> "A . . . review of acupuncture research reports showed that most acupuncture research [has] been undertaken to prove the therapeutic efficacy of acupuncture rather than generate knowledge that could be used to inform clinical decision-making" [25].

1. **Random assignment:** Reductionist models assume that patients are more or less interchangeable once a similar disease condition label has been assigned. For example, patients with pancreatic cancer, or arthritis of the knee, are alike in biomedically relevant ways, such as their disease state and the standard interventions to be used. Starting with a processual model, one would not make these assumptions. First, patients would be seen as individuals – one would be interested in how pancreatic cancer expresses in *this* patient, how the knee has gone bad in *this* case, as well as how the individual is *experiencing* their condition. Secondly, the processual model assumes that patients are responsive not only to medical care but also to the environment in which it is delivered including the person of the practitioner. For example, people who eagerly anticipated 'trying out' acupuncture would be disappointed – liable to *nocibo* effects – if assigned to nonacupuncture treatment, and the issue could go the other way round as well.

2. **Placebo control:** The reductionist idea is to minimize the effects of expectation in the patient *and* the practitioner, so one divides the research population into two groups, one of which receives the test pharmaceutical, while the other receives a pharmaceutically inactive 'placebo' that looks, feels and tastes just like the 'active' test drug. Both participating patients and physicians are 'blind' to which group they belong to. Then, if a significant (or in drug

assessment even a small) difference in response appears, the difference between the placebo and active group represents the active potential of the test drug. This model has been made to work pretty well for drugs, and has worked very well for the pharmaceutical industry [27].

It cannot work for hands-on medical practice, be this surgery, massage therapy or acupuncture care. First, it is very difficult to 'blind' hands-on practitioners, though there have been sometimes comical efforts to do so. Secondly, most acupuncture patients quickly learn whether a needle has been 'active'. Thirdly, if the practitioner is involved in following energy, and especially if the practitioner is involved in encouraging participation by the patient, one cannot possibly create a successful 'placebo'. Again, though there have been some ingenious, and many lamentable, efforts to create placebo needling, in fact – if the whole body is responsive – there cannot be 'sham' (placebo) points. Furthermore, if *qi* is present not only inside the body but surrounding it, and actively exchanging with the practitioner and 'universe', then again one cannot create a functional sham merely by holding the needle away from the body. Indeed, many historical and contemporary observations indicate that even non-contact 'needling' is an 'active intervention'.

3. **Set protocol designs:** A set protocol is a set of actions that are repeated the same way each time. Taking a daily pill at breakfast is an example of a set protocol, and with pharmaceutical research a pill protocol is easy to set up. However, it is difficult in a processual model like AOM because (a) it is 'hands-on' – treatment is delivered during the visit, not afterwards via a pill; (b) if practitioners follow the movement of *qi*, they may need to change intervention pattern (protocol) in the midst of a treatment or from treatment to treatment, and this is not permissible in a set protocol-based research design.

More subtly, clinical research typically depends on static, biomedical disease diagnoses, whereas the diagnosis in AOM often yields variability where biomedicine sees sameness (e.g. Schnyer and Allen [28]). In any case, AOM prefers to give moving diagnoses, descriptions of what is happening *now*, rather than settled states of being like diseases.

Each of these issues can be accounted for in a high-quality scientific research design [29–32]. Accounting for them yields a desired methodological end, *model fit validity*. But before one can account for them, one has to be aware of them – and raising awareness has been one of the pragmatic goals of writing this chapter.

CONCLUSION TO PART 2

Key points made in part 2 include:

- Metaparadigm positions markedly affect the practice of medicine and scientific research. Yet because such assumptions are largely out of awareness, they easily spring methodological traps on unwary researchers.
- The random-assignment placebo-controlled clinical trial design (RCT) was built according to the reductionist logic of biomedicine, and presents numerous challenges when applied to assessing 'holistic', 'hands-on' or 'energy-based' medical practices.
- Acupuncture is one such practice. Its logic is different from that of biomedicine since its focus is on flow, movement and dynamic change in whole body-persons (verbs) rather than on objects and states of being (genes, cells, microorganisms, tissues, diseases, pills, nouns). To study acupuncture accurately demands that research designs integrate the explanatory model of acupuncture.

- The best way to find out how the explanatory model of acupuncture is actualized in practice is to work with actual practitioners via interview, observation, even video-taping. Though more research is needed, rich data presented in this chapter are sufficient to identify several distinctive effects of applying an energy-based 'whole systems' logic to the delivery of medical care.
- Scientific methods appropriate to the assessment of energy-based 'whole systems' medical practices exist and are ready to be applied to the appropriate assessment of acupuncture as we move toward building a scientific evidence base for energy-based medicines. All that is required is to realize that medical paradigm matters and to perceptively account for it in research design.

ACKNOWLEDGMENTS

My special thanks to participants in the Acuperceptions Project for their insightful words and thoughts. A second warm round of thanks to Lisa Taylor-Swanson LAc, Dan Ebaugh LAc and Mimi Malfitano for their helpful guidance when prereading this manuscript, and to the editors of this text for suggestions to strengthen it. Finally, a special thanks to the whole of Canaan Valley WV for providing a superb environment in which to think, analyze and write this chapter.

Evidencing energy: experiences in acupuncture and therapeutic bodywork (Zero Balancing)

14

Tim Newman

❝ *There is no sanctuary from the inclusiveness of nature.*

Arnold Berleant [1]

INTRODUCTION

Advances in technology have a tendency to result in disembodied learning, estranging us from instinctive connections with the natural environment. This estrangement even causes distrust of the very elements that constitute our material and spiritual origins and our own innate abilities to sense them directly. With loss of such contact and trust, we have developed a culture of dislocated function at many levels. In particular, instead of art, philosophy and science being three complementary notes of the same chord, we have allowed and sometimes encouraged them to become polarized in antagonistic and destructive oppositions.

Here, I want to encourage a more broad-based (anthropological) approach to evidencing energy [2], which I find the most natural way to make science from our senses.

In this chapter, I intend:

— to confirm the human being as a supremely skilled and artistic sensory instrument

— to demonstrate how the apparently vague and elusive term 'energy' can have a real and tangible existence in our lives – and how its profound effects are evident through matter-of-fact, everyday examples

— to describe how, through our senses (touch in particular), what science still finds difficult to measure is available to us through our own direct experience

— to challenge the notion that the contribution made by subjective or artistic evidence is secondary to laboratory or clinical investigation

— to counter the negative attitudes to personal anecdote that distort proper appreciation of holistic approaches

— to indicate that science is a human endeavor (arises out of humanity), not inhuman. As such, it requires art and heart and humor, as well as information. The apparent split between Newtonian (object/particle) and quantum (process/wave) physics is an appearance but not reality.

'ENERGY' AND THE SPACES BETWEEN

A group of diners, deliberately falling silent and unobtrusively holding hands under the tablecloth, creates a focus of attention and stillness, a lacuna or void in the general chatter of the room. Even though entirely unconscious of why it is occurring, other diners too suddenly grow quiet . . . recognizing this 'dip' with slight unease, and then plunging back into their conversations having acknowledged . . . what?

Whether we listen for it deliberately, as with music, or just through sheer immersion in an 'ocean of connectedness' in which we live and move and have our being, this 'gap', 'pause', 'nothing' is precisely what gives any sequence of moves its particular effect – whether in music, painting, reading, conversation – yet allowing individual interpretation so that there are infinite varieties of expression. This echoes the passage in Chapter 11 of the *Daodejing* where it is only the emptiness of space within a room that makes its structure useful [3,4] (although the *dao* itself is not simply the void between things, according to Zhuangzi (Chuang Tsu) [5]).

Could these gaps or 'nothings' actually be something to do with this thing called 'energy'? Could the invisible and apparently undetectable and unmeasurable meridians of acupuncture in fact be the essential organizing pauses between the atomic pulsings of organs, body tissues and functions in the 'on/off' reality of the material world?

When I asked Edzard Ernst, the first full-time professor of Complementary and Alternative Medicine (CAM) in the UK, whether he believed in the existence of energy of any kind being involved in acupuncture and other healing, he shook his head and said 'no'. In my experience, the moment you mention the word 'energy', even to some experts in CAM, people feel wrong footed, even disturbed, especially if confronted by foreign terms such as '*qi*'. They assign such talk to intangible or fanciful realms where you have to believe in some exotic model, perform daily ritual practices, or subscribe to cultish or religious philosophies.

During my training in traditional acupuncture it was the quality and presence of most of my teachers that convinced me of a reality behind and beyond the words and information being presented – together with the fact that it was based on their experience. Subsequently I met another therapeutic method – Zero Balancing (ZB) – whose founder–instructor doctor and osteopath Fritz Smith MD (b. 1929) had the gift of making things simple, tangible and usable.

ZERO BALANCING

In 1976, at a holistic health conference in San Diego, Fritz Smith witnessed a man fire-walking unharmed and, having examined him before and after, he realized that any explanation for this would not be found within the tradition of Western medicine [6]. Rather than turning his back on his own medical training, he decided instead to *expand* his theoretical and conceptual framework to admit other ideas and possibilities, and in so doing learned to straddle the gap between the comforting regularity of Newtonian laws and the apparent randomness of quantum principles. The ZB method Fritz Smith created is a form of body-handling therapy using 'conscious touch' [7] based on an inspired integration of Western medicine, acupuncture, osteopathy, meditation and yoga. It has been taught for nearly 40 years as an adjunctive skill to health practitioners across the board, and indeed to interested members of the public who found themselves intrigued by their experience as receivers and fascinated by some of the principles used to 'explain' the method and its effects.

In particular, Fritz Smith turned the idea of 'energy' into something we students all understood, recognized and felt – immediately – and without being asked to believe in anything other than our experience through touch and sensation. I never forgot the impact of those classes, nor the expressions of discovery and surprise as my colleagues and subsequently my own students went through a similar process. The bridging of worlds through a neatly defined vocabulary of structure and energy (form and function – mass and movement – body tissue and tension – wind and sail) became for many of us an instinctive window on the way things happen or unfold in daily life, whether in our perception of it, or our engagement and interface with it – or our self-awareness in our moment-by-moment experience. In ZB, all these combined, in a broad relaxed attention to the flow of the present moment, are defined as the 'witness state'.

This apprenticeship in consciousness and touch fundamentally affected the practice and performance of all my therapies (acupuncture, massage, ZB), and later my own instructing of them, including my subsequent practice as an artist. When I belatedly took evening classes in art theory, I was amazed at the overlap of terms used to describe energy bodywork and the mind of the artist. My therapeutic trainings had equipped me for life and art in a way that neither my culture nor schooling had achieved.

The remainder of this chapter presents examples from my ZB training/teaching and from everyday occurrences that are all ordinary, common sense experiences; any reader can resonate with or verify them themselves – they do not need an expert or an '-ology' to authenticate them or give them authority. Whether talking of heat, gravity, vibration or simply the energy of held tension, I hope to convey something meaningful about 'energy'.

We humans are the skilled and artistic sensory instruments 'par excellence' for scientific exploration. In these days of quantum entanglement and ordered chaos, it is precisely our combination of simultaneous sensory awareness – in normal and expanded consciousness – that gives us the edge in holistic and holographic perception, so far unmatched by any objective device however sophisticated.

ZB: FEELING THE FLOW IN BONE

❝ Unless I am stimulated, I don't know who I am.

Fritz Smith [8]

At a recent ZB workshop [9] I was demonstrating how to make an energy/structure evaluation of the forearms by introducing a slight bowing or bending (microflexion) movement, feeling in my hands for the quality of elasticity in the bones' response. The following exchange took place:

Tim: How does it feel when I gently bow the forearm bones? Can you tell any difference between the feel of them?

Lisa: Yes. The right one feels OK, and the left one feels different – sort of . . . gritty?

Tim: . . . and my experience of the two forearms is that the right one felt bendy and the left one felt harder.

(After Tim passed a held stretch, combining traction, bowing and rotary forces through the 'gritty' forearm – the site of a previous fracture – Lisa was asked to describe how the left forearm felt.)

Tim: Any difference in how it feels now?

Lisa: Yes – the pressure feels smoother.

Tim: . . . and to me it feels more elastic or yielding.

In this experience, Tim had speculated that there might or might not be a palpable 'read-out' in a forearm with a fracture history. Although Lisa's forearm was biologically healed and radiographically normal, she still experienced occasional sensations in it that were 'odd' rather than painful. The difference in evaluation of each forearm was a subjective sensory one, felt as the bony structures of each forearm transmitted the tension of the testing movement (bowing) – and both Lisa and Tim experienced the arm's resistance to being flexed, using the vocabulary that sprang to mind in the moment.

In terms of ZB theory, the combined forces (fulcrum) were applied and held momentarily as a 'working field of influence' directed through the site of injury. In turn this helped the structural/cellular (tensile) constituents of the forearm bones to 'line up' in a more organized way along the direction of flow, bridging the site of the fracture and integrating it within the form/function of the whole forearm. In a much milder way, this is comparable to the weak electrical field that is applied clinically to speed/stimulate healing in fractures [10].

This account is offered as personal anecdotal evidence for the experience of energy in the body, although it begs many questions.

This process is illustrated in Figure 14.1. The flow of energy in an uninjured arm (A) is contrasted with the diminished (B) or distorted (C) flow in an arm that has an old fracture. Flows (B) and (C) might give the experience described by Lisa as 'gritty'. Part (D) shows the disturbed area held under tension for a few seconds. If the flow has normalized or harmonized to feel 'smoother' it might now look like (E). You cannot change the trauma history, but the experience, meaning or interpretation of it can change, and the way it becomes isolated or integrated into the fabric of the person's body-being.

SYNCHRONICITY AND THE FLOW OF CONNECTEDNESS

In another workshop at the same conference [11] a participant asked to remember an 'energy' or '*qi*' experience recalled a time when, following an acupuncture treatment, she had spontaneously begun to see little dots or particles moving in everything she looked at – the 'atomic' reality, as it were, underlying the usual appearance of things. While she was at the beginning of her story, even before she reached this description, there suddenly popped into my head an experience recounted by a student of mine who had wandered outside during a ZB training seminar morning break. She had spoken of 'suddenly seeing worms' wriggling in and through everything – spontaneously interpreted by her as a unifying, connecting movement that permeated all space and matter as part of a universal field or medium.

What are we to make of such experiences? Were these 'dots' or 'worms' purely meaningless projections of the mind/brain into the visual field, masquerading as external phenomena? Or, like the forms of bluish spiraling 'orgone' energy that Wilhelm Reich (1897–1957) perceived in a healthy, vibrant atmosphere [12], was this a glimpse of the pulse of life in space-time? Were these individuals momen-

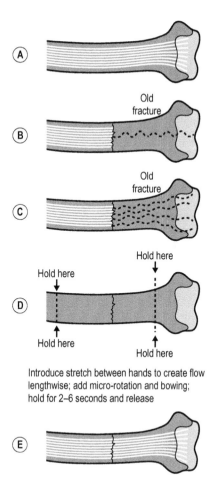

FIG 14.1 Energy flow through bone. (A) Normal flow through bone prior to fracture. (B) Diminished flow some time after bone healing. (C) Distorted flow some time after normal tissue healing. (D) Combined energetic forces (straight traction, rotation, bowing) directed through site of trauma and held for 2–6 seconds. (E) More normal flow re-established through bone tissue.

tarily sensitized to the usually invisible 'nature of things', suddenly seeing without the usual filters and able to perceive invisible wavelengths like ultraviolet – as with people who claim to see auras and *chakras*? Why are these experiences so often dismissed as delusion, rather than being explored as extra antennae or capacities of human instrumentation – sometimes referred to as 'extra sensory perception' (ESP)? Indeed, was my memory of a similar experience triggered by her knowing what she was about to say?

Even though I have not had their particular experience, it is a given to me that there is a connectedness to life, and that within that connectedness many synchronicities occur of an entirely unexceptional nature, however surprising or delightful we may find them in the absence of any demonstrable paths of connection. As Father Claude Larre (1919–2001) said, speaking on the manifestation of life through the interaction of *yin* and *yang*, to the Chinese mind this is 'so obvious as to need no explanation' (C Larre, personal communication, 1983) – except of course to minds that have forgotten or not been awoken to perceive

SOME OBSERVATIONS ON THE BONE FLOW EXPERIENCE

—— Evaluations were quite inexact at one level, involving both forearm bones together, in more or less the same way. However, this did not seem to matter in terms of evaluation or outcome.

—— The balancing force was applied to both bones in the forearm, through the area of previous trauma (but not limited to that), so situating its influence within the whole anatomical/functional context of the injury.

—— The three applied tensile forces (traction/rotation/bowing) were all related to the leverage forces that normal activity directs through the forearm. However, Lisa was in a relatively neutral position when I applied pressure, so the bones of the forearm received these forces with the arm in a passive and supported state.

—— Although no outcome was predicted or assumed – ZB simply introduces a 'clearer stronger field' and accepts both 'no change' and 'change' responses as equally valid – it was evident that, in the experience of both parties, something had happened that suggested a change in the way the 'gritty' arm had become 'smoother'.

in this way. None of this is 'secret wisdom' or elitist knowledge; direct access to the connectedness of life occurs simply through alertness of being or an ability to notice what is in front of you. Our inability to evidence the energetic reality of our world is partly also due to our failure to think and question in the right way – just as standard science throws out all the 'useless water' from a cell and centrifuges the residue imagining that this will lead to discovery of its inmost secrets [13].

As minute dots living on the surface of our planet, we are usually unaware of the many forces and influences at work in our environment as well as within us, the micro- and macrocycles of circulation that sustain our cells, us and the earth itself. Until the 1920s, for instance, no one knew of the existence of the jet stream in the upper atmosphere [14] while, in the oceans, currents of different temperature, such as the Gulf Stream, maintain identity for centuries despite shifts of shape within the whole, and despite not having a discreet envelope to house them.

Indeed, Theodor Schwenk (1910–1986) postulated that the simplest forms of life itself originally evolved by forming cellular membranes around organized flows, and these flows evolved to become themselves the vessels for circulation of food and waste that had previously been absorbed or excreted across the cell membrane. Such flow lines are visible bridging the femur and the pelvis in human anatomy [15].

Water and wind are both prime forces for the shaping of our environment and for the creation and transport of nutrients. In Jan DeBlieu's image, wind is 'an organic force that binds all humankind together . . . When I think of the global winds, the bands of air that surround the whole earth, it is as something more complex, yet at the same time singular and whole. The wind is a membrane that pulses and shifts and fastens us inside a life-sustaining vessel' [16]. It seems reasonable to me that the energy pathways of acupuncture are a similar organizing system of communication and maintenance at a prestructural/pre-body-tissue level – and that they themselves are involved in delivering the information necessary for growth and homeostasis. If the energy of wind and the charge of water are so integral a part of our planet's circulation, why would we not be subject to an internal energy weather system for the health and intercommunication of our little human worlds?

INTRODUCING THE EXPERIENCE OF ENERGY

As previously stated, the word 'energy' seems often to wrong-foot either or both parties in a conversation. There is no such difficulty if one simply describes 'what is happening' or 'what I saw or felt' in everyday language. Energy appears to be an abstract idea only when conceived as an intangible substance or force – although nothing can happen in fact unless energy is involved, regardless of whether we can see it. This becomes obvious to anyone, of any background or intelligence, once they focus on their sensory experience – and allow their own spontaneous poetic language or unexpected imagery to stand in for more sober descriptions.

However, following the guidelines of my own training, I try to use neutral or purely descriptive words to keep discussion in the realms of everyday speech and common sense: hot and cold, loose or tight, light and heavy, free and stuck, moving or still. I still remember a student who, asked to write up his case studies using this kind of language, described the movement in a person's left and right sacroiliac joints as 'The left felt like riding a bicycle over sand, the right felt like riding over solid ground'.

John Hamwee writes in his book on ZB: 'You can have a subjective experience of the flow of energy through a vertical structure. Stand under the spire of a church or cathedral, and it is a remarkable sensation . . . as if all the separate parts of you are lined up harmoniously.' He compares this feeling of a 'flow of energy' with the pattern of iron filings created by a magnet, 'as though all the "filings" that make up my own body have become aligned to some hidden pattern' [10, p 30].

When first introduced to the idea of feeling a person's aura (or the boundary/limit of their personal energy field), my mind scorned the obvious contradiction of sensing manually something invisible and without apparent structure – it equated to 'feeling nothing' – which was clearly impossible. However, instructed to feel my own energy field, bringing my two hands together from shoulder width to about 8–10 inches (20–25 cm) apart, I discovered there was something palpable between them. Furthermore, as my hands approached and parted, this sensation was as clear as if I was pressing a balloon lightly. Now, in a more curious and intrigued frame of mind, I attempted the same with another person, and both of us could verify the moment when we 'touched' – although we were not doing so physically.

This is very similar to the sense of engagement or connection felt in an exercise designed to help ZB students get to know the structural and energetic bodies through *sensation*, prior to evaluating or balancing tensions (energy) held within the bony anatomy (structure). Students are instructed to hold a short length (two to three connected sheets) of toilet tissue lightly, so that it dips between them rather than being straight. In this state of looseness, they are only connected *structurally* through the paper, but lack a felt sense of this connection. They then slowly 'take out the looseness' in the tissue until they first feel the connection between them as the tissue becomes taut and slight traction is transmitted through it as a perceptible 'tugging'. If done with attention, and not suddenly or excessively, the tissue does not break (Fig. 14.2).

A further aspect of this exercise is that it is carried out with whole body awareness rather than being 'done from the hands and wrists'. This means that effectively the two partners become finely supported through the delicate fulcrum of their connection – and in such cases will usually report distal or global body sensations as well as those felt at the fingers. For example, in the first conference presentation mentioned above, participants reported feeling: 'warmth in my hands' – 'a sense of electric current in my arms' – 'an awareness of flow down my legs' – 'a realization of distress in my partner' (suffering from toothache) – 'a stillness and a coming to centre'. Ironically, when I tried this demonstration with Professor Ernst

Evidencing energy

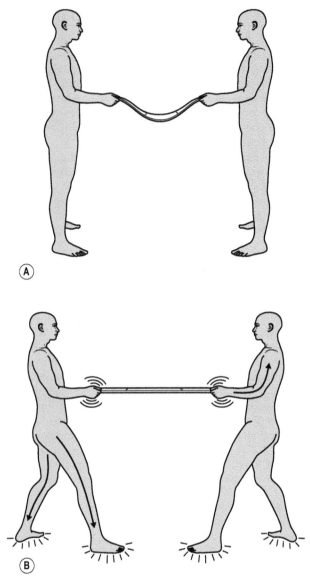

FIG 14.2 (A) Taking out the looseness in structural (paper) contact. (B) Holding the energetic contact (tension) with awareness. Felt connection: structure and energy are now experienced together with secondary sensations such as warmth, flow, electricity, stillness, etc., as described in the text.

and asked what difference he felt between the loose and the taut states, he could only see it as 'pulling' and was not able to make any of the conceptual or sensory links that others have reported when trying it.

The skill of developing simultaneous consciousness of self and other – or of physical and energetic boundaries – as epitomized in this exercise is of primary importance for any professional who is handling another person, with all the implicit trust and permission dynamics this involves. It can also be vital within families where assumptions, or ignorance, about personal energetics result in frequent trespass, insult or overriding of individual tolerances.

Yet it is a conundrum of ZB practice that someone performing an action for the first time can be as effective as someone with years of experience. There is a sensitivity – an innocence and purity of attention – in the beginner's touch that it is an art to retain when repeatedly performing similar sequences over years of practice.

EXPERIENCES IN RECEIVING AND LEARNING ENERGY MEDICINE (ACUPUNCTURE AND ZB)

When I first dipped a toe into the waters of CAM, I had no particular concept of energy except as something belonging to an 'impossible subject' (physics). I would say I was pretty earthbound as well as relatively uninformed. I tried acupuncture treatment for a number of reasons – and had no idea it would lead me into what I regard as being 'properly educated about life', nor that it would become my means of livelihood and introduce me to another training that became my chief practice. I chose to train at the College of Traditional Acupuncture founded by J R Worsley (1923–2003) because I had observed over time how a group of acupuncture students improved in themselves as they learned. They seemed to take better care of themselves, got to grips with their life issues and became 'happier and healthier'. It was ultimately their 'radiance of spirit' and personal transformation that determined me to begin training – not because I understood or even believed in energy.

A lot of the training was taken on trust while we recovered lost sensitivities or awoke new ones. I did not really believe I could feel energy, but acted as if I did (this turns out to be a viable strategy), backed up in the meantime with other diagnostic skills that involved seeing, hearing, asking, smelling and touching. My early patients clearly benefited from what I was doing, and I had sufficient confidence instilled by encouragement from more experienced practitioners to believe that my ability to feel/see energy would improve over time.

I also benefited from osteopathy (traditional manipulation as well as cranial), which I experienced as a purely physical handling, but my first ZB session during a class with Fritz Smith was altogether different: although clearly being engaged physically, there was a strange detachment to it – and a startling experience of energy release.

The short 'intake' before working with me was instructive. After taking note of some recent elbow surgery and a history of bone trauma, Fritz Smith asked if there was anything else he could do for me. Somewhat apologetically, and acknowledging the previous benefit of osteopathy, I mumbled something about my trousers not 'hanging comfortably' on my waist/hips – that they were never really a 'good fit', and that I was always aware of a place where they rubbed on the right side of my low back. (I later discovered this was over my sacrum at the level of the sacroiliac joint.)

I can now see my description as an energetic evaluation of how bone and cloth (structure) were integrated with gravity and movement (energy) in a less than optimum way. Despite feeling a complete idiot for mentioning the way my clothes did not fit, I then received a session where the feeling of pressure or stretch in my body evoked sensations for which I had no vocabulary, in parts of my body that I was not used to feeling (consciously, anyway).

In the middle of wondering what was being touched and sometimes feeling quite hard sore points in my back, Fritz Smith found a spot in the lumbar area. Probing it with his fingers, he began to recount an anecdote to the class about another time and another place to the extent that I started to wonder if he was paying any attention to me (although, importantly, his touch did not waver a jot). But then, without warning, there was a terrific rushing feeling up my spine and out of my head and ears, and a wave of grief or sadness (without any associated memory), accompanied by a roaring in my ears. I felt utterly at the mercy of the flow until it dropped in intensity and then stopped quite quickly. This remains a 'peak experience' in my life and I have no doubt that it was real – neither hallucinated nor imagined, and originating as a release within my body (i.e. it was my energy and not Fritz Smith's).

In my second session – a year later – I had a similar but minor rush very early in the session, and the rest of the session was pleasant but not dramatic – until I sat up. Then I felt immensely powerful and heavy – as if just resting my hand upon Smith's head would have pushed him down through the floor like a comic book character. I also felt as though I could have walked through the wall, which would have just broken effortlessly before me. This feeling of buzzy weight calmed down within a few minutes. More long term – and this lasted for months – was that whenever I came to rest, whether sitting or standing, I felt as though I was 'plugged in' to the ground or earth – experiencing the connection as an active current. As the skeleton acts as a conductor or 'lightning rod' for gravity, I interpreted this as the effect of better posture and transmission of gravity through my structure into the supporting structure of the ground (my own version of the experience of flow in the John Hamwee quote above).

I also came to understand these powerful sensations in my own and other people's bodily experience as the provoking of tissue resistance to suddenly increased flow of energy/blood or whatever through it; this causes intense pressure as the surge begins, but becomes less noticeable once the initial wave or 'bore' has passed through.

CONCLUSION: THE INTERPERSONAL DYNAMICS OF ENERGY

Fritz Smith noted that, as well as being able to observe energy directly through sensation, when a person is in response to an energetic modality such as ZB or acupuncture there may be a number of unconscious and involuntary responses: eyelid/eye movements, changes in breathing pattern, borborygmus (tummy rumbles). Even in the toilet tissue experiment, some people may show these responses once the connection has been made – and in acupuncture practice, when taking the pulse, palpating for a point and needling, these same signs are frequently observed, in a way not elicited by less engaged touch. For example, one of my own acupuncture patients responded so strongly, just to the feeling of connection on having her wrist held for pulse taking, that she asked, startled: 'Has the treatment begun already?'

If they find they are not seeing such signs as these regularly in their practice, ZB students are asked to focus on and sense the quality of their energetic engagement with the receiver's bone and ligament structure. This can also be a useful tool for any practitioners training in the touch professions – together with an understanding of how, when two or more people are closely connected through touch, energetic changes can happen very fast.

Fritz Smith has identified four main ways that energy behaves through contact (Interface – Blending – Streaming – Channeling), and has made a significant contribution to therapeutic training and awareness by highlighting the potential for projection, 'pick-up', exhaustion and confusion particularly, but not only, in the helping and caring professions.

I began this chapter by extolling the virtues and capacities of our amazing human sensitivities, and pleading for the human science value of what they register. However, just because we are sensitive instruments of healing and restorative care, we can also be imposed upon, confused, overloaded, even abused, either for fear of hurting people when we say 'no', or because of a learned self-sacrificing ethic, or because we have not acquired the skill of establishing meaningful boundaries that enable us to assist intimately without being overwhelmed by the demands and distress of those we assist.

Unawareness of such interpersonal energy dynamics can compromise relationships (therapeutic or otherwise). For instance, it can be very helpful to recognize through body signals and cues when you are maintaining a clear boundary or distinction between you and your client, and whether you have made a clean disconnect from this interaction before moving on to another client or going home after work. For this reason, I have taught workshops across Europe on 'The art of meaningful conversation through touch' that foster awareness of boundary changes and energy dynamics, and I would dearly like to see an awareness of energy boundaries and behavior incorporated in standard training throughout the health professions – and beyond. As we incorporate new ideas into our overburdened health services, it is vital that we develop ways of service that are less destructive to both providers and carers, and more respectful all round.

I have been active for more than 25 years as an artist and as a therapist and teacher of ZB, and I believe I have enough knowledge and experience in my head and in my being to affirm that the evidence for energy is in and all around us – overwhelmingly so. Our current science may not be able to explain 'life' or 'consciousness' [17], but anyone who has received acupuncture or ZB and experienced the consequent feelings and sensations engendered, or who has practiced them 'nonmechanically', is left in no doubt that there is an 'energy' component to their experience. For those to whom energy is a word for the unreal, none of this can make sense, but for those who marvel at our sensitivities, the world itself does not make sense without some universal connecting action/fabric – whether innate and neutral – or creative and godlike.

Everything . . . is eternal, alive, and evolving: not just animals and plants, but rivers and clouds and, planets, electrons, even light and energy itself. . . . The whole universe is a living, remembering, self-revising process [18].

Eight modalities for working with *qi*: *chakra* acupuncture, with *qigong*, meditation and the five sources of energy

Gabriel Stux

INTRODUCTION

This chapter draws on more than 30 years of experience in acupuncture and Chinese medicine and 20 years of experience in working with different modalities of energy medicine. New methods of energy medicine are described that have been developed and put into practice in a large acupuncture clinic. Of these eight modalities, different ways of using *qigong* and meditation are the most essential. Special attention is given to conscious breathing with regard to different parts of the body, and the *chakras*, and to using the hands to help bring increased awareness to these spaces within the body. This approach facilitates the interconnections between the Organs by drawing on their five sources of energy (*qi* or *prana*) and circulating this in the nourishing Mother–Child (*sheng,* 生) cycle of the Five Elements (*wuxing,* 五行).

The main intention of this work is to bring soul and body together and connect the soul with the heart space by opening the crown *chakra*. Additionally,

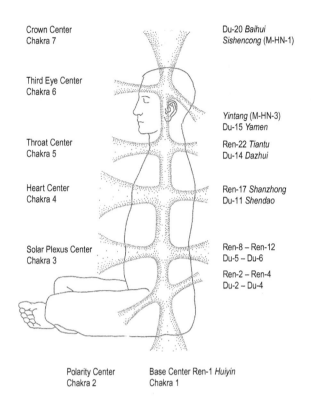

Crown Center
Chakra 7

Du-20 *Baihui*
Sishencong (M-HN-1)

Third Eye Center
Chakra 6

Yintang (M-HN-3)
Du-15 *Yamen*

Throat Center
Chakra 5

Ren-22 *Tiantu*
Du-14 *Dazhui*

Heart Center
Chakra 4

Ren-17 *Shanzhong*
Du-11 *Shendao*

Solar Plexus Center
Chakra 3

Ren-8 – Ren-12
Du-5 – Du-6

Ren-2 – Ren-4
Du-2 – Du-4

Polarity Center
Chakra 2

Base Center Ren-1 *Huiyin*
Chakra 1

FIG 15.1 Locations and openings of the *chakras*. *(Figure supplied by Gabriel Stux.)*

awareness is directed to the flow of energy, focusing on the *light* level of the life force. When the crown *chakra* has been opened, light and energy can flow from the soul (the eighth *chakra*) into the heart space and thence through the whole body (Fig. 15.1). This awareness exemplifies the spiritual application of the different modalities.

THE *CHAKRAS*

The word '*chakra*' is derived from a Sanskrit word meaning 'wheel'. *Chakras* are experienced as constantly moving currents of energy. They play an important role in Indian medicine and yoga and also correspond to the system of the Chinese Organs, especially the *sanjiao*.

There are seven primary or main *chakras* and dozens of smaller secondary ones, most of which can be related to significant acupuncture points. The *chakras* correspond to five spaces within the body: the pelvic cavity, abdomen, chest, throat and cranium. The seven main *chakras* are located along the spine from the perineum in the lower pelvis to the top of the head. Five of the primary *chakras* have a ventral and a dorsal opening and two – the first and the seventh – have one opening. The first opens toward the Earth, the seventh toward the sky (Fig. 15.1). Each *chakra* is related to specific emotional, mental, physical and spiritual levels of existence, and is associated with a certain color, sound, symbol and frequency of vibration (such associations vary according to different authorities).

The *chakras* receive, assimilate and transform the life force (termed *prana* or *qi*), regulating its flow through our energy system and thus keeping our mental and physical health in balance. As the *chakras* progress from the lowest to the highest levels, they govern increasingly spiritual functions.

THE EIGHT MODALITIES

The methods used in this approach are described as:

1. CROWN *CHAKRA* OPENING FOR EXPANSION AND CONNECTION

The point *baihui* (百會, Du-20) is of particular relevance when it comes to opening the energy field to light. *Baihui* opens and enlightens consciousness. It also opens the inner spaces of the body to the direct influence of the soul.

The session begins with needling *baihui*. Then a further 4 (+4), 8 (+8) or 12 (+12) needles are inserted concentrically around it to open the crown *chakra*. The four points surrounding *baihui* are the *sishencong* (M-HN-1) points. An additional circle of four needles, *baihui* +8, will lead to a further opening of the crown *chakra*. The third circle of four needles, baihui +12, leads to an even more significant opening of the *chakra* and helps to release deep tensions on top of the skull, as several points are located near the Gall Bladder channel. The application of needles to all these points leads to an extraordinarily wide opening of the crown *chakra*.

The 12 points, which surround *baihui* in *three concentric circles*, have been named '*Treasure Points*' by one patient. We are in the process of collecting feedback on the effects of these points, which have also been also named '*The Twelve Light Points of the Soul*'.

To a lesser degree, the 'enlightening' effect can also be noticed from inserting a needle into *baihui* only, although all points that activate the crown *chakra* have this enlightening effect. When we include more points, however, the flow of light and energy into the Heart *chakra* and the whole body is much stronger and much more noticeable for the patient (*baihui* +8, +12). The result is a more extensive and conscious connection between body and soul.

2. GROUNDING AND ACTIVATING THE BASE, STRENGTHENING THE KIDNEY

After opening the crown *chakra*, the *yang* pole of the body, we turn to its opposite, the *yin* pole, to strengthen the Kidney and activate the first and second *chakras*. Needles are inserted into the points *taixi* (KI-3), *sanyinjiao* (SP-6) and *taichong* (LIV-3). The 'NADA points' of Michael O Smith (auricular Heart, Kidney, Liver, Sympathetic and *shenmen* points) are particularly relevant when activating the Kidney and the base. They have a calming and grounding effect on the Kidney energy.

The auricular Heart and Kidney points harmonize relations between the two Organs. As a result, a strong connection between the Heart and the pelvis – where the Kidney energy is centered – develops over two or three sessions. It is recommended that the patient should sit upright in the second half of the acupuncture sessions, as this activates the flow of light and life force from the crown to the Heart and base even more.

3. HEALING MEDITATION PRACTICE DURING ACUPUNCTURE SESSIONS

The meditation practice introduced here consists of three steps building on each other:

Deep conscious breathing

Breathing is the first and main source of our life force. We *breathe in* vital energy, the life force. Whenever we breathe in deeply and relax, our vital energy is activated. The word *inspiration*, from the Latin *inspirare* 'to breathe in', is consistent with the idea that breathing is the gateway to our creativity and spirituality. We talk about feeling energetic and inspired. Conscious breathing is to be understood as a bridge between the soul and the physical body, thus helping to connect body and mind.

After the acupuncture needles have been inserted, awareness should be focused on the breath, so the patient is asked to observe their breathing. The first step is to *inhale deeply* for about 5 to 10 minutes. Deep and continuous inhalations charge and strengthen the life force. The therapist may support the patient by saying:

'Breathe deeper, breathe deeply into the chest', or
'Breathing deeply activates and strengthens your life force and gives you more energy', or
'Breathing deeply makes you feel more alive'.

The last two affirmations help the patient to develop a stronger motivation.

Then the patient turns his attention to breathing out. Here, the emphasis lies in a *prolonged and complete exhalation*, relaxing more and more with each outbreath. The therapist may say:

'Breathe out slowly and deeply', or
'Take more time to exhale', or
'Let your tension go with the exhalation', or
'Each breath helps you to relax more and more'.

Conscious and prolonged exhalation helps the body to relax and release tension, thus harmonizing the life force and allowing for more *flow of qi*. Health is characterized by a free-flowing *qi* and pulsing of the breath and vital energy within the body's Organs, channels and energy centers. Focusing the awareness on the breath is an essential way to enhance the healing effect of acupuncture.

Awareness of the body

Once the breathing technique has been established – usually during the first acupuncture session – and the patient feels comfortable with it, the therapist introduces the patient to increased body awareness. The patient is asked to close his eyes, feel inside the body and to become aware of bodily sensations and emotions while *consciously watching the breath* at the same time.

In the course of treatment, the therapist encourages the patient to go deeper and deeper into the body, while mirroring the process by doing the same and directing his awareness inside his own body. This approach helps the patient to focus his awareness and feel increasingly relaxed. He may also experience slight tingling sensations and a *gentle flow of energy*.

Qigong

Qigong is one of the modalities of Chinese medicine, the results of practice being to harmonize and energize the life force. It is a way of *cultivating qi*, working with and becoming aware of *qi* by using the breath and certain positions of the hands, gently and slowly. The breath and the hand positions help to focus awareness and direct the flow of the life force.

During the acupuncture session, the patient holds his arms in a circle in front of the different regions of the body, the hands facing the body as usual in *qigong*, beginning with the chest area and then moving the hands downward to the abdomen, and later further down to the region of the pelvis. The distance at which the hands should be held from the body can slowly be expanded. However, the ideal distance comes about naturally and is determined by the patient himself.

The hand positions together with breathing technique help the patient to direct awareness to particular areas and hold it there, consciously perceiving the flow of energy inside the body. Blockages are loosened and will eventually dissolve. A deep relaxation is felt after a few sessions.

4. HEART *CHAKRA* HARMONIZING THE CENTER

When working with the seven *chakras* and the different modalities of using *qi*, the centrality of the Heart *chakra* is emphasized. It is the fourth *chakra* down from the crown or up from the base. It is also located in the center of the chest, and is the one with exceptional healing energy. It harmonizes and balances, its main qualities being *compassion*, *love* and *tolerance*.

The associated acupuncture point is *shanzhong* (Ren-17). Adding four surrounding points at a distance of 1 *cun* from *shanzhong* intensifies its effect, just as with *sishencong* and *baihui*. Furthermore, *shendao* (Du-11) on the back can be chosen as a supplement. These six points help to activate and open the Heart *chakra*. Additionally the patient holds his hands in a circle in front of the chest and uses the breath to focus awareness there. The therapist may support the patient by saying: 'Allow your heart to open.'

The combination of acupuncture, awareness of the breath, and *qigong* hand positions leads to a further opening of the heart, an expansion and strengthening of its energy, so that eventually the patient experiences a widening of the heart space and will feel more joyful and humorous. This in turn helps him to become more conscious of this *chakra*.

A further opening of the Heart *chakra* can be achieved during an acupuncture session when both the therapist and patient direct their awareness to the Heart *chakra* and hold it there. Happy thoughts or childlike play also activate this *chakra*, bringing about a compassionate and healing energy. The Heart's warmth and joy expand and flow into the Lung, and from there into the whole body. The Heart also warms regions of the body that are cold, such as the Lung or Kidney. The way in which the *'warm heart'* supports the flow of *qi* has a particularly healing effect, because it activates the *shen* (神) or Spirit by which all the other Organs are invigorated.

5. FIVE SOURCES OF THE LIFE FORCE, THEIR QUALITIES AND THE METHOD OF ORGAN FLOW MEDITATION

Organ flow meditation (Fig. 15.2) follows the principles of the nourishing Mother–Child cycle of the Five Elements and strengthens the five inner Organs. These Organs are the sources of the life force in our body. The *'Mother–Child law'* states that each Organ in the *sheng* cycle strengthens the next one, as a mother nurtures her child. The sequence of Organs and Elements in the nourishing Mother–Child cycle is:

Metal – Water – Wood – Fire – Earth
Lung – Kidney – Liver – Heart – Spleen.

The meditation begins the cycle with the Lung (Metal) and continues from there. In this way, the Lung (Metal) nourishes the Kidney (Water), the Kidney nourishes the Liver (Wood), the Liver nourishes the Heart (Fire) and the Heart nourishes the Spleen (Earth). The nourishing Mother–Child cycle, or cycle of enhancement, supports the flow of energy between the five *zang* (*yin* Organs). Organ flow meditation is a simple and effective method to strengthen these and harmonize their energies: the activating energy of the Lung, the tranquil, regenerative energy of the Kidney, the vibrant, moving energy of the Liver, the joyous, expanding energy of the Heart and the nourishing energy of the Spleen.

Lung to Kidney is the first and most important part of the meditation and consists of two steps. Each one should be practiced for 5 to 10 minutes. The first step is to breathe deeply but gently into the chest, filling the lungs completely (Fig. 15.2A). In the second step we send the breath down into the centre of the pelvis – the region of the Kidney – and then deeper, until the connection to the Earth is felt through the pelvic floor and in the whole pelvic area and lower back. Practicing diligently leads to a distinct awareness of the pelvic region, which will feel warmer and more alive. Even the feet will feel warmer after a few sessions.

The importance of the first part is that it provides the necessary conditions for the other four parts to happen naturally. The two steps charge the Lung and the base

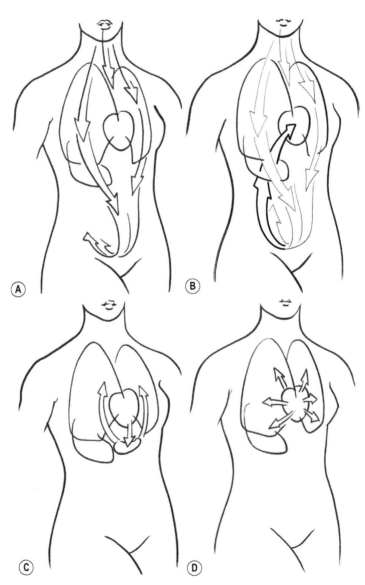

FIG 15.2 Organ flow meditation. (A) First part – Lung, and Lung to Kidney. (B) Second and third parts – Kidney to Liver, and Liver to Heart. (C) Fourth part – Heart to Spleen, and Spleen to Lung. (D): Fifth part – Heart to Lung. *(Figure supplied by Gabriel Stux.)*

with energy, building up a fullness from which the energy can then move effortlessly from the base to the Liver and from there to the other Organs one by one.

Breathing should be done consciously but without any kind of force. Each breath should be taken deeply yet gently, allowing the breath to flow easily through the Organs and the whole body. Organ flow meditation should be practiced in this way from beginning to end.

Kidney to Liver is the second part of the meditation. By breathing deeply the energy moves from the pelvic region to the right upper abdomen, filling this region with the now strong *qi* of the Kidney (Fig. 15.2B). Strong Kidney *qi* is the prerequisite for a strong and free-flowing energy of the Liver, which enables appropriate emotional expression as well as movement and strength of muscles and tendons. Deep breathing should be maintained for another 5 minutes. Practicing this part frequently will lead to a sense of action, orientation and drive, which is contained until needed.

Liver to Heart is the third part of the meditation. The energy that has gathered in the Liver now moves to the Heart (Fig. 15.2B). The flow of *qi* strengthens the charge and movement of the Heart, which is the foundation for appropriate emotional expression and a lifting of the spirit. Here, too, we maintain deep breathing. The breath is sent into the chest, the area surrounding the heart, for about 5 minutes. This leads to an expansion of the chest, an opening; tension or tightness in this area is loosened. The Heart will feel softer and there may be a feeling of fullness and peaceful joy

Heart to Spleen is the fourth part of the meditation. The *qi*, which has gathered in the Heart, now flows into the area of the upper left and mid abdomen (Fig. 15.2C). The energy has a grounding and nurturing quality, and strengthens the Spleen and Stomach, which aid in digesting food as well as ideas. Breathing deeply into the area of the abdomen for 5 minutes releases anxiety and worry. The region feels relaxed and comfortably filled, as after a good meal. Gathering energy through deep breathing into the Spleen area increases the awareness of what is truly nurturing and appropriate for the body to function in the best possible way. The Heart energy expands directly into the Lung, warming the chest (Fig. 15.2D).

The fifth and last part of the meditation happens by itself when the *qi* gathered during the previous parts moves from the *Spleen to the Lung* (Fig. 15.2C). This brings the nourishing Mother–Child cycle, the cycle of enhancement of the Five Elements, to a close and completes the Organ flow method.

Organ flow meditation can be practiced in a one-to-one session as well as in small groups during seminars. The therapist starts by practicing each section of the Organ flow individually during the acupuncture session. Once the patient is able to perceive each part distinctly, he moves on to practicing the whole cycle. Disorder in one of the parts of the cycle may supply significant therapeutic information; blockages can be treated with additional methods.

Qualities of the Five Elements

The qualities of the Five Elements are a most helpful tool in diagnosis. They help us to use the energy of the patient and therapist, thus improving the results of the treatment. We are able, for example, to show greater consideration to the particular sensitivity of Metal-type people or motivate Water types to become more active by making use of their strength and stability. The qualities of the Five Elements help us understand the patient's constitutional potentials as well as his weaknesses.

Metal element (the Air quality)
The major signs of Metal are small bones, very fair skin, aquiline features and broad shoulders. Metal is a dual element: Metal people are visionaries and idealists, yet they have a sense of practicality. They love both luxury and simplicity. They are very sensitive and are often considered aloof and distant; they need to

maintain their boundaries because they feel easily overwhelmed. They are particular, detail oriented and perfectionist. They are subject to health problems involving boundary violations but have strong immune systems. Even though they may fall ill frequently, they recover quickly. People who are Metal types are susceptible to skin and respiratory system allergies. They easily get sunburned, and prefer to stay indoors. They prefer to be in environments they consider safe, with a minimum of dust or clutter and a maximum of beauty and stylish design. Signs of Metal deficiency include the slow healing of skin and chronic respiratory and skin conditions, including recurring bronchitis. The Metal element is more mental than physical and requires refinement, cleanliness, tranquility and space to thrive.

Water element

The major physical signs of Water are big bones or wide hips – Water people carry weight in their hips and thighs. They are prone to shadows around the eyes. Water people are quiet and obervant, and may appear mysterious or secretive. They are good listeners and give sound advice because they have an innate wisdom. They appear to be easygoing, but when working they are very persistent. They require a lot of sleep, rest, meditation or time just to 'be'. They are strong both physically and emotionally, and handle catastrophes and emergencies calmly. They need to watch being too willful or stubborn. Their main health problems come from the frozen state of Water, a condition that encourages tumors or high blood pressure from a lack of flow of the emotions. Deficiency occurs when their lifestyle is too active and Water is not replenished. This causes aging and degeneration of the body as well as problems with infertility and impotence. Strong Water energy usually leads to longevity when life is lived wisely and energy is conserved rather than spent. Water deficiency is reflected in conditions such as loss of bone density, deafness, thinning hair, osteoarthritis and weakness of the bladder.

Wood element

The major physical signs of Wood are sinewy tendons and a hard body. Wood people constantly need to be 'doing' something. They enjoy argument and discussion. They feel compelled to exercise and love to work hard. They are seen as aggressive and assertive and tend to clench their fists. Wood people are action oriented and quick to take offense. Their rashness can lead to accidents. They are also prone to stress injuries such as strained, pulled or torn muscles and tendons. The other scenario that occurs with Wood deficiency is various forms of exhaustion including chronic fatigue. Wood people have very strong livers and enjoy processing toxins, whether emotional – caused by anger – or chemical, as in drugs and alcohol. However, the latter can create Wood stagnation, especially when old anger and resentments are not released. This makes Wood people susceptible to environmental toxins or problems like headaches. They are also prone to addiction. Wood people resist aging and fight the weakening of their bodies, trying to maintain their previous levels of physical and emotional activity. They need to develop flexibility instead of rigidity.

Fire element

The major physical signs of Fire are slim hips and shoulders, mobile hands, *sparkling eyes* and redness in the throat and neck areas. Fire people tend to be small in stature and very lively. Their main goal in life is to play. They love new experiences and communicating – whether verbally or through body language. Fire people are changeable and often erratic. They are also very charismatic and charming. They tend to flourish in warmer climates as they dislike wearing much clothing and have a naturally high body temperature. They are *full of ideas* and prefer starting to finishing. They enjoy excitement and can become thrill seekers. They are naturally attuned to rhythm and love to dance. Their biggest health problems come from inflammation, which is caused by unrestrained Fire and an overactive nervous system. Fire people are prone to disturbances in speaking and thinking caused by an overactive imagination. These include stuttering, phobias and mental illnesses. The Fire element's primary Organ is the Heart, which controls and regulates the expression of all emotions. Suppression of emotions can therefore cause problems with the heart including arrhythmia, tachycardia and heart disease. Fire people maintain a youthful persona, but their erratic lives may cause burnout and ultimately bring sadness.

Earth element

The major physical signs of Earth are plumpness in the abdominal area, the jowls, upper arms and calves. Earth people tend to be sedentary and enjoy sitting a lot. They value comfort, consistency and pleasure. They thoroughly enjoy food and companionship. They are the collectors of the world and love to accumulate possessions and people, becoming very attached to their loved ones as well as things. They have a fondness for sweets and starches. They are often considered warm and affectionate. When the Earth element is in excess there is a strong tendency to overeat and gain weight to the point of obesity. Earth people tend to worry and become overly involved in the lives of others. They feel excessive sympathy for those they care about. Earth stagnation is shown in the tendency for the circulation of lymph and blood to coagulate causing such problems as varicose veins. When the Earth element is deficient there are problems with the Stomach and the ingestion and digestion of food or ideas. Conditions that are related include anorexia, bulimia, diabetes and flatulence. Earth deficiency is common when too much nurturing is given to others at the expense of the self. Earth people move slowly and can become habit bound. Movement and change is to be encouraged for a more balanced Earth element.

6. PERCEIVING VITAL ENERGY WITH THE THIRD EYE FOR DIAGNOSIS

The Third Eye is the sixth *chakra* and closely connected with the crown. The ability to perceive energies is an important prerequisite for energy diagnosis and a successful treatment. Here the Third Eye plays an essential role: it is the 'seat of insight'. The Third Eye and the Heart *chakra* play a vital part in energy medicine.

The Third Eye has three functions: receptive insight, perceiving energies and an active, clarifying function.

Receptive insight of the Third Eye means the ability to look into the nature of things (e.g. diseases) and understand how they are interrelated. Every kind of visual recognition, of seeing – including the ability to perceive energies – is a function of the Third Eye and belongs here. It means looking beyond the surface of things and realizing the meaning of a piece of art, for example, or of dreams. The ability to perceive energies can be directed toward energy fields that are stable, radiant and healthy as well as to blocked and stagnant energy fields.

When the ability of receptive insight is strongly developed, it raises awareness, heightens intuition and enhances visionary abilities. Thinking is then characterized as clear understanding and concise discernment.

The active function of the Third Eye helps to clarify diffuse energy patterns, which are found in many diseases, and to open them out. Dysfunctional patterns may become more apparent. As a result, the patient may find it easier to appreciate the causes underlying a particular disorder, becoming aware of the sensations, emotions and thought patterns underlying a headache, for example, or any other chronic condition.

The Third Eye's clarifying function can be used during the session by either the therapist or the patient, when he starts to open his Third Eye. We talk of 'the opening of the Third Eye' when the area of the forehead comes increasingly into focus and the awareness stays there. Third Eye energy has a subtle quality and a *gentle, clear* and *cool character*.

In no way does the above give a full account of the Third Eye's practical implication. Only by practicing the relevant exercises to develop its potential will this 'organ' be fully experienced and available for therapy.

7. *CHAKRA* ACUPUNCTURE

The author has developed *chakra* acupuncture as a method of energy medicine that extends and supplements Chinese acupuncture, joining both approaches into one practice as well as integrating the Indian concept of the *chakra* system.

The basic concept of Chinese acupuncture is to dissolve blockages and stagnation in the channels and Organs by *harmonizing the flow of qi*. Conditions that are either deficient or excessive are balanced by achieving a harmonious interplay of *yin* and *yang*.

Chakra acupuncture uses traditional acupuncture points and complements them by adding the so called '*chakra* points'. These are points that lie near the *chakras*. Stimulating these points and spaces through acupuncture is called 'opening of the *chakras*' because it *activates* them and increases the flow of vital energy within them.

It is not recommended to start treatment by working on the actual illness. Rather, we begin by *opening* the *chakras, increasing the flow of life force*, and letting a high charge *build up* within them. This helps the patient to become aware of the *chakras* and the energy inside his body. In the beginning, it is important to start the *chakra* acupuncture treatment with the crown, Heart and base *chakras* and to establish a strong and constant flow of energy within them.

First, the needles are inserted into the traditional acupuncture points as well as the *chakra* acupuncture points. The points used most frequently to open the *chakras* are *baihui* (Du-20), in the centre of the crown *chakra*, and *sishencong* (M-HN-1) surrounding *baihui*. Further relevant *chakra* points are *yintang* (M-HN-3) and *yamen* (Du-15) for the sixth *chakra*, *shanzhong* (Ren-17) and *shendao* (Du-11) for the Heart *chakra*, and *taixi* (KI-3) and *sanyinjiao* (SP-6) for the base *chakra*.

Secondly, the patient is asked to place his awareness on the *chakras* one by one, starting with the crown *chakra*. After a while the patient may feel a slight tingling or a gentle flow of energy. These indicate the opening of the *chakra*. The sensations should be observed during the entire session. Should the patient not feel the opening, he should start breathing deeply into the *chakra*. Breathing deeply furthers the opening of the *chakra* and intensifies the flow of life force through it.

Thirdly, the therapist directs his awareness to his own *chakras* simultaneously. He repeatedly reminds the patient to be aware of the crown *chakra*, to:

'Open this area', and to
'Observe the flow of energy from the top of the head downwards'.

When the patient feels a distinct flow of energy through the crown *chakra* he should move to the Heart *chakra* and proceed in the same way as described above. He focuses awareness on the Heart *chakra* and breathes deeply until the opening of the *chakra* is felt, mostly as a widening, a charge, a flow of warm energy in the area.

The combination of acupuncture and awareness is important and makes the treatment more efficient.

The chakras *and how they are related to acupuncture points and Chinese Organs*

(See Fig. 15.1, and compare with Table 4.1.)

First or base *chakra, muladhara*

Location:	perineum
Opening:	one opening, downwards
Function:	connection to the Earth
Chinese Organ:	Kidney *yin*
Acupuncture points:	*huiyin* (Ren-1)

The position of the base *chakra* corresponds to the point *huiyin* Ren-1, 'meeting of *yin*', where the *yin* qualities of the body gather.

Second or polarity *chakra, svadhisthana*

Location:	pelvis
Opening:	two openings, one to the front, one to the back
Function:	sexuality
Chinese Organ:	Kidney *yang*, Bladder, Large Intestine
Acupuncture points:	front: *qugu* (Ren-2) to *guanyuan* (Ren-4)
	back: *yaoshu* (Du-2) to *mingmen* (Du-4)

The polarity *chakra* balances *yin* and *yang* inside and outside the body; a balanced polarity *chakra* is the basis for harmonious sexuality – that is, *yin* and *yang* in balance and exchange with another person. The first and second *chakras* form a unit and correspond to the Kidney and the lower *jiao* of the *sanjiao*.

Third or solar plexus *chakra, manipura*

Location:	abdomen
Opening:	two openings, one to the front, one to the back
Function:	personal will and emotional expression
Chinese Organ:	Spleen, Liver, middle *jiao* of the *sanjiao*
Acupuncture points:	front: *shenjue* (Ren-8), *zhongwan* (Ren-12)
	back: *xuanshu* (Du-5), *jizhong* (Du–6)

The *manipura chakra* regulates personal will in the upper part of the body and emotional expression in the lower part. When imbalanced it is responsible for striving for power, anger, rage and addiction.

Fourth or Heart *chakra, anahata*

Location:	center of the chest
Opening:	two openings, one to the front, one to the back
Function:	harmonizing, balancing, integrating, healing
Chinese Organ:	Heart, upper *jiao*
Acupuncture points:	front: *shanzhong* (Ren-17)
	back: *shendao* (Du-11)

The Heart *chakra* is the most important healing *chakra*, much more so than all the others. Its main qualities are compassion, love, tolerance and joy. Being located between the three upper and the three lower *chakras*, it forms the center from which the energies of all other Organs are influenced. This makes it the essential *chakra* for integration.

Fifth or throat *chakra, vishuddha*

Location:	throat
Opening:	two openings, one to the front, one to the back
Function:	strength and expressiveness of speech
Chinese Organ:	Lung
Acupuncture points:	front: *tiantu* (Ren-22)
	back: *dazhui* (Du-14)

Strength and expressiveness of speech and creativity are related to the throat *chakra*.

Sixth or 'Third Eye' *chakra, ajna*

Location:	forehead, between the eyebrows
Opening:	two openings, one to the front, one to the back
Function:	intuition, clairvoyance, ability to discriminate, understanding, focus of the mind
Acupuncture points:	front: *yintang* (M-HN-3)
	back: *yamen* (Du-15)

Seventh or crown *chakra, sahasrara*

Location:	at the vertex of the cranium
Opening:	one opening, upwards
Function:	understanding the higher aspects of being, connection to the soul
Acupuncture points:	*baihui* (Du-20), *sishengong* (M-HN-1)

8. SPIRITUAL ACUPUNCTURE

This approach integrates the modalities described above, especially modalities one to four: opening the crown, strengthening the base, expansion of the Heart through conscious breathing, increased awareness and *qigong*.

Spiritual acupuncture focuses on the light level of energy, starting by activating and opening the crown *chakra*. It focuses on the *flow of energy and light* from the eighth *chakra*, the soul (situated above the crown *chakra*), to the Heart and base, bringing a luminous quality of consciousness to the practice of acupuncture.

An increasing flow of light can be felt when putting the hands around the space of the crown *chakra*, holding them like a funnel. This helps the body to open upward towards the soul, which provides the inner light of consciousness. The soul, above the crown *chakra*, can be perceived as a ball of light by the Third Eye when the light of the soul moves down through the *chakras* into the body. When the patient feels the crown *chakra* distinctly open, the therapist moves on to the next *chakra* until reaching the base *chakra*, thus helping to connect with the energy of the Earth.

NOTES

The locations and functions of the *chakras* described here are based more on my own therapeutic observations and experiences rather than the manifold literature on this subject, which is often contradictory. Additional material used in the preparation of this chapter can be found in the References and further reading section at the end of the book.

In my experience over more than 20 years, these methods have not resulted in any adverse effects, as may occur with some types of *qigong* with less emphasis on strong 'grounding' as central to the work.

Anyone using these modalities is invited to send me their feedback at: stuxgabriel@me.com.

Ki in *shiatsu*

Patrizia Stefanini

16

CHAPTER CONTENTS

INTRODUCTION

To provide a simple definition for the Japanese word *ki* (氣; in Chinese *qi* or *ch'i*) in the context of *shiatsu* is not easy. Generally translated as 'energy' or 'life-force', it is used to indicate one of the five Vital Substances (the other four being *jing*, *shen*, *xue* and *jin ye*, respectively Essence, Spirit, Blood and Body Fluids), which according to traditional Chinese medicine represent all aspects of human form and function (see also Chs 4-6, 10, 20). The Vital Substances have varying degrees of 'materiality', ranging from the most rarefied to those that are entirely substantial. Together they form the ancient Chinese conception of body-mind [1].

Lifebreath, from the ancient Indian *prana*, also provides an adequate translation of *ki*, and a concept that highlights an ability to sustain life through the movement that it brings from its flow in man.

> *The Chinese character for Ki contains the radicals for both 'steam' and 'rice'. In its refined forms Ki moves and flows almost invisibly, like steam. In its denser aspect it slows or coalesces into form, such as rice [2]. (Fig. 16.1)*

In philosophy and traditional Chinese medicine *qi* is divided into three qualitative aspects: *shao* (少), lesser, intermediate, young, meaning an energy with potential for growth, the energy of youth; *tai* (太), greatest, maximum, adult, that which is the strong energy of maturity; and *jue* (厥), complete, minimum and elderly. It is very much in the nature of Chinese thought to divide and reunite. Thus these three energies then divide into their *yin* and *yang* components, and from these arise a further six energies, cosmic expressions of the single *ki* force.

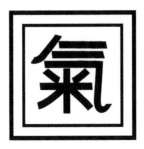

FIG 16.1 The classical Chinese character for *ki* (*qi*), showing the characters for 'steam' and 'rice'.

In Japanese the term *ki* is used daily, often linked to other different ideograms, providing different meanings depending on their context, for example in describing someone's character [3]:

> *ki ga chiisai* (気が小さい) = 'small *ki*' = timid, apprehensive
> *ki ga yowai* (気が弱い) = 'weak *ki*' = weak, hesitant
> *ki ga tsuyoi* (気が強い) = 'strong *ki*' = strong
> *ki ga mijikai* (気が短い) = 'short *ki*' = impatient, choleric
> *ki ga nagai* (気が長い) = 'long *ki*' = patient.

Also:

> *kiryoku* (気力) = *ki* + strength = dynamism
> *genki* (元気) = origin + *ki* = health, wellbeing
> *seiki* (生気) = life + *ki* = vitality, vigor
> *konki* (根気) = root + *ki* = patience.

Man, placed between Heaven and Earth, represents the unification of the *ki* of Heaven and the *ki* of Earth, in a close relationship with nature. *Ki* therefore has a central role in *shiatsu* (literally 'finger pressure', 指圧); pressure exerted from different parts of the practitioner's body is applied along the channels (meridians) that are said to be the preferential pathways for *ki* flow in the human body. Meridians are also a means for *sensing* the expression of vital functions on different levels (physical, emotional, mental and spiritual). In these places of interaction and exchange, the *shiatsu* practitioner can support and enhance the life quality of the client. Shizuto Masunaga, the originator of *zen shiatsu* (禅指圧), made use of the amoeba, a unicellular organism, as a metaphor to introduce a new way of understanding the meridians; he described them as vital functions in a process of continuous transformation and change (the ancient Greek word *amoibè* – αμοιβή – means 'change'). The quality of change is a fundamental aspect of this system, envisaged as the precious gift of life itself. Masunaga speaks of a cyclical activation of the life functions to allow birth, development and the very act of living life. Each meridian provides a sort of 'specialization' of *ki* or ability to behave in a specific manner. *Ki* is dynamic, interactive, flowing and transforming to sustain the quality of life.

The above concepts fit very well with the results of a modern approach to life science developed by a number of pioneers. As far back as 1957 Albert Szent-Györgyi, recipient of the 1937 Nobel Prize in Medicine, wrote that the inability of biologists to define animate matter in comparison with inanimate matter depends on their neglect of the two most important ingredients of living matter: water and electromagnetic fields [4] (and in particular the electromagnetic properties of water). He pointed out that excitation of the electron clouds of the biomolecule and their consequent chemical activation depend on the ordered, quasi-crystalline structure of layers of water close to the cellular membranes and some hundreds of water molecules thick. The *ordered structure* of this 'interfacial' water was in turn the consequence of an electromagnetic field trapped somehow in the water layers.

While this topic was the subject of as many as 175 articles produced before 1957, this wisdom has not been utilized by mainstream molecular biology in the ensuing decades. However, some physicists, foremost among them Herbert Fröhlich, took up the suggestion and developed the concept of *coherence* (namely the oscillation in unison of a large ensemble of particles) as a possible source of the trapped electromagnetic field (see also Ch. 9). As described below, the energy stored in coherent water structures may well correspond to *ki*.

THE HISTORY OF *SHIATSU*

Shiatsu originated indirectly from acupuncture, the ancient Chinese healing art, from which principles were applied in the traditional form of Japanese massage called *anma* (按摩). Its ancient origins are related to other training practices for the *do* arts in the *dojo* (道場) training halls (*do* = 'way', *jo* = 'place', so literally 'place of the way'). It would appear that *anma* was informally practiced from 200 BCE [5].

In the early 1900s, *shiatsu* developed as an independent system equipped with its own theory and technique, and became acknowledged in Japan for its therapeutic qualities. The profound and dramatic changes in Japanese society during the American occupation immediately after the Second World War almost resulted in *shiatsu* and other traditional practices being prohibited by law. However, fortunately this did not happen, and by the end of the 1940s Tokujiro Namikoshi had established the Nippon *Shiatsu* School, the first official training school for *shiatsu* practitioners. In the 1950s the Japanese Ministry of Health officially recognized *shiatsu*. Subsequently this spread the world over, with the resultant generation of numerous styles. The most widespread style by far in the Western world originated in Tokyo, in the *Iokai* School (医王会, literally, 'Association of the King of Medicines') founded by Shizuto Masunaga who, in the 1970s, proposed *shiatsu* as a way ('*do*') for the personal development of both giver and receiver. Furthermore, he recovered many concepts from Far Eastern healing traditions, combining aspects of Shintoism (*shin do*, 按摩, way of the spirit) and Buddhist philosophies in his teachings [6]. An analogous process was undertaken more or less at the same time when Morihei Ueshiba founded the martial art *aikido* (合気道, 'the way of unifying (with) life energy'). Masunaga's *shiatsu* shifted the focus from the static aspect of the human form to its more interactive and dynamic characteristics, giving the practitioner the prospect of adventuring into the realms of energy with an approach that is both practice based and intellectual, and in which meridians are no longer considered as structured energetic channels but rather as dynamic pathways of life function expression, which together determine the 'being' of a human. In particular, he affirmed that meridians have a variable nature and depth: how they will manifest depends both on the treatment given and on the nature of the interaction between practitioner and receiver.

Prior to his death at the age of 56, Masunaga left personal tasks to a few of his immediate students who further developed his system in the 1980s. One of these in particular, Pauline Sasaki, perceived that aspects of the universe envisaged in quantum physics have parallels in *shiatsu*, just as many others have sought 'quantum' explanations for the type of subtle vital energy encompassed in the concept of *ki*. She sought further associations and correspondences, and applied these principles to her own style of working, using the name 'quantum *shiatsu*' to symbolize this perspective and technique. In her form of *shiatsu*, the physical body and energetic body are both considered as resonating energetically but do so differently, and so manifest as distinct entities. This approach suggests a way of resolving the paradoxical dichotomy of energy and matter (wave and particle).

SHIATSU **AND SCIENCE**

I studied for many years with Pauline Sasaki, finding inspiration and ideas for personal evolution in applying her *shiatsu* method From this experience, and fostered by my university studies in physics, came a gradual formulation of my own thoughts on the dynamics and organization of *ki*. These in turn provided an explanation of what I perceived whilst treating clients.

Referring back to Masunaga's system, I have found in practice that the meridians (when perceived during *shiatsu* contact) do not keep to their exact locations as shown on his meridian charts; rather they deviate from their original pathways, reflecting differences in individual conditions. Moreover, the information they hold is not always limited to the present condition of the individual.

These observations become clearer if we focus on the meridian in its vibrational aspect of continuous change and movement. In this light the pathway indicated on the meridian chart can be redefined as the *most likely* location for the *ki* expression of the meridian, rather than its *exact* location. Developments in modern physics provide a model for resolving this apparent uncertainty. On pressing, I seek a precise vibrational quality of the meridian as a wave, with a range of vibration frequencies that describe the different levels of *ki* expression. From this concept came the theory of meridians as 'wave packets' [7]. If we choose to describe reality in this way as wavelike, we must consider the likelihood (probability) of being able to recognize the spatial location of each entity in question. In this case, the 'wave packet' is a reasonable description, where no single frequency value holds true, but rather a probable range of frequencies that express the various properties of the meridian. Supported by the quantum model in which observer and observed *together* determine the result of a given experiment, I believe it is possible to define the subjective experience of *shiatsu* more carefully than previously. The vision of the meridian system as a network is very appropriate as it is not tied to the four-dimensional reality of space and time.

In a previous article [8], I pointed out many of the similarities in worldview between *shiatsu* and quantum physics. It received interesting comments. Among them, one from Andrew May, physicist and *shiatsu* practitioner, was quite appreciative and at the time he suggested I read a study by Cyril W Smith (see Ch. 9) entitled 'Is a living system a macroscopic quantum system?' [9] where he writes that 'the secret lies in the fact that the body is predominantly composed of water'. I later used this idea for further development of my own vision of the energetic dimensions of living beings. To do so I delved into some new aspects of biophysics of which I will give a description in the following pages. Here I owe much to the physicist Professor Emilio Del Giudice, one of a highly specialized group at the Institute of Biophysics in Neuss (Germany), who included me on his research team.

The living system can be considered a macroscopic quantum system, which well describes its properties. One of these is '*coherence*', a concept related to the dynamic nature of reality. Matter is not inert; it is in perennial fluctuation. Even a vacuum fluctuates, being packed with fluctuating fields. It is due to the properties of coherence, in the presence of a large number of atoms, that fields can fluctuate in harmony amongst themselves – as if atoms are dancing in unison. This establishes a dynamic order that is fundamental for equilibrium in living beings.

In this coherent state, an electromagnetic field is held within the fluid (matter) of the body: it cannot radiate outwards. The wave has become the prisoner of matter.

> In living systems, water takes part in the dynamics of life, not only because it accounts for 99% of all the biomolecules but also because it provides energy to living matter. Water has the ability to achieve an extended form of organization and provide an ensemble of different Coherence Domains which have phase locked, thus maximizing their ability to 'look for' energy from the environment. This 'coherence of coherences' of 'biological water' in living systems corresponds to a sort of higher organization. An efficient mechanism of energy transformation from Coherence Domains to biomolecules in living matter guarantees the transfer of biochemical energy necessary for the maintenance of life cycles [10].

In living matter coherence domains, atoms and molecules share a dialogue because the various coherence domains are in phase one with another, or rather, they are correlated. We can consider the degree of coherence in a living system as a measurement parameter for health, it being related to the efficiency of energy transfer and use of the system's resources to carry out its vital functions. Given the particular properties of coherent domain chains, strongly linked with the peculiar nature of biological water, energy can travel through them and is available for the body's vital activities. A human being is in a healthy condition when this flow occurs consistently. To be healthy does not require much energy, given that an excess would extinguish the system's coherence, its dynamic passing rapidly from one of ordered movement to chaos. Illness may ensue when, on losing coherence in the system, energy fails to move and becomes blocked. It is not the quantity of energy but its coherence that allows it to flow through our being. These concepts can be seen as analogous to the understanding of *ki* flow in *shiatsu*.

In the last two decades a viable framework for a coherent dynamics in living organisms has been worked out by a number of scientists such as Giuliano Preparata, Emilio Del Giudice, Giuseppe Vitiello, Fritz-Albert Popp, Vladimir Voeikov, Enzo Tiezzi, Larissa Brizhik, Gerald Pollack and others. The essence of this approach is contained in the following points:

1. A large ensemble of N water molecules, when its density N/V in a volume V exceeds a critical threshold and its absolute temperature T lies below a critical value, undergoes a phase transition from an original gas-like configuration where all the molecules are uncorrelated to a coherent configuration having a lower energy where all the molecules move in unison. This transition implies a sharp decrease of 'entropy' (measuring the system's disorder); as a consequence the newly coherent system releases energy outward, resulting in an increase in its entropy larger than that lost by the system. In the coherent system water molecules oscillate between a configuration where all electrons are tightly bound to an excited configuration where one electron is so weakly bound as to be quasi free (Fig. 16.2).

2. In normal bulk water at nonvanishing temperatures the collision of the system with external molecules may push a fraction of the coherent molecules out of tune so that a flickering situation occurs, with molecules continuously transiting from coherent to noncoherent and vice versa. However, molecules near a surface are attracted to it (as in 'surface tension'), stabilizing the system and shielding it from the disruptive effects of collisions. Consequently water at interfaces with membranes, microspheres or biomolecule backbones could be considered fully coherent in a particularly stable way. According to the electron properties of coherent

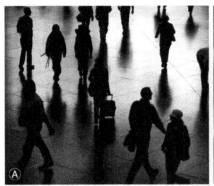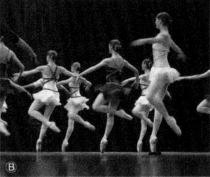

FIG 16.2 Visual impression of coherent water and its electron properties: (A) figures walking noncoherently; (B) coherence in a dance sequence. *(Courtesy of Fotolia; (A) ©Dmitry Nikolaev/Fotolia, (B) ©jeancliclac/Fotolia.)*

water listed above, interfacial water is a donor of electrons whereas normal water is an acceptor of electrons. The interface between coherent and normal water therefore acts as an electric battery whose electromotive force (the 'vital force'?) has been estimated as around 100 millivolts, in good agreement with observed cell membrane potentials.

Points (1) and (2) accord well with the findings of Szent-Györgyi.

3. The presence in the coherent region of a large reservoir of quasi-free electrons makes it possible to excite them easily with tiny amounts of energy, resulting in the creation of electron vortices that, because of coherence and the consequent lack of collisions, are virtually frictionless, do not lose energy, and can continue to exist for a long time. During this time additional excitations may occur so that large amounts of energy can be stored in the water's coherent structure. This property makes it possible to collect large amounts of low-grade (high-entropy) energy from the surroundings and transform it into high-grade (low-entropy) energy capable of performing electron molecule excitations within living systems.

This low-grade energy flowing within the body is a good potential candidate for identification with *ki*.

COHERENCE AND MERIDIANS

The following citations present interesting and relevant ideas produced by scientists at the Institute of Biophysics at Neuss, founded by Professor Fritz-Albert Popp in 1996, where there is an ongoing encounter between modern science and traditional therapeutic arts, providing a way for both toward mutual enrichment.

> *Here we suggest that self-organization of the living organism implies the appearance of an array of quasi-one-dimensional coherent domains that behave as the pathways where a flow of matter, Energy and information is self-confined. This array is dynamically maintained and disappears when the organism dies so that it cannot be detected in any [anatomical–pathological] investigation post-mortem. This array can be linked with functioning of energetic channels known as meridians in . . . Eastern medicine [11].*

Moreover, the organism can be represented as a liquid crystalline continuum, which can carry the signals for intercommunication in a way, similar to liquid crystals . . . Such systems are highly nonlinear optical media and can support the existence of specific pathways for the propagation of electromagnetic signals. . . . Therefore the above described hypothesis that an organism represents a liquid crystalline continuum, similar to liquid crystals, opens the possibility to describe the meridians as optical pathways along which electromagnetic signals propagate in the form of nonlinear soliton-like packages [12].

In this context, it makes sense to look at the collective behavior of the system's components rather than at the single part. When I envisage the meridians as a particular form of coherence domain within the connective tissue, I see them as a sort of watery sheath encasing molecular chains. It is within this fluid that energy captured by the molecules is channeled.

Energy is delivered to the molecules by what is called a *soliton* – a localized wave packet that does not dissipate energy in its movement. When it encounters a 'metabolic situation' that requires just the amount of energy it holds, the soliton gives up this energy and ceases to exist.

Coherence is not just the subject of scientific discourse, but is also central to particular life experiences that most of us have (or witness), sooner or later. Situations manifesting a 'sense of coherence' are those that we may define as 'being in the zone' or 'going with the flow' – life movements where, thanks to an intrinsic state of harmony and wellbeing, everything seems easy.

> Solitons were first described by the hydrodynamic engineer John Russell Scott on the basis of his observations in a canal near Edinburgh in 1834 (Fig. 16.3) [13]. The soliton concept can be applied in various scientific contexts, and was first introduced in biophysics by A S Davydov.

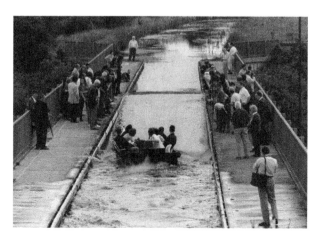

FIG 16.3 The 'solitary wave', as first observed by John Russell Scott, recreated in the Union Canal near Edinburgh, 1995. *(Courtesy of Larissa Brizhik.)*

HADO SHIATSU

The development of a system I call *hado shiatsu* has grown out of the aforementioned concepts. In the Japanese spiritual tradition '*hado*' (波動 はどう) is the innate transforming power of each thing and each living being. The literal translation of its ideogram is 'wavelike movement, vibration'. The word *hado* is currently also used by Masaru Emoto in his research on the characteristics of water. Dr Emoto describes himself as 'not so much as a scientific researcher but more from the perspective of an original thinker' [14]. His photographs of water molecule crystals, showing different formations in different exposure situations, have stirred interest the world over and have become part of an ongoing debate on the so-called 'memory of water'.

The modern biophysical idea that quality of life is closely linked to the *degree of order* within our energy system is intriguing. This order is tied to the way in which energy is used, rather than its quantity. There is also an association here with *light*. A ray of light can stimulate the formation of solitons, an extremely efficient way of utilizing available energy to sustain functional order within a system. Indeed, Hugo Niggli has suggested that melanoma cells and the fibroblasts involved in carcinogenesis may lose the ability to capture sunlight [15]. As a result their coherence, or consequent degree of order, diminishes and their chaos level increases, along with increased cell proliferation and the onset of various other dysfunctions. Research on this possibility is ongoing.

> *Preliminary observations confirm the suggestion that the MLC (meridian-like channels [see Glossary]) and perhaps even the meridians/channels of Chinese medicine are non-local, morphologically non-fixed. Along them, the electronic excitation may propagate most likely in the form of optical solitons. These pathways may actually coincide with the zone of the body surface which is favourable to ordinary reflection [16].*

Under specific conditions it is possible that, as with light, *shiatsu* pressure can also produce solitons that donate their energy to sustain life processes. The first hypothesis of *hado shiatsu* has to do with the prospect of stimulating soliton production in the receiver's system during treatment using the meridian system as the preferential pathways for creating such soliton events. Relaxed perpendicular pressure on the privileged access points of the meridian network (the so-called personal *tsubo*, 壷 or ツボ) provides a gentle, system-efficient stimulation (in Oschman's words, 'cells answer to whispering' [17]).

Several scientific studies support the hypothesis that a 'therapeutic' touch on the human body produces an electrical charge that then passes preferentially into the meridian-like channels, which act as ideal low-impedance transmission pathways. The particular stimulated meridian 'lights up' with the production of 'coherent photons' [18–20].

After years of refusal by Western medicine to countenance an energetic basis for therapeutic practices, we now envisage the eventually rich and increasingly vital comparative investigation of different approaches worldwide. Indeed it has been shown that with the movement of electrical charge in the human body (which we can consider as equivalent to the movement of *ki* in the context of *shiatsu*) an electromagnetic field is established [21]. This field can be of varying shapes and dimensions, and is quite individual (Fig. 16.4). However, it appears to take on a form that remains more or less the same, and interestingly expresses mainly in the infrared and visible frequency range. Seto et al [22], for example, have found that 'an extraordinary large biomagnetic field' can be detected from the hands of practitioners of a variety of healing and martial art techniques, including *qigong*, *yoga* and meditation, although their findings have not been fully replicated.

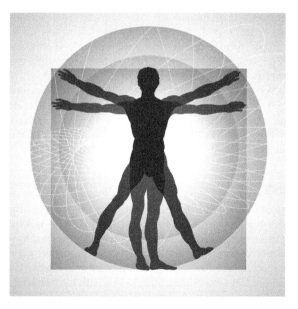

FIG 16.4 The human field (artist's impression). *(Courtesy of Fotolia; ©ag visuell/Fotolia.)*

Light – and the colors that are its different vibrational components – transforms into life. This ancient and well-known equation now takes on a certain depth and resonance, given new scientific knowledge of how life manifests and is self-generated.

Light emission by living organisms has been investigated now for nearly a century, with intensive study of biophotons by Popp and his colleagues since 1972 [23]. It would appear that the information carried by emitted biophotons could indeed tell us much about the quality of life of a living being.

The *hado shiatsu* hypothesis is also sustained by Oschman's contemplation on the cell. In his influential book on energy medicine [17], he asserts that the cell is not merely a bag filled with solution and that it does not have the inner structure we usually find in biology text books. Such descriptions may be appropriate for the anatomical–pathological study of dead cells, but the living cell has a quite different internal structure, involving a cellular matrix that is connected, across the cell surface, with the connective tissue system or extracellular matrix. The shift here is from a mechanical viewpoint to a model of the 'living matrix' that is functional and dynamic; such a model legitimizes the concept that the cell's architecture and biochemical functionality are intimately related. In this light, if *shiatsu* pressure can alter the form (architecture) of tissue, why can it not also determine the complex inner functioning and diverse behavior of the cells of which it is composed?

Time is another aspect important as a direct consequence of considering the human being from a quantum perspective. Of all the definitions in quantum physics, that of time is one of the most bizarre. In nonrelativistic coherent systems, in fact, communication occurs at virtually infinite velocity – a characteristic of communication between objects in phase. We speak of synchronous events or, better, of events occurring simultaneously. Such synchronicity belongs implicitly to a holistic system such as the human being. Therefore, *shiatsu* based on the linear cause-and-effect approach is reductive and no longer adequate, the therapeutic dyad being a feedback system where the course of time is not so much linear as circular. Simply put, 'everything is':

Real processes . . . are not experienced as a succession of instantaneous time slices like frames of a moving picture. Nor can reality be consistently represented in this manner [24].

I believe this concept of time is very appropriate to the *shiatsu* experience where, by means of the meridian network, space-time opens up to new dimensions and meanings. Through touch I have often perceived clues revealing information about my receiver's life that are not set in present time and so logically should be completely inaccessible to me.

We also have the daily experience in *shiatsu* that changes occur in parts of the body quite remote from the part that is touched. Without the Japanese theory of *ki* and the insights of quantum physics, living systems are far more difficult to understand, thus helping to account for the widely observed limitations of the twentieth-century reductionist, materialist biomedical paradigm.

APPLICATIONS

Purely anamnestic information is not enough for the *hado shiatsu* practitioner. Further information arising from resonance with the receiver is required, and it is touch that provides this most adequately. Once we have listened to what the client says about their motivation and to their particular requests we will then meet that person through *contact*, in other words, making our own energetic field resonate with that of the client. This experience supplies us with the nonverbal information we need to be able to express our own healing intent in a gesture that is therapeutically effective. How? Contact with the coherent system of the practitioner may help to restabilize coherence in the system of the client who – for whatever reason – has lost it. Noncoherence may manifest in terms of symptoms or malaise. However, to be truly effective the practitioner must be in a state of coherence greater than that of the client. As *hado shiatsu* practitioners, we must therefore look after our own health, or the degree of our own system's coherence. Only in this way can the treatment be effective and attain the desired increase in coherence in the receiver's system, meaning an increase in *ki* dynamics, synonymous with self-healing.

In November 2008, I took part in an as yet unpublished research project headed by Professor Emilio Del Giudice in Tuscany to monitor the *ki* field in the human and how it changes during a *shiatsu* treatment. Previous studies by Dr Klaus Schlebusch and colleagues [16] using an infrared camera (ThermoCam) had already provided strong support for the hypothesis of *ki* flowing in meridians considered as dynamical pathways. This camera is sensitive between 3.4 and 5μm in the temperature range 10 to 450°C. As the biomagnetic field extends some distance from the body surface (see Fig. 16.4), the fields of two adjacent organisms interact with each other.

It was interesting to observe in this experiment how the field structures of both practitioner and receiver became more and more evident as the session went on. At one point field lines became visible between the two people on the camera screen, demonstrating the energetic communication between them and persisting even after the end of actual treatment, in witness of the continuing relationship that is set up between giver and receiver once a therapeutic connection has been established.

If we can envisage the meridians as impermanent and dynamic structures that in their manifestation become tools in the service of life, perhaps we can also affirm that the process of healing may itself change the properties of space and time forever. Correspondingly, human matter may change its form when it resonates with the healing field that develops in the therapeutic encounter.

In practice, after the *shin* (神) or 'data collection' phase, I begin the actual treatment, into which I weave some working hypotheses – the first being that it is possible to stimulate soliton production in the meridians. Mindset as technique in *hado shiatsu* further allows me to use an imagined ray of light, and then to vibrate this intention in my field and feel how my receiver's energy responds to this stimulus. A key factor is being aware of the range of visible light frequencies that naturally exist in our energy field. Focusing on these frequencies allows the receiver to recognize them in their own field and thus to resonate with them. Using this strategy, and after only a few sessions, there is a notable increase in the vitality of the receiver. Vitality is also expressed in behavior that demonstrates a changed relationship with the self and the beginnings of a renewed approach to difficulties that were previously experienced as overwhelming. During treatments I select the appropriate places and moments to enter into resonance with the receiver's energetic field. The range of imagined light rays emitted will vary, with varying qualities, depending on how my interaction with the receiver is initiated and develops. This interaction is perceivable through touch and observation, is unique every time and always contributes towards enriching my understanding of the therapeutic relationship and of life itself.

In summary, *ki*, nourished by such energy offerings from the light spectrum, contributes to the vital functions of the body, defined by Masunaga as manifesting in the meridians (*keiraku*, 経絡) as the way of *ki*. Also relevant here is the second working hypothesis outlined above, that *shiatsu* pressure can modify cellular architecture (its form), and consequently that it can also influence cell behavior and function. Often at the end of a treatment I receive verbal feedback from my clients that indicates their feelings of 'expansion and brightness', or they report images occurring during the session that have to do with light. *Hado shiatsu* works well in allowing positive self-recognition and an ability to contact potential inner resources for change, translating as a general sensation of enhanced movement/vibration and vitality.

For myself as practitioner, the feeling is one of global connection with my own energy field, allowing me to 'tune in', respond and change as appropriate, resonating moment by moment with my receiver. Therefore I try to 'whisper to the cells', without forgetting that the largest part of any object, including the human body, is empty space! Energy medicine is based on playing with such energetic interactions.

CONCLUSION

It is never possible to draw final conclusions. I am traveling, and my journey is long and varied. I respect life, and learning about it is enriching. I meet, I experiment and I research. For sure my research on *ki* has given me ideas in this personal journey that have become a key to understanding life, both my own and my clients'. In my travels I carry with me a holistic and interdisciplinary model of human functioning, as well as the belief that the traditional Oriental ways of investigating life and those of the new science of life look like coming together at a core point: the way of communication between the energetic fields of different human beings. In modern scientific terms this entails exploring biophoton function, namely the photons that comprise the fields of living system fields and how the information they convey is connected to health. I also recognize that the healing process is complex and involves many factors, including for example the individual choice to become well again or to hold on to patterns of illness, a choice that is not always easy to make.

ACKNOWLEDGMENTS

With acknowledgement to Professor Emilio Del Giudice for his support and inspiration, and to Elaine Wright for her assistance in translating this chapter.

Bioelectricity and *qi*: a microcurrent approach

17

Darren Starwynn

INTRODUCTION

Microcurrents are low-intensity electrical currents of less than 1 milliampère (mA), measurable in millionths of an ampère (microampères, µA). This chapter examines the role of therapeutic microcurrent and 'color light' in supporting pain relief as well as functional and energetic balance in the body. In principle, gentle, well-chosen energies are ideal for these purposes since they so closely match the body's innate activity and can help the body heal, balance and detoxify itself. We will start with some current understandings of how microcurrents relate to *qi* and subtle energy fields in the body, and then examine some powerfully effective treatment techniques based on these understandings.

Our bodies are totally wired for energy. Every function, from digesting our lunch to thinking about a big meeting tomorrow, is inextricably related to energy fields and currents in our organs, fascia and nervous system. This wiring makes sense when you think about the trillions of cells that make up our bodies. Each of these cells is a bioelectric organism whose functions are based on transfer of charged molecules (ions) within its organelles and across its membranes.

It has been well established in Western science for over a century that electrical activity governs most of our vital functions. This activity includes the electrical pacemaker that keeps the heart beating, brain waves that support consciousness and digital transmissions through our nervous system.

PHYSIOLOGY AND SUBTLE ENERGY FIELDS

Contemporary research has revealed more about possible physiological roles of subtle energy fields. Some of this research indicates that subtle energy fields not only emanate from the physiology of our life functions but may actually help to create and govern them. This idea of a conscious, formative energy field which acts as a template for the physical body goes back to ancient China, and is echoed in the modern work of Sheldrake [1], Nordenström [2] and Burr. In his book *Blueprint for Immortality* [3], for example, Burr stated:

> *This field is electrical in the physical sense and by its properties relates the entities of the biological system in a characteristic pattern and is itself, in part, a result of the existence of those entities. It determines and is determined by the components.* More than establishing pattern, *it must maintain pattern in the midst of a physio-chemical flux. Therefore, it must regulate and control living things. It must be the mechanism, the outcome of whose activity is wholeness, organization, and continuity.*

Burr's description sounds a lot like two interdependent bases for life spoken of by ancient Chinese Daoists – *qi* (氣) and *li* (理) (see Chs 3 and 11). *Qi* is the motivating energy behind life and *li* is the etheric template from which life's structure and form arises [4].

Research from Russia and Germany suggests that our bodies circulate not only electrical energy but also photons of light, much in the same manner as fiberoptic cables [5]. The pioneering scientist Fritz-Albert Popp, for example, has conducted extensive experiments into how living things communicate through light emitted from their cells and tissues (see also Ch. 16). He has confirmed that living organisms can create coherent light (the form of light produced by lasers). Popp also considers that 'DNA in the active state of a living cell is one of the most essential sources of biophoton emission' [6].

Music and sound therapies may affect and regulate the body similarly, through 'phonons', the equivalent particles of acoustic energy that transmit though the living crystalline matrix of the body described below.

This remarkable, complex and interwoven network of energy fields and transmissions in our bodies has been called the 'living matrix' by a number of contemporary scientists. In his book *Energy Medicine: The Scientific Basis* [7], James Oschman states:

> *The living matrix is a continuous and dynamic 'supramolecular' webwork, extending into every nook and cranny of the body: a nuclear matrix within a cellular matrix within a connective tissue matrix. In essence, when you touch a human body, you are touching a continuously interconnected system, composed of virtually all the molecules in the body linked together in an intricate webwork.*

He goes on to suggest how this understanding can enhance the healing arts:

This is an important image of the structure of the living body. Our images shape our therapeutic successes because they can give rise to specific intentions. Intentions are not trivial, because they give rise to specific patterns of electrical and magnetic activity in the nervous system of the therapist that can spread throughout their body and into the body of a patient.

POLARITY AND POTENTIALS OF THE HUMAN BODY

After a distinguished medical career during which he developed the needle biopsy now used in hospitals internationally, Bjørn Nordenström dedicated over 20 years to studying human bioelectricity. He concluded that the body's complex electrical system of 'biologically closed electric circuits' regulates all its organs and tissues. Nordenström wrote that this electrical system works to balance the activity of internal organs and, in the case of injuries, represents the very foundation of the healing process. Significantly, disturbances in these fields may lead to the development of cancer.

The theme of changes in the electrical potentials of the body in response to disease and external stimuli runs through much recent research. Hiroshi Motoyama, a Japanese scientist and Shinto (神道) priest, has also made great contributions to our understanding of the electrical nature of the body and acupuncture systems [8]. His AMI device ('apparatus for measuring the function of the acupuncture meridians and the corresponding internal organs') effectively assesses meridian energy by sequential electrical measurements of the *jing* (井) acupoints at the distal end of each meridian (*sei* points in Japanese). This device can be used to indicate the body's energetic responses to many forms of stresses and therapies in real time. Motoyama has shown that changes in current levels in response to a 3-volt stimulus depend on the polarization of certain levels of the epidermis: the current *before* polarization occurs is an indicator of meridian function; that *after* polarization reflects activity of the autonomic nervous system (ANS), in particular of the sympathetic nervous system.

In general, when a stimulus is systemic, that is, from overall body or emotional reactions and increased ANS activity, measured areas become more negative in electrical potential compared with surrounding tissues (this is the galvanic skin response, or GSR). However, Motoyama confirmed that local stimulation (not sympathetic in origin) has the opposite effect. When *mild* mechanical, electrical or thermal stimuli are applied to a local area the electrical resistance will be lowered, and the positive potential of the area in relation to surrounding areas will increase. This is associated with transfer and accumulation of ions within the body fluids in the area.

As you will see in the description of the treatment techniques that follow, the ability to accurately balance positive and negative electrical fields of the body is crucial to good clinical results.

So how do these findings support the value of microcurrent therapies? To answer this we need to understand that our body can be viewed as composed of living crystals.

CRYSTALS, SEMICONDUCTION AND PIEZOELECTRICITY

Semiconduction and piezoelectricity are two electrical qualities of the crystalline substances that occur prolifically in the human body. Both are highly relevant to understanding the electrical qualities of the meridian system and why microcurrent and light therapies provide such impressive results.

Semiconduction is the only known mode of conduction outside of metal wires capable of transmitting very small currents over long distances, but this transmission is possible only in substances with very orderly molecular structures, such as crystals. Many crystals are semiconductors, able to both conduct and resist electrical flow, so are somewhere between insulators (such as rubber) and conductors (such as copper wires). Semiconduction allows for many activities vital to both computer technology and life processes. Computer microprocessors use specially created semiconductors to produce desired functions, and our bodies similarly use semiconduction to transmit subtle electrical energies and information throughout the body.

The Hungarian Nobel laureate Albert Szent-Györgyi was the first to point out [9] that the molecular structures of the human body are sufficiently well organized to support semiconduction through passing information along chains of protein molecules. Robert Becker, an orthopedic surgeon, conducted many experiments to test this principle, and concluded that energy transmission and communication of the meridian system is based on semiconduction along the perineural glial cells that support the nervous system. Semiconduction also occurs in other connective tissue, bone and the lumen of blood vessels, allowing subtle currents to be transported over long distances without losing charge. Becker demonstrated that these semiconducted currents are completely different from electrical activity within the nerves themselves. Nerves transmit relatively high-frequency electrical action potentials, whereas glial cells transmit slower direct currents of much smaller amplitude. He postulated that such direct currents represent the more primitive aspect of our electrophysiology, which support healing and regeneration, and that acupuncture points are in effect 'way stations' that boost the charge along the pathways [10].

Many allegedly 'primitive' creatures such as salamanders and lizards can regenerate whole limbs and organs whereas 'higher' creatures such as human beings can do this only in very limited ways. Becker was able to induce limb regeneration in both frogs and rats by applying direct microcurrents in experimental settings – feats these species cannot accomplish on their own.

According to physicist Dwight Bulkley [11] (cited by Gary Buchanan [12]):

All therapeutic techniques may be understood as reversals of state of 'polarization' in a three-dimensional, crystalline network. The human mind-body, considered as an oscillating flexible crystal, may be 'poked' in many ways, at many points to change its mode of oscillation, to affect the quantitative 'deconditioning', by inducing realignment and reversals within the total structure.

For me, this further confirms the great importance of correct use of polarity agents in legitimate energy therapies. Electrical polarity reversals in the body can be considered a prime cause of pathogenic states, and are likely results of a degradation of proper balance and regulation of *qi* in the body.

A pioneer in understanding and utilizing the power of electrical polarity therapies was Yoshio Manaka, a Japanese physician and acupuncture researcher. To explain the body's sensitivity to energy stimulation, he postulated an 'X-signal' system consisting of immeasurably small charges in and around the body that ultimately regulate all life processes [13]. Although the X-signals cannot be measured with currently available tools, their effects can be clearly observed through changes in pressure pain at acupoints, pulse diagnosis and kinesiology in the form of muscle testing.

Manaka showed how this X-signal system is exquisitely sensitive to polarity agents such as magnets, 'ion-pumping cords' or polarized electrical probes. I am highly indebted to Manaka for this knowledge, and have adapted his principles with use of polarized microcurrents through probe electrodes. This has shown excellent results for pain relief and many other powerful therapeutic effects.

Piezoelectricity is another inherent electrical quality of the body. This is the tendency of a crystalline structure, when deformed or struck, to release an electrical charge. The forces of movement and gravity on human and animal bodies are constantly triggering such releases. Becker measured this activity in bone, and showed that bone regeneration is turned on by these endogenous charges. However, in the body this phenomenon is not limited to bone. Connective tissues of many kinds and even blood vessels possess piezoelectric properties. The fascia in particular can be compared to a complex, stretchy network that is constantly releasing and circulating subtle charges, literally interconnecting every part of the body with every other part [14].

The 'living matrix' is closely associated with semiconduction and piezoelectricity, and is highly responsive to low-intensity energies. Oschman [15] sums this up as follows:

> The most exciting property of the living matrix is the ability of the entire network to generate and conduct vibrations. Modern biophysical research is revealing a wide range of properties that enable the body to use sound, light, electricity, magnetic fields, heat, elasticity, and other forms of vibrations as signals for integrating and coordinating diverse physiological activities, including those involved in tissue repair.

APPLICATIONS FOR THERAPY

There are well-established therapeutic energy applications to the body in both Western medicine and most complementary and alternative medical systems. Allopathic medicine uses lasers for surgery, ultrasound and electrical stimulation for physical therapies, and light therapies for treating psoriasis and depression. Alternative healing arts have long used magnets, music, colored light, gemstones and various types of electrical devices for treating a wide range of disorders of the body and psyche.

Microcurrent therapy has emerged as one of the most useful and versatile energy therapies, and has valuable applications for pain relief, assisted rehabilitation, nonneedle acupuncture and esthetic rejuvenation services. Just as semiconduction is a middle ground between conduction and resistance, microcurrents are currents with intensities somewhere between conventional electrostimulators and the subtle innate energy fields of the body. For this reason microcurrents are gentle enough to act in harmony with the body's own electrical activity but are a strong enough intervention to cause rapid effects that the body would not produce on its own.

Following extensive experiments with various instrumentation and treatment techniques in an effort to learn how to produce the most effective therapeutic results using microcurrent, I have found the greatest successes using a combination of microcurrent and various therapeutic colors of light applied through acupuncture points. I have named this combination therapy 'Microlight therapy™' [16]. The great value of Microlight for healing arts and esthetics has now been confirmed by large numbers of practitioners and doctors in the US and elsewhere.

DEVELOPMENT OF EFFECTIVE TREATMENT TECHNIQUES

Many medical techniques and drugs used in past centuries seem quaint, antiquated or just plain dangerous from the perspective of modern medicine. So it should and will be for most electrotherapeutic techniques used today. It is dismal to see how poorly and inconsistently so many impressive-looking devices work for long-term relief of pain and disease. You will rarely hear a physical therapist or chiropractor come home from a day of work and enthusiastically rave about their experiences with conventional electrical stimulation. Practitioners using micro-current electroacupuncture methods do often get excited about the results. What is the difference?

The difference is mainly due to a lack of understanding of bioelectricity. Sadly, this ignorance carries over to very limited and incomplete information about energy medicine being taught in schools of the healing arts.

As described above, the living matrix of our bodies is exquisitely sensitive to subtle energies. Indeed, as long as they are not overbearingly strong, the amount (intensity) of electrical current or light applied is much less important than the correct choice of treatment techniques and its other parameters. (One exception to this 'less is more' principle is acute inflammatory pain: in some cases, high-intensity milliampère currents can more quickly sedate the inflammation, reduce edema and relax muscle spasms. However, even in these cases I advocate following the high-intensity stimulation with microcurrents for a 'cool down' period.)

There are many vital aspects of the body's response to energy that need to be understood before good treatment techniques can be selected. Let us take a look now at the most important principles that underlie good microcurrent and Microlight techniques.

RESONANCE

The 'law of resonance' concerns how vibrating energy fields interact with and influence each other. In particular, pulse rates, or frequencies, of microcurrents and wavelengths (colors) of light each resonate with various body systems and tissues. In my experience, proper selection of colors and frequencies has had a big impact on what tissues are affected and how effective treatments have been. In treating Liver imbalances, for example, I have observed that some patients respond better to green light with polarized microcurrent, whereas others respond better to microcurrent with red or violet light. Good responses are determined by improvements in symptoms and stronger muscle test indicators on the test point for the Liver.

POLARIZATION

The 'law of polarity' (*yin–yang* or positive–negative duality) applies to all matter, including the human body. In my experience, not knowing how to apply positive and negative electrodes to appropriate zones on the body is probably the biggest reason for poor results and aggravations. As already mentioned, Manaka developed many practical systems using polarity agents to balance *qi* throughout the body.

RESISTANCE (AND ITS INVERSE, CONDUCTANCE)

Resistance is what slows the transmission or penetration of energy. Good technique requires getting therapeutic energies through the skin's electrical barrier. This in turn promotes circulation of energy by reducing resistance at therapeutic acupuncture points associated with injured or diseased tissues.

A justification from those advocating the use of high-intensity electrotherapies and intense therapeutic lasers has been the need to use high energy to overcome skin resistance [17]. Although it is true that higher voltages will more efficiently reduce resistance in inanimate objects, this perspective is not usually the most useful for treating living organisms. Many researchers have shown that acupuncture points have less resistance than surrounding tissues, and are in effect bioelectric 'windows' into the inner body. Treating such less resistive 'open' acupoints therefore allows low-intensity or subtle energies to engage the inner workings of the body more efficiently. High-quality microcurrent equipment usually includes a point location feature that measures differences in electrical skin resistance to locate these points.

'LESS IS MORE'

In the world of energy medicine, smaller amounts of energy seem to promote the most profound healing results. As mentioned above, Yoshio Manaka's 'X-signal' theory is based on his extensive research in applying very low-level stimuli to acupuncture points and observing profound changes and reactions in the body. His experiences and my own confirm that lower levels of energy applied to the body frequently produce superior benefits over higher, more invasive energies.

LAW OF SPECIFICITY

This law follows the 'less is more' principle: the more specific are the treatment sites, the less stimulus is needed. Playing all the keys on a piano at once creates jarring noise, whereas playing selected keys can produce beautiful music. This same principle applies to microcurrent and light stimulation. Applying gentle stimulation through appropriate acupuncture points, including auricular, hand and other microsystems, produces far more powerful clinical effects that flooding larger areas of the body with high-intensity electricity and light. There are some microcurrent techniques that do involve flooding large areas using pad electrodes that can be valuable for acute pain relief, tissue healing acceleration and assisted rehabilitation. Yet in my experience these techniques rarely deliver the dramatically rapid results with pain relief that point-specific treatments do.

Another system of microcurrent therapy called *frequency specific microcurrent* (FSM) does mainly rely on flooding regions of the body with microcurrent. FSM is usually used with little to no point specificity. But it is based on using sequences of specific electrical frequencies for therapeutic effects, and so is a different fulfillment of the laws of specificity and resonance. (See Ch. 23.1 for more details.)

ACCOMMODATION

Living systems do whatever they can to tune out repetitive, intrusive stimuli. This is 'accommodation'. Modulations are changing patterns of stimulation that reduce accommodation by keeping the attention of the mind/body, so to speak. Using appropriate modulations in microcurrent or other energy medical devices can extend the effectiveness of therapy.

PROPRIOCEPTION

This refers to the marvelous feedback system between peripheral muscles and nerves and the central nervous system. Injuries, strokes and some diseases can interfere with proprioception, causing difficulties in movement and other bodily functions. Good technique should aim to augment and help restore this feedback system to healthy functioning.

Wing and Goodheart developed valuable microcurrent techniques based on proprioception. One such is the treatment of the Golgi tendon organs in the origins and insertions of injured muscles with manual pressure and microcurrent probes [18].

MICROCURRENT THERAPY AND *QI*

It could be said that the bioelectric principles just discussed are based on universal laws of physics and metaphysics that govern how the body actually works, in an unbroken continuum with the Earth and the Universe. Treatment techniques that are not based on these principles will not deliver good, consistently effective results and may produce aggravations of pain and discomfort. These principles can also be viewed as descriptions of various aspects of the movements and transformation of *qi*, a premise I have confirmed through a great deal of testing using the pulse and *hara* (腹, abdominal) diagnoses of classical acupuncture.

According to the classics of Chinese and Japanese traditional medicine, changes in the pulse and abdomen reflect the quantity, qualities and location of *qi* and Blood in the body. In the tradition of Manaka, I have checked pulse positions and abdominal regions before and after application of microcurrent and Microlight treatment techniques and noted the changes. The most effective techniques are those that rapidly balance the pulse and alleviate abdominal tension or weakness. Pulse and abdominal changes have been most significant when applying optimal frequencies and colors (law of resonance), correct polarities (law of polarity) and minimal intensities of current (less is more). Applying microcurrent and light through acupuncture points (law of specificity) increases effectiveness even more.

Ted Kaptchuk introduced valuable understandings about *qi* in his seminal book *The Web That Has No Weaver*. Through careful study of Chinese acupuncture sources he concluded that *qi* is a term that cannot be accurately translated into English. Rather than just equating *qi* with energy he states: 'Chinese thought does not distinguish between matter and energy, but we can perhaps think of *qi* as matter on the verge of becoming energy, or energy at the point of materializing' [19].

Kaptchuk describes the five major functions of *qi* in the body. Three of these are strongly affected by microcurrent stimulation: promoting movement, warming the body and holding tissues in their proper place (preventing prolapses). The microcurrent rehabilitation techniques described below do help promote freer range of motion and improved gait after injuries. The rapid pain relief produced by these therapies most likely stems from improved circulation of *qi* through previously blocked areas. Microcurrent therapies, especially when using warm adjunctive colors of light (such as red, orange and yellow), often trigger noticeable warming of the tissues. Series of Microlight facial rejuvenation sessions have been documented to tighten and lift sagging facial muscles.

These effects indicate that gentle electrical stimulation, especially when applied with appropriate techniques, can have powerful effects on *qi*.

MICROCURRENT AND LIGHT TREATMENT TECHNIQUES

Here are descriptions of treatment techniques based on the bioelectric principles just described. They have been extensively used and refined by myself and hundreds of doctors and practitioners using the Acutron system and Acutron Mentor device [20]. The power of these techniques derives from how they work in harmony with the living matrix and the laws of energy. They are divided into two categories: probe and pad therapies.

MICROCURRENT PROBES

These probes are handheld wands that pass electrical microcurrents through their tips (Fig. 17.1A). In many quality microcurrent devices, the probe electrodes can perform two functions: searching and treating. In search mode, the probes act as point locators, and give visual and audio indications when they are over maximally conductive treatment sites. The associated meter can display a numerical reading expressing 'excess' or 'deficiency'. When the probe button is pressed, the probes switch over to treatment mode, in which currents are passed through the probe tips into the body for the length of time set on the device timer. This rapid alternation between searching and treatment is very useful for accurate, effective pain relief treatments.

In the protocols that follow, I will be referring to two main forms of probe treatment: 'biphasic' and 'polarized'. These refer to the electrical polarity orientation of the probes, an extremely important factor in producing good results. The probe may be negative (stimulating, putting electrical energy into the point), or positive (sedating, drawing electrical energy out of the point).

Biphasic means that the polarity of the probes alternates, or switches back and forth every few seconds. Polarized means that the probes stay fixed in their polarity positions, with one staying negative and one remaining positive, throughout application of the technique.

PAD ELECTRODES

These electrodes are the more traditional electrostimulation pads that have been used with TENS (transcutaneous electrical nerve stimulation), interferential therapy and other such methods. Pad electrodes apply therapeutic currents to a larger region of the body than do probes. Figure 17.1B shows their use in interferential therapy. This very useful method involves two pairs of pads with the pairs set to different frequencies that, when mixed in the body, are thought to produce deeply acting interference fields.

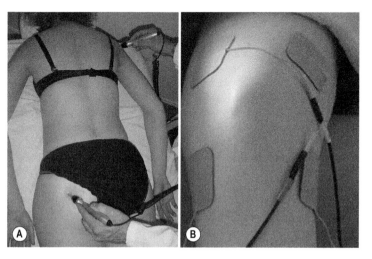

FIG 17.1 (A) **Microcurrent probes.** Polarized probes, placed locally and distally – here for a shoulder problem. The switch on the lower probe is used to start and stop the flow of treatment currents. (B) Pad electrodes around the knee, showing their use in interferential treatment.

Bioelectricity and *qi*: a microcurrent approach

Pads can deliver either high-intensity milliampère currents that produce noticeable tingling or muscle pulsations, or low-intensity microampère currents (microcurrents), which are generally below the threshold of sensation.

In many of the protocols that follow, brief probe treatments for rapid pain relief or other acupuncture-style treatments are used, followed by longer periods of pad stimulation. Pad treatments can be attended or unattended.

COLOR LIGHT THERAPY

I have found a significant advantage in adding color light therapy to acupuncture or microcurrent treatments. Visible light represents a much higher frequency level of electromagnetic energy than that of electrical stimulation or needles, and can evoke much more targeted effects. Color therapy also often offers greatly increased pain relief over acupuncture or microcurrent alone. Color light can be added to treatments as a separate step, or can be applied simultaneously through the Microlight (microcurrent and color light) combination probe system developed for the Acutron system.

PROBE TECHNIQUES

1. **'Circling the dragon'**: This technique is the use of two microcurrent treatment probes set to *biphasic* (back and forth) polarity, placed close together on the body to bracket areas of localized pain. Typical treatment time per body area is 1–3 minutes to relieve pain, release trigger points and improve range of motion.

2. **Polarized probes:** This technique is the use of treatment probes with *fixed* polarity for local and distal acupuncture point placements, including stimulation of auricular or Korean hand points. This technique can cause dramatic pain releases and is useful in meridian balancing treatments for systemic effects.

   The main difference between the use of these techniques is that 'circling the dragon' uses probes that are close together for local treatment only, whereas polarized technique is about local and distal placement, in the manner of good acupuncture treatments (see Fig. 17.1A).

3. **Microcurrent *mu–shu* technique:** *Mu* (募), or Alarm (or Collecting) points, are diagnostic and treatment points on the front of the body (Fig. 17.2A). Each *mu* point registers disorders of an associated Organ (*zangfu*, 臟腑). *Shu* (輸), or Associated (or Transporting) points, are acupoints on the back, on both sides of the spine, that also directly connect with associated Organs and can be used both diagnostically and for treatment in acupuncture practice (Fig. 17.2B). Because they connect directly to Organs, *mu* and *shu* points can provide optimal treatment of visceral disorders, particularly when treating both together in the '*mu–shu* technique'.

   To apply Microlight *mu–shu* treatment, polarized probes with color light are applied, the positive probe to the front-*mu* point of the targeted Organ, and the negative probe to its associated back-*shu* point. Treatment time is about 30 seconds per set of *mu–shu* points. Colors are selected based on the Organ correspondences of the Five Element (*wuxing*, 五行) theory of Chinese medicine, for color is literally food for the *zangfu* (this is not considered the case, of course, in Western medicine). I have experienced remarkable responses when adding a few minutes of this technique into pain, addiction or internal disease treatments.

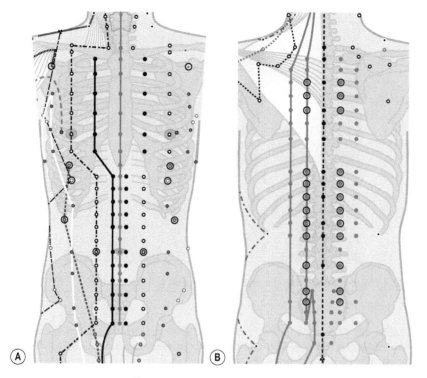

FIG 17.2 (A) The front-*mu* (募, Alarm/Collecting) points and **(B)** the back-*shu* (輸, Associated/Transporting) points. *(After Kubiena and Sommer [21] with permission.)*

4. **'Reverse body image'/'great loops':** Also using polarized probes, the positive probe is applied on a local area of pain, and the negative probe on a tender point on the opposite aspect of the body. For example, in shoulder pain, the former is positioned on the shoulder and the latter at a tender point on the opposite hip (see Fig. 17.1A).

PAD ELECTRODE TECHNIQUES

1. **Interferential:** This creates a much broader stimulation pattern for large joints and body regions. It is used for acute or chronic pain, neuropathy or postexercise soreness. Interferential treatment can be applied with high (milliampère) or low (microcurrent) treatment currents. High currents are generally used for acute pain and injuries and edema, and microcurrent for subacute or chronic pain and peripheral neuropathies (see Fig. 17.1B).
2. **Kinetic electrotherapy:** This is another of the favorite microcurrent therapies, again because it is simple, elegant and works well. Four pad electrodes are placed around an injured or painful area, the current flow is started, and then the area is mobilized. This maneuver can be accomplished in many ways, for example:
   a. Patient moves joint through range of motion (active motion).
   b. Practitioner moves area for them or uses rehabilitative exercise equipment to do so (passive motion).
   c. Bodywork is administered, such as *tuina* (推拿) (see Ch. 5), *sotai* (操体), manipulation, traction, etc.

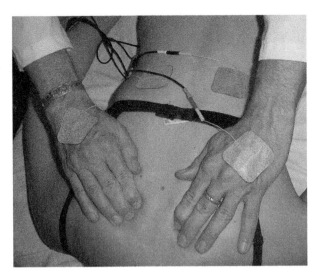

FIG 17.3 Electromassage with the practitioner's hands as living electrodes.

Again, all of these maneuvers are applied *while* the current is flowing through the muscles and fascia. This technique is a prime rehabilitation therapy applicable for a wide range of conditions.

3. **Electromassage:** In this method the practitioner's hands become living electrodes (Fig. 17.3). A four-pad interferential treatment is set up by placing one pad from each pair on the patient's body to bracket the region of pain or dysfunction, the other pad from each pair being positioned on the back of the practitioner's hands. The body should be moistened where massage is to be applied, the current is started, and then massage, trigger point release, acupressure, friction or any other applicable bodywork style is used. This can accelerate the results of bodywork, and tight and restricted areas release more quickly and easily – a labor-saving technique!

ROOT, BRANCH AND SEQUENCE THERAPY

The terms Root (*ben*, 本) and Branch (*biao*, 標) originated in ancient Chinese divination methods. They were eventually adopted in Chinese medicine as terms to differentiate between causal and symptomatic therapies. A *Root* treatment is one that improves overall health or treats chronically weak Organs. *Branch* treatments focus more on alleviating painful or distressing symptoms. A skilled acupuncturist will offer treatments as needed to address both Root and Branch.

Another contribution made by Manaka, whose work with polarity agents and subtle energy acupuncture was mentioned earlier, was his 'four-step treatment system' [13]. Based on his understanding of the movements of *qi* and the 'less is more' principle, he developed a system that offered the benefits of both Root and Branch treatment in the same session. This treatment was done by performing a sequence of techniques along the following lines:

Step One. Root treatment to address constitutional issues and structural imbalances by balancing the body's electrical/meridian system with polarity agents.

Step Two. Neuromuscular treatment through the *yang* meridians.

Step Three. Applying proprioceptive Asian bodywork to correct structural imbalances – analogous to manipulation or physical therapies in Western healthcare.

Step Four. Symptomatic treatments, usually through auricular or Korean hand microsystem points.

Each of these steps directly responds to imbalances of *qi*. Treatment is not selected theoretically, but always through pragmatic testing and observation of the patient's body and meridian status.

In my own adaptation of Manaka's four-step system for use with microcurrent electroacupuncture [22], I have found that applying sequences of brief treatments has been highly effective and versatile. The following case study offers an example of this approach.

CASE STUDY: CHRONIC LOW BACK PAIN AGGRAVATED BY EXERCISE

Patient:

A 53-year-old male with a long history of lower left congenital back pain at L5–S1 level. He had a tendency to be overweight and worked very hard at exercise to control this. His intense exercise routine was aggravating his back pain. He had had long-term pain relief after two previous Microlight treatments given a year earlier.

Energetic evaluation:

Kidney and Liver test points were weak. Patient showed marked pain on pressure in lower left back and significant pain on walking. He was still exercising, including some dead lifts. I instructed him to stop those for at least a month, but continue with other exercises.

Technique sequence used:

- **Technique 1:** Circling the dragon local probe therapy with purple light, lower left back.
- **Technique 2:** Polarized probe therapy with positive probe on center of pain area and negative probe on a sequence of distal acupoints on the right hand and left leg. This was followed by placing the positive probe on the pain area and the negative probe on tender points on the upper chest (reverse body image).
- In addition to the Microlight therapy the patient received a few acupuncture needles on distal acupoints *ling ku*, *zong bai* [23] and KI-3.
- **Technique 3:** Microcurrent interferential pad therapy was applied on the lower back while *sotai* Oriental bodywork was performed. Patient lay prone on a treatment table and was asked to perform straight backward leg raises with pressure against my hand while holding his breath, then releasing the leg.

The patient's pain was dramatically reduced after this treatment. He had good relief for 5 days and then reinjured his back after doing more intense exercise. He returned to my clinic and I reviewed his exercises.

His second treatment was similar to the first one except that I added the Root element of strengthening his Kidneys. I did this by applying the *mu–shu* technique with scarlet light. The positive probe was applied to acupoint KI-16 on the front while the negative probe was applied to BL-23 on his back, using bilateral stimulation. I also gave him adrenal glandular supplements.

The patient's pain was totally eliminated after the second treatment. He did not seek further treatment.

CONCLUSION AND FUTURE DIRECTIONS

The current debate on redefining many aspects of healthcare is largely based on the realities that costs must be contained and efficiency of many treatments improved. Energy medicine offers valuable solutions for clinically effective and cost-effective care – with few negative side effects. Microcurrent and light therapies are practical, highly effective methods to support pain relief, rehabilitation and esthetic rejuvenation. Energy therapies can also be a valuable support for healing of many internal conditions.

Although *qi* cannot be precisely defined in any language, it can be observed indirectly and is clearly affected by good microcurrent and Microlight therapies. The techniques described in this chapter have been developed through the experiences and trials of the author and many dedicated practitioners, and are those that work in harmony with and respect the laws of energy movement governing the body's bioelectricity.

The success of these techniques in practice indicates that further fruitful applications of microcurrents for healing and regeneration will surely be developed in the fullness of time.

Energy psychology: working with mind–body synergy

Phil Mollon

18

CHAPTER CONTENTS

INTRODUCTION

Energy psychology is a vibrant and evolving field of highly effective procedures for the deep and rapid relief of emotional disorders. The evidence so far strongly suggests it is superior to traditional cognitive, behavioral and psychodynamic approaches – particularly in so far as it subsumes and builds upon all of what is valuable in those earlier methods. Whereas most psychological therapies for the past 120 years have worked predominantly with the *mental* phenomena of thoughts and emotions, as if these can be addressed separately from the body, energy psychology engages the synergy of the informational fields of both psyche and soma. Emotions are, after all, partly bodily events – and our thoughts are partly determined by these bodily events and our interpretation of them, which in turn influence what happens within the body. The crucial observation that opened the window to these new therapeutic possibilities was that distress is expressed and encoded not just in bodily attitudes and armoring (as realized by Wilhelm Reich and many others subsequently), but also as information in the body's 'energy' fields – a discovery first made by psychiatrist Dr John Diamond when building upon his earlier studies of Applied Kinesiology (AK) and traditional Chinese medicine. It is important to note that energy psychology is not based upon any theory, but rather upon

237

such observations of reality, of replicable phenomena. Any practitioner who has learnt to work with the basic principles and procedures can verify these 'thought field' phenomena [1–3].

ORIGINS

In 1964, a Detroit chiropractor called George Goodheart was puzzled by the condition of a woman patient with a protruding shoulder blade. He noticed some nodules around the area where the muscle ligaments attached to the bone. On massaging these, he found to his surprise that the shoulder blade position became normal. Although this event was of no particular psychological significance in itself, it formed the basis of Goodheart's interest in muscle function. He began to study what literature was available on testing muscle function and to explore the link between muscle abnormality and bodily sickness states. What he found was that different diseases may cause specific muscles in an individual to test weak. A treatment that causes these muscles to test strong would tend to have a positive effect on the person's health. Muscle responsiveness could thereby be used to select an appropriate treatment. It was also clear that these phenomena are subtle: muscle bulk seemed irrelevant to whether it would test weak or strong – and muscle strengthening exercises had no effect on such tests.

For Goodheart, the chiropractic 'triad of health' was particularly relevant: disease could result from structural, chemical or mental problems, and the interaction between these. For example, certain foods or environmental pollutants may generate both physiological and mental disturbance; anxious thoughts about the physiological disturbance leads to more release of stress hormones generating more physiological disturbance; resulting muscle tension, perhaps in the chest, spine or neck, then causes further stress. Goodheart began to use muscle testing to explore therapeutic procedures in all three realms of the triad of health, identifying those that were helpful and detecting their effects.

Structural therapeutics may include chiropractic, massage and osteopathy; *chemical* therapeutics include nutrition and medication; *mental* therapeutics include various forms of psychotherapy. By 1970, he had begun to explore links between the muscle–organ–gland correspondences that he had noted in his own work, and the acupuncture *meridian*–organ associations described in Chinese medicine. Techniques that corrected certain meridian imbalances had a beneficial effect on the organs and glands he found associated with that meridian – and were also observed to strengthen the muscles associated with them. In turn, Goodheart noted that techniques that caused the muscle to test strong also had a positive effect on the associated meridians. There were thus clear observable bidirectional links between organs/glands, muscles and meridians. The meridian energy realm could be viewed as an additional dimension mapping on to the triad of health. This whole field of inquiry and treatment, based on muscle testing, became known as Applied Kinesiology [4,5].

In addition to the interplay between mind, body (structural and chemical), and the meridian energy system, Goodheart found another phenomenon of particular psychological interest. When someone makes a statement they believe to be true, the tested muscle appears strong – and similarly when they think of someone or something emotionally positive for them. However, when thinking of something emotionally negative, or when making a statement they believe to be false, the muscle tests weak. It seems that negative emotions and lies are weakening. The stronger muscle response to true, versus false, statements has been verified objectively using computerized measures of muscle strength [6].

John Diamond built on Goodheart's work, applying muscle testing to explore people's responses to a wide variety of visual, auditory and chemical stimuli.

He found rather consistent results in terms of which visual and auditory stimuli (e.g. facial expressions, symbols and line drawings, music) and nutritional samples tested 'strong' and which tested 'weak'. This work was summarized in his 1979 book *Behavioral Kinesiology* (subsequently retitled *Your Body Doesn't Lie* [7]). His findings can easily be verified by readers since he provides many of the visual stimuli in the book. It appears that some part of our being has access to information that is not available through our normal senses, and this knowledge can be communicated via the muscle signaling system.

METHODS OF MUSCLE TESTING

There are different ways of muscle testing. It is very much an art, and like any other mode of communication it can be prone to error. Nevertheless, it can provide useful hypotheses to guide therapeutic work. Although testing the absolute strength of a muscle through exerting maximum pressure against resistance can provide information, in practice this would be tiring and physically stressful. In the field of energy psychology, most experienced practitioners aim to exert the minimum pressure necessary to reveal differences between 'strong' and 'weak'. Often the technique is to apply light pressure to the wrist of an outstretched arm. What we look for is a sense of the muscle 'locking' versus a 'spongy' feeling. It can take very little pressure to detect this. However, some people are difficult to muscle test, whereas others are very easy. Sometimes it is necessary to coach people into allowing their body to respond appropriately; for example, sometimes it is helpful to explain that some tension is required in the muscle (some people just hold their arm in a floppy manner with no muscle tone) whereas with others there is the opposite problem and it has to be explained that 'If you feel your arm giving way, it is ok to let it go'.

Diamond [8] used muscle testing to detect which meridians were out of balance by pressing on the client's outstretched arm while the latter put the fingers of the other hand on various meridian test points (the acupuncture 'Alarm' or 'Collecting' points – see Fig. 17.2A). The muscle would register weak when an out-of-balance meridian was stimulated. Diamond then found that a meridian that was out of balance could be restored by the use of a particular affirmation specific to that meridian. Thus, for example, the Lung meridian would respond to 'I am humble', the Gall Bladder meridian to 'I reach out with love' and the Large Intestine to 'I am clean and good'. Different meridians were also linked with different emotions and moods. For example, the Triple Warmer (*sanjiao*) meridian that Goodheart linked to thyroid function might be linked with depression, the Heart meridian with anger, the Gall Bladder with rage, the Large Intestine with guilt, the Conception Vessel (*renmai*) with shame – and so forth. These are not fixed or absolute links. A particular state of mind might consist of layers of these emotions, which could be detected and corrected through the Diamond method. The significance of Diamond's work is that he extended the scope of muscle testing, discovered links between emotions and meridians, found a way of muscle testing to identify, in sequence, the meridians that were out of balance and was able to use forms of words to correct these imbalances. Words, the body, emotions and energy meridians were thus seen to be intimately, precisely and complexly related.

DR ROGER CALLAHAN: THOUGHT FIELD THERAPY (TFT)

In 1979, Californian clinical psychologist Roger Callahan took a further crucial step. Callahan had been working for about 18 months with a patient, Mary Ford, who suffered from a long-standing phobia of water (drinking and bathing little, and avoiding rain, rivers and the ocean). A cognitive therapist and colleague of Albert Ellis (the developer of rational emotive therapy), he had tried various behavioral and cognitive methods, but with only modest success. Mary was able to sit with her feet dangling in the water on the side of Callahan's swimming pool, but still experienced considerable discomfort when doing so – she still had the phobia. Callahan used AK and detected a disturbance in Mary's Stomach meridian. Acting on a whim, he asked her to tap under the eye, where the meridian starts. To his astonishment, after just a few seconds Mary leapt up exuberantly declaring 'it's gone' and ran toward his swimming pool. Alarmed that she was going to jump in, Callahan called after her shouting 'Mary, you can't swim'. Fortunately, she was fully aware of this, and explained that the anxious tension she had experienced in her stomach had suddenly gone and she was excited to feel free of this at last. The phobia she had suffered as long as she could remember was gone in that moment – and never returned [1].

Callahan had never encountered or heard of a result like this before. Fortunately he did not discount it as merely a one-off fluke, but continued to explore. His early success rate was, however, very poor. Most people did not recover from their psychological difficulties simply by tapping under the eye, and Callahan found that *sequences* of meridians usually needed to be tapped. Using a modification of Diamond's method, he could find the precise sequence of meridians that underpinned the person's particular problem. He would ask the person to think of the problem whilst muscle testing. The arm would go weak. He would then ask the person to touch different meridian test points ('Alarm points') until he found the one that made the arm strong. This would be the first meridian in the sequence. After treating this meridian, he would then look for the next one that would make the arm strong – and treat that one. He would continue in this way until the arm remained strong when the person thought of the problem. The arm remaining strong at this point would correspond to a subjective cessation of anxiety or other distress associated with the thought of the problem. Callahan called this his 'causal diagnostic procedure'. It is precise yet subtle, and the phenomena are easily verified and replicated by anyone who properly learns this technique from Dr Callahan or an authorized teacher. As Callahan points out, the energetic underpinning of the 'thought field' is both visible and palpable: shifts in muscle tone can be clearly seen and felt [9].

These observations have far-reaching implications. That a precise sequence of meridians underpins the experienced disturbance indicates that some *information* is encoded energetically. Callahan [1] compares this with a combination lock. Tapping the wrong sequence will not free the lock, but the precise correct sequence will; tapping randomly on the lock buttons might take a long time to find the correct sequence. With muscle testing, Callahan was able to locate the sequence easily. Moreover, he found that recurrent sequences were found with many patients to underpin common states of mind. For example, anxiety would often be encoded as Stomach meridian, Spleen and Kidney, and the associated tapping points would be under the eye, arm and collar bone. Claustrophobic anxiety might involve the same meridians but in a different order: under arm, eye and collar bone. Depression might relate to the back of the hand (*sanjiao* meridian) and collar bone, trauma to the eyebrow (Bladder meridian) and collar bone, and so on. These regularly occurring sequences he termed 'algorithms' [1]. Many practitioners of Callahan's Thought Field Therapy just rely on these without recourse to muscle testing and get good results – but his causal diagnostic procedure (taught like much of this material only in his workshops and home study DVD courses) is more precise, allowing for the idiosyncratic encoding of each individual.

PSYCHOLOGICAL REVERSALS

Callahan encountered a further problem in work with some of his clients. In most cases, if a person is muscle tested to the statement 'I want to be well', or 'I want to be over this problem', the muscle will register strong (an affirmative answer). However, in some cases, the muscle would register weak – indicating that the statements were not registering as true. In such circumstances, the statements 'I want to be sick' or 'I want to keep this problem' might register as true, and the person would not respond to subsequent meridian tapping. Callahan noticed that these same people had also not responded to conventional psychotherapy.

He called this phenomenon 'psychological reversal' since the muscle signaling system was giving a precise reversal of the expected response. Initially he did not know what to do about this. However, by trial and error he discovered three simple procedures that would often 'correct' the reversal [10]. One was to have the person make a statement of self-acceptance (e.g. 'I completely accept myself even though I have this problem'). Another was to have the person tap the side of the hand, a point on the Small Intestine meridian (there is no obvious reason why – it just has this effect). A third way of correcting reversals was to have the person ingest a little of the Bach Flower 'rescue remedy', a now well-known preparation based on principles similar to those of homeopathy. Mostly, Callahan relied on a combination of tapping the side of the hand and the affirmation of self-acceptance. In these ways, through finding precise meridian sequences and by neutralizing psychological reversals, Callahan was able to achieve good results in a high proportion of cases [1].

When reversals are present, nothing will be achieved using Thought Field Therapy procedures – but when they are corrected, the same patient will rapidly resolve their problem. Tapping a sequence when the person is psychologically reversed will result in no change. Once the reversal is corrected, the same sequence may bring about a marked drop in subjective distress.

Callahan has identified several levels of reversal. The most pervasive would be identified by a weak muscle response to the statement 'I want to be well' or 'I want to be happy' or 'I want to be alive' (and strong to 'I want to be sick', etc.). More specific reversals relate to a particular target problem, and are revealed by a weak muscle response to 'I want to be over this problem' (and strong to 'I want to keep this problem'). A mini-reversal occurs when most of a problem has cleared with a tapping sequence, but a little of it seems to persist; this mini-reversal will be revealed by a weak response to 'I want to be *completely* free of this problem' (and strong to 'I want to keep *some* of this problem'). A 'level 2' reversal relates to the future: a weak response to 'I *will* be completely free of this problem'. A 'level 3' response is shown by a weak response to 'I want to be *even better*'.

Callahan himself does not particularly relate the reversals to motivations or psychodynamics. However, many practitioners, including this writer, have found that reversals express quite specific motivations or anxieties, except when they are caused directly by 'energy toxins' such as foods, grooming products or environmental substances that disorganize the person's energy field. The main motivations, concerning safety, deservedness and identity, can be revealed by muscle testing in turn each of the following statements: 'It is safe to be over this problem', 'I deserve to be over this problem' and 'I will still be me if I am over this problem'. The value of being able to pinpoint rapidly these internal objections behind psychoenergetic reversals is immense, allowing a precision and clarity of work not possible in traditional talking therapies. We can also usefully test other statements, such as 'All parts of me want to be over this problem'.

NEUROLOGIC DISORGANIZATION

Another obstacle that Callahan identified was termed 'neurologic disorganization', and was inherited from the earlier field of AK [5]. Although this can include phenomena of a neurological nature, such as left–right confusion, clumsiness, and so forth, it is also encompasses energetic phenomena. It is best revealed by the 'palm over head' test. When the palm is down the muscle should test strong, but palm up the muscle should test weak. If there is no difference or if the response is reversed (palm down is weak and palm up is strong), neurologic/energetic disorganization is indicated. I am inclined to think that the 'strong in both palm positions' response indicates an energetically locked system; in such a state the system cannot release stress since the bioelectrical (positive/negative) polarization necessary to allow an in–out flow of subtle energy is absent. Several methods of correcting this reversal have been found [5], the earliest being 'cross crawl' whereby the person marches on the spot, smacking the knees with opposite hands alternately. A method of sitting with ankles and hands crossed, known as 'Cook's hookups', also works well. Dr Callahan's own technique is called 'collar bone breathing', a sequence of holding first the fingers, and then the knuckles, against the ends of the collar bones, whilst tapping an acupressure point on the back of the hand and undertaking a controlled breathing pattern. I have found that the following simpler variant of this technique works well.

Modification of Callahan's collar bone breathing exercise

Cross your hands over the upper chest, with your fingertips resting on the collar bones. Then go through the following breathing sequence, holding for about 5 seconds at each point: breathe in all the way (through the nose); then breathe out half way; then breathe out all the way; then breathe in half way; then breathe normally. Then change the hands to knuckles (still crossed); breathe in all the way; breathe out half way; breathe out all the way; breathe in half way; breathe normally.

Having worked with the client's system to the point that it is 'ready' (correctly polarized and not disorganized) and 'willing' (not showing a psychological reversal against resolving the target problem) [11,12], the practitioner then has the task of addressing the problem directly as expressed in the energetic thought field. When a person thinks of a troubling experience, his or her muscle will test weak. The Callahan 'diagnostic' method (described above) is used to locate the sequence of meridians that will cause the muscle to test strong when the client continues to think of the problem (i.e. whilst the 'thought field' is activated). The procedure is followed until the muscle remains strong when the client thinks of the problem 'in the clear' (without touching any meridian Alarm point). This will correspond to a subjective experience of no longer feeling troubled by thinking of the target problem.

EMOTIONAL FREEDOM TECHNIQUES (EFT)

Callahan refined and simplified his procedure. Now it is elegant, rapid and efficient, free of superfluous elements. When used properly, it produces clear, predictable and replicable results [13]. Nevertheless, a simplified derivative, called Emotional Freedom Techniques (EFT), has been popularized by one of his students, Gary

Craig. This added nothing new to Callahan's procedure, but simply removed the more complex components of muscle testing and concern for the sequence of meridians. In 'EFT', the meridians can be tapped in any order. Whilst lacking the precision of TFT, it is still surprisingly effective. However, without a working knowledge of the energy system, how to test it and how to correct its dysfunctions, the EFT practitioner may be somewhat in the dark, so to speak. An EFT client may repeatedly tap rounds of meridian points with limited effect. In contrast, a TFT practitioner would expect a significant drop in subjectively experienced distress after a single sequence of taps – normally a drop of at least 2 units on a scale of 0 to 10; if this does not occur, then something is blocking the process, which needs to be identified and corrected. Dr Callahan considers that EFT may be suitable for amateurs, or as a self-help strategy, but that TFT is the procedure that professional practitioners should follow.

ENERGY TOXINS

Because of the rapid, clear and predicable effect of TFT, Callahan was also able to identify some unexpected factors that may impede recovery. The notion of 'individual energy toxins' can initially seem strange. Sometimes a person may repeatedly display energetic disorganization or psychological reversal, such that after these have been corrected they reappear a few moments later. It has been found that these effects are often due to environmental pollutants such as grooming products and perfumes, detergent smells, air 'fresheners', fumes, certain foods or other ingested substances, electromagnetic disturbance or energetic disturbances inherent in the ground (sometimes called 'geopathic stress'). The strongest clue to their action is that when they are identified and avoided or neutralized then the subsequent TFT procedure is effective. Callahan developed a '7-second treatment' for energy toxins [14]. This is extremely effective in temporarily neutralizing energy toxins so that reversals or disorganization are dissipated and TFT can proceed successfully. (The method involves a combination of a breath pattern and subtle pressure on the head; although very effective, it should be learned from a licensed TFT teacher.) Of course, energy toxins are likely to affect other aspects of the person's life and interfere with other forms of psychotherapy, but with less efficient methods they would not be detected.

EXPANDING THE APPLICATION OF THOUGHT FIELD THERAPIES

Through the 1980s, Callahan was working largely alone. To have persisted when many of his colleagues regarded him as either mad or a charlatan (or both), with his referral sources drying up, resulted in significant financial challenges. Dr Callahan has alluded to the hardship of those years. He wrote a book called *The Five Minute Phobia Cure* [15] and presented his methods on TV programs, demonstrating treatments with members of the audience. By the 1990s he had extended his approach to trauma and other conditions [2,16]. Others were beginning to learn and develop TFT – not always with his approval – and some were independently developing similar methods, such as James Durlacher [17]. Fred Gallo, a psychologist, coined the term 'energy psychology' [18], which is now widely used to refer to the broad range of applications of the principles developed by Diamond and then Callahan and others – although neither of these men would endorse that term and tend to be critical of the field. In the United States, some of the leading figures in energy psychology have been accomplished people in their core professions of psychology, psychiatry or social work [3,19]. As a result, in 1998 the Association for

Comprehensive Energy Psychology was established, an organization devoted to promoting research, sharing ideas and developing ethical standards for this lively emerging approach. Amongst the many diverse approaches of energy psychology [20] I regard the following as some of the more important: Tapas Acupressure Technique (TAT); Seemorg Matrix/Advanced Integrative Therapy; Healing from the Body Level Up; Reed Eye-movement Acupressure Psychotherapy (REMAP).

Dr Callahan is inclined to consider attempts to improve on his TFT techniques as being 'like drawing a moustache on the Mona Lisa'. Whilst I do not offer a modification of his basic method, I have found it possible to use the principles of TFT in relation to the deeper psychodynamics of the mind – which I call Psychoanalytic Energy Psychotherapy (PEP) [21,22]. The main points of this are as follows:

- The work can be free-associative, the practitioner asking the client 'What comes to mind now?' By following trains of association, enhanced by energy procedures, it is possible to access the core issues that are troubling the person very rapidly.
- We can 'allow the meridians to speak'. This can be done in two ways. One is to identify the sequence of meridians involved in a problem, or even just underpinning the person's current state of mind, and as each meridian is tapped the person is asked to say what comes to mind. The second approach is for the practitioner to voice the likely emotions linked to each meridian as the sequence is tapped. For example, as a client is working through a pattern of injurious criticism by her mother, the practitioner might comment as the Gall Bladder meridian is tapped 'all the rage you felt when your mother humiliated you', and then, as the Large Intestine meridian is tapped, 'and all the ways you turned that rage on yourself, intensifying your feelings of guilt and badness' – building up an emotional narrative as the meridian energy sequence is worked through. This depends on the therapist being readily able to discern the meridian sequence, either through skilled and rapid muscle testing, or through trained intuition.
- If muscle testing/body signaling is used, this can be a direct and very precise route to the unconscious and the person's deeper attitudes and anxieties, revealing the psycho- and energy dynamics of their system … Psychological reversal phenomena provide crucial information about unconscious conflict and motives for retaining the problem. As a reversal is identified – for example, to do with safety or deservedness – the client is asked 'So why might you feel it is not safe to be free of this problem?' Typically, the person's immediate reply is 'I've no idea', which is then followed by telling you exactly why!
- It is possible to address the more hidden perturbations in various layers and structural components of the person's mind–body–energy system; we can check for perturbations at the level of 'conscious mind', 'unconscious mind', 'all parts of me', 'my body', 'my meridians', 'my *chakras*'. There are other, less well-known parts of the energy system that can also be checked, in addition to meridians and *chakras*. I usually find that after perturbations have been cleared from *chakras* there may be a need to return briefly to the meridians, which are nearer to the surface of the system, in order to clear any energetic 'debris' that has now floated up from the depths. I call this 'multilevel clearing'.
- The multilevel work can include the 'shadow self'. This Jungian concept alludes to all that is at odds with the conscious personality – yet also suggests more of a structural dissociative quality than is implied by the Freudian unconscious. Probably we all have a shadow self as a normal structural component of our full identity – but the shadow can itself be in a state of health or sickness. It can be filled with rage, or used as a psychic dumping ground for unwanted 'outlaws' from the conscious personality, thereby acting as a source

of self-sabotage. This is revealed, for example, by muscle testing the statement 'A part of me wants to sabotage my life'. On the other hand, it can be healed with energy psychology just like any other component of the personality.
- A further highly effective application is to focus on disturbance generated by internal figures. For example, a critical and rejecting mother may form the basis of an internal mother who is even more harsh and critical (since internal figures/objects are often distorted, imbued with the person's own emotions in addition to the actual characteristics of original external figures). There are two steps to this process. One is to have the person tap the specific sequence relating to a phrase such as 'all the times and ways my internal mother has attacked me' (the phrase 'all the times and ways' derives from Seemorg Matrix/Advanced Integrative Therapy). The second step concerns the healing of the internal figure itself. Thus the person can tap the specific sequence for 'all the traumas of my internal mother'. This procedure can have far-reaching positive effects, transforming internal relationships in remarkable ways.

CLINICAL EXAMPLES

The rapid and deep processes of change described here depend upon considerable fluency in reading the client's energy system as the thought field layers are accessed. They are not based upon the use of TFT algorithms or other 'ready made' tapping sequences.

The following examples are all composites, combined from different clients. None corresponds exactly to any specific person. However, the essential clinical processes and outcomes are accurate.

CASE STUDIES

A lady with severe body dysmorphia

Sally was a lady in her early 30s who had suffered from a severely negative body image since age 9. There had been a moment at that age when she had looked at some nude magazines at a friend's house and had suddenly been overwhelmed with the thought that she would never be pretty like the girls in the pictures. Subsequently, she had reached puberty early and this had evoked teasing from classmates. Later she had suffered bullying at secondary school, where she was called 'fat'. At age 17 she was raped, told no one at the time, blamed herself, felt filled with shame and resorted to a period of heavy drinking, taking drugs, and promiscuity. When seen for an initial consultation she reported feeling 'ugly, hairy, spotty and fat', obsessed with minor imperfections in her skin, and phobic of TV ads or other images involving attractive women. She was, however, happy with her husband and children, and had also experienced her parents as supportive.

During the first treatment session, TFT was combined with Eye Movement Desensitization and Reprocessing (EMDR), focusing on her general rage and fury with men and with pornography and those who make and watch it, and her envy of attractive women. Following this she reported feeling somewhat amused by the thoughts that between us had been voiced as she tapped – for example, to do with the stupidity of men, etc.

At her next session, 2 months later, she reported having felt rather better, not blaming and criticizing herself so much, and not so 'self-obsessed'. We then targeted the rape at age 17, again using a combination of EMDR and TFT. Strong feelings were expressed, of shame, rage and guilt. Remaining dysphoric feelings about herself were also targeted.

When we met for the fourth time, a further 2 months later, she reported feeling very well – no longer obsessed with her appearance, more assertive, no longer experiencing nightmares, no longer troubled by disturbing and shame-laden memories from the past and generally more able to be appropriately assertive. Her CORE (Clinical Outcomes in Routine Evaluation) score had dropped from an initial 18 to a very low 3. We agreed to stop. A follow-up a few weeks later indicated that she was still feeling very well. Her CORE score had dropped even further to 2.

Fibromyalgia

Selena, a woman in her 40s, had been suffering from debilitating fibromyalgia (weakness and pervasive muscle pains) for some years following a previously very stressful life and a viral infection. She had experienced abusive relationships and rape in childhood and as an adult.

Muscle testing revealed a clear psychological reversal against being well, also indicating her belief that it was not safe to be well. Selena associated to the idea of being 'invalid', of being invalidated by others and by herself. She thought it probably felt unsafe to be well because being unwell gave her some protection against being available sexually. Since this was a high-level reversal, we took this itself as the target issue – and began to explore the meridian sequence underpinning the phrase 'The origins of feeling it is not safe to be well'. As Selena tapped on the emerging sequence, she was asked to report whatever came to mind. This led rapidly to angry thoughts of being assaulted as a child, of being unprotected, along with sensorimotor memories of being violated – deepening to alternating feelings of black despair and intense overwhelming rage. The perception of her *illness as a kind of sanctuary* came to her mind. With further multilevel clearing, including of the shadow self, Selena reported feeling 'Like something has stepped out of me' and adding 'I can't remember the last time I felt like this, I can't believe how much better I feel'. A few weeks later, She wrote to me saying her fibromyalgia had been much improved since this session.

Freedom from childhood distortions

Aleisha, a woman in her 40s, told me a complex story of career success and relationship unhappiness. She was aware of a chronic difficulty in expressing herself in intimate relationships. Her mother had died when she was age 14, leaving her having to assist her father in looking after several younger siblings. As we explored psychological reversals, an issue of not feeling it was safe to be well became apparent (when muscle testing weak to 'It is safe to be well'). Her associations were to the image that people have of her of always coping, having to be strong and never relying on others. She feared that if she became completely well her own needs and vulnerabilities would be overlooked and she would have to continue looking after others. As she then focused on a current relationship dilemma, the first meridian was the *dumai* (Governor Vessel), which is often linked with issues of control and autonomy. She associated to how she can be very controlling. Next the Large Intestine meridian came up, and she commented that she sometimes suffered from irritable bowel. Then the throat *chakra* (often linked with expression) came into focus; this led her to talk of many aspects of her difficulties in expressing herself, particularly her ambivalence towards her father, as well as blocked feelings about her mother's death.

When Aleisha came for a second session a couple of weeks later, she reported feeling 'really good', with more energy, more positive feelings for her father and increased enjoyment of her current partner. A second session worked through more of her anger and sorrow about losing her mother, layers of different emotions emerging as she tapped on the sequence of meridians.

Subsequently Aleisha reported having felt transformed by these two sessions, released from the pains and traumas of her childhood. This was the end of the therapeutic work.

RESEARCH AND EVIDENCE BASE

Taken as a whole, the evidence base for energy psychology methods is substantial. The forms of evidence include randomized controlled trials (RCTs) [23–25], thousands of brief single case studies [26], field data from use with posttraumatic stress disorder (PTSD) in disaster zones [27], brain scan data showing before and after treatment images and the brain effects of stimulating specific acupressure points [28,29], audiovisual recorded examples showing behavioral change, studies of effects on heart rate variability (HRV) [30–32], systematic clinical observation studies [33,34] and uncontrolled pilot studies. Internationally, the numbers of practitioners and clients treated are enormous. Relevant neuroscience and biological models are provided by Pert [35], Oschman [36] and Ruden [37], whilst the physics is offered by Tiller [38].

One large audit and preliminary trial of TFT-type methods in South America over a 14-year period involved 36 therapists treating 29 000 patients at a number of centres [39]. Since this study received no funding, the data do not meet the rigorous standards required for formal research. Nevertheless, randomization and control were used, along with double blind assessments and standardized measures – and the results were remarkable. In a subgroup of 5000 patients, positive results were found in 90% of those treated with TFT, but only 63% of those treated with Cognitive Behavioral Therapy (CBT) and medication. 76% showed complete relief from symptoms with TFT, but only 51% of those treated with CBT and medication. At 1-year follow-up, patients in the TFT group were less prone to relapse than those in the CBT and medication group. Positive results were also quicker with TFT. In 190 phobic patients, positive results were obtained with 69% using CBT and medication, over a mean of 15 sessions. The other group, using TFT combined with a visual–kinesthetic dissociation technique, produced positive results with 78% in a mean of three sessions. Functional brain imaging supported these findings – which were sustained, and even improved, at 12-month follow-up.

In a commentary, Aalberse and Sutherland concluded:

No reasonable clinician, regardless of school of practice, can disregard the clinical responses that tapping elicits in anxiety disorders (over 70% improvement in a large sample in 11 centres involving 36 therapists over 14 years) [40].

Interestingly, Joaquin Andrade, the lead author of the research study, no longer uses the 'energy' theory of TFT. Instead, he hypothesizes that results are due to neurobiological effects of sensory–kinesthetic stimulation, acupressure points being hypothesized as dense concentrations of mechanoreceptors.

SOME RANDOMIZED CONTROLLED STUDIES OF EFFICACY

Wells et al [25] carried out a well-designed study of the use of EFT with people who were phobic of small animals (e.g. spiders, rodents, cockroaches). A 30-minute treatment with EFT was compared with a similar length control session of diaphragmatic breathing known to produce physiological effects associated with deep relaxation. Moreover, the control condition also contained all the elements of EFT except for meridian tapping. EFT produced significantly greater drops in fear, shown on both self-report and behavioral measures – and these were sustained at follow-up.

Baker and Siegel [24] undertook a replication and extension of the study by Wells et al, but using a 'no treatment' control, with another comparison group receiving Rogerian counseling. Participants in the EFT group improved significantly, whereas the other two groups showed no change.

Another RCT [23] reported on the use of TAT as an aid to weight loss mainte-nance, compared with *qigong* and CBT. The TAT group gained no weight, but the other two groups did.

Waite and Holder [41] conducted a study purporting to debunk EFT. They assigned participants suffering from anxiety to one of four groups: a standard EFT protocol, tapping on the arm using EFT verbalizations, tapping on a doll with the fingertips (yes, it is rather odd!), or making a paper toy. Two minutes of each treat-ment were given. All three tapping conditions produced a drop in anxiety of 18%, whereas the paper toy condition produced no drop in anxiety. It has been noted that a drop of 18% after a couple of minutes of any kind of treatment is a remark-able result – and one that lends support to those who argue that it is tapping on mechanoreceptors (distributed all over the body) that produces the effect. My own additional hypothesis is that tapping the fingertips actually stimulates a deeper part of the energy system than the meridians alone.

Feinstein [26] and Mollon [22] have summarized in detail the available evi-dence for energy psychological procedures.

CONCLUSION – AND A WORD OF CAUTION

The chiropractor George Goodheart in the 1960s allowed himself to be led and informed by his observations, no matter how seemingly strange, thereby discover-ing the links between muscle tone, illness and the energy meridians of traditional Chinese medicine. Building on his foundations, psychiatrist John Diamond and then clinical psychologist Roger Callahan found ways of working with the mind–body–energy system to relieve all manner of emotional distress. Callahan dis-cerned most clearly that information characterizing the 'thought field' is encoded in the subtle energy system of the body. Many others have explored further, devel-oping the field now known as 'energy psychology'. All the colleagues I know who have taken the trouble to learn to use energy psychology methods have been impressed by the results. However, this work does take effort and dedication to learn – it is neither easy nor simple.

One note of caution may be of relevance. The immediate positive effects of energy psychology approaches can give rise to undue optimism. Energy psy-chology is not itself a panacea for the ills of humanity. There are inherent mor-phic field distortions in the human energy anatomy that are difficult to heal, and which give rise to profound conflicts and contradictions within the psyche and 'human nature'. Deep species-wide energetic reversals exert a continual pull away from the value systems of love, truth and health. In working with clients I have become aware of a common – possibly ubiquitous – unconscious sense of guilt about belonging to the human species. This primal guilt may form the core around which more individual feelings of guilt and 'badness' later form. The tragedy of the human condition is that we are, in part, truly malignant, destructive of other species, the planet and each other – whilst at the same time capable of a sense that this is not how it should be. Although work with the energy system can help to reorient a person's system towards the values of health, these same distortions will oppose the potential benefits of energy psychology. Knowledge of the energy fields, and how to work with them, has always been 'forbidden'.

Craniosacral biodynamics

Franklyn Sills

CHAPTER CONTENTS

INTRODUCTION

In this chapter, I describe a particular paradigm of life energy and healing work called *craniosacral biodynamics*, or *biodynamic craniosacral therapy*. In this approach, the practitioner's principal orientation is to the forces at work within and around the human system. Although this concept is age old, the origin and particulars of this orientation have their roots in the work of an osteopath, William Garner Sutherland (1873–1954). Over the course of his career, Sutherland shifted from a predominantly biomechanical orientation to one that appreciates the interplay of the primary forces at work in the human system. These creative forces underlie and precede biomedical understanding of genetics and are an expression of the most fundamental ordering matrix of life itself. This viewpoint acknowledges that life is a mystery, that all forces and forms originate in an infinite present, that healing is a function of these forces at work within and around the human system and that healing can therefore occur only in the present moment.

Clinical work in craniosacral biodynamics is largely perceptual in nature. The heart of clinical practice is one's own state of presence, the clarity and safety of the relational field one generates, and the ability to orient to and perceive the underlying forces and processes organizing the human system and to be in right relationship to all of this. This work entails an intimacy of contact and communication, which demands both stillness and humility on the part of the practitioner. The awareness of one's own interior world is critical in the creation of a safe and efficient healing relationship. In this process, we inevitably meet our own human condition and our own suffering. This is a huge undertaking. It means truly inquiring into and taking responsibility for the nature of our own suffering and ego processes. From this ground of awareness, it is possible to form clear and healing relationships with others. One truly learns what it means to meet another person deeply in their joy and suffering. Indeed, we learn within the clinical context that we can explore deeply what it means to be a sentient human being.

As an osteopathic student at the beginning of the twentieth century, William Garner Sutherland was fascinated by the bones of the cranium. He was taught that they are fused by adulthood, but could not understand this as skulls can be disarticulated and cranial bones have sutures that seem to be designed for movement. His investigations proved to him that the living skull expresses motion and that this motion is physiologically important. While looking at a temporal bone, he described how the thought struck him that it was 'beveled like the gills of a fish for *primary respiration*' [1, p 3]. This thought led him on a lifetime journey to discover its nature.

Sutherland, being an osteopath, began by describing the subtle inherent motions and pulsations he could feel in biomechanical language and used motion testing and various techniques to release what he experienced as resistance and patterning in tissue relationships. In 1945, however, he had an extraordinary experience that transformed his understanding, his approach to healing and the language he used. He was called to the bed of a dying patient who was in great pain. As Sutherland accessed the man's system through holding his head, a depth of stillness arose and he had a direct experience of what he called the *Breath of Life* as the man comfortably and peacefully passed from this life. Sutherland's language now shifted as he focused on primary respiration and its inhalation and exhalation phases. His approach became one where no force is used from without, but rather the unerring potency (life force) within is trusted to initiate and carry through the healing process. What needs to happen cannot be learned through analysis or motion testing, but is a factor of what Sutherland called the *intelligence* of the system and the intentions of the Breath of Life (see below).

POTENCY

Sutherland perceived that the cerebrospinal fluid becomes potentized with this life principle – a process he described as one of *transmutation*, or a *change in state*. The primary respiration is a field phenomenon that, through transmutation, generates an ordering force within the fluids of the body, and it is this that he called *potency*. This life force first manifests within the fluids of the conceptus, orchestrates embryological formation and maintains physiological order throughout life. The transmission of the potency of the Breath of Life into the cerebrospinal fluid became the most fundamental concept in his treatment modality. We will discuss the nature of potency in greater detail later.

Sutherland experienced primary respiration as a subtle, stable tide-like respiratory motion. The underlying field phenomenon he thus called the *Tide*. The Tide can be sensed as if moving from the horizon towards the midline of a person's system and then, through transmutation, as the potent ordering force within the body. Here we have a concept of the human system based on an understanding of the dynamic of an inherent life force. We also have the revolutionary concept that it is the fluid systems of the body that convey this ordering principle to all of its parts. Sutherland discovered that the fluid dynamic of the body is essential to its expression of health [1,2].

There are similar concepts in many forms of traditional ethnomedicine that place the main healing focus on life energy or life force. In Chinese medicine, for instance, the emphasis is on the balance of *qì* and the potency of *jīng* in the body. Interestingly, *jīng*, or Essence, is similarly sensed as an inherent ordering principle that is intimately related to the body's fluid systems. Along with *qì* and *shén*, *jīng* is considered one of the 'Three Treasures' of traditional Chinese medicine (see Chs 4,

6 and 10). In some systems it is said to be the subtle material basis for the physical body and is *yin* in nature, which means it orders, nourishes, fuels and regulates the body and its functions. In Ayurvedic medicine there is a similar concept, namely *ojas*, which is seen as an essential ordering force, again manifesting in the fluid systems of the body at a cellular level (Dr Trivedi, personal communication, 1981) [3].

THE BREATH OF LIFE

As already mentioned, in the latter part of his career Sutherland stressed that the human system is ordered by what he called the Breath of Life. In the last 10 years of his clinical practice he became especially attuned to its action and mysterious *Presence* within the human system. This also coincided with the shift in his language from a predominantly biomechanical orientation based on analysis and technique to a more fully biodynamic one focusing on the inherent forces that facilitate healing. Increasingly he both spoke and wrote about the Breath of Life and its unerring potency, as he realized that it is the Breath of Life and the intelligent forces it generates that make the healing decisions and carry those decisions out.

My first clinical experience of the Breath of Life took me totally by surprise. I was in the early days of my clinical practice and was working in a London health center with an excellent mix of practitioners from different healing traditions. We were all actually talking to each other about our perspectives and our work, and cross-referring clients. An older woman was referred to me by a homeopath. When I first met her, she was an imposing figure, large and solid. She dressed eccentrically and had a will, a determination that gave out the message 'Don't mess with me'. I discovered that I was just one of a long list of practitioners she had seen over the years. She had experienced almost every form of therapy and healing art imaginable. At first I could not orient her to working on a treatment table. She just needed me to hear her story, and as she sat in the chair opposite me, for five or six sessions I experienced an overwhelming wave of painful history. She had been a Jewish teenager during the Second World War and was trapped in the Warsaw ghetto with her family. She had many relatives and friends there. Just before the ghetto was closed down, her family made her leave. She packed a bag and, in the middle of the war at the age of 15, literally walked across Europe. After a period of struggle and danger, she reached the French coast and talked a kindly and courageous French fisherman into sailing her across the English Channel to safety. She spent the rest of the war with relatives in London and was currently living in a modest woman's club. She held a huge amount of guilt and shame for leaving her family in Warsaw, all of whom had subsequently died in concentration camps.

When I was finally able to place her on the treatment table, I discovered the most defended system I had ever encountered. No expression of primary respiration was apparent and her system was rock solid. I knew many ways to initiate change in a person's system and, over many sessions, tried all of them to no avail. Her suffering had brought me to my knees, as with so many practitioners before me. This went on for at least 6 months and, although I sometimes wondered why she was still coming, I also knew that she found the work supportive and of benefit. Then in one very special session, something happened.

As in most sessions, she spent 10 minutes or so recounting her week to me and we moved to the treatment table. As usual, there was little evidence of tidal motion in fluids or tissues. I settled into my listening and for the first time was struck by the reality that there was little I could do to make any difference. Before then, I had hope that my intentions and skills could help, but now everything seemed futile. I settled into this realization and, in a state of despair, literally let everything go. All that I knew went into a darkness, a literal cloud of unknowing. As I let myself settle into this darkness, my tension and fear subsided and I could maintain a still

Craniosacral biodynamics

and receptive state. Over some time, we entered stillness together, a stillness much deeper than I had ever yet encountered in clinical practice. It was way beyond my experience of stillpoints or neutrals (for meanings of these terms, see Glossary).

Gradually, we settled into a timeless, totally present-time state. Suddenly, seemingly from nowhere, yet present everywhere, a Presence came to the forefront. I sensed something moving through me and it was as though my heart was burst open with love and joy. There is simply no other way I can describe this. Both my client and myself were deeply moved. As the intensity subsided, I sensed radiance permeating the client's system and it was as though multiple issues were safely attended to all at once. Soon after, the fluid tide surged, the tissue field reorganized and the session came to a close. This process marked a dramatic change in both our session work and her life. This experience also marked a major change in my understanding of the work I do, the nature of healing and, indeed, life itself. I have never forgotten it.

Over time, I have come to understand that the Breath of Life is a divine presence only appreciated in a state of stillness and unknowing. It appears everywhere all at once and is numinous, nonlinear and radiant. It arises out of a profound *Stillness* that lies at the heart of all form and is the fulcrum from which all form arises. Unlike the Tide it generates, it has no rhythm, yet is at the heart of all rhythms. It cannot be manipulated or used by the practitioner in any way. One can only humbly witness its creative action within and between human systems. Clinical work in its presence is about stillness, resonance and cooperation. This is a humbling and joyful process to witness. The direct presence of the Breath of Life is not an everyday clinical experience. It emerges as a state of grace, and this cannot be controlled or manipulated in any way.

DYNAMIC STILLNESS

The Breath of Life arises from profound Stillness. As practitioners deepen their relationship to client's systems, over time, Stillness becomes a direct clinical perception and is found to lie at the heart of all clinical process. Because of the direct perception of Stillness in clinical work, there is a clear tradition of its appreciation in the cranial field. Sutherland encouraged practitioners to sense the Stillness at the heart of the Tide. Here he was not talking about a simple ceasing of tidal motion, but was pointing to a much deeper truth. Rollin Becker DO, a disciple of Sutherland's, called the Stillness at the heart of all life 'dynamic and alive'. Following on from Becker's insight, this implicate ground of emergence is commonly called the *Dynamic Stillness* in the cranial field [4].

This appreciation of Stillness is seen in all the great spiritual traditions. Commonly, the first stage of contemplative practice is to drop beneath the conditioned movement of the conceptual mind and to enter Stillness. As this process deepens, the meditator or contemplative discovers that Stillness is an omnipresent ground of emergence for all of life, a gateway to its deepest mysteries and the root of our human condition. In the *Straightforward Explanation of the True Mind*, the Zen Buddhist Chinul (1158–1210) states:

> ...the basic substance [essence] of the true mind transcends causality and pervades time. It is neither profane nor sacred; it has no oppositions. Like space itself, it is omnipresent; its subtle substance is stable and utterly peaceful; beyond all conceptual elaboration. It is unoriginated, imperishable, neither existent nor nonexistent. It is unmoving, unstirring profoundly still and eternal....Neither coming nor going, it pervades all time; neither inside nor outside, it permeates all space...all activities at all times are manifestations of the subtle function of true mind [5, p 245–247].

This is the best description of the Dynamic Stillness that I have ever encountered. It speaks to the root of my condition. In Zen, true mind is the heart of awareness itself, an omnipresent and vibrantly still ground from which our very being arises. Profoundly still, it is yet dynamically present and all function arises from it. It permeates all space, and all activities and forms are manifestations of its subtle function and action. The power of the Breath of Life is rooted in Dynamic Stillness as it manifests *Creative Intelligence* throughout space and time. An awareness of Dynamic Stillness thus brings the practitioner to the center of things, the basic essence of life itself.

THE LONG TIDE AND DYNAMIC EQUILIBRIUM

In his work, Sutherland became more and more aware of subtle, stable tide-like phenomena within and around the human system. Over time, he realized that these tidal motions at the level of primary respiration were direct expressions of the creative intention of the Breath of Life, the *Tide*. Becker preferred to call this the *Long Tide* to differentiate it from other tidal motions and this is the term that is now commonly used. The Long Tide, the direct expression of the creative intention of the Breath of Life, is the most formative level of primary respiration. It seems to arise from 'nowhere', manifests like a great wind arising within a vast field of action and radiates through everything. It is the Long Tide that generates the potency of the local ordering fields.

The Long Tide is very stable and is the most inherent constitutional resource of the system. It manifests as a stable primary respiratory cycle of 50-second inhalation and 50-second exhalation (100 seconds in all), commonly perceived as a streaming of radiance that seems to move through both practitioner and client all at once. People speak of a sense of awe, and of stillness, light and great space in its presence. A deep sense of interconnection and support is also commonly experienced. What Buddhists call the mutuality or co-arising nature of all things becomes more self-evident. Patients begin to feel that there is something much deeper supporting their human condition than mental–emotional states, physical structure, function and physiology. Practitioners commonly sense that it moves from the outside in, manifests through the midline, makes healing decisions and maintains the coherency of the human system. Indeed, some people call it a *coherency wave*, as it functions to maintain the coherency of the human system in the midst of all conditions.

Viktor Schauberger (1885–1958) was an Austrian scientist whose research is relevant to our discussion [6]. From a family of foresters, he spent much time in nature, and in his observations of the natural world he came to recognize a subtle, yet powerful, ordering force that he called the *Original Motion*. As did Sutherland, he perceived that this is a manifestation of what he called Creative Intelligence, the divine creative intention in action, and, like Sutherland, he perceived that it transfers its ordering intentions to the waters or fluids of the world. Again like Sutherland, Schauberger noted that the Original Motion (the Long Tide in biodynamics) acts from the 'outside-in'. Locally, forces seem to arise 'from nowhere' and spiral from outside in to generate stable fields of action. These, in turn, organize cohesive living structures.

Schauberger perceived that the Long Tide manifests locally via spiral-like centrifugal and centripetal motions, a universal principle at work on all levels of creation, equally present in the creation of stars and galaxies and in the generation of microscopic plants and animals. He maintained that, when a *dynamic equilibrium* is established between these centripetal and centrifugal forces, a stable ordering matrix is generated that in particular underlies the organization of the human system. This dynamic field of action is continually being renewed and re-established in every moment (Fig. 19.1).

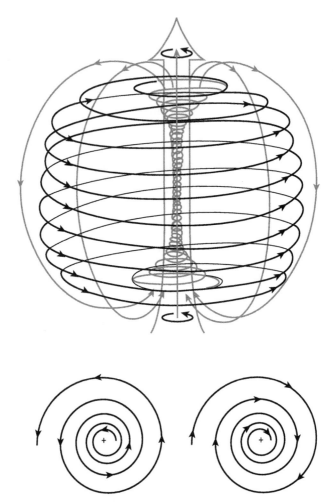

FIG 19.1 Schauberger's 'Original Motion', an expression of dynamic equilibrium between centripetal and centrifugal forces.

Dynamic equilibrium is a state in which all the forces involved in the generation of form are in balance. Becker noted that is a dynamic state in which there is a *rhythmic balanced interchange* between those forces present [4]. It is not static, but an alive and dynamic state of interchange and balance with stillness at its heart. As the forces in play achieve this state of dynamic equilibrium, potency is concentrated and form is generated. This concept of dynamic equilibrium is fundamental to craniosacral biodynamics. The healing processes in our clinical work at a Long Tide level are accessed through practitioner attunement and resonance, and via deepening states of stillness and dynamic equilibrium.

THE HUMAN ORDERING MATRIX

The local field of action generated by the Long Tide is called the *ordering matrix* or *ordering field*. When the centrifugal and centripetal winds of the Long Tide enter dynamic equilibrium locally, a stable field is generated. This matrix can be sensed as a subtle energetic field within and around the human system. It manifests at conception and functions as a formative ('quantum-level') primal template that orders embryological development and maintains the coherency of the body-mind system throughout life. As we shall see, the ordering matrix is directly expressed as an organizing force within the fluids of the body that maintains cellular order and generates inherent motions in both fluid (the *fluid tide*) and body tissue (*tissue motility*).

In classic yogic teaching this level of field-matrix organization is called the *chakra* system, with its field pulsations. In this tradition, the life force (*prana*) is organized in very discrete ways. Like the Long Tide, *prana* is not just a local phenomenon but emerges from a vast field of action. In a similar way, the Chinese speak of organizing centers called *dantian* (*tan t'ien*) that are energetic fulcrums for different functions in the body-mind. Particularly significant are the umbilical and abdominal centers, the heart center, and the upper *dantian* in the third ventricle of the brain (seat of the spirit, *shén*). I believe that all these ways of describing reality, whether in terms of quantum fields, holographic principles, potency and the Breath of Life, the *chakras* and *prana*, or the *dantian*, *jīng* and *qì*, point to the same truth. The human system is organized within subtle quantum-level, dynamic bioelectric–biomagnetic fields that are expressions of a deeper *Creative Intention* at work. When practitioners hold a relatively wide perceptual field and allow their minds to become still and simply listen, these phenomena can actually become discernible. Awareness of this level of organization has very important clinical implications. Healing processes can be initiated from the depths of the creative principle, which underpins all of the biodynamic interchanges within the human system.

In recent years the wisdom of this understanding has been described in scientific terms by researchers in biology and biophysics. Biophysicist Mae-Wan Ho discusses this in her groundbreaking book, *The Rainbow and the Worm* [7]. In her research, she found that microscopic invertebrate animals are organized in quantum fields of light. These are responsive to the environment, have an orienting midline (a literal shaft of light at their center) and clearly maintain the order of the organism. She calls them *coherent quantum electrodynamic fields*, and she and other scientists believe that these may be responsible for the organization of all of life (see also 'Coherence and meridians' in Ch. 16). Dr Sutherland's images of potency, liquid light and the radiance of the Tide are reflected here. In terms relevant to body-oriented therapies, this implies that there is a level of organization within the human system that is always coherent and whole, based upon quantum interplay of biodynamic phenomena and perceived in the living system as bioelectric/biomagnetic forces within a unified field of action. Becker even calls palpation at this level *quantum touch* [8].

TRANSMUTATION, IGNITION AND INCARNATION

For order to be maintained, the forces and organizational principles of the ordering matrix must directly manifest as life force within the body-mind system. As mentioned above, Sutherland thought of this as a process of transmutation (Randolph Stone, founder of Polarity Therapy, termed such changes in state 'step-downs' [9]). One important transmutation is from the field forces of the matrix to the fluids of the body. Think of the ordering matrix as a precise multidimensional quantum form within which the human body is suspended and sustained. There is a transmutation of potency from this matrix, via its midline, into the fluids of the body. Potency then manifests directly as an ordering and orienting principle in the body's fluids. Sutherland described this occurring via what he called *ignition*, with the Breath of Life manifesting its creative intentions as a 'spark' within the body's fluids. This spark moves through the quantum midline of the ordering matrix and generates a force or potency within the body's fluids that maintains order and generates the inherent motions of the fluid tide and tissue motility. This embodied level of life force conveys the intentions of the Breath of Life, the Long Tide and the ordering field it generates.

THE MID TIDE

As transmutation occurs, an embodied force within the fluids called *tidal potency* is generated. This allows the forces of the Long Tide, as primary respiration, to manifest as an embodied principle. With this, a tidal rhythm called the Mid Tide is also generated. The Mid Tide has three fields of action: *potency, fluids and tissues.* Potency is the organizing factor, fluid the medium of exchange, and cells and tissues organize around its action. Within the Mid Tide, potency, fluids and tissues are perceived with a tide-like motion at a rate of anywhere from 1 to 3 (commonly around 2–2.5) cycles per minute. This is a direct expression of the change in state of potency as it shifts from the ordering matrix through its midline into a physiologically functioning principle within cerebrospinal fluid. As potency moves, fluids and tissues pulsate as a unified field. As mentioned above, fluid motion is called the fluid tide and tissue motion is called motility.

The tidal potency is an energetic field sensed both within the fluids and locally around the body as a driving and ordering force (up to 10 inches, or 25 cm, off the body). Its field of action is sometimes called the *fluid body*. It can be literally sensed by the practitioner as a tidal drive within the fluids that generates the fluid tide. This tide is perceived as both longitudinal and transverse fluctuations throughout the body. The action of the tidal potency also generates tissue motility – an inner respiratory motion within cells and tissues – and acts to order the fluid–tissue field. This can be sensed as an inner welling up and receding within the tissue field and within individual tissue structures. At the level of the Mid Tide, the human system is perceived to be whole. Tissues are experienced to be a unified tensile field of action that expresses motility as a whole, rather than simply as separate parts in motion.

These seemingly abstract ideas have physiological reality. Recently it has been found that the water molecules within all connective tissues form discrete hydrogen bonds. These bonds literally create a unified fluid matrix throughout the body. Furthermore, the connective tissues of the body have peptide side chains that bond with these water molecules. A unified fluid–tissue field results, which exhibits phenomena that Ho likens to liquid crystalline structures. The body is literally a unified fluid–tissue crystalline whole of tissues, fluids and bioenergetic phenomena exhibiting discrete quantum effects and waveforms within its matrix [7]. At a Mid Tide level, inertia and resistance within the system are experienced as distortions within whole tensile fields of action, rather than just resistance between separate parts. The potency within the fluids acts to center and contain the unresolved experiential and conditional forces met in life (from trauma, accidents, environmental conditions, toxicity, genetics, etc.). Becker called this the 'centering action' of the potency of the Breath of Life [8]. Clinical work at this level orients to both the universal and conditional forces in the body, and acts to liberate the potency centering the unresolved conditional forces generating pain and pathology, so that these can be resolved in present time. Commonly, clinical work at a Mid Tide level involves an appreciation and augmentation of the action of tidal potencies within fluids and tissues. The practitioner's attitude is one of attunement, resonance and appropriate response to the conditions present.

CRANIAL RHYTHMIC IMPULSE

Another rhythm within craniosacral therapy is the *cranial rhythmic impulse* (CRI), later shortened by some practitioners to the *cranial rhythm*. It commonly manifests at rates of 8–14 cycles a minute. The CRI is the most common rhythm discussed in many cranial courses, and is a conditional rhythm that expresses historical forms and central nervous system and autonomic nervous system activation. Whereas the Long Tide is totally stable, and the Mid Tide is relatively stable, the CRI is highly variable in its expression. It is first and foremost an expression of the conditions of our lives as these conditions are met and centered in some way. It is relatively super-ficial and generated as tidal potencies act to center (neutralize, contain and compen-sate for) the unresolved inertial forces of trauma, toxins, pathogens and experience in general. The level of the CRI is one within which effects and affects, such as tissue resistance, fluid congestion, emotional charge and psychological form, are more eas-ily perceived than the underlying tidal forces that order them.

Whereas tissue motility within the Mid Tide is sensed as a unified and holistic dynamic, in the CRI the tissue structures may seem to be separate in their expres-sion of motion. Because of this, the CRI has become associated with what is known as *craniosacral motion*: the individual and particular motions of tissue structures sensed within its faster rate. Sensing the CRI is like looking at things from the out-side in, through a very small window. These externalized CRI motions are com-monly *flexion/external rotation* and *extension/internal rotation*. At this level, inertia within the system will be perceived as tissue resistance within and between sepa-rate structures. Information at this level is commonly gained via motion testing and by the application of palpation methods such as fluid direction and traction-ing or compression–decompression of tissues and tissue structures.

When relating to the CRI, you are in direct relationship to the suffering of a per-son within this human form. This must be appreciated and respected. Witnessing and acknowledging suffering at this level *can* have a profound effect. It can allow the person to be heard within his or her experience of suffering and can facilitate a reconnection to the deeper tides and the inherent healing forces at work within the system. In biodynamic terms, clinical work at the CRI level is via recognition of suffering and a reorientation of the system to primary respiration, deeper tidal forces and Dynamic Stillness.

INHERENT TREATMENT PLAN

One of the great strengths of craniosacral biodynamics is its orientation to health. There is an understanding in our field that the underlying health of the human system is a principle that is with us from the moment of conception, is never lost and always at work. In this understanding the potential for healing, and the knowledge of what needs to occur, is already enfolded within the illness and suffering present. Becker called this territory the arising of the *inherent treatment plan* [4]. This plan orients the practitioner to the knowledge that the arising and sequencing of what has to happen within any given healing process is a function of primary respiration, not of practitioner analysis, and will unfold in its own way. The practitioner does not have to analyze or diagnose to learn what needs to happen, nor is it necessary to decide what to do or how to intervene. The practi-tioner does, however, have to develop an inner state of stillness, orientation and listening that opens a perceptual doorway to this intrinsic process.

I once heard Becker, on a recorded tape, say, 'Trust the Tide and get out of the way!' That certainly sums it up. As one listens to the human system with a wide and still perceptual field, needing and expecting nothing, and learns to orient to primary respiration and the stillness from which it arises, something begins to emerge. A clarification of intention begins to happen. It is not my intention, or your intention as practitioner; it is the healing and centering intention of the Breath of Life. Clinical method is then a matter of practitioners' orientation and their abil-ity to attune and resonate to the intentions of primary respiration and the nature of the arising process. Work then centers on supporting the healing process in any way that is clinically appropriate without obstructing the inherent forces acting to resolve the issue. This process is humbling, and a great gratitude to the Intelligence inherent within all conditions, the Health that is never lost, inevitably arises.

PHASES OF THE INHERENT TREATMENT PLAN

There are many ways to orient both to a biodynamic approach to craniosacral therapy and to the arising of the inherent treatment plan. Although healing processes may take a multitude of forms, as the inherent plan unfolds a number of common phases emerge. Within the clinical context the nature of this unfolding is dependent upon certain practitioner skills. The first and most basic skill to develop is the ability to allow one's mind to still, to shift out of self-forms and ego states and enter a state of presence, the being-state outlined earlier. From this state of inner stillness, the practitioner then learns to orient to the Source and the forces of creation that emerge from it. In a craniosacral biodynamic context, the first step in this shift in orientation is to learn to sense the presence of primary respiration within and around oneself. From here, the task is then to sense primary respiration in relation to the client's midline, body and arising process, and to learn to negotiate a clear relational field and holding environment.

In developing these skills, students of a biodynamic approach learn to establish a wide perceptual field and to negotiate both the quality of their physical contact and the distance of their attention from the client's system and midline. As they come to hold a respectful and appropriate listening field, the next step in the emergence of the inherent treatment plan is the settling of this relational field. Until basic trust is established, nothing of any depth can occur. Practitioners may sense, as they deepen into a still state of presence, that the conjoined practitioner–client field seems to settle and deepen, with qualities of stillness and expansion. Most pointedly, practitioners may perceive that their own field settles and a quality of mutuality or nonseparateness emerges. By this I do not mean a merged state, but a state where there is both differentiation *and* a sense of direct knowing, being to being.

The next phase in the inherent treatment plan arises as the practitioner settles more deeply into a receptive being-state, while oriented to primary respiration in relationship to the client's midline, body and local biofield. Here a resonance occurs between them, with an emerging shift to the primary respiration. I call this the *holistic shift*. With this the practitioner notices a shift from conditioned patterns, nervous system activation, historical patterns and so forth to a quality of wholeness as primary respiration begins to manifest. When the shift deepens, the client's body is perceived as a unified fluid–tissue whole. Commonly there is also a shift from the more superficial CRI level of rhythm to the Mid Tide or Long Tide level of primary respiration. Once the holistic shift deepens then healing processes naturally begin to emerge. These are not factors of practitioner analysis, but of decisions made by the potency of the Breath of Life. Healing intentions may emerge from the Mid Tide level of expression, or from the Long Tide, or more directly from Dynamic Stillness. Once conditional forces have been resolved, then a process of reorganization and realignment to natural midlines also occurs.

Practitioner skills appropriate at a CRI level are not helpful at a Mid Tide level. Likewise skills that may be helpful within the Mid Tide will get in the way as the healing process deepens and the Long Tide manifests healing intentions. All of this is a deeply personal learning, which is not just about outer forces or another's pain and healing process, but also entails our own healing at the deepest levels of our personal and interpersonal wounding. As one of my teachers told me, 'the Breath of Life leads us into our deepest places of pain as the potential for healing is initiated'. In my personal experience, as I deeply attend to a client's pain and healing needs, I find that we are both cast into the mystery of life itself.

SECTION 5
CLINICAL APPLICATIONS OF *QI* AND ENERGY-BASED MODALITIES

SECTION CONTENTS

SECTION INTRODUCTION

Different fields of scholarly study, academic approaches and clinical practices have been divided by somewhat arbitrary boundaries placed upon expertise, knowledge and specialization. However, insights from these different fields have been converging on a new, central understanding of energy in human physiology as related to health and healing. Aspects of *qi* have been central to Asian and ethnomedical practices in the East. In the West, a new mosaic of understanding *qi* or bioenergy in its various interpretations is emerging in clinical fields as diverse as pediatrics, immunology (in HIV), neurology, the difficult conditions of chronic fatigue and fibromyalgia, and cardiology. Here a number of very different *qi*/energy-based approaches used in these fields are outlined. That such a variety of clinical tools can be seen as influencing the energy of the body surely demonstrates that the nature of human physiology is inherently and fundamentally energetic in nature. As fresh insights converge in the practice of energy medicine, we can hopefully look forward to a new era for a more complete kind of health and healing in the twenty-first century.

Qi in children

May Loo

CHAPTER CONTENTS

INTRODUCTION

Chinese pediatrics is an ancient healing art mentioned as early as the first century BCE in the *Huangdi Neijing, The Yellow Emperor's Inner Classic* (or *Classic of Internal Medicine*). The child, as much as the adult, is an individual, an energetic, physical, emotional and spiritual being. In addition, pediatric patients have very specific *qi* states that define their unique physiology and characterize their pathophysiology, and in children of the twenty-first century both of these may differ from earlier times. Children also have unique developmental and specific Organ *qi* characteristics. By understanding their distinctiveness, practitioners can promote health and overcome illnesses in children of various ages and developmental stages.

THE BASIC PHYSIOLOGY OF CHILDREN – *YIN* AND *YANG* IN THE YOUNG

The basic physiology of children encompasses three general *qi* states:

1. 'pure *yang*' (*chun yang*, 純陽) (maximum *yang*)
2. young *yang* (*zhi yang*, 稚陽) and young *yin* (*zhi yin*, 稚陰)
3. 'clear visceral *qi*' (*qing zang qi*, 清臟氣) (modified in the modern child).

PURE *YANG*

All Chinese pediatric textbooks list 'pure *yang*' as the foremost characteristic of children. The term is misleading, as the word 'pure' does not imply that the child is devoid of *yin*. *Yang* signifies both *yang* or Fire and the *qi* of physiological processes. Kidney *yang*, the basis of all *yang*, is the most *yang*. Although Essence (*jing*, 精) is a *yin* substance, it is the most *yang* of the *yin* (and so often called 'fiery Water'). The newborn has maximum Kidney *yang* and pre-Heaven (prenatal, congenital) Essence (先天之精), both of which decrease with age. The child would therefore have maximum *yang* in the usual categorization of *yin* and *yang*. However, there is another *yang* that is not included in adults: that of the process of growth and development. Pure *yang* refers to the fact that the child has pure or maximum potential for growth. Just as a seed or a young tree has the full potential of becoming a fully grown tree, the zygote has the fullest potential of becoming a human being. The younger the child, the more rapid is the growth and development. This is most evident in the first year of life: birth weight is doubled by 6 months, when the child sits up, and tripled by the time the baby becomes upright. Therefore, 'pure *yang*' is not interpreted as absolute *yang*, or as '*yang* without *yin*' but rather describes how the child is exuberant and full of life, with the maximum potential of becoming a being between Heaven (*tian*, 天) and Earth (*tu*, 土). The categorization of *yin* and *yang* for children would be more accurately shown as in Table 20.1.

YOUNG *YANG* AND YOUNG *YIN*

Children have young *yang* and young *yin*. The *yang* here refers to *qi* and *yang* functions, and the *yin* refers to Blood and Fluids (see Table 20.1). The child's skin is tender and *wei qi* (衛氣) – the protective or defensive *qi* that circulates

Table 20.1 *The categorization of yin and yang for children*		
	Yang	**Yin**
Maximum *yang*	Kidney *yang* (basis of all *yang*)	Essence (most *yang* of the *yin*)
Pure *yang*	Growth and development Qi (氣) yang functions	Blood (*xue*, 血) Fluids (*jin ye*, 津液)

under the skin – is weak. The Internal Organs are delicate and immature and *qi* within them is insufficient. The physiological functions, both *yin* and *yang* processes of the Internal Organs, are not well developed. The corresponding Western medical principle is that the child has an immature physiology and weaker immune system. The child is *yin* deficient, meaning that the Blood and Fluids are insufficient and are in a delicate balance. The famous Qing dynasty physician Wu Jutong (1758–1836) pointed out in his classic *Detailed Analysis of Warm Diseases* (*Wenbing Tiaobian*, 温病条辨/溫病條辨) that the growth process of the child is one of 'the development of *yang* and *yin*'.

CLEAR VISCERAL *QI*

The Chinese pediatric classics further state that children have 'clear visceral *qi*', which in ancient times meant pure and strong *qi* uncontaminated by improper diet or emotions. This condition holds less true for the modern child. With administration of medications, even in utero, in the neonatal period, and in infancy; with additives in foods and improper diet; with environmental toxins; with increased emotional stress – with all these, the 'visceral *qi*' is becoming less 'clear' as evidenced by an increasing incidence in children of adult illnesses such as cardiovascular disease and type II (adult onset) diabetes. Nonetheless, compared with the modern adult with so much toxic and emotional 'baggage', the 'clear visceral *qi*' in children can still be modified as 'relatively clear' visceral *qi*.

THREE PATHOPHYSIOLOGICAL CHARACTERISTICS OF CHILDHOOD ILLNESS

The interplay of physiological factors predisposes the child to three unique pathophysiological characteristics of childhood illnesses:

1. easy onset – fragile and immature Organs; pathogenic evils (*xie*, 邪) enter easily
2. rapid transformation – disease progression and changes occur quickly
3. rapid recovery.

EASY ONSET

Children are more vulnerable to illness because they have tender and delicate skin, their pores open more readily, and their level of defensive *qi* (*wei qi*) is low. Pathogens can enter easily via the skin to obstruct the flow of *wei qi*, and via the nose or mouth to invade the fragile and immature respiratory and digestive systems, especially after the period of passive immunity acquired from the mother.

RAPID TRANSFORMATION

The rapid onset of illnesses is followed by rapid change and transformation. Once the pathogen enters, because of the delicate balance of *qi* and Fluids, 'young *yang* and young *yin*', disease processes undergo easy and rapid transformation from Cold to Hot, Hot to Cold, Excess to Deficiency, Deficiency to Excess, or even the simultaneous exhaustion of both *yin* and *yang*. Take the case of the Western diagnosis of upper respiratory infection (URI) and the Chinese diagnosis of invasion of Wind-Cold: initially the child develops simple common cold symptoms. However, because the body has so much *yang*, so much 'Fire', the body responds to the cold by raising the body temperature, which in turn consumes *yin* so that the body in turn has less Fluid, and high fever ensues. Since the child's *qi* is already low, there is insufficient *qi* to fight off pathogenic influences, which can quickly obliterate *qi* and render the child *qi* deficient. The child becomes simultaneously exhausted of both *yin* and *yang*. Western pediatricians are trained to be apprehensive of a 2-week-old infant with URI symptoms, because that child can look robust one minute, but can quickly become septic with fever and lethargy – a *yang* collapse picture that is compatible with meningitis – and may even develop seizures with high fever. As children become older, there is gradual increase of *yin* and of *qi*, fevers do not run so high and URI does not quickly turn into meningitis.

Even after the symptoms of an illness resolve, pathogenic *qi* may still linger in the body, causing further injury to and transformation within the child. Acute illness weakens the child's body, diminishes *qi* and injures *yin*, further predisposing the child to acute illness. Lingering symptoms such as persistent dry cough, or recurrent sore throat in spite of negative streptococcal cultures, point to the energetic residuals of pathogens.

RAPID RECOVERY

In spite of the above pathophysiological characteristics, children tend to recover rapidly from illnesses. Most pediatric conditions are acute illnesses due to an attack of exogenous pathogens or improper diet, involving relatively superficial responses without complex Organ or emotional involvement. The relatively clear *qi* in the *yin* and *yang* Organs further enables children to recuperate quickly.

These general physiological and pathophysiological characteristics are rooted in ancient times and have been used to describe children since the Ming Dynasty (1368–1644). As already mentioned, modern lifestyle and its effects on the state of children's *qi* are now quite different: stress, the lingering bioenergetic effects of illness, environmental toxins and medication, increasing exposure to electromagnetic fields, and unhealthy dietary habits all share responsibility.

ORGAN PHYSIOLOGY AND PATHOPHYSIOLOGY IN CHILDREN

Children also have specific Organ physiology and pathophysiology. Three major constitutional states affect the *yin* Organs: Lung *qi* deficiency, Spleen *qi* deficiency and Liver vulnerability.

THE LUNG

The Lung in Chinese medicine is akin to the 'minister' in charge of government; it governs *qi* and respiration, controls dispersing of *qi*, defends the body, regulates water through sweat and controls skin and hair. The Lung in children is considered 'immature' and vulnerable to Cold and Dryness, thereby predisposing children to frequent respiratory problems. Pediatric Lung *qi* is 'young', meaning weak and insufficient and often unable to carry out the Lung function of moving *qi* downward. Reversal of *qi* flow (*qi* flow opposite to the normal direction, or *jue qi*, 厥氣) manifests as cough and wheezing. When the *qi* is insufficient to move Blood, respiratory distress may be accompanied by cyanosis, agitation and cold limbs – the clinical picture of status asthmaticus. Lingering pathogenic Lung *qi* can manifest as a persistent dry cough with minimal sputum; persistent *qi* depletion can manifest as fatigue.

THE SPLEEN

The Spleen in Chinese medicine is really the incorporation of both Spleen and Pancreas as one entity. It is the *yin* Organ of the digestive couplet, the Stomach being the *yang* Organ. Together they function as the granary official of the body. Food 'rots and ripens' in the Stomach, while the Spleen/Pancreas has six major physiological functions:

1. The Spleen governs transformation and transportation of *qi*. Spleen has the important function of transforming food into Food *qi* (*gu qi*) (穀氣), which combines with *kong qi* (空氣 or air, the basis for Lung *qi*) to form *rong qi* (營氣), the Nutritive *qi* (often known as *ying qi*, 營氣), which is the basis for *qi* and Blood. Spleen directs *gu qi* to the Heart to form Blood. Spleen then transports *gu qi* and other refined parts of the food to all parts of the body – Organs, muscles and limbs. Because the *gu qi* extracted by the Spleen is the material basis for the production of *qi* and Blood, the Spleen together with the Stomach is often called the Root of Post-Heaven (Postnatal) *qi* (後天之氣).

2. The Spleen also separates 'clear' (*qing*, 清) from 'dirty' (*zang*, 髒) Fluid, moving the former to the skin via the Lung and the latter downward to the Intestine. Since the Spleen usually sends *qi* upwards, it has an 'uplifting' effect to hold Organs in their place and prevent prolapse.

3. The Spleen/Pancreas corresponds to the Earth element, as Mother Earth is the provider of nourishment to all living beings. Spleen controls Blood both in production and in prevention of hemorrhage. Food *qi*, assisted by Original (*yuan*, 原, or Prenatal) *qi* from the Kidneys, forms Blood in the Heart. Blood circulates in the blood vessels, and it is the Spleen that 'holds' the Blood in the vessels and prevents hemorrhage.

4. The Spleen opens into the mouth and manifests in the lips, and is responsible for taste, for chewing and preparing food for further digestion, and for moistness of the lips. The flavor associated with the Earth Organs, the Spleen and Stomach, is sweetness. Children naturally develop a preference for sweet tastes as early as 1 month of age. Sweet is the predominant flavor in fruits and vegetables. Eating normal amounts of naturally sweetened food is healthy, whereas consuming an excess of sweet foods, especially the artificially sweetened foods that are major constituents of a modern child's diet, can induce digestive imbalance. Early introduction of solids has been associated with abdominal discomfort and allergic gastrointestinal symptoms.

5. The Spleen influences the capacity for introspection, for thinking, studying, focusing and memorizing data. Overwork can be injurious to Spleen *qi*. When this is deficient, children do not feel centered, cannot think clearly and have difficulty with concentration and schoolwork.

6. The emotions associated with Earth are sympathy and worry, characteristics of the mother. When Spleen *qi* is in balance the child is capable of giving and of being sympathetic. When it is out of balance the child may worry excessively, and even become obsessive in extreme circumstances.

The Spleen/Pancreas in children is 'immature' and constitutionally weak. There is impairment of all of the above six functions, but especially in the transforming and transporting of food and fluids. Insufficient nutritive *qi* and Blood may be formed, along with a tendency toward accumulation of Phlegm. These account for the predominance of digestive symptoms in children. The diet of the modern-day child further contributes to Spleen deficiency, as it is rich in Phlegm-producing foods, such as milk products, ice cold drinks and foods such as ice cream, and unnecessarily artificially sweetened foods, such as candies, cookies and cakes. Children's stressful lifestyle and excessive school pressure cause further deterioration of Spleen function. The vicious cycle of Spleen *qi* deficiency and digestive symptoms begins with colic in infancy, and includes a wide range of symptoms: poor appetite, indigestion, abdominal pain and distension and loose stools; fatigue, paleness and Blood deficiencies such as anemia. Whereas Western medicine considers poor appetite in toddlers as a normal phase, Chinese medicine attributes it to insufficient and immature Spleen *qi*.

LUNG AND SPLEEN

The digestive system is closely linked to the respiratory system, and the most common disorders in children are respiratory and digestive illnesses. Children with Spleen deficiency often become ensnarled in a Spleen–Lung deficiency cycle, especially with unhealthy modern-day lifestyle and diets. Both Organ systems have orifices that are in direct contact with the external environment. Pathogens can easily and directly enter the respiratory and digestive systems via the nose or mouth, and invade the fragile Organs internally. Fluid in the Lung accumulates and transforms into Phlegm, which in turn blocks airways – bronchi and bronchioles. The child has more difficulty getting air in and out, resulting in signs of respiratory distress such as nasal flaring, tachypnea (rapid breathing) and intercostal retractions (pulling in of muscles in the rib cage.) Children's 'young *yin*' further predisposes them to become Fluid depleted easily; the Phlegm becomes thicker, the fever tends to rise higher and in turn causes more *yin* deficiency. Since the Lung breathes in Heavenly *qi* to form Nutritive *qi*, when the Lung function is compromised all the other Organs, especially the Spleen, are also affected.

THE STOMACH

The Stomach, coupled with the Spleen/Pancreas, is the most important *yang* Organ. It 'rots and ripens' food, a process which needs sufficient Fluids derived from food and drink. The Stomach is therefore vulnerable to Dryness. The Spleen–Stomach couplet together is responsible for all the *qi* produced after birth (後天之氣).

Ingested food and fluids must move downward in the gastrointestinal tract. Therefore, Stomach *qi* must flow downward. When the Stomach is healthy, food and *qi* move from the stomach to the Small Intestine, and then to the Large Intestine. When the Stomach is unbalanced, the downward *qi* movement is poorly directed and there may be a reversal of *qi* flow upward. This may result in symptoms such as burping, regurgitation, nausea, vomiting and a sense of fullness. Regurgitation is a common symptom in infants, owing to immature and insufficient Stomach and Spleen *qi*. Conventional treatment with upright positioning in effect engenders a gravitational downward pull of *qi* flow. Regurgitation can be treated simply with tonification of Stomach and Spleen.

THE LIVER

The third constitutional weakness in children is Liver vulnerability. The Liver is called the 'general' of the *qi* system. It directs smooth and proper *qi* movement in all directions, and profoundly influences digestion, secretion of bile, and emotions. When Liver *qi* flow is smooth, Stomach and Spleen can carry out digestive functions harmoniously, with Stomach *qi* flowing downward and Spleen *qi* flowing upward. Liver *qi* also affects the flow of bile. Chinese medicine associates Liver *qi* stagnation (*qi zhi*, 氣滯) with frustration, irritability and anxiety – the emotions of an impatient child. When the Liver *qi* is out of balance, these emotions become exaggerated. Smoldering anger is most characteristic of Liver, and can be accompanied by resentment and even withdrawal (the Yellow Bile of the *choleric* in Greco-Roman-Renaissance medicine, see Ch. 2). Accompanying physical symptoms may include a heavy sensation in the chest, a 'lump' in the throat, and abdominal distension.

In Chinese medicine, the Liver stores Blood, regulates the quantity of Blood and Fluids according to activity and also regulates menstruation. It is a Wood Organ, represents youth, and springtime and is also the Organ associated with the longest period of childhood development. All the Liver's metabolic processes are essentially for pediatric growth and maturation, just like a seedling blossoming into a tree.

Vulnerability of the Liver in children means it is prone to develop disorders, generally manifesting as Liver *yin* deficiency and Liver *qi* stagnation (*qi* not moving) or *yang* excess. Since children are constitutionally *yin* deficient, a growing 'Wood' child is more prone to have Liver *yin* deficiency. Liver Blood and Fluid deficiency can manifest as dizziness, muscle spasm and weakness. Since Liver *yin* nourishes and lubricates tendons and ligaments, deficiency can manifest as both gross and fine motor incoordination, which can affect children's athletic abilities. The Liver is susceptible to Wind. When Wind combines with Liver Fluid deficiency, young children are prone to develop febrile seizures in which Heat from febrile illnesses dries up the Liver *yin* and stirs up Liver Wind, resulting in contraction and tremor of the sinews. A more serious Liver *yin* deficiency would manifest as disturbance of the Ethereal Soul (*hun*, 魂), so that the child may appear confused, impulsive or unable to focus.

However, Liver *qi* and *yang* usually become stagnant rather than deficient. In these circumstances, children would manifest physical symptoms such as headaches (*yang* rising upward) and behavioral symptoms such as low frustration tolerance, proneness to anger and aggressiveness. Medications, which are metabolized in the liver, can result in various Liver imbalances. As the Liver opens into the eyes, jaundice in liver disease first manifests as yellowness in the eyes.

A 'FIVE ELEMENT' MODEL FOR THE DEVELOPMENTAL STAGES OF CHILDHOOD

A thorough understanding of children requires consideration of the developmental stages through which they pass. Childhood is a wondrous progression of acquiring new skills, and especially of achieving a new understanding of oneself, and of one's relationship with the world, with nature and the universe. Children develop by assimilating the world into their own mental and physical frames of reference, which in turn change over time as they progress through the different stages of development. A 'Five Element' developmental theory developed by the author provides one way to identify vulnerable Organs in different age groups, and the Organ of origin in chronic illnesses, which can facilitate the practitioner's assessment and treatment of children.

This theory correlates well with the theory of cognitive development in children created by Jean Piaget (1896–1980), briefly described in the appendix to this chapter. Interested readers are referred to Chapter 5 in *Pediatric Acupuncture*. (See Note at end of chapter.)

Childhood is divisible approximately into four developmental stages that can be correlated with the Five Elements (*wuxing*, 五行):

Phase I. Infancy to early childhood: birth to 2–3 years, Metal (Mother of Water), transition into Water phase
Phase II. Early childhood: 2–3 to 6–7 years, Water transition into Wood phase
Phase III. Early childhood to preteenage: 6–7 years to 12 years, Wood phase, transition into Fire phase
Phase IV. Teenage and early adulthood: Fire phase, transition into Earth phase

Phase V. Adulthood: Earth phase, transition into second Metal phase (middle age), and second Water phase (old age).

It is important to note that the transition from one stage to another is not abrupt or sharply demarcated. One Element is predominant in each phase, and gradually transitions into another Element but never completely disappears, resulting in each phase containing characteristics of at least two Elements simultaneously.

PHASE I. INFANCY TO EARLY CHILDHOOD

This phase can be characterized metaphorically as the Metal transition to the Water phase of development, Metal being the 'Mother' of Water in the creative (*sheng*, 生) cycle of Elements. The vulnerable Organs during this phase are Lung and Kidneys, as respiratory illnesses are prevalent in the infant and young child, and the marrow, the brain (associated with the Kidney), is sensitive to nourishment and any form of insult. Since the Mother is in symbiotic relationship with the Child, the digestive system, the Spleen, is also susceptible to insult and injury.

PHASE II. EARLY CHILDHOOD

This next phase is Piaget's 'preoperational phase' of cognitive development. Many characteristics correspond metaphorically to both the Water and Wood Elements. The identity of the Water child is still very much defined by mother, as all bodies of water are defined by Mother Earth: lakes, oceans, rivers. The corresponding Water Organ is the Kidney, the foundation of all the *yin* and *yang* of the body, of the marrow and the brain, and of Essence (*jing*) – the ultimate life-defining force that determines development, sexual function and aging. Life begins with the Water, with Kidneys. The corresponding emotion is Fear. When the child is not overcome by Fear, his Willpower, the emotion of the healthy Kidney, helps him to decide when to let go and when to hold on.

The vulnerable Organs in this Water to Wood phase are the Kidney and the Liver. Congenital and developmental anomalies are often genetic, transmitted through the Kidney *jing*. The brain is considered as marrow (controlled by the Kidney), so that nervous system development is most vulnerable during this stage, when any severe illness can result in mental retardation. In particular, young children prior to age 6 are susceptible to seizures, which are 'internal Wind' disorders.

PHASE III. EARLY CHILDHOOD TO PRETEENAGE

The child between 6–7 years and 12 years of age is Piaget's 'concrete operational phase' child with reasoning abilities. From the Five Element perspective, the child in this stage is like a young tree, growing above ground, the tree being the Daoist symbol for man – rooted in Earth, reaching upward toward sky, coming into being between Heaven and Earth. Heaven is symbolic of the father, providing guidance and direction for the child, the tree, to grow straight and upward. Thus, nourished by Mother Earth and guided by Father Heaven, the child learns *yin* and *yang*, right from wrong, which correlates to the rationalization process of concrete thinking.

The corresponding Element is Wood, and the Organ is the Liver, associated with emotions such as frustration, irritability, smoldering anger, and anxiety – the emotions of an impatient, operational child. Healthy Liver *qi* enables the child to understand and take proper directions for growth so that the tree grows straight and upward. The child's increasing motor activities are also associated with the Liver, which rules the tendons and sinews and controls movement.

Balance is an essential aspect of *qi*, and excess (*shi*, 實) and deficient (*xu*, 虛) and *yin* and *yang* may interact. For example, when Liver *yin* is deficient, Liver *yang* may become excessive (Fig. 20.1) with physical symptoms of excess such as

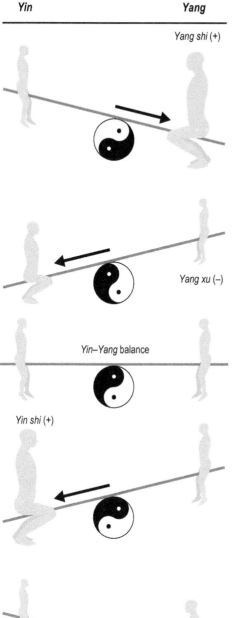

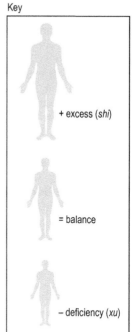

FIG 20.1 **Balance is an essential aspect of** *qi*. This simplified illustration shows how excess (*shi*, 實) and deficient (*xu*, 虛) *yin* and *yang* interact. From top to bottom: *yang* excess, *yang* deficiency, *yin-yang* balance, *yin* excess and *yin* deficiency. Note that these differences are dynamic and relative, not absolute. (*Figure supplied by David Mayor.*)

hyperactivity, or excess emotional symptoms such as increasing irritability, frustration and anger. The child may also manifest cognitive difficulties and appears to be impulsive and 'out of it', inattentive, unable to focus, follow directions or think clearly. A well-balanced Liver enables the child to make decisions (the function of the coupled *yang* Organ, the Gall Bladder), to take more charge of his life, to become his own 'general'.

This is the crucial moment of establishing equilibrium between *yin* and *yang*. The father becomes an important balance for the mother. From each parent, the child obtains both masculine and feminine perspectives, and incorporates the *yang* and the *yin*. The Wood child still has a very close relationship with mother, needing nurturance and foundation for 'growing roots', and looks to the father, to Heaven, for direction and guidance.

PHASE IV. TEENAGE AND EARLY ADULTHOOD

Teenagers and young adults in their early twenties correspond metaphorically to the Fire element. The predominant emotion that corresponds to the Heart is passion. As teenagers develop their sexual identity, they enter into intimate relationships (if so favored) that are in reality infatuations, and are consumed by 'Fiery' passion. This is the archetype of romantic love, exemplified by Tristan and Isolde, or Romeo and Juliet: young, passionate love with life-and-death intensity.

The teenage Fire child establishes himself as the 'emperor' of his being, no longer dependent on Heaven or Earth, father or mother. He is rebellious, scorching Mother Earth and following his own directions, rejecting Heaven. When the Fire child is out of control he behaves recklessly, sending sparks flying everywhere, igniting whatever they touch. He feels fearless, indestructible – the exact opposite of the fearful Water child. When he is in a state of balance, he can provide warmth to others. He contributes to the future by providing nurturing ashes for the Earth.

Whereas the Water child is in a state of symbiotic oneness with mother, and the Wood child reflects the dyad of mother/child and father, the Fire child is one of a triad: mother, father, himself.

The vulnerable Organ during this phase is primarily the Heart. However, if the previous developmental phases were well balanced, with the appropriate amount of Wood for a warm Fire, or appropriate rational preparation for what Piaget calls the 'formal operational stage', the teenager though driven by passion is still able to distinguish right from wrong. However, if the previous phases were not well balanced the Fire child goes out of control, and sexual exploitations and reckless behavior may lead him into compromising situations with serious consequences.

From the Fire phase, the teenager progresses to the Earth phase of adulthood, when he can himself become the nurturer. The middle years of life correspond to a second Metal phase, while old age declines into the Water phase. The life cycle begins again.

USING FIVE ELEMENT DEVELOPMENTAL THEORY

Modern psychology posits that most adults are essentially grown-ups who are still 'stuck' at various ages in childhood when they experienced times of physical or emotional trauma. Freudian psychology considers the first 5 years as being crucial for adult behavior and personality formation. The Five Element developmental theory provides another perspective on the possible origins of physical and emotional disorders. It has been the author's experience that adults who manifest certain Elemental characteristics would often relate a trauma experienced during that phase of development. For example, some adults traumatized in the Wood phase of development may have difficulty determining right from wrong, and may be more prone to develop anxiety disorders.

Therefore, the Five Element developmental theory can be useful in two areas:

1. to identify the vulnerable Element according to the age and development of the child
2. to provide a means to trace the Element of *origin* of a chronic illness – this is especially helpful in sorting out which Element to treat in complex disorders with multiple symptoms, such as Attention Deficit Hyperactivity Disorder (ADHD).

Childhood illnesses are simple yet complex: simple because the majority of pediatric disorders are acute, fairly straightforward conditions; complex because children have different physiology and pathophysiology at different ages and at different stages of development.

When working with the *qi* in children, the *qi* state of the practitioner is of the utmost importance for successful treatment because children, even babies, remain very intuitive and sensitive to the physical and emotional states of people around them. At the time of treatment, the practitioner and the child share a *qi* 'field'. When the practitioner is in a good state of *qi* balance, having a healthy lifestyle and dietary habits and participating in *qi*-enhancing activities such as *qigong* or *taiji quan*, positive *qi* will be directed to the child, making treatment more effective. In the author's experience, children are receptive and responsive to a variety of treatment modalities for *qi* balance, including Chinese medicine (CM) treatment with needle and nonneedle acupuncture, acupressure and *qigong*, and non-CM practices such as homeopathy, chiropractic, massage and herbal medicine.

A CASE EXAMPLE

JM is a 6-year-old boy who has experienced recurrent wheezing episodes/ asthmatic attacks since 9 months of age, when his parents divorced. He is now on two bronchodilators and periodically requires treatment with steroids. An acupuncturist using CM assessment determines that he is Lung *qi* deficient. Since his symptoms began when he was an infant in the Metal/Water phase, and since he is now in the Wood phase of development, the practitioner (with strong *qi*) balances his Lung, Kidney and Liver *qi* using the following acupoints:

SP-3, LU-9 (tonification)

LU-10, HT-8 (sedation)

KI-3, KI-6, KI-7 (tonification)

LIV-3, LIV-13 (neutral stimulation).

The child experienced rapid improvements, and his medications were tapered off. He still has occasional flare-ups, which seem associated with being emotionally upset with his parents.

In this case, as so often in pediatrics, the child is the identified patient (IP) whose symptoms manifest dysfunction in the family. It is imperative to point out that, although the goal of treatment is toward balancing the child's *qi*, assessment of any child should encompass an evaluation of the child's *qi* and symptoms in relation to the parents' *qi* and overall family dynamics.

I. SENSORIMOTOR STAGE (0 TO 2–3 YEARS)

Children at this age perceive reality by what they can see, grab, touch, or put in their mouths. Objects are initially perceived as extensions of themselves – that is, objects are spatially related to the body. Mother, the warmest and most perceived 'object', is a part of the self.

II. PREOPERATIONAL STAGE (2–3 YEARS TO 6–7 YEARS)

During this period, the child manifests specific cognitive characteristics: egocentrism, illogical transformations, vivid imagination and animism. This magical, egotistical, illogical thinking is one dimensional: everything revolves around the child, the self. When there is only one point of view and all other perspectives are not being taken into account, reality is distorted and the child does not understand right from wrong.

III. CONCRETE OPERATIONAL STAGE (6–7 TO 11–12 YEARS)

During this developmental stage, the child learns to operate mentally on a concrete rational basis. The child is capable of two-dimensional thinking, learning right from wrong, and of relating to the world on a more realistic level defined by time and space. However, the operational child needs direction and information to negotiate in the real world.

IV. FORMAL OPERATIONAL STAGE (11–12 YEARS TO YOUNG ADULTHOOD)

This is when the child progresses from linear to abstract thinking. He can now ponder over hypothetical problems that are beyond his concrete realm of experience, such as ideas, philosophies or abstract events. He becomes increasingly aware of his possible role in society and makes plans for work, for the future, and possibly for college, marriage and family.

NOTE

This chapter is based on material from the author's textbook on pediatric acupuncture:

Loo M 2002 *Pediatric Acupuncture*. Churchill Livingstone, Edinburgh.

Additional material relevant to this chapter can be found in the References and further reading section at the end of the book.

Qigong, taiji quan (*tai chi*) and HIV: the psychoneuroimmunology connection

Mary Lou Galantino • Laura Muscatello

INTRODUCTION

Treatment for HIV and AIDS has improved in the last decade. The success of highly active antiretroviral therapy (HAART) makes decreased viral loads, increased CD4+ cell counts and prevention of opportunistic infections (OIs) possible [1,2]. HAART is an effective strategy for preventing disease progression of HIV infection, particularly when patients adhere closely to their treatment regimen. However, due to the powerful drug combinations, there are still side effects and other related symptoms including asthenia, anorexia, cough, pain and fever [3]. Additional side effects include metabolic complications that can impact patients' adherence levels. Selected chronic complications associated with antiretroviral therapy (ART) include lipodystrophy, hyperlipidemia, insulin resistance and diabetes, peripheral neuropathy and bone disorders such as osteopenia/osteoporosis [4].

As a result of these side effects, recent studies show that 53–84% of HIV positive individuals have reported using at least one form of complementary and alternative medicine therapy (CAM) to manage these symptoms and improve quality of life (QOL) [5–7]. This makes those with chronic conditions, including HIV and cancer, the second-largest group to use CAM [8]. Patients have reported learning about various therapies from friends, family and media [9]. Primary reasons for use include decreasing pain from direct effects of HIV on the peripheral or central nervous system, immune suppression (OIs) and side effects of HAART [5]. Other reasons include stress reduction, depression, anxiety, fatigue, nausea, insomnia, night sweats, dizziness, prevention of weight loss or gain and weakness, dermatological problems and boosting immunity [1,5,7]. Common forms of CAM used by people living with HIV include nutritional supplements, massage, acupuncture, meditation, yoga, aerobic exercise and other movement therapies [6]. Exercise and movement therapy can improve QOL without compromising immune function [10]. Most recently, the use of *taiji* and *qigong* have been the subject of popular discussion for their positive benefits with symptom management and decelerating disease progression to AIDS. In a recent study it was found that 3.8% of HIV positive individuals use *qigong* regularly [6]. A loss of body and muscle mass, a common symptom of people living with HIV, can cause a decrease in physical, metabolic and immune function [8] and one goal of these therapies is to counteract such side effects. Effectiveness of therapies can be measured based on QOL, symptom management, disease deceleration and CD4+ T lymphocyte levels [11]. Research on movement therapies (including *taiji* and *qigong*) can provide evidence of fostering maximum QOL in chronic HIV disease.

TRADITIONAL EXERCISE

Substantial evidence suggests that traditional exercise provides considerable physiological and psychological benefits for people living with HIV disease [12]. Exercise training in particular may help alleviate some of the metabolic adverse effects associated with HAART by favorably altering body composition and patterns of body fat distribution. Studies have shown that aerobic training can help reduce total body and visceral fat, as well as normalize lipid profiles in HIV-infected patients [13]. A systematic review examined the effectiveness and safety of progressive resistive exercise (PRE) interventions on immunological/virological, cardiopulmonary, weight and body composition, strength and psychological outcomes in adults living with HIV. Results indicated that PRE, or a combination of PRE and aerobic exercise, may lead to statistically significant increases in weight and arm and thigh girth among exercisers versus nonexercisers. Trends toward improvement in submaximal heart rate and exercise time were also found. Individual studies suggest that PRE contributes to improved strength and psychological status. This approach appears to be safe and may be beneficial for medically stable adults living with HIV [14].

Challenges remain, however, regarding the mode, duration and intensity of many traditional standardized exercise programs as these may vary during a chronic illness. The chronic course of HIV disease is frequently associated with various OIs that may impact cardiac and respiratory systems. Although patients with HIV infection of course share many cardiovascular risk factors with the general population, HIV infection itself may increase cardiovascular risk [15]. Therefore, individuals may not be physically able to maintain an aerobic fitness level sufficient to sustain a significant change in the immune system. The stage of disease and the type of illness involved may preclude more strenuous exercise activities at various times. During these times, less traditional movement therapies may be more appropriate and efficacious. In fact, movement therapy includes a number of constructs that are similar to those used in physical therapy, and it can complement an individual traditional exercise program.

BACKGROUND ON MOVEMENT THERAPIES: *QIGONG* AND *TAIJI*

The US National Center for Complementary and Alternative Medicine (NCCAM) defines movement or mind–body therapies as various modalities that foster healing of the entire person and that may take the form of interventions such as a dance therapy program, a particular technique (e.g. Feldenkrais, Alexander) or a martial art-related approach such as *taiji* or *qigong*. 'Biofield' therapies are, according to the NCCAM, intended to affect energy fields that purportedly surround and penetrate the human body but are as yet scientifically unproven (in contrast to 'bioelectromagnetic-based' therapies, which involve unconventional use of known electromagnetic fields). Some forms of energy therapy manipulate biofields by applying pressure and/or manipulating the body by placing the hands in, or through, these fields. Examples include approaches such as *reiki* and Therapeutic Touch (see Chs 12, 22) and also some forms of *qigong* – a component of traditional Chinese medicine that combines movement, meditation and controlled breathing (see Chs 6, 7). The effects of these energy therapies are considered to include improving the flow of blood and *qi,* so enhancing the health of both body and mind (or spirit) [16]. This chapter will focus on the use of *qigong* and *taiji* with HIV/AIDS patients.

Taiji and *qigong* differ from other conventional exercises in their slow speed, use of full concentration, and the importance of breathing and relaxation – all of which result in increased blood and *qi* flow [17]. By developing and consolidating *qi* (which we interpret as 'bioenergy', or the 'energy of life'), miscommunications between internal organs, tissues and cells are corrected and rejuvenated. Focus is on the regulation of the mind, breath and body [18], with the eventual desired outcome being the prevention and healing of diseases [19].

Qigong is an energy-based mind–body movement therapy used for healing, preventing diseases and improving quality of life. It mostly focuses on meditation, stretching and fluid movements [19,20] (see Chs 6 and 7 for more information). Based on integrating mind, breath, posture and movement by using visualizations and rhythmic relaxation sequences [21], it has been reported to reduce anxiety, depression, blood pressure, oxygen demand, total cholesterol and blood lactate levels, while improving mood levels, sleep quality and duration, heart stroke volume and brain synchronization [21–27].

Taiji quan has been practiced for over 700 years as an 'internal martial art' (*wushu*) that is based on developing and using 'internal' (*qi*) rather than 'external' (muscular) force. Since the early twentieth century its long movement sequences have also been widely utilized as a health and 'moving meditation' exercise, as it focuses on maintaining balance and calmness. In addition it encourages proactive responses rather than reactive responses to stress [28,29]. The five traditional schools of *taiji* share three essential features quite similar to those mentioned above for *qigong*: (1) the body is naturally extended and relaxed, giving priority to lissomness, (2) the mind is tranquil but alert and (3) body movements are slow, smooth and well coordinated throughout the exercise period [30] (See also Ch. 6).

TAIJI AND THE HIV/AIDS LITERATURE

Taiji intervention for HIV patients has shown results in significantly higher quality of life, greater emotional and social wellbeing, lower physiological distress, enhanced appraisal-focused coping abilities, and stress management, and impacts positively on immune function and neuroendocrine responses [28,31–33].

In a Cochrane systematic review, four randomized controlled trials and controlled clinical trials of 206 patients with rheumatoid arthritis were included to examine the benefits and harms of *taiji*. Practicing *taiji* for 8 to 10 weeks demonstrated decreased stress, increased muscle strength in the lower body and improved balance, posture and ability to move in the experimental group. In addition, one study showed significantly greater selected upper extremity range of movement (ROM) outcomes, self-reported frequency and enjoyment of exercise 4 months after treatment than those that participated in a relaxation program control group. These findings have implications for patients living with HIV who encounter HIV-related rheumatological complications [34].

The impact on balance and posture has also been studied. *Taiji* practitioners were compared with nonpractitioners on five balance tests and performed significantly better on three of them [35]. Landmark studies have also shown that *taiji* can prevent falls in elderly patients [36,37]. In an aging HIV population, and with the variety of central and peripheral nervous system dysfunction that may occur with HIV disease, *taiji* may be a useful option. Cardiorespiratory responses to *taiji* training have also been investigated. One comparative study examined ventilatory and cardiovascular (CV) responses to *taiji* and found significantly lower ventilatory frequency – suggesting a better use of ventilatory volume than was anticipated from comparable exertional levels on a cycle ergometer [38]. *Taiji* practice resulted in findings of decreased depression, fatigue and state anxiety. This result was demonstrated in a study of 96 experienced *taiji* practitioners that compared *taiji* with meditation, brisk walking and neutral reading [39]. Compared with a sedentary control group matched for age and gender, *taiji* participants had a significantly higher VO_2 (oxygen consumption), O_2 pulse (oxygen uptake per heartbeat at rest) and work rate during *taiji* exercise.

A recent randomized study conducted with a sample of people living with advanced HIV disease compared a no-treatment control group with groups using either traditional aerobic exercise or *taiji*. Outcome measures included the medical outcomes short form MOS-HIV health survey, and physical tests including functional reach, sit-up and sit-and-reach tests. The MOS-HIV survey showed a significantly greater perception of overall health after the intervention. Significant differences were demonstrated in all functional measures compared with the control group. Both aerobic and *taiji* exercise interventions benefited this group of AIDS patients [31].

QIGONG AND THE HIV/AIDS LITERATURE

Qigong is one of the four core aspects of Chinese medicine (along with acupuncture/moxibustion, herbal medicine, and *tuina* and other forms of massage – all of which have been used with people living with HIV disease – and is believed to foster a spontaneous balancing and enhancing of the natural healing resources in the human system. From a psychoneuroimmunological (PNI) perspective, however, it is important to recognize that there are physiological similarities between these East Asian movement therapies and the traditional use of aerobic exercise. The physiological mechanisms of *qigong* are listed by Roger Jahnke, an experienced master *qigong* and *taiji* practitioner and teacher, in Table 21.1 [40]. The three main areas he considers to be enhanced through the practice of *qigong* are: (1) oxygen metabolism, (2) the lymphatic system and (3) the nervous system. The activities involved can be broken down as follows: (1) relaxation, (2) meditation, (3) concentrated movement, (4) various postures, (5) breathing practice, (6) visualization and (7) self-massage.

Table 21.1 *Physiological mechanisms of qigong*

Physiological mechanisms	Structures and substrates	*Qigong* activity
I. Oxygen		
1. Energy generation	Oxygen uptake	Movement/breath
2. Aerobic water	Oxygen uptake	Movement/breath
3. Immune enhancement	Oxygen uptake	Movement/breath
4. Free radical neutralization	Oxygen uptake	Movement/breath
II. Lymph		
1. Aerobic generation	Oxygen	Movement/breath
2. Propulsion		
(a) Aerobic	Oxygen	Movement/breath
(b) Intrinsic contraction	Interstitial fluid volume	Breath/relaxation
(c) Muscle pump	Muscle contraction	Movement
(d) Gravitational	Body position	Postures/movement
(e) Breath apparatus	Lungs, diaphragm, cisterna chyli	Breath activity
3. Immune function	Propulsion	Breath, movement, and posture
4. Cerebral fluid flow	Propulsion	Breath, movement, and posture
5. Nutritive function	Propulsion	Breath, movement, and posture
III. Nervous System		
1. Autonomic	Brain, neurochemistry, nervous system	Relaxation and breath
2. Neurotransmitter profile	Hypothalamus	Relaxation and visualization
3. Microcirculation	Hypothalamus	Relaxation
4. Immunity	Macrophages, leukocytes	Relaxation, meditation
5. Brain hemisphere control	Brain, nervous system	Alternate nostril breath and right and left side movement
6. Brain wave frequency	Brain, nervous system	Meditation
7. Neuroreflex stimulation	Neuroreflex system	Rubbing points
8. Brain structures	Hypothalamus, pituitary, pineal gland, third ventricle	Intention, meditation, and visualization

From Jahnke, 1996,40 with permission.

Relaxation (in the form of 'progressive' relaxation) and meditation alter heart rate, brain wave activity, neurotransmitter profile, skin temperature and muscle control [41–43]. Both are activities integral to *qigong*, and both are processes influenced by voluntary control of the body's self-regulating mechanisms. Moderate body movement that occurs within a context of deep relaxation is also common in *qigong*. Research on exercise, relaxed states and other triggers of specific physiological responses is clearly implicated as a useful resource that may help build a scientific foundation for *qigong* and other self-applied health maintenance methods of the Asian systems of traditional medicine [40].

However, a major challenge to modern science is the traditional explanation of *qigong* in terms of *qi* flow. Can there indeed be a scientific interpretation of the *qi* of Chinese medicine and philosophy and the *prana* of Indian Ayurvedic medicine and yoga (see, for example, Chs 10-12, 16)? Despite this fundamental problem, the literature of bioenergetic research is prolific. In particular, biofields are often interpreted in terms of electrical models, and electrodynamic fields have been studied by several researchers [44–46]. Nordenström [47], for example, has described the vascular interstitial closed circuit as a system of preferential ion conductance pathways comprising a network of biological circuitry.

Qigong itself clearly has exciting applications in the management of HIV disease and, even if the traditional model may resist scientific reinterpretation, further research is warranted to evaluate the physiological underpinnings of *qigong* in terms of immunological markers, physical improvements and QOL outcomes.

INTERCONNECTION OF THE NERVOUS, ENDOCRINE AND IMMUNE SYSTEMS: *QIGONG* AND *TAIJI* IN HIV/AIDS

In the body, sufficient communication between systems is essential to maintain homeostasis. The limbic–hypothalamic–pituitary–adrenocortical system coordinates three major systems: the nervous, immune and endocrine. More specifically, the neuroendocrine system links the psychological state and the immune system via signaling by chemical hormones or neuronal impulses in pathways arising in the central nervous system. In a complementary way, the immune system communicates with the nervous system using cytokines [23]. Because both hormones and cytokines in the blood are such a major part of this communication, good circulation is ideal. Movement therapy, including *taiji* and *qigong*, is helpful since the muscle contractions involved improve circulation. In addition, meditation influences neural impulses within the cerebral cortex, causing secretory cells in the hypothalamus to release hormonal messengers whose active sites are in other parts of the body [21,22]. The combination of movement and meditation is potentially powerful.

THE NERVOUS SYSTEM

Movement therapies such as *taiji* and *qigong* have been found to regulate the autonomic nervous system (ANS) [21]. This is made up of a sympathetic division, which mobilizes body systems (during 'fight or flight'), and a parasympathetic division, which conserves energy to promote homeostasis (during 'rest and digest'). Movement therapy down-regulates the activity of the sympathetic division and up-regulates the activity of the parasympathetic division, thus favoring relaxation and energy conservation [48].

Movement therapy also affects brain wave activity, specifically by increasing alpha wave amplitude and so enhancing relaxation [22,27]. This allows improvement in anxiety and mood status. Furthermore, during relaxation the body can repair damaged cells and intercellular communication pathways. This is essential for people living with HIV, in whom the virus attacks the immune system, disrupting communication and function.

THE ENDOCRINE SYSTEM

Hormones are the chemical signals that allow the nervous and endocrine systems to communicate with the immune system. Melatonin in particular, secreted by the pineal gland and commonly known for regulating circadian rhythms, has been a hormone of interest for its influence on cytokine production. In one study, *taiji* and *qigong* sessions increased melatonin levels, enhancing cell-mediated immunity and antibody production [22]. This can be explained because it is the psychosensitive pineal gland that activates the neuroendocrine axis, with melatonin modulating hypothalamic function in particular, the hypothalamo-pituitary axis (HPA) [22].

THE IMMUNE SYSTEM

One of the most profound effects of HIV is depletion of the immune system. With disease progression the immune system weakens, becoming susceptible to OIs. One of the main goals of treatment is to decelerate this depletion. *Qigong* has been found to increase the numbers of white blood cells and complement C3 concentration [21,23].

Depletion of CD4+ T lymphocytes is one of the most common characteristics of disease pathogenesis and progression. Two causal hypotheses have been considered. The first focuses on the *destruction* of mature CD4+ T cells due to apoptosis (programmed cell death), autoimmune reaction and disruption of the cell membrane. The second hypothesis considers that T cell *production* is impaired, owing to infection-mediated death of progenitor cells, cytokine dysfunction, OI, vitamin deficiency and lineage-restricted hematopoiesis [49].

Mindfulness meditation akin to the methods used in *qigong* and *taiji* has been found beneficial in keeping CD4+ T lymphocyte counts unchanged. Two theories have been presented to explain this phenomenon. The first is that it has a positive effect on hematopoiesis, so that turnover and redistribution cancel each other. Meditation training also reduces stress, thus reducing HIV viral replication and therefore HIV ribonucleic acid (RNA) levels in addition [50]. Significant improvement in the ratio of CD4+ and CD8+ cells is also a benefit of these movement therapies [51].

As already mentioned, cytokines are the messengers that the immune system uses to communicate with the nervous system. They are effector glycoproteins that modulate both pro-inflammatory and anti-inflammatory regulators. There are two types of cytokines. Type 1 cytokines, which promote cell-mediated responses, include interferon gamma (IFN-γ), tumor necrosis factor alpha (TNF-α) and interleukin 12 (IL-12). Type 2 cytokines, which include interleukins IL-4, IL-6 and IL-10, are anti-inflammatory regulators favoring humoral responses [51]. Cellular immunity involves the T lymphocytes, whereas the humoral immune response is mediated by secreted antibodies produced in the cells of the B lymphocyte lineage. *Qigong* increases the number of cytokine-secreting cells, and thus benefits the immune response [23]. *Taiji* has been found to reduce depressed mood and fatigue states, so decreasing hypothalamic–pituitary–adrenal (HPA) axis stimulation and resulting in lower levels of TNF-α [28]. Activation of TNF-α and TNF-γ cytokines in turn leads to enhancement of natural killer (NK) cell activation and cellular immunity [23]. In addition, reduced physiological stress raises levels of IL-2, which is instrumental to the immune system in helping distinguish between self and foreign antigens, so resulting in enhanced cellular immunity [28].

Activation of the class of lymphocytes called NK cells is important as they are the first defense against invaders; they are often impaired or decreased in chronic HIV disease. Other studies have shown that participation in movement therapies and mindfulness meditation has a positive effect on NK cell numbers and cytotoxicity, as well as improving neutrophil function [22,50].

STRESS

Researchers have known for many years that immunity is affected by psychological conditions, and that depression or stress may exacerbate certain diseases. The well-known relationship between stress and immune functioning [52,53] suggests that both acute and chronic stress can impair or alter the immune response in those affected with HIV.

Stress has been defined as the body's nonspecific response to a demand placed on it and the consequences of the failure to respond appropriately to emotional or physical threats [54]. The dynamic of stress involves social–environmental factors, stressors and the individual. Stress activates the HPA axis as follows: the paraventricular nucleus of the hypothalamus secretes corticotropin releasing factor (CRF); this stimulates release of adrenocorticotropic hormone (ACTH) from the pituitary into the bloodstream; in turn, this cause secretion of cortisol and other glucocorticoids from the adrenal cortex [55]. Chronic psychological stress activates not only the HPA axis but also the sympathetic–adrenomedullary (SAM) system, with secretion of norepinephrine and epinephrine [29,56,57]. Other neurotransmitters involved in the stress response include melatonin, anandamide and nitric oxide [56].

There are many harmful effects of stress. Their summation leads to a weakened immune system and impaired communication throughout the body. First of all, stress causes oxidative damage, adversely affecting cellular repair and function [58]. Next, there is an inverse relationship between NK cell activity and cortisol levels. In most disease conditions – including HIV – increased cortisol levels are seen with decreased NK cell activity, thus weakening the immune system [22]. Cortisol is also a known inhibitor of type 1 cytokine production [22,51], although stress-impaired memory – as in the AIDS-related dementia complex – may be associated with increased levels of interleukin 1 (IL-1, a type 1 cytokine) in the hippocampus [56]. In general, when stress is sensed by the brain, the body responds with allostasis or adaptive responses that maintain balance. Over time, maintaining this can cause an accumulation of neural, immune and stress mediators that have an adverse effect on organ systems, leading in the HIV patient to disease progression [56]. In particular, increased levels of norepinephrine and epinephrine also result in immunosuppression, with HIV disease progression via viral replication [29,56,57]. In one study, patients received comprehensive medical, neurological, neuropsychological and psychiatric assessments every 6 months, including an assessment of stressful life events. In 42 months, results demonstrated that the more severe the stressful event, the greater was the risk of early HIV disease progression. For every severe stress episode reported during a 6-month period, the risk of early disease progression doubled, with higher levels of severe life stress increasing the odds of developing HIV progression nearly fourfold among the 66 patients who were monitored for 2 years or more [59].

Thus, stress is a pathogenic factor accelerating HIV pathogenesis, impairing the impact of HAART and worsening symptoms [50].

STRESS MANAGEMENT AND THE RELAXATION RESPONSE

Stress management can effectively reduce anxiety and thus increase quality of life by modifying stressor appraisals, enhancing spirituality and fostering inner strength [7,29]. In addition, altering one's perception of stress can impact neuroendocrine immune responses [29].

The relaxation response is a physical state of deep rest that changes the physical and emotional responses to stress and is the opposite of the 'fight or flight' response [41]. It is made up of physiological mechanisms that are active in repetitive mental or physical activity. When the relaxation response is elicited, sensitivity to the stress hormones norepinephrine and cortisol can be reduced, thus decreasing sympathetic nervous system reactivity during stressful situations. Levels of the neurotransmitters serotonin (5-hydroxytryptamine, 5-HT) and dopamine may also be increased in the brain [56]. *Taiji* and *qigong* are both examples of movement therapies that elicit the relaxation response.

Physiologically, they cause decreased oxygen consumption and carbon dioxide elimination, and reduced metabolism, heart rate, arterial blood pressure and respiratory rate [56]. Furthermore, *qigong* and *taiji* not only help with stress management and lead to physical improvements, but can also specifically decrease levels of cortisol [22] by reducing signals to the limbic system and so decreasing HPA axis activity. In addition, *taiji* and *qigong* are reported to increase nitric oxide levels nonspecifically, which may also counterbalance norepinephrine and other monoamine neurotransmitter activity. [56]

MOVEMENT AND MOOD

Movement therapy for mood disturbances has been advocated since the time of Hippocrates, and more particularly since the early twentieth century, although empirical evidence of its beneficial effects on mood has accumulated slowly. Most of the relevant data come from studies on the effect of exercise on depression [60,61].

The research literature that links movement and mood tends to focus on vigorous movement, such as aerobic exercise [62], although studies conducted with patients who were not institutionalized but who met the diagnostic criteria for major or minor depression found a comparable reduction in depression for both aerobic and anaerobic movement, compared with sedentary controls [63]. This finding is significant because individuals suffering from chronic diseases are less likely to engage in vigorous aerobic movement because of their symptoms and loss of energy for everyday activities [64]. Therefore, *taiji* and *qigong* are movement therapies that are potentially useful alternatives to vigorous activities for individuals suffering from chronic diseases including HIV.

Taiji and *qigong* are often practiced in a group setting. Professionals in clinical psychology and occupational therapy have studied group intervention from a psychosocial perspective [65,66]. Although many studies have documented patterns of emotional distress in persons with HIV disease, few controlled evaluations of group therapy outcomes exist. Most of the reported studies concerned depressed HIV positive individuals and the evaluation of a specific drug intervention, but, in one group therapy study, symptoms of depression decreased and skills in active behavioral coping were noted [67]. In another report, cognitive–behavioral and social support group therapies produced reductions in depression, hostility and somatization. Tests for clinical significance of change underscored the benefits of social support group intervention and long-term follow-up [68].

Despite this paucity of studies, literature on long-term AIDS survivors is replete with anecdotal evidence linking survival to one or more of the following: (1) having a positive attitude toward the illness, (2) participating in health-promoting behaviors, (3) engaging in spiritual activities, and (4) taking part in AIDS-related group activities [69–71]. Positive relationships have been demonstrated between hardiness and perception of physical, emotional and spiritual health, participation in exercise and the use of special diets [72–74]. Such conclusions would indicate that *taiji* and *qigong* may well be beneficial in part because they involve participation in a group exercise program.

DEPRESSION

One of the main symptoms of chronic conditions, including HIV/AIDS, is depression. Depression has been linked to accelerated CD4+ T cell decline, mortality, increased viral load and disease progression to AIDS [57]. It is now understood that one possible mechanism is that depression can be linked to a chemical deficiency of the neurotransmitter 5-HT and disturbances in the metabolism of its precursor, the amino acid tryptophan. Immune-mediated catabolism of tryptophan by tryptophan 2,3-dioxygenase (TDO) may also impair serotonin synthesis, by decreasing levels of the precursor. TDO is up-regulated by increased cortisol levels due to stress. Thus, levels of tryptophan are regulated by TDO in response both to stress and to immune responses. HIV patients have been found to have decreased levels of both tryptophan and 5-HT. One of the effects of HAART is to inhibit tryptophan degradation in addition to halting viral replication and slowing down the chronic cellular immune response [2]. *Qigong* has been claimed to have similar effects to antidepressants such as the serotonin selective reuptake inhibitors (SSRIs), thus decreasing depression [55].

Tryptophan also affects other processes besides serotonin synthesis. There is a positive correlation between tryptophan and hemoglobin levels, indicating that tryptophan catabolism may impair hematopoiesis. Decreased levels of hemoglobin have been used to predict fatigue and depression. Conversely, there is a negative relationship between CD4+ cell counts and tryptophan, indicating that decreased leukopoiesis may be linked to enhanced tryptophan degradation [2]. In summary, stress-induced increases in cortisol level up-regulate TDO so reducing levels of tryptophan and 5-HT, as well as hemoglobin and leukocyte counts, which result in depression, fatigue and weakened immunity respectively. Use of *taiji* and *qigong* can increase levels of tryptophan, resulting in greater synthesis of 5-HT. These movement therapies have considerable impact on the intricacies of the central, peripheral and immune systems, thus regulating and balancing the ANS and improving overall quality of life. Clearly further research needs to be undertaken on the complex role of psychoneuroimmunological systems in the support of HIV/AIDS patients using these methods.

CONCLUSION

The HIV epidemic in the United States continues to affect racial/ethnic minorities disproportionately and is increasing among men who have sex with men. Late HIV diagnosis remains common. To reduce HIV transmission and facilitate early linkage to care and antiretroviral treatment, the Centers for Disease Control and Prevention recommend universal voluntary HIV screening for all persons aged 13 to 64 years in public and private care settings. Recent studies demonstrate dramatic reductions in morbidity and mortality with widespread use of HAART, and some document improved outcomes when HAART is initiated with CD4 cell count ≥ 350 cells/mm^3. As people with HIV live longer, they are increasingly affected by chronic diseases, notably cardiovascular and renal disease, diabetes and non-AIDS-defining cancers. Providers should ensure that patients undertake preventive lifestyle changes (e.g. smoking cessation, exercise, weight loss, dietary modification) and undergo recommended screening tests to reduce their risk for these important comorbidities [75]. *Taiji* and *qigong* are among various CAM modalities that can reduce the stressors of the initial diagnosis and aid in long-term management of HIV disease.

Energy-based therapies in neurology: the example of Therapeutic Touch

Eric Leskowitz

THE MULTIDIMENSIONAL MODEL OF HUMAN FUNCTION

This overview is designed to emphasize the multidimensional nature of human beings and the importance of having a full spectrum of therapeutic approaches to deal with illness and health. This perspective is particularly important in considering therapies that may at first appear to have no basis in scientific fact, according to the Western medical model.

It is helpful to think of human beings as having four main levels of function and structure. The most concrete level is physiology. The biomedical model focuses all its treatments, whether pharmaceuticals, surgery, radiation or genetic manipulation, on this concrete level.

Emotions and thoughts constitute the next important levels. Here the realm of thoughts, beliefs, attitudes and emotions are considered as one level. This dimension is addressed by psychotherapy and other mind–body techniques.

The last dimension is the spiritual. The most lasting value of holistic medicine may be that it finally bridges the long-standing gap between religion and science. We now have scientific data validating the clinical efficacy of interventions like prayer [1] and the laying on of hands [2] – two approaches that were formerly taboo for medical researchers to investigate, let alone prescribe. What these and other spiritually based therapies have in common is an insistence that human beings are animated by a special type of vital energy.

283

This vital energy fills individuals up with health when they are inspired, and is drained when they are ill. Many cultures speak of the phenomenon in their own language. In China, the energy is called *qi*; in India, yogis call it *prana*; in Hebrew mysticism, it is called *ruach*; in Western medicine, however, there is no word or concept for this vital energy. The end result is called *homeostatic balance*, the name for a process whose mechanism is not well understood.

A wide range of alternative medicine therapies deal with this dimension of subtle energy. These therapies tend to be the ones that are most controversial and the most difficult for mainstream science to comprehend. Some of the most prominent energy-based therapies and practices are addressed elsewhere in this book, including acupuncture, *qigong*, homeopathy, *shiatsu* and *taiji quan*. The focus in this chapter is on one of the few Western-based techniques that acknowledges and harnesses this so-called subtle energy: Therapeutic Touch (TT).

HISTORIC PRECURSORS OF THERAPEUTIC TOUCH

To be fair, some of the medical renegades of the Western medical tradition did try to characterize this subtle life energy. Sigmund Freud talked of *libido*, his onetime close colleague Wilhelm Reich researched orgone, Henri Bergson wrote of *élan vital* and, most importantly for this chapter, Franz Mesmer tried to harness 'animal magnetism'. Although widespread opinion holds that Mesmer was a charlatan, his technique was actually a precursor of TT and was more valid than mainstream medicine could ever credit. In addition, the reception he was given by the medical establishment of his time has interesting overtones with respect to the once hostile reaction of the American Medical Association (AMA) to CAM and the recent controversy over a widely publicized attempt to debunk TT.

Austrian physician Franz Anton Mesmer (1734–1815) participated in the intellectual ferment that swept Europe in the late 1700s, in particular the interest in the newly discovered forces of electricity and magnetism [3]. He developed a wildly popular form of magnetic therapy that used magnets supplemented by his own personal store of so-called 'animal magnetism' to heal his wealthy aristocratic patients. The wide range of disorders that he healed would probably mostly be labeled as conversion symptoms today. However, because the medical establishment in France was threatened by his runaway success, both medical and financial, King Louis XVI asked the French Royal Society to investigate the claims of Mesmerism. The eminent scientists appointed, including Antoine-Laurent de Lavoisier, Joseph-Ignace Guillotin and Benjamin Franklin, found that his patients did, in fact, get better, but only through the powers of imagination and suggestion. They discounted the existence of a magnetic *'fluidum'* that Mesmer claimed to transmit to his patients by making his famous Mesmeric passes. These passes consisted of stroking the air several inches from the patient's body in repeated downward movements. The fact that a separate commission vindicated Mesmer after his death was no solace, as he had effectively been run out of town, never again to recover his reputation or influence.

Two hundred years later, the tide has turned. Modern biomagnetism has documented that there *is* an energy field surrounding the human body [4]. Purported energy healers have been shown to emit measurable negative body potential surges of up to 90 volts under experimental conditions [5]. Other evidence that supports the involvement of subtle energy in healing is discussed elsewhere in this book.

THE TECHNIQUE OF THERAPEUTIC TOUCH

In the early 1970s, a team consisting of nurse Dolores Krieger and medical intuitive Dora Kunz developed the standardized treatment known as Therapeutic Touch [6]. TT was designed to be acceptable in medical settings and was built on the nursing tradition of compassionate hands-on caring while at the same time allowing medical professionals, particularly nurses, to harness some of the same subtle energies that saints, mystics and healers had been working with for centuries.

The standardized TT treatment protocol involves five steps [7]. The first and most important step is centering, in which the nurse healer takes a moment to quieten her mind and focus on a heart-centered wish to be of service to the patient. The second step is known as the assessment, in which the nurse scans the patient's external energy field by placing the palms of her hands several inches away from each part of the patient's body in turn. The nurse tries to sense alterations in the subtle perceptions of tingling or temperature that are typically experienced in this process. These alterations are thought to reflect underlying physiological problems and indicate the regions to be addressed in step three.

In the third treatment step, the nurse tries to 'unruffle' and clear these apparent energy blocks with a series of slow, stroking movements down the patient's energy field. The nurse does not actually make any physical contact. These movements are identical in form to Mesmer's passes. In the next step, the nurse focuses his or her hands on one particular region and directs and modulates the flow of energy there. This balancing phase may also involve direct physical contact with the patient's body. In the final phase, the nurse evaluates any changes in the patient's energy field hoping to detect the symmetric and open flow that marks a successful treatment.

SCIENTIFIC STUDIES

In the past 20 years, a large amount of clinical literature has built up around TT (see also Ch. 12). By 1998, an article in the *Journal of the American Medical Association* (*JAMA*) that sought to debunk TT listed 129 references [8], and as of November 2009 Medline gave 525 TT citations. The technique has been applied to a wide range of conditions, from preoperative anxiety to osteoarthritis, not only measuring subjective variables such as pain, anxiety and self-esteem, but also TT's effects on general medical conditions and objective physiological processes, including immune function and wound healing. Experimental rigor, in particular the double blind research protocol, is inappropriate for TT, in part due to the nature of TT itself. A sham TT technique has been developed in which patients can be blinded to TT. In this technique, nurses move their hands in the typical downward strokes of TT, but occupy their minds with mental arithmetic rather than the attitude of compassionate caring that marks true TT. Unfortunately, the nurse cannot be blinded to the treatment being given because, by definition, he or she is aware of which of these two states of mind is being used. Hence, TT research can at best be only single blind (the patient), rather than double blind.

Because of such methodological difficulties, some TT studies have been marred by controversy, perhaps befitting TT's place as the most prominent energy modality during a time in the 1990s when many reports on newly emergent methods of alternative medicine were met with an aggressive backlash of skepticism. For example, the *JAMA* article mentioned above has been shown by the present author to be methodologically unsound and politically driven [9]. These caveats aside, TT has now been taught to over 100 000 nurses in North America, and is available in many major medical centers.

Two key physiological studies are now discussed, followed by some case vignettes that illustrate how TT has been integrated into the Pain Management Program at Spaulding Rehabilitation Hospital in Boston.

Stress is known to inhibit numerous physiological processes. One such process that is susceptible to objective monitoring is wound healing – that is, the rate of repair of damaged skin. For example, the skin of people under high stress, such as caregivers of Alzheimer's patients, heals much more slowly from punch biopsies than does the skin of matched controls [10]. One well-known and seemingly well-controlled study by Daniel Wirth [2] appeared to show dramatic benefits to TT in wound healing. However, subsequent research was unable to verify the reported experimental protocol or to gain access to the original raw data; details of this story are available online, but the underlying conclusion is that Wirth's research is likely fraudulent [11]. Significantly, though, his protocol is amenable to replication, and such a study would provide definite proof of TT's purported physiological impact on the healing response. Along these lines, an in vitro study has shown that TT enhances the rate of cell growth in a test tube, a protocol that eliminated the confounding psychological factors of expectation and placebo [12]. Research may eventually demonstrate the ability of TT to enhance the body's healing response after surgery or injury via a similar mechanism of blast cell stimulation.

Another important study [13] showed that stress-induced immunosuppression could be reversed by TT, as measured by serum levels of immunoglobulins A and M in medical students during final exam time. Again, a clinically important physiological variable was affected in a positive manner by a relatively brief course of TT. The potential clinical applications are intriguing, especially given the wide range of medical conditions that are characterized by immune dysfunction.

THERAPEUTIC TOUCH IN NEUROLOGY: SOME EXAMPLES

PERIPHERAL NEUROPATHY

A clinical vignette from Spaulding Rehabilitation Hospital highlights potential applications of TT to peripheral neuropathy (although no formal research studies have yet been conducted with this specific syndrome). Lillian was a 68-year-old woman who had developed neuropathic pain in the distribution of her femoral nerve, which had been accidentally injured during vascular surgery several years earlier. She was able to obtain only slight relief with standard medications for neuropathic pain. In addition, her allodynia was so severe that she could not participate in any form of rehabilitation that involved direct physical contact, including physical therapy manipulation and tactile thermal desensitization. However, during the course of a TT treatment she felt the sensitivity decrease to such an extent that she allowed the TT practitioner to touch her leg, the first time she had allowed another person to touch her. This decreased sensitivity opened the door to a range of other standard pain management approaches, which were able to decrease her discomfort significantly. During psychotherapy she was – again for the first time – able to express her rage and disappointment at the trusted surgeon who had damaged her nerve.

MULTIPLE SCLEROSIS

Several reports in the nursing literature describe the use of TT in the care of multiple sclerosis (MS) patients. One case study [14] highlights the adjunctive role of TT in MS care, noting in particular its benefits for such subjective symptoms as mood and comfort. Another paper [15] emphasizes the high rate of use of various alternative therapies by MS patients and indicates that TT is one of the most popular. Results are reported in terms of quality of life but are not quantified by using more specific validated measures. This could greatly strengthen the TT literature on MS. In addition, given the current conceptualization of MS as an autoimmune disorder, the above-mentioned demonstration of enhanced immune functioning following TT takes on added significance.

DEMENTIA

No studies exist concerning the use of TT to reverse the degenerative process underling dementia, but several papers describe its use in bringing about behavioral changes in Alzheimer's patients. In one naturalistic study [16], TT was introduced as a stress-management technique. It was found to induce a relaxation response in dementia patients who had a history of agitated behavior, but it was not effective in decreasing the actual levels of these behaviors. Direct physical contact, as in hand massage, proved more effective than TT in reducing agitation in these patients – suggesting that when brain damage exceeds a certain threshold, the effects of TT may be too subtle to translate into overt behavioral changes.

HEADACHE

One of the best-designed TT studies so far performed looked at the effects of TT on tension headache pain [17]. By using the sham TT intervention mentioned earlier, expectancy and placebo factors could be taken into consideration. A matched group of 60 headache patients was studied, all of whom were naive to prior TT treatments; 90% of the members of the active treatment group experienced improvements in symptoms following TT, averaging a 70% decrease in degree of symptom intensity. Of the control patients, 80% reported pain reduction that averaged only 37% in degree. It should be noted that both groups practiced deep breathing. Therefore the placebo group was actually receiving a treatment known to be somewhat helpful in itself for mild headache symptoms, and the treatment group in fact received two treatments: TT plus breathing. Furthermore, this differential benefit was even more pronounced 4 hours after the initial treatment, again favoring TT over sham TT controls.

POSTOPERATIVE PAIN

In a single blind clinical trial that measured postoperative pain in 108 patients [18], a single TT treatment reduced their need for analgesic medication, although reported pain levels were similar between patients who received genuine TT and those who received a sham TT control intervention. Presumably, the untreated patients used additional analgesics to make up for the differential impact of TT. The author cautiously notes that TT may be best conceptualized as an adjunctive pain therapy rather than as a primary treatment modality.

BURN PAIN

Pain, anxiety and impaired immune function are all known to follow burns to a significant area of the body surface. One study [19] measured the impact of regular TT treatments on these three variables in patients in a hospital burn unit. Again using sham TT as the control intervention, this single-blinded randomized clinical trial determined that 5 days of regular TT caused statistically significant reductions on self-reported pain (McGill Pain Questionnaire Rating Index) and anxiety (Visual Analog Scale). Immune function was also altered, as reflected by a 13% decrease in CD8+ cell concentration, although the clinical significance of this cellular change was not clear. Again, the authors call for more studies to look at the long-term effects of ongoing TT and to control more tightly for behavioral variables that might influence outcome.

OTHER PAIN CONDITIONS

TT has been successfully used to treat several cases of phantom limb pain at Spaulding Rehabilitation Hospital [20]. Further studies are planned to validate its efficacy, and to explore further the finding that both the patient and the therapist reported energy-like tactile sensations when the therapist's hands were 'smoothing out' the contour of the phantom limb, despite lack of proximity to any physiological tissue at the time these sensations were being experienced.

CONCLUSION

For years the medical establishment has shown a good measure of resistance, often well deserved, to novel energy-based therapies like TT, but the tide is turning. The field of biomagnetism is documenting the existence of subtle human electromagnetic energy fields. A rapidly growing body of evidence is proving that TT and its relatives can be effective in a wide range of clinical situations. This includes most prominently a variety of pain conditions, as research on TT in other neurological conditions is still in its infancy. Further research is needed to move beyond the description of subjective variables into the realm of measuring functional outcomes and biological parameters. The current situation is full of promise for future discoveries in the application of energy-based therapies to the problems of medicine, in general, and neurology in particular.

Qi in chronic fatigue syndrome and fibromyalgia

Carolyn McMakin • Peter H Fraser

CHAPTER CONTENTS

23.1 FREQUENCY SPECIFIC MICROCURRENT AND OTHER INTERVENTIONS

Carolyn McMakin

MEDICAL MODEL OF CHRONIC FATIGUE SYNDROME (CFS) AND FIBROMYALGIA (FM)

Chronic fatigue syndrome is a complex psycho-neuro-endocrine-immunological condition consisting of a range of symptoms that include fatigue, impaired cognitive function, nonexudative pharyngitis, swollen tender lymph nodes, depression, loss of energy, sleep disturbance and some degree of body pain [1]. The Centers for Disease Control and Prevention (CDCP) defines CFS as a complex illness characterized by prolonged debilitating fatigue and multiple nonspecific symptoms including headaches, recurrent sore throats, fever, muscle and joint pain and neurocognitive complaints [2,3]. Some patients have elevated titers of various infections including the viruses Epstein–Barr (EBV), enterovirus, parvovirus B19 and bacterial infections *Coxiella burnetti* and *Chlamydia pneumoniae* [4,5]. In addition to the fatigue, some patients have cardiac symptoms including sinus tachycardia and cardiac wall abnormalities that improve with antiviral treatment [6].

Many patients mark the onset of the condition to the sequelae of some flu-like illness or to immunizations received prior to overseas travel. It has been challenging to determine whether the viral portion of the immunization or their mercury-based (thimerosal) preservatives have contributed to the symptoms, or whether the patient acquired some hard-to-detect parasite during the overseas travel.

There has been no satisfactory answer to whether viral and other infectious agents cause the onset of CFS or are opportunistic once the hypothalamic–pituitary–immune axis is compromised.

It has been demonstrated that EBV elevates levels of the inflammatory peptide interferon gamma (IFN-γ), resulting in degradation of serum tryptophan in CFS patients but not in normal controls [7]. IFN-γ and other inflammatory peptides have been shown to interfere directly with cognitive function and may be responsible for some complaints of impaired memory and concentration. Inflammatory peptides such as IFN-γ can also stimulate class C pain receptors and create generalized widespread aching. Tryptophan being the immediate precursor to serotonin, its degradation may be responsible for reduced levels of serotonin and complaints of depressive mood, sleep disruption and pain, all of which are serotonin mediated. This cascade of viral residuals involving inflammation and leading to reductions in tryptophan and serotonin, with sleep disturbance and pain, could reasonably be linked to the disruptions in neuroendocrine processes found to be dysfunctional in CFS, and argues for a viral onset hypothesis.

However, *any* initiating insult that up-regulates cytokine-mediated inflammation specifically in the nervous and immune systems and causes disruption of neurotransmitter and immune function could cause the complex of symptoms associated with CFS [1]. Serotonin and its precursor tryptophan are known to be impaired by inflammation. Dopamine and acetylcholine can also be disrupted by neuroinflammation and reductions in these neurotransmitters would disturb mood, sleep and cognitive function. Histamine is released by white blood cells as part of the immune response to allergens, food or environmental sensitivities, parasitic or viral infestation, and interferes with cognitive function, creates fatigue and activates class C pain fibers. Some CFS and FM syndrome patients have a history of exposure to environmental toxins such as organophosphate chemicals and heavy metals known to interfere with cell membrane, immune and neurological function and synthesis of neurotransmitters. These patients have the characteristic symptoms of CFS and FM but may or may not have increased viral titers.

Physical pain does not predominate in CFS as it does in FM. Substance P, a pain-mediating peptide elevated in the spinal fluid and blood of FM patients, is not elevated in CFS [8,9].

FM is diagnosed when the patient has full body pain, fatigue and sleep disturbance lasting more than 3 months and 11 of 18 tender points are tender to less than 4 kg of pressure, indicating central pain sensitization. It lacks the symptoms of viral infection, general inflammation and cardiac irritability that characterize CFS. However, both conditions share aberrations in tryptophan, serotonin metabolism and neuroendocrine function [10–12].

In both FM and CFS, pain, sleep disturbance and fatigue elevate stress levels and the neuroendocrine system changes its function altering both regulatory hormones from the brain and peripheral hormones from the gonads, adrenals, liver, pancreas, kidneys and thyroid. The chronic stress response becomes maladaptive when hypothalamic–pituitary–adrenal (HPA) axis disruptions create endocrine symptoms for both FM and CFS in addition to the complaints of pain and fatigue found in these populations.

Circulating cortisol levels from the adrenals are typically mildly reduced in CFS and FM patients and the adrenals do not respond normally to stimulation by corticotropin releasing hormone in laboratory testing [11–14]. Reduced circulating cortisol levels produce fatigue and inability to mount an appropriate stress response. These patients also reverse the normal high-in-the morning, low-at-night diurnal variation in cortisol secretion making them very fatigued in the morning and more alert at night, which interferes with sleep onset.

In an adult, growth hormone mediates amino acid transport across the cell membrane that is required for tissue repair. Most growth hormone is produced during stage IV sleep, which is not achieved in patients with CFS and FM. Growth hormone is reduced centrally by suppression of growth hormone releasing hormone (GHRH) in response to chronic stress [15]. Normal patients produce a spike in growth hormone following exercise that enhances muscle repair and recovery from exercise. FM and CFS patients have impaired growth hormone production from all of these mechanisms and, in combination with the inability to produce a postexercise spike in growth hormone, they become intolerant to even minimal normal levels of exercise [16].

CLINICAL CONSIDERATIONS IN CFS AND FM

The tidy statistics in the results section of a published peer-reviewed study cannot begin to describe the clinical picture confronting the clinician who sees a patient with chronic fatigue syndrome or fibromyalgia. The CFS patient often presents with nonspecific symptoms and a life in shambles due to disabling fatigue, inability to concentrate or think clearly, chronic sore throat and swollen lymph glands, depression, unexplained weight gain or weight loss, exercise intolerance, depression and malaise and often the loss of employment and relationships caused by these symptoms. The fibromyalgia patient presents with intolerable unrelenting body pain in addition to fatigue, sleep disturbance, cognitive dysfunction and a host of neuroendocrine abnormalities.

Depending on chronicity they may have been told more than once that the symptoms are psychosomatic, 'all in their head', and that they should just 'get over it'. Even if the patient had previously been healthy, productive, employed, happy, active and positive, a few months or years of debilitating symptoms, combined with the judgments rendered on their character by the medical profession, leave many with battered self-esteem and without help for their symptoms. Patients who have a history of depression, low self-esteem and childhood physical or sexual abuse have emotional and nervous system predispositions that may contribute to their susceptibility and may, justly or unjustly, be blamed for the entire syndrome. Once the label of incurable, crank, depressive, problematic CFS/FM patient has been internalized, recovery becomes an emotional as well as physical challenge.

Even on the most superficial level the complexities of treating CFS are related to the complex interactions between the activated, up-regulated immune system, the inflamed nervous system, the dysfunctional HPA axis and the impact of emotions and psychological state on all of the above systems. As if this is not enough, 85% of the immune system surrounds the digestive system, bringing the gut and digestive function inevitably into the picture.

On a deeper level the question arises for the practitioner of Oriental medicine, or any practitioner treating CFS and FM patients, about the impact of *qi* on all of these systems and the impact of all of this dysfunction on the available amount and flow of *qi*. We will return to this consideration shortly.

PHARMACOLOGICAL AND MICROCURRENT TREATMENTS FOR CFS AND FM

The real tragedy in CFS and FM patients is that treatments found to be effective in the literature do not seem to have made much of an impression on the general practitioners who first receive these patients into the medical system. The most ubiquitous and least expensive source of information about treatments comes from sales representatives sent out by pharmaceutical companies. Physicians are more likely to hear about various therapies being promoted according to company sales goals and marketing calendars than they are to hear about complex therapies for complex conditions like CFS and FM. Physicians must seek out the research, be willing to think through a complex condition and its treatments, and understand at the same time that the model for the illness being used in the study in front of them may or may not match the next CFS or FM patient they see (a similar situation will confront the average CAM practitioner).

Complex, multifactorial conditions like CFS and FM are completely unsuited to the double blind, placebo-controlled, single agent studies currently preferred by the 'evidence-based' medical model. It is highly unlikely that any *single* intervention will produce long-term overall improvement in symptoms, much less resolution of the condition. It is far more likely and reasonable that a *complex* of interventions will be required for resolution of such complex conditions. Lifestyle changes and pharmacological/nutritional interventions could include the following:

- Low-dose physiological cortisol replacement reduces fatigue and may be helpful until other strategies normalize adrenal function [17].
- Long-term antiviral therapy with valaciclovir has shown significant reductions in all CFS symptoms including fatigue, cardiac irregularities and sleep disturbances, with patients returning to normal activities [6]. Intravenous vitamin C is a potent antiviral and may be helpful for patients and practitioners who prefer not to use antibiotics or antiviral medications.
- Antiseizure medications such as Lyrica® (pregabalin) and Neurontin® (gabapentin) have been used to reduce pain successfully in FM but have no approved use in CFS [18]. These medications offer some pain relief but have side effects such as sedation and impaired memory and cognitive function, which many patients find objectionable. Often the benefit of pain relief outweighs the inconvenience of the side effects and a balance can be found.
- Serotonin selective reuptake inhibitors (SSRIs) are used as antidepressants and may be useful in low doses to alleviate the reductions in serotonin caused by cytokine-mediated disturbance in tryptophan metabolism [19].
- Tryptophan and 5-hydroxytryptophan (5-HTP) are available as supplements and may be used with fewer side effects than SSRIs to improve serotonin levels and function at a dose of 100 mg two to three times daily. This will improve sleep, pain and mood but will not affect viral loads, inflammation or immune system activation [10,20].
- Treatments such as mild aerobic exercise [21] and low-dose tricyclic antidepressants [22,23] improve mood, sleep and alleviate some symptoms in both FM and CFS.

- Omega-3 fish oils (EPA/DHA) are useful in reducing inflammation and may improve cognitive function but have no known effect on viral infections [24–26]. Intravenous vitamin C may reduce viral load [27,28] and inflammation [29] but has no known effect on serotonin levels or pain.

A very different approach is frequency specific microcurrent (FSM), which has been shown to reduce pain and levels of all of the inflammatory cytokines including IFN-γ, with recovery from fibromyalgia in 58% of patients in a collected case report [9]. FSM has also reduced symptoms of chronic fatigue in unpublished cases.

Microcurrent is a battery-operated physical therapy modality providing current in millionths of an ampère (μA). This physiological current is the same as that which flows normally through the body and cannot be felt because it is not sufficient to stimulate sensory nerves. Microcurrent between 50 and 500 μA increased energy (adenosine triphosphate, ATP) production in rat skin by 500% in one unreplicated study. Current levels above 500 μA caused ATP production to level off and current levels above 1000 μA actually reduced ATP production [30]. Standard electrotherapy delivers current in milliampères and, according to this research, reduces ATP production.

FSM uses frequencies that were developed in the early 1900s for a completely different electrical modality. The list of frequencies thought to 'remove pathologies' and to 'address specific tissues' was obtained in 1996 from an osteopath who bought a practice in Canada in 1946 that came with one of these antique devices manufactured in 1922. The frequencies were taken at face value and first applied in 1995 using a two-channel microcurrent device. The frequencies appeared to have the effects described on the list provided with the antique machine.

The frequency for reducing inflammation does reduce pain and all of the inflammatory cytokines in FM patients and both lipoxygenase and cyclooxygenase inflammation in mice, but is not useful for any other condition. No other frequency tested reduced inflammation [9,31]. The frequency to reduce scar tissue both reduces scar tissue and increases range of motion in patients with mature burn scarring, but does not change inflammation (R Huckfeldt et al, unpublished presentation, 2003). There is one frequency that eliminates the symptoms of both shingles and herpes infections in a 20-minute application. Treatment with this – and only this – frequency combination for 2 hours aborts the viral attack and the symptoms do not return. The treatment protocols for myofascial pain, fibromyalgia, shingles, adrenal support, wound healing and other clinical applications have been developed by trial and error in a clinical setting [32–34] (Fig. 23.1).

QI IN CFS AND FM – *QIGONG*, ACUPUNCTURE AND FSM

Practitioners of Chinese medicine consider that CFS and FM reflect a disharmony and depletion in the supply and flow of *qi* in the body [35]. These patients present as qi deficient, *yin* deficient and so *yang* deficient as to be intolerant of *yang* interventions, food or situations. In the author's experience, pulse diagnosis consistently reveals CFS patients to be Spleen, Lung and Kidney deficient with Damp (*shi*, 濕) and congestion predominant in the other pulses. Experience with a CFS patient population suggests that Western medical acupuncture may have as much difficulty as Western medicine in sorting out the complexities of CFS symptoms. FM patients are usually as *yin* deficient and depleted as CFS patients but because of higher pain levels may have excess Heat (*re*, 熱) in some meridians. *Qi* has been described and defined in many ways, from literal and well defined to poetic and metaphorical (see Chs 1, 3, 5 and 11, for example). Here it is considered as the energy behind all energies, the basic stuff from which both particles and waves

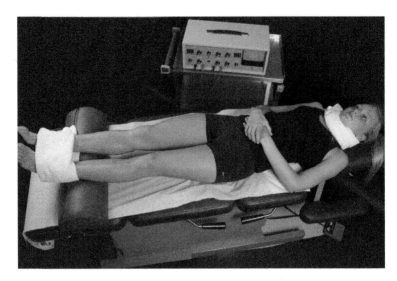

FIG 23.1 Frequency specific microcurrent treatment of fibromyalgia caused by spine trauma. One frequency combination (40 Hz and 10 Hz) was found to reduce substance P and all inflammatory cytokines and to increase endorphins in FM associated with spine trauma. Pain was reduced from an average of 7.3/10 to 1.3/10 in 90 minutes. The patient is treated with positive contacts at the neck and negative contacts at the feet using pulsed polarized positive DC current. 58% of patients recovered from FM within a 4-month period. The treatment has not been studied in chronic fatigue.

arise, providing both essence and form in the manifestation of all life and matter. As such it pervades and sustains life and the universe, and in particular is the spark of life that dims in patients who are chronically ill. There is no really satisfactory description of this in either Newtonian or quantum physics, and readers are welcome to their preferred and most comfortable appreciation of *qi*, based on their own experience and understanding.

For purposes of this discussion, optimal health requires that adequate amounts of *qi* move in a smooth and balanced way through the meridians. Its flow can be disturbed by various physical, mental and emotional factors including but not limited to inflammation, allergies, physical and emotional stress, anger, fear or grief, infections, toxins and trauma. Its flow, in short, will be disrupted by any and all of the conditions associated with CFS and FM.

The question becomes, 'Does CFS create the *qi* deficiency and block its flow or does the deficiency and disrupted flow of *qi* contribute in some way to the onset and perpetuation of the illness?' As with every other question that arises when considering this complex condition the reply must be, 'It depends'. Etiology will vary from patient to patient and practitioners are challenged to relinquish attachment to a preferred model that does not match the particular patient being treated. CFS and FM are unsuited to a reductionist approach to health and illness – regardless of the model used.

Qigong is a traditional intervention used to strengthen *qi* through self-practice and to improve its flow in order to prevent and even cure disease. In one trial, 18 female patients were taught a *qigong* routine during weekly classes over 6 months and asked to practice it daily for 15 minutes while continuing to take prescribed medication and keep medical appointments. Patients completed a medical outcomes questionnaire and a sleep diary during a 2-week baseline control period and at 3 and 6 months following the start of the trial. Parameters assessed included:

vitality, sleep problems, social activity limitation due to ill health, health distress, mental health, psychological wellbeing and pain. All parameters changed significantly over the 6-month trial, although pain was reduced the least and was the last parameter to change. No patient withdrew due to adverse effects [35].

There is some epidemiological evidence that *qigong* can produce significant and positive changes in the neuroendocrine and immune systems and in psychological state [36–38]. If *qigong* has the effects on *qi* that it is presumed to have then it could be said that improving the strength and flow of *qi* will improve the symptoms of CFS and probably FM.

Acupuncture improves the flow of *qi* and so has been useful in the treatment of CFS and FM. In one randomized controlled study of electroacupuncture for FM, outcome parameters showed significant improvement in the active treatment group (50% showed satisfactory improvement, 25% dramatic improvement with almost complete disappearance of symptoms), but no patients improved in the sham group. Points treated included ST-36 and LI-4 (bilaterally), with six other points not described but chosen depending on the patient's pain pattern and according to the empirical efficacy of the sites in the treatment of pain [39,40]. In the author's clinic, microcurrent probes have been used to stimulate acupuncture points on the Stomach and Bladder meridians, producing excellent, consistent but temporary symptomatic improvement.

Using FSM to increase ATP production has been observed to change the dynamic of acupuncture pulses: frequencies for 'vitality in the spleen' improved the strength and quality of the Spleen pulse, but without affecting any other pulse; frequencies to 'remove paralysis and restore vitality in the kidney' improved the Kidney pulse. These changes occurred within seconds (P Lollis, personal communication, 2003).

If one thinks of *qi* as energy, flow and information then it is possible that FSM may be useful within an acupuncture model for improving *qi* and its flow in CFS and FM patients. It may be a stretch to equate the increases in cellular ATP production due to current flow with increases in *qi*, but some patients respond as if this is exactly what happens as their general energy levels improve with regular use.

The FSM frequencies can be seen as supplying corrective information in the form of resonance patterns that remove tissue pathologies such as inflammation or scarring that impair cellular function and the flow of *qi*. Another scenario is that the atoms in every bond and molecular structure oscillate slightly at a characteristic frequency and every molecular bond has a resonant frequency that will amplify these oscillations, eventually causing them to come apart.

The reductions in inflammatory cytokine levels and lipoxygenase- and cyclooxygenase-mediated inflammation induced by FSM could be seen as improving intracellular communication through resonance [9,31]. The changes in viral symptoms seen in shingles and herpes – the same class of virus as EBV – are most likely the result of frequency resonance disrupting the bonds that hold the viral capsid together. This is currently the only model that accounts for the speed with which symptoms abate and lesions disappear. The frequency combination for shingles and herpes has been useful clinically in the treatment of CFS patients although no formal trials have been done to confirm the effect. FSM may eventually prove useful for improving CFS symptoms within both the biomedical and acupuncture models.

SYNTHESIS OF THE TWO MODELS

The patient sitting before any practitioner is not the illness with which he or she presents. The patient is a living complexity comprising simultaneously body, soul, energy field, meridians, chakras, *prana*, breath, emotions and the neurological, endocrine, immune, digestive, respiratory, cardiac, reproductive, urologic, fascial and epithelial systems, as well as the biochemicals, neuroelectrical system and neurotransmitters that allow them to interact and communicate.

Intellectual honesty requires the admission that we can only appreciate small parts of this hologram at any one time and so we operate, at any given time, from a partial model for convenience and not because it is the only model, or even the best one. That said, any analysis of FM and CFS and suggestions for effective treatments must be approached with humility and the certainty that all models, even ones with which we do not agree, are simultaneously true to some extent. CFS patients are *qi* deficient and retain Damp *and* they have increased viral titers, reduced levels of cortisol, tryptophan and serotonin. FM patients are *yin* deficient *and* they have increased substance P, central sensitization, neuroendocrine and immune dysfunction and elevated cytokines. Both states, all models are simultaneously true.

It is as though the condition and the patients are a loosely woven delicate fabric that can best be seen by standing back to appreciate the multiple strands creating the complexity of the weave, paying attention to detail and patterns. Any intervention that tugs on one thread will influence the whole fabric but one thread is only one thread and cannot be confused with the multiple strands creating the weave. It is unreasonable to proceed as if the fabric were made of only one thread just because that one thread is our favorite color and one that we understand and prefer.

CFS and FM patients need the hope and relief that can only come from an integrated, team approach to treatment that places all helpful interventions on an equal footing depending on the patient's history, presentation and treatment preferences. The physician's own treatment preferences and model for the condition cannot be the only consideration. Acupuncture, *qigong*, FSM, prescription medications, diet, supplements, exercise, sleep, stress reduction and lifestyle changes all have value in the treatment of both fibromyalgia and chronic fatigue. The practitioner skilled in only one intervention can refer the patient to practitioners skilled in the other interventions creating a team of resources for the patient to choose from. An educated, informed, empowered patient is a powerful ally in the journey towards recovery.

A wise physician once said, 'It is the physician's job to see the patient as healed until the patient can see it for himself' (C Novak, personal communication, 1988). Perhaps the most powerful therapy available for CFS and FM is the belief and determination that it can be cured.

23.2   HEALTH AND THE HUMAN BODY-FIELD

Peter H Fraser

THE NUTRI-ENERGETICS SYSTEMS THEORY

Before discussing the constellations of symptoms identified as chronic fatigue syndrome and fibromyalgia, I will outline my theory of the human body-field and my approach to addressing these and similar illnesses. This comprehensive theory – the NES (Nutri-Energetics Systems) theory [41,42] – ranges across many disciplines, from biology to quantum physics, so discussion here is by necessity somewhat simplified.

Nearly 30 years ago I left a post as professor of acupuncture in my native Australia to begin investigating the physical reality of *qi*. I suspected that, whatever *qi* is, it is not some still unknown and quasi-metaphysical energy but a known energy of physics, albeit one that had not yet been reliably measured in the human body. However, although there are findings on the electromagnetic characteristics of acupuncture points and meridians, it was my belief that the larger body-field, and thus *qi*, cannot be restricted to the electromagnetic spectrum of energy. I therefore decided to look deeper into physics and biology to try to address the question of what natural, known energies might account for the human biofield. I concluded that *qi* is in the realm of quantum physics. The results to date of this investigation offer enhanced understanding not only of such illnesses as CFS and FM, but of the bioenergetics of most other diseases as well.

THE MERIDIAN SYSTEM UPDATED

After decades of research, I have uncovered a structure to the human body-field that goes further than traditional Chinese medicine (TCM) and integrates it with modern biology, anatomy and physiology. This body-field is more than the aura, *chakras* and meridians – it is a highly structured, systems level network of information and energy that is intimately linked with the physical body. The body cannot function without the body-field as its underlying information template, and that template itself could not arise without the dynamical processes of physical growth and metabolism. The body-field drives physiology at the subcellular level and is inextricably linked to and affected by internal and external fields of energy and information.

The body-field has several substructures. In NES theory, its main components are:

- **Interactional fields:** Relating to the interaction of the body-field with the natural fields of the Earth and cosmos (such as the magnetic polar and gravitational fields), and its orientation to them (particularly that of the spinal column subfield).
- **Energetic driver (ED) fields:** Subfields correlated to the organs that arise during fetal development and that 'power' them. When an ED becomes distorted or blocked, the correlated organ begins to lose function. Fatigue is a classic sign of an ED distortion, which is why it is also often the first sign of physical illness. The EDs have affinities with the TCM idea of the *zangfu* acting as power sources for the meridians.
- **Energetic integrator (EI) fields:** Nonlinear energy and information pathways in the body-field (not the physical body) that are similar to meridians in that they regulate many disparate aspects of the body (mineral, cellular, tissue, organ, endocrine, even emotional). They may be represented mathematically over a wide frequency range and according to particular 'phase wave' relationships. Like the body-field itself, they are best read or scanned and then treated in preferred logarithmic frequency sequences. When these are followed, clinical results are enhanced. To my knowledge, only NES theory has identified these sequences.
- **Energetic terrain (ET) information sequences:** Complex energetic and information structures representing emotional states and other energy configurations that I call 'emotional oscillators', also correlated to the brain and linked to past traumas. ETs appear to link bioenergetically to blocks of genetic code for protein replication, but discussion of this is beyond the scope of this chapter. ETs appear to play a significant bioenergetic role in CFS, FM and indeed all illnesses.
- There are other structural aspects to the body-field, but these are beyond the scope of this discussion.

A strong point of NES theory is the level of detail that can be demonstrated in correlations between the body-field and body. For example, let us compare NES EI 8 (Liver Integrator) with the Liver meridian of TCM, which has an internal channel that links to the eye. In TCM, not much more is known about this connection to the eye, but using NES theory we have discovered that EI 8 communicates not with the entire eye but only with the iris and retina. Beyond the iris and retina, the EI 8 information pathway also communicates with the hypothalamus, supraoptic nucleus and visual cortex, with the maxillary sinus, and with the myocardium, mediastinum, diaphragm, corpus luteum and the nerves of the liver (but not generally with the liver cells themselves, which are linked more robustly to the Liver ED field). EI 8 also correlates to calcitonin, adrenalin, prolactin, estrogen and estrone in terms of endocrine connections, and to the mineral chromium.

My own research dovetails with that of others, particularly in the following three fields, which each have a bearing on understanding how the body functions.

1. The connective tissue matrix

Several frontier biologists have shown that the body's connective tissue network has a fluid crystalline composition and appears to be a high-speed, superconductive network for transmitting information throughout the body [43]. For this reason and others, the 'living matrix', as this is sometimes called, has been identified as the primary correlative to the Chinese meridian system, the *jingluo* (see also 'Coherence and meridians' in Ch.16, and Ch.19). Like the network of meridians, it is a system of *preferred* pathways for energy and information. From a bioenergetic perspective, distortions in the flow of information through the connective tissue matrix must be considered as part of the root cause of most illnesses.

2. Cavity dynamics

At all levels, the body is made up of resonating cavities. There are obvious major ones – cranial, thoracic and abdominal – but also myriad smaller cavities such as the eye sockets and nostrils, sacs and hollow spaces in the sinuses, ears and elsewhere, and those in the organs themselves. There are also myriads of microtubules and nanotubes throughout the body, especially within the brain, lungs and kidneys. From physics we know that cavities attract, store and resonate with energy, and yet for some reason conventional biologists almost completely ignore the body's cavities (which often only exist as potential spaces defined by their outline rather than as actual spaces). In contrast, I have come to understand that one of the primary bioenergetic functions of body cavities is collecting Source energy, a kind of overall constitutional energy that excites the body at all levels, from the cell-field through the organ-field to the whole body level (at which the holistic organizing field is called the 'morphic field' in NES theory).

But what is this Source energy, or *yuan qi*? To my mind, a possible explanation is the energy generated by magnetic pulses in free space [44]. To understand this connection, some quantum physics background is necessary. The space resonance theory of astrophysicist Milo Wolff predicts that quantum reality is wave dominated, rather than particle dominated, and that when two spherical standing scalar waves interact, the resonance characteristics of quantum space change [45–47]. According to Wolff, what scientists identify as the different particles of quantum mechanics are really interactions of different kinds of space resonances. For Wolff, there are only three 'real' particles (the electron, proton and neutron), and other quantum particles are only 'appearances' caused by these varying characteristics of space, which themselves are determined by interactions of quantum spherical standing scalar waves. These wave interactions may also cause the appearance of magnetic pulses, and the energy from these pulses may collect in body cavities, such as the *sanjiao* in TCM, as a kind of Source energy that contributes to 'powering' the physical body. Thus, a fundamental aspect of the breakdown of body function may be at the level of cavities and their ability to attract and store Source energy. In any bioenergetic therapy for any chronic disease, the cavities would need to be addressed. Methods of clinically addressing Source energy depletion include using NES 'Infoceuticals', going out of doors in the sun, deep breathing, walking barefoot on the earth and so on.

3. Beyond bioenergetics to bioinformation

Other forms of *qi* inside the body are also of interest (see for example Chs 4, 5 and 20), but first we need to distinguish between energy and information. Energy is fundamental to the workings of the material universe – that is why it is a primary focus in physics: for anything to happen in this universe, particles/waves must interact, and in those interactions, energy is always exchanged. However, in the last few decades physicists have begun to recognize that information may be more fundamental than energy – a 'thing' unto itself and the core substance of the cosmos [48]. This makes sense for without an organizing force, or forces, energy moves chaotically or randomly. The organizing forces of nature appear to be various types of fields, derived from the interactions of Wolff's three basic particles.

In the 1920s, physicist Louis de Broglie produced a mathematical theory that suggested that all nature consists of 'matter waves'. He was proved correct and received a Nobel Prize for this work. Other physicists, including Milo Wolff in the 1980s, agree with this general premise. It seems that a matter wave is the actual energy wave on which information *acts* (to organize the energy into a unique pattern) and also on which it can be *carried* (just as radio waves carry information, the patterns that encode the meaning in a song or a voice).

According to my research into Chinese medicine, *qi* does not correlate with any specific energy in physics. In trying to find a relevant model of how a fundamental wave pattern might encode information, I turned to European radionics, but found that its number system is similarly unable to correlate to electromagnetic or other real frequencies. So after a decade of reading and research, I turned to the field of quantum electrodynamics, as developed by Richard Feynman and other leading physicists. At last I could explain some of the odd features that I had found with electrodermal testing. Moving on from Feynman, I encountered Wolff's theory of space resonances. This predicts that matter waves will be found with frequencies of about 10^{24} Hz, making them a perfect network for carrying information through space.

In terms of the human body, the *qi* of each organ may actually be a whole group of matter wave frequencies that arise as a result of the dynamics of what is called 'global scaling'. This is a mathematical construct describing space resonances caused by interactions of Wolff's basic particles (electrons, protons and neutrons). Since 1967, global scaling theory has been applied to the sizes and masses of living things, to embryology, to the patterns of chemical physiology and even to the arrangement of the planets in the solar system [49–52]. A basic premise of the theory, even as it was applied to astrophysics by physicist Hartmut Müller [52,53], is that space – including all energy and matter – is organized logarithmically, not linearly, by scale. Information is carried within standing waves (stationary waves through which energy moves) whose nodes are scaled logarithmically, not linearly, so that in the material universe even if these nodes are physically distant, in logarithmic space they are adjacent. This means, essentially, that everything is connected and information can travel instantaneously. Furthermore, standing waves and their nodes in logarithmic space are scaled over a range of frequencies, and they can carry messages that are created by sets of vectors that are self-arranging in space. In NES theory the EIs of the human body-field are arranged in a similar logarithmic fashion, as discussed briefly below.

Thus the *qi* of each organ may have a relationship to a block of frequencies that are not electromagnetic in character but which instead can be described according to global scaling and worked out via its special mathematics. My own research has also shown that the body-field can be 'tagged' with messages imprinted onto these scaled-down matter waves. This may sound like science fiction, but work with NES 'Infoceuticals' does appear to show it is possible. These are liquid remedies of purified water and a small quantity of plant-derived minerals. Each Infoceutical is imprinted with information that is correlated to specific aspects of the body-field and its substructures (with that information being forced into the electron structure of the microminerals using a proprietary process). Currently, there are 66 Infoceuticals, grouped into several categories (Drivers, Integrators, Terrains, etc.) and they are taken as drops in water. The information they hold is designed to correct distortions in the body-field (there is no claim of any direct effect on the physical body).

So what does all this have to do with CFS and FM, or with any illness or disease for that matter? It sets the stage for an entirely different view of pathology: one that is not biochemical and that goes beyond even bioenergetic approaches. It is purely bioinformational.

CHRONIC FATIGUE SYNDROME (CFS) AND OTHER SUPPOSEDLY VIRAL DISEASES

Because many people have reported a bout of flu-like symptoms or a general immune suppression before they came down with CFS, orthodox medicine has focused on a viral connection. However, even the connection between viruses and more specific diseases is not absolute in microbiology. And, although microbiologists describe the human immune system as based entirely on cellular and humoral activity, disregarding its bioenergetic dynamics, no one seems able to make it work better when it is not functioning correctly. In contrast, if we consider all disease as a corruption or even starvation of information and energy, we do obtain more sensible therapeutic outcomes. Bioenergetically, CFS is simply a corrupt message resembling that of a virus – which after all is just DNA and RNA information that is foreign to the body.

The proven mathematics of global scaling can also help us to understand what may be going on in conditions that appear to be viral but where no virus is ever found. As previously mentioned, global scaling theory predicts that quantum space is logarithmic in nature, not linear, and that energy and information can scale up in nature via the dynamics of standing scalar waves. These insights dovetail with the NES theory of the body-field's EIs, whose structures are arranged via a logarithmic scale of quantum field frequencies extending from 10^1 to 10^{16} Hz in the human body-field. In recent investigations, we observed that in every person tested who suffers from a disease attributed to a virus but in which the virus cannot actually be found in laboratory tests, there is a similar bioenergetic pattern – a pattern of what I call 'scaling drop-out'. I also suspect that ETs play a major role. In part, these are bioenergetic environments in the body that can attract and host viruses, but the viruses do not have to be actually present to have an impact. As farfetched as it may seem, there is evidence that viral families each have their own biofield template (a kind of species/family-level morphic field), and the human body may react to exposure to the energetic field of a virus without ever having been in contact with or infected by the actual virus [41]. NES research carried out since 1998 has verified that ET 7 has a specific bioenergetic effect on the body-field that appears to successfully address the correlated physical symptoms of CFS. This is where theory meets practice, and we are extremely hopeful about this approach.

THE PATTERN OF 'SCALING DROP-OUT'

In tests on this population of clients, I noticed distortions in the function of the following sequence of Energetic Integrators (the meridian listed in parentheses after the EI is a partial correlation only):

EI-6 (Kidney meridian)
EI-7 (Gall Bladder meridian)
EI-8 (Liver meridian)
EI-9 (Thyroid/*sanjiao*)
EI-10 (Pericardium/Circulation meridian)

The frequencies of these EIs range from 10^6 Hz to 10^{10} Hz, the range where I believe information 'drop-out' is happening along the continuous global scaling wave. In principle, we should be able to devise a NES Infoceutical that could provide a bioinformational correction for this massive drop-out. This would work informationally and energetically in the body-field, as when rebooting a defective computer operating system. However, this project has yet to be undertaken.

A surprising correlation to the scaling drop-out hypothesis is that a bioenergetic 'match' is found not only between this sequence of EIs and CFS, but also between it and the bioenergetic signatures of multiple sclerosis, HIV/AIDS and some cancers. Of course, this says nothing about treatment or cure at a physical level, but is additional data that suggests that many seemingly incurable diseases may be correlated to information drop-out following the collapse of scaling. I say 'seemingly incurable' because these diseases may not respond well to chemical treatments. Their response to bioenergetic and bioinformational clinical approaches remains to be seen.

PARALLELS WITH THE DISCOVERY OF REVERSE TRANSCRIPTASE

In 1975, Howard Temin and David Baltimore shared a Nobel Prize for their discovery of reverse transcriptase, modifying the so-called 'central dogma' of biology with their work on how retrovirus family viruses can alter ribonucleic acid (RNA) by polymerase activity. In effect, they showed how information can flow in *both* directions between deoxyribonucleic acid (DNA) and RNA – a radical revision of genetics, but one that fits exactly with my own observations and theory (Fig. 23.2A, B). (In Figures 23.2 and 23.3, arrows indicate the direction of information flow.) The result is that certain types of viruses, such as retroids like HIV that encode reverse transcriptase, can mutate quickly and evolve different forms. This has direct relevance to the ETs in NES theory, which correlate bioenergetically to families of microorganisms (although this is not their only correlation). The link to the ETs means we have a third biological model (Fig. 23.2C).

Figure 23.3 shows in more detail the flow of information from the genetic level to the bioenergetic/bioinformational level of the correlated EIs and ETs. For the sake of simplicity, the diagram begins with the flow of information at

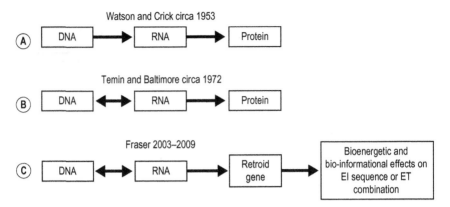

FIG 23.2 Comparison of: (A) the Watson and Crick model of information flow between DNA, RNA and protein, and (B) the more recent model of Temin and Baltimore; (C) the NES model of information flow between DNA, RNA and protein.

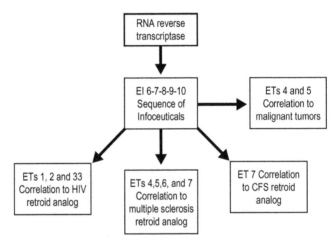

FIG 23.3 The NES model of information flow between RNA and the body-field Energetic Integrators (EIs) and Energetic Terrains (ETs).

the biochemical level, although I am *not* saying that genetic information is the most fundamental level of communication in the body indeed (this entire chapter argues against that view).

STRESS AS A CAUSATIVE AGENT

It would be premature to make any clinical treatment claims for these insights, but the apparently strong correlation between one prominent line of modern molecular biology and the latest bioenergetic and bioinformational research is cause for excitement. I sense that there will be a great deal more to this story as it unfolds. The big question, however, is not about the bioenergetic effect of viruses or their information fields, but about what manner of stress upsets the sequence of the five EIs that are correlated to seemingly viral diseases. This question is a huge research subject on its own and awaits further investigation.

On the basis of NES theory, it seems highly likely that the use of the EI 6 through EI 10 Infoceuticals might serve as a reconnector of information flow in the body-field after mental stress has upset the scaling process that affects the entire physical body matrix and the body-field itself. As such, this sequence of Infoceuticals is merely a bioinformational antistress therapy. More research must be done to verify this before it can be used clinically. What is true of CFS and all other diseases, however, is that bioenergetically and bioinformationally, it is always efficacious to address stress, as well as the other factors previously mentioned (the connective tissue matrix, cavities of the body) and one not yet mentioned – the heart.

RETROID DISEASES AND THE HEART

On the basis of my research into the traditional meridians, I believe that the only ones that link energetically to human DNA and RNA are the divergent meridians (*jingbie*, 經別), of which there are 12. All of these also link to the heart organ (in addition to certain types of purely energetic Heart fields). So, for the clinically minded bioenergetic health worker, it has to be said that in treating this group of diseases the energetic function of the heart must be supported as a matter of priority. The heart is of supreme importance not only as an organ/muscle but also as an imprinter of information in the body. In NES theory, the heart is truly the 'emperor' of the body (as it is in TCM) in that it is the major processor and generator of the information that cells need to function. I consider it highly likely that through the heart's myriad energy dynamics – the pressure and sound waves, electrochemical signals, cavities and resonances, and other mechanisms – it imprints information primarily onto the lipids in the blood, which then carry the information to all the body's cells for their use. In this model the information breakdown between the living matrix and central nervous system is mediated by the heart as imprinter, and such a breakdown contributes to the formation of retroids that may actually be manufactured by the body under the influence of stress. Therefore, I do not believe that CFS or other similar illnesses, and perhaps any chronic illness, can be effectively treated without addressing the heart at a bioenergetic and bioinformational level.

The electrical heart: energy in cardiac health and disease

Alan Watkins

CHAPTER CONTENTS

❝ *All forms of healing are ultimately modifications of time and energy.*
Helen Graham [1]

THE SPARK OF LIFE

A female friend recently sent my wife a text message full of excitement announcing her first pregnancy. She came round a few weeks later to give us a blow-by-blow account of her 18-week ultrasound scan. Like many mothers to be, she became quite emotional when she described seeing, for the first time, the baby's heart beating. This really brought home to her that the baby was alive.

In fact the first beat of her baby's heart occurred much earlier than the day she witnessed it. That first spark of life, that first heart beat, is detectable in an embryo just 21 days after conception. We still do not know why the muscular tube that folds in on itself and becomes the human heart suddenly starts beating. Although we have discovered the source of the beat – a cluster of electrically excitable cells nestling in the upper chamber of the heart – why they suddenly start beating in a regular fashion is still a mystery.

The heart contracts about 100 000 times each day, pumping blood around the body. Each contraction starts with an electrical spark from the heart's built-in pacemaker, which is then conducted to the rest of its muscle cells causing them to contract.

In the last 130 years we have been able to measure this 'spark of life'. The first reported recording of the electrical current surging through the heart was made in Britain in 1872 by Alexander Muirhead (1848–1920) [2]. A few years later John Burdon-Sanderson (1828–1905) created an image of the heart beat [3], and at the turn of the twentieth century a British doctor called Augustus Waller (1856–1922) working at St Mary's Hospital in London recorded the image of the heart beat using a capillary electrometer fixed to a projector [4]. The image was projected on to a photographic plate pulled by a toy train.

It was not until 1903 that a Dutch doctor, Willem Einthoven (1860–1927), developed a more sensitive technology capable of generating a more reliable image of the heart beat. Einthoven's first machine weighed 600 lb (272 kg), required five people to operate it and used powerful electromagnets that generated so much heat they needed to be cooled by water. His machine converted the electrical current that surged through the heart into a simple deflection of a recording needle on a piece of paper. This device was the first ever electrocardiogram (ECG). He labeled the first deflection with a letter from the middle of the alphabet and called it the 'R' wave. Einthoven later received the Nobel Prize for his work in creating the prototype of the modern-day ECG machine.

JUST ONE BEAT

Einthoven's nomenclature remains today with the R wave of the ECG occurring when the heart contracts. Since then five other needle deflections have been detected during a single heart beat, giving rise to the P, QRS, T and U waves (Fig. 24.1). The P wave occurs when the two upper chambers of the heart contract and is followed quickly by the first heart sound as the valves of the upper chambers of the heart close behind the ejected blood. The shape of the P wave can reveal information about the health of the upper heart chambers.

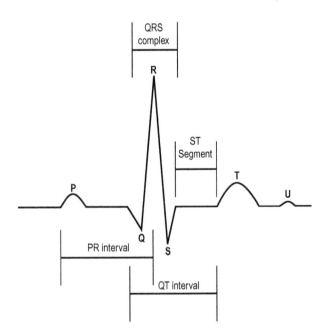

FIG 24.1 The different deflections in a single heart beat.

The QRS complex is made up of a downward, an upward and then a second downward deflection, and occurs when the two lower chambers of the heart contract. The QRS is followed by the second heart sound as the valves close behind the blood that is ejected on its way to the lungs (from the right side of the heart) or the body (from the left side of the heart). Thus the heart makes two discrete noises as it beats – 'lup-dub'. The quality of these sounds and any additional noises can reveal information about the integrity of the values of the heart.

The flickering changes of direction that the needle makes, first noticed by Einthoven, simply reflect the direction the electric current takes as it navigates its way through the conducting tissue within the heart itself. It initially moves away from the recording electrode on the front of the chest (giving rise to the Q wave), then toward the recording electrode (the R wave), and then away again (the S wave). The shape of the QRS complex can reveal information about the health of the main pumping chambers of the heart.

After the heart has contracted, it then has to relax to allow time for it to fill back up again before its next contraction. This relaxation is called 'repolarization' and is when the chemical balance in every heart cell resets. It also causes a deflection of the ECG needle, giving rise to the 'T' wave. After the T wave it is sometimes possible to see an additional 'U' wave, which, if present, is not thought to be very clinically important.

The gap between the 'S' and 'T' waves, called the 'ST segment', is used to determine whether there is any blockage in the arteries supplying the heart muscle with oxygen. If the ST segment is elevated, this suggests the patient may be having a heart attack. If the ST segment is 'depressed', this suggests that there is insufficient blood getting to the heart muscle and the coronary arteries supplying the heart muscle may be partially blocked. The depression in the ST segment is an important indicator of heart disease during the treadmill exercise stress test.

So the shape of the beat itself can reveal a great deal of information about the health of the heart, whether its arteries are blocked and whether electrical currents are being conducted normally within it. For example, if the spark from the heart's electrical pacemaker is poorly conducted around the heart then the shape of the beat is likely to become abnormal. Occasionally, excitable cells outside the heart's pacemaker will 'cluster fire' (fire closely together) and provoke a contraction. Such an abnormally shaped QRS complex is called an 'ectopic' beat (i.e. it is generated by cells outside the normal location for heart beat generation). Everyone generates ectopic beats, and they become more frequent as we age. Strong coffee can also increase the number of ectopic beats generated. As a rule of thumb, up to 10 000 ectopic beats a day are permissible before any medical involvement is necessary. Most people have only a handful of ectopic beats, which they usually do not even feel.

The regular rhythmic beating of the heart can also become disordered leading to a loss of the synchronized contraction of the upper and lower chambers of the heart or an 'arrhythmia'. When the source of this arrhythmia is in the upper chambers (atria) of the heart it is relatively benign. However, when the source of the arrhythmia is in its lower chambers (ventricles) it is very serious and usually a sign of advanced heart disease.

THE ENERGY OF THE HEART

One of the apparent differences between Western orthodox medicine and Eastern or alternative medical philosophies is the notion of 'energy'. This idea is central to Chinese medicine and is also a key focus among the disciplines of complementary and alternative medicine (CAM). Orthodox medical practice generally dismisses energy as simply a concept and claims that acupuncture meridians, the energetic imprints of homeopathy and the subtle body of 'integral practice' [5] have no anatomical basis and therefore are not real in any sense.

Ironically, orthodox medicine tends to think that the energy in which it is interested is somehow different from the energy of Chinese medicine or CAM. In fact orthodox medicine has developed a number of highly sophisticated ways of measuring the energy patterns of a number of bodily systems. For example, the aforementioned ECG is a measure of the heart's electrical energy; the electroencephalogram or EEG is a measure of the brain's electrical energy; the electromyogram or EMG is a measure of a muscle's electrical energy.

In addition to electrical energy seen in an ECG the heart also produces electromagnetic and chemical energy, as well as sound waves and blood pressure waves. All these frequencies and forms of energy convey information [6]. The heart's sound energy can be measured using a sonogram or cardiac ultrasound. The force of the heart's contraction produces an energy wave that can be measured as blood pressure. More recent research has demonstrated that the heart actually produces chemical energy in the form of hormonal signals such as oxytocin [7]. Often known as the human *bonding hormone*, oxytocin was previously thought to be produced only in the brain. However, the heart also generates such signals and so may have a role to play in human bonding and helping individuals connect with each other. When the heart contracts it also sends a pulse of information along the artery walls in the form of a pressure wave. This wall distension wave is conducted to every bodily organ, and in a way resembles what is described as the flow of *qi* ('energy') around the body. This pulse pressure wave reveals important information about the health of the cardiovascular system.

There is evidence to suggest that the energy and information flow patterns of the heart may have an integrating effect on the energy patterns of all other systems. Recent research on complexity and emergence has revealed that clusters of oscillating energy sources, as generated by different bodily nerve networks, can synchronize when connected with each other. This phenomenon, called *entrainment*, was first described by the Dutch physicist and inventor of the pendulum clock, Christiaan Huygens (1629–1695) [8]. It is as though these systems are connecting with each other and harmonizing their functions. Thus the ECG and EEG may start to generate very similar waveforms. The biological and performance benefits of such coherence are yet to be fully explored.

Western medicine does indeed measure all sorts of subtle and gross energy patterns generated by the body and mind. For example, cerebral blood flow studies have identified specific areas in the brain that become active when we feel pleasure or fear or when we concentrate or meditate. Some studies have even suggested that energy patterns change when we experience God [9]. Similarly, a magnetic resonance imaging (MRI) scan can show changes in the electromagnetic energy fields of any body organ and so detecting these changes in the energy field can be a key weapon in the battle against cancer.

The Western scientific concepts involved in these findings are really not far from the Eastern notion of *qi* flowing around the body. While language and nomenclature may differ between East and West, between orthodox medicine and CAM, both are intimately concerned with understanding energy, energy flow and their contribution to health and disease.

HEART RATE VARIABILITY (HRV)

In addition to looking at the shape of the beat, the rhythm of the contractions and the sound of the heart, it is possible to study changes in the heart rate, or its *variability*. When the pulse is taken in orthodox medicine it is usually to determine the average heart rate (the number of beats per minute), often based on counting the number of beats felt in 15 seconds and multiplying by four. What is ignored in obtaining this average is the fact that the heart rate changes repeatedly during those 15 seconds. In fairness, though, it would be difficult to detect this variability just by feeling the pulse.

If you actually record the changes in someone's heart rate for 4 minutes you will see that it may fluctuate between 60 beats per minute (b.p.m.) and 120 b.p.m. So when you report the average heart rate you essentially ignore all this variability and the information it contains. Taking an 'average heart rate' is the equivalent of listening to a Chopin piano concerto and saying the average is 'F sharp'. Thus there is a massive loss of information in taking an average. In fact we now understand that the variation in the heart rate is critical and reveals vital information about your heart and your entire body.

The reason the heart rate varies over time is that the distance between one beat and the next is constantly changing (Fig. 24.2). Sometimes the beats are close together, in which case the heart is going fast, and sometimes the beats are further apart, in which case the heart rate is slower. So it is possible to calculate an individual's heart rate based on the distance between two beats. This perpetual change in the inter-beat interval is known as heart rate variability – or HRV for short.

So if your heart beats were 0.859 seconds apart for the rest of your entire life, your heart rate would be stuck at 70 b.p.m.; if the beats were 0.793 seconds apart the heart rate would be stuck at 76 b.p.m. However, if you look at anyone's heart rate over time, you can see that it is constantly varying.

The recording of the changes in someone's heart rate is called a 'tachogram'. This term literally means 'speed picture' – that is, a picture of how the speed of the heart rate changes over time. Such recordings or HRV traces can reveal considerable information about an individual's actions. For example, heart rate speeds up when a threat is perceived.

In Chapter 10, Chris Low emphasizes the role of *subtle* energy as 'information exchange'. In fact *all* energy provides information and HRV is a particularly powerful source as it reveals information about many aspects of an individual's health and vitality. Clearly a low level of variability yields less information than a high level of variability although a low level of HRV does suggest that the system is in a poor state and likely to break down.

An example of information generated from a simple tachogram is seen in Figure 24.3A. While this executive was in meetings his heart rate was fluctuating around 65 b.p.m. Then he left work and started walking quickly toward the train station. His heart rate leapt up almost immediately, reaching 105 b.p.m. before it started to fall as he reached the station.

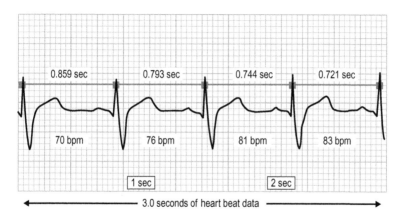

FIG 24.2 Variability in the inter-beat interval.

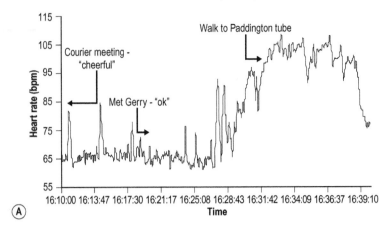

Heart rate (30 mins)

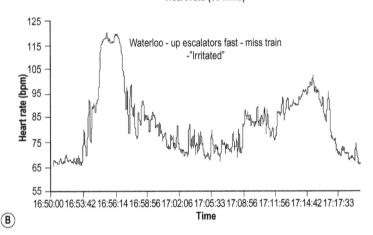

Heart rate (30 mins)

FIG 24.3 Changes in heart rate with increased activity and stress. Changes when someone: (A) starts walking fast, and (B) runs up an escalator and is under mental stress, having missed a train.

In the tachogram in Figure 24.3B are shown the effects on the heart rate when the executive runs up an escalator. Again the heart rate nearly doubles from a steady 65 b.p.m. to 120 b.p.m. before dropping back to a higher resting level of 75 b.p.m. But then something interesting happens. The executive realizes that he has missed his train. For the next 10 minutes his heart rate remains elevated, reaching up to 100 b.p.m. This rise in heart rate occurred while the executive was standing still. You would expect his heart rate to have continued to drop to his normal resting rate of 65 b.p.m. But his heart rate is racing at a speed that is akin to his walking fast again. Missing his train clearly has a direct biological effect, causing him to burn energy at a much higher rate than necessary for at least 10 minutes. This observation helps explain why people who have had a very difficult, but largely sedentary, day come home exhausted.

Watching an individual's tachograms during a normal working day reveals that, for most people, the normal pattern of HRV is far from a state of equilibrium.

In fact the normal pattern is a chaotic HRV trace all day. Changes in an individual's external environment, whether they are a therapist or a patient, result in almost instantaneous changes in their internal physiological environment. These internal changes – most of them unconscious – in HRV and other physiological signals result in different actions being taken and ultimately a change in the external environment. Thus there is a bidirectional interaction, with both internal and external environments affecting each other. Such interactivity may, as Chris Low suggests, be at the core of the therapeutic relationship.

WHY HRV IS IMPORTANT

HRV tachograms can reveal sudden changes in individuals' physiology of which they may or may not be aware. Although such analysis is useful it does not tell the whole story. It is now possible, in addition to just looking at HRV on a tachogram, to quantify the amount of variability in a number of ways. There are now some 15 000 scientific papers published that have looked at HRV and why it is important.

Why is HRV so important?
- It predicts death and illness.
- It reveals biological age.
- It quantifies energy levels.
- It alters brain function.

HRV PREDICTS DEATH AND ILLNESS

Dublin Hospital Obstetric Department has one of the lowest emergency cesarian section rates in the world (about 5%). As a result the infant mortality rate and the number of birth complications are amongst the lowest in the world. Why? The simple answer is that Dublin pioneered the 'active management of labor'. They could pretty much guarantee that once you entered the labor ward you would have a healthy baby in your hands within 12 hours. The John Radcliffe Hospital obstetric ward in Oxford, where I worked, followed their protocols carefully.

A key part of the active management of labor was continual monitoring of the baby's heart rate during labor. We looked at the baby's tachogram and were particularly interested in the baby's heart rate variability. If we started to see a loss in the amount of HRV we would then stay with the mum to be, watching the trace like a hawk. Sometimes this loss of variability was temporary and was simply due to the fact that the baby had fallen asleep despite being squeezed by regular muscular contractions every 4 minutes. If the HRV tachogram did not recover we would start to get concerned that the baby was in trouble. If this concern mounted we would consider more invasive measures and obtain a sample of the baby's blood from its scalp. We would test this blood to determine whether there was too much acid in the bloodstream, as indicated by a low pH level. A low blood pH would confirm that the baby was indeed in real danger and would trigger a rush to the operating theater and an emergency cesarian. Since 1965 it has become common obstetric practice around the world to watch a baby's HRV during labor for early signs of fetal distress, and to prevent death [10].

In 1978 Dr Graeme Sloman, an Australian physician, reported in the *Medical Journal of Australia* that HRV can also predict adult mortality after a heart attack [11]. He noticed that some heart attack victims had a degree of variability whereas others' hearts ticked like a metronome. Those with little HRV died right on the ward. None of the traditional risk factors such as age, cholesterol levels or smoking predicted the outcome. Since then there have been many studies demonstrating the ability of HRV to predict death from heart disease [12–14]. Some studies show that a combination of different HRV parameters is more predictive than is a single measure, and HRV analysis based on nonlinear dynamics may be even better at risk stratification [15,16].

The role of HRV in predicting death took another significant step in 1997 when Dekker and colleagues discovered that HRV predicts death, not only in babies or heart attack victims but also 'all cause mortality' [17]. In other words, HRV could predict the demise of anyone from any cause [17–19]. Why can HRV, a measure of cardiovascular flexibility, predict death from noncardiovascular disease? [18] The answer is that HRV is a measure of *overall* system flexibility. A loss of flexibility means a brittle system unable to adapt to physiological stress. Such a brittle system is likely to break.

Unfortunately, poor HRV cannot be fixed with a pill. It is, however, possible to improve the HRV with lifestyle changes (see below).

BIOLOGICAL AGE

In addition to predicting illness and mortality, HRV can tell you about your energy and dynamism. HRV can in fact be used as a measure of biological age – that is, the actual age of your body rather than your chronological age in years [20]. The general rule is that HRV declines each year by approximately 3% from about the age of 30 until you have no more variability. So if your HRV is assessed for 24 hours it is possible to tell roughly how old you are to within about 1 year, based on the decline in your heart rate variability. When you reach the point of zero variability, your system becomes brittle and likely to break. The decline in HRV over time can be seen as similar to reports of how *qi* declines with age.

The good news is that HRV can increase with the right kind of lifestyle adjustments. For example, exercise [21], omega-3 intake [22], emotional self-management [23], breathing practices [24,25], *yoga* [26] and *qigong* [27,28] have all been shown to improve HRV. In fact HRV is increasingly being used as a methodological tool to test the biological effects of a wide variety of therapeutic interventions such as acupuncture [29]. In one acupuncture study the increase in parasympathetic tone in the autonomic nervous system, which is often thought to be indicative of relaxation, was correlated with increased activity in various regions of the brainstem involved in memory and emotion processing [30]. However, not all studies have been so well controlled. Some have used HRV inappropriately in an attempt to validate less scientifically tested approaches such as thought field therapy (TFT) [31](see Ch. 18).

The examples shown in Chapter 10 (see Fig. 10.1) illustrate the difference in HRV amplitude with normal aging in two individuals with a 58-year age difference. Clearly, the 80-year-old has much smaller HRV amplitude compared with that of the 22-year-old.

TIME MANAGEMENT OR ENERGY MANAGEMENT?

Most people working today live hectic lives. They often complain that they never have enough time and are 'time poor'. Many companies even run 'time management' courses in an attempt to help their employees with this affliction. But it is not possible to 'manage' time. Time does not change and is not amenable to management. In fact it is not even the problem.

The real issue is energy [32]. If you are overworked, overwhelmed and exhausted, then giving you more time to complete a task will not help you. You simply do not have the energy to get it done. Conversely, if you have boundless energy you can get through large volumes of work in double quick time. So time and energy are intimately related [1] – but the key is energy, not time. Companies would be better placed running energy management courses, not time management courses. Again this is very similar to the concept of *qi* and loss of *qi*.

Companies need people, and particularly leaders, with fantastic energy reserves, great dynamism and an ability to renew their energy levels easily, but how do you know whether your energy levels are above average or below average? How do you know if you have a full tank or are running on empty? You may have a vague subjective sense of your own energy levels and vitality, but how accurate is your assessment really?

An ambulatory 24-hour HRV assessment can objectively quantify your energy levels. In fact HRV can be used to determine who has the energy to keep going all day responding to job demands and who is likely to run out of steam at lunchtime.

In the early stages of exhaustion there is often an excessive increase in epinephrine levels and an increased activation of the sympathetic nervous system (SNS). This state can go hand in hand with agitation and hypervigilance, and is often the picture seen in individuals with chronic fatigue [33]. Such excessive arousal can ultimately lead to sympathetic exhaustion. Thus people under excessive stress who are constantly pumping epinephrine into their system as they fight or flee from pressure will often exhaust their adrenal glands' ability to produce sufficient epinephrine to cope with the demand. The degree of exhaustion of the SNS can be quantified using HRV analysis.

Furthermore HRV analysis can be used to determine whether a low level of energy in the SNS is matched by a similarly low level of energy or vitality in the counterbalancing parasympathetic nervous system (PNS). Obviously exhaustion of the PNS as well as the SNS/adrenals is of more concern than just SNS exhaustion. Fortunately, appropriate intervention can help improve energy levels. For example, we have been able to demonstrate an average 30% increase in PNS and SNS energy within 6 months with a tailored coaching program (A D Watkins, in preparation).

Crocodiles and wildebeests

The value of HRV in quantifying levels of energy and dynamism is easily seen if you compare mammals and reptiles and their ability to respond to a threat or rise to a challenge. Reptiles, because they are cold blooded, do not have much HRV. They can lower their heart rate, but they cannot do it quickly. In contrast, all warm-blooded mammals have a lot of variability. In fact, it is what helps make them responsive and dynamic.

So if you watch a deer in the forest, with its ears up it responds to every single noise and potential threat. It is finely attuned to its environment. In contrast, a reptile is not that dynamic. So when mammals meet reptiles you see a clear difference in their dynamism and energy.

A good example is when a crocodile attacks a wildebeest. The crocodile sneaks up on the wildebeest like a stealth machine. It floats like a log in the water, with a heart barely ticking at four beats per minute. When the crocodile gets to within a foot of the wildebeest, it stops. You may wonder why. What is the crocodile doing? Why doesn't it just grab the wildebeest, only a couple of feet away? The answer is that it can't because its heart is beating too slowly. It simply does not have the energy just to jump out of the water. So it makes no move while it gradually pumps up its heart rate until it has sufficient energy to leap out of the water and lunge at the wildebeest.

By comparison the wildebeest is very responsive, within one heart beat. As soon as it sees, out of the corner of its eye, that something is lunging out of the water, its heart rate shoots up and the wildebeest jumps backwards.

If the crocodile's lunge fails to grasp the wildebeest, it will back down into the water and wait. It needs to gather energy for a second attack. What it will not do is chase the wildebeest up the bank. With little HRV, it cannot change its heart rate quickly enough. The crocodile is biologically constrained and reptiles have slowly, over centuries, yielded much terrain to more rapidly adaptable mammals.

Humans may be seen on a continuum between the mammalian wildebeest and the reptilian crocodile. Some people may seem a bit more reptilian, with little dynamism, while others appear highly reactive or sensitive with plenty of HRV.

Thus it is possible to use the 'variability' of the heart's electrical signal to quantify the 'vitality' of the human system. HRV could be considered a way to measure our ability to respond flexibly to our environment, our aliveness, or in other terms 'vital energy'.

THE DIY LOBOTOMY

HRV, in addition to predicting health and being able to quantify energy levels, can tell us something about brain function. In fact HRV can affect the ability to think clearly.

At rest, most people's HRV pattern is relatively chaotic, fluctuating between 60 and 100 b.p.m., meaning the heart basically sends the brain an erratic signal. When someone is put under pressure, the signal becomes even more erratic and starts to fluctuate wildly. It looks like a 'mini-earthquake' (Fig. 24.4). One of the reasons that people stop thinking clearly when they are put under pressure is that their frontal lobes stop working properly. Stress causes a 'DIY lobotomy'. This process, in which the frontal cortex is inhibited, is called *cortical inhibition*. It is the reason why smart people do stupid things.

This functional lobotomy is why some people go blank in an exam; it underpins stage fright and is at the core of much human error. Many TV programs are built around the phenomenon. Under the glare of the studio lights many people's physiology becomes chaotic, brain function is inhibited and they blurt out silly answers that make everyone laugh. The quality of an individual's physiology when under pressure can determine the quality of their answers when being interviewed by the media. In fact an individual's ability even to understand the questions being asked of them can be impaired by their chaotic physiology.

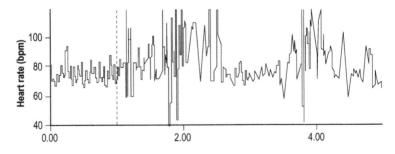

FIG 24.4 Chaotic HRV signal sent to the brain.

Similarly, if you approach children in a classroom and put them under pressure by asking them a question you will often flip their physiology into chaos and shut their brain down. They will then be unable to answer the question even if they really know the answer.

What causes the physiology to become chaotic is the perception of threat. Whenever any of us perceive that we are under threat, or feel overwhelmed or even mildly stressed, we will often inhibit our own frontal cortex. For example, a man in a meeting with his boss may find himself saying irrelevant or even stupid things that he had not planned to say. If his frontal lobes are completely inhibited he may not be aware his performance is way off the mark. Our brain can be so inhibited and perception so impaired that we do not even realize that we have underperformed. In this example, the man may come out of the meeting thinking he did well when he actually did very badly.

Such brain shutdown is an inevitable consequence of being put under pressure.

Frontal lobe shutdown

Shutting down the frontal cortex impairs a whole variety of different brain functions. Impaired brain function is often seen in individuals who have suffered frontal lobe damage as a result of traumatic brain injury. Individuals with post-traumatic stress disorder (PTSD) have similar problems [34]. In fact one recent study demonstrated that HRV could be used to determine the degree of impairment in individuals with PTSD and another suggested that HRV biofeedback could be used to improve physiological and psychological health in individuals with PTSD [35,36].

Individuals with frontal lobe impairment find it extremely difficult to plan, organize and sort information. They are unable to stick to time lines and find it very difficult to sequence tasks correctly. They can behave inappropriately, are often excessively aggressive and can be antisocial. They tend to take much greater risks and have a disregard for safety. They also find it very difficult to concentrate and their ability to shift their attention is impaired, leading them to get stuck on the first answer they come up with. Frontal lobe impairment also adversely affects working memory and the ability to learn.

The frontal lobe impairment that occurs transiently when chaotic HRV signals are sent to the brain is not an all-or-nothing phenomenon. The frontal lobes can be partially impaired. However, most people are experiencing some degree of frontal lobe inhibition most of the time. In other words, everyone is trying to perform with partially impaired frontal lobes, although most of us tend to think that our own function is fine most of the time. We often believe that the

Frontal lobe impairment
- Planning and organization are severely impaired.
- Individuals are unable to inhibit their responses.
- Individuals take much greater risks.
- Individuals exhibit more aggressive, inappropriate and antisocial behavior.
- Timelines and sequencing are disrupted.
- Attention shifting is impaired leading to perseveration on faulty answers.
- Working memory is impaired.

problems we experience are attributable to someone else's impaired performance, and that it is their responsibility to fix a situation rather than recognizing our own contribution and taking responsibility for improving matters.

Binary thinking

Why are we humans permanently on the edge of shutdown? The answer to this question, as with so many questions about why human beings operate in a certain way, is 'survival advantage'. Hundreds of thousands of years ago, when human ancestors became bipedal and started to walk upright, survival was the only imperative. Physiological processes and responses that promoted survival persisted over time whereas those that did not were lost. So the ability to shut your own brain down used to confer an advantage under the simple survival scenario. Imagine for example that you are wandering across the North American plains some time after the last ice age. A bear appears from behind a thicket, sees you, and immediately considers you to be fair game.

Right at that moment you do not need sophisticated thinking. In fact, if you stand still and try to be clever, pondering whether you are looking at a North American black bear or a grizzly bear, whether the bear looks hungry or is able to run fast, then the chances are that the bear will eat you. What is required, at that moment, is for you to shut down all complex thought processes and for your thinking to become binary. Your brain creates just two binary options for you; fight/flight or play dead. So brain shutdown saved your life.

Unfortunately, survival in the modern world requires the exact opposite response. When you are under pressure from your boss, a client or even the media, you absolutely need your smart thinking. What you do *not* want to do is become very aggressive (fight response), and you are unlikely to be able to run away by changing the subject or avoid the issue (flight response); nor can you look like a startled rabbit or a deer caught in the headlights (play dead). Such unfortunate binary brain function can now have career-limiting consequences.

So today we are operating with software in our brains from 200 000 years ago and we have never had an upgrade. Frontal lobe impairment no longer has survival advantages. Most of the time this physiological phenomenon largely just impairs performance.

CARDIAC COHERENCE

As the pressures of modern life increase, our ability to respond (our 'response-ability') to the demands we face is a key to our success. With a brain that is shut down by the simplest of threats our chances of performing at our best are easily impaired. Thus one of our primary tasks in the modern world is to take response-ability and learn to manage our responses to the demands we face better, so limiting frontal lobe shutdown.

Fortunately, challenge and threat do not have to lead to the chaotic HRV signals that cause a functional 'lobotomy'. The human system has evolved a mechanism for *enhancing* brain function that also involves HRV. Individuals can learn to generate a very different type of HRV signal when they are under pressure. Rather than it fluctuating wildly in a chaotic way, the electrical input to the brain can be varied in a much more stable and orderly fashion. Such a harmonious signal is known as *cardiac coherence*.

Cardiac coherence means that the heart rate still varies, but in a much more stable and orderly fashion. For example, it may vary between 60 and 80 b.p.m. in a consistent repeating pattern with the distance between the heart rate peaks or troughs remaining constant. This stable pattern gives rise to the classic

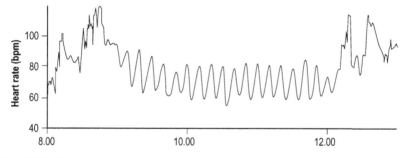

FIG 24.5 Moving from chaos to coherence.

'sinusoidal curve' (Fig, 24.5). There remains variability but it becomes predictable and rhythmic compared with the unpredictable erratic variability seen in a chaotic heart rate pattern.

It appears, from our own studies conducted over the last 14 years [37] (A D Watkins, in preparation, 2010), that such coherence enhances brain function and enables the frontal lobes. Learning how to switch physiology from chaos to coherence can help move from a lobotomized position to one where smart thinking is enabled.

CONCLUSION

The *degree* of HRV reflects youth, vitality and can predict a healthy long life, whereas the *pattern* of HRV can determine the quality of brain function at any one moment.

HRV provides useful objective measures of vitality, predictors of mortality and illness, and has repeatedly been shown to improve a wide variety of medical conditions. HRV feedback, for example, has been shown to improve HRV and symptomatology in depression [38,39], fibromyalgia [40], heart disease [41] and asthma [42], as well as reducing blood pressure [43,44], improving quality of life [45] and even enhancing physical (dance) performance [46].

Much remains to be explored, but initial evidence suggests that understanding the energetic interplay between different bodily systems, and the heart energy in particular, may contribute significantly to improving health and quality of life.

The electrical heart: energy in cardiac health and disease

SECTION 6
CONCLUSION

Themes of *qi* and a dozen definitions: content analysis and discussion

David Mayor • Marc S Micozzi

CHAPTER CONTENTS

> ❝ *Practitioners of most alternative healing believe that one source of their intervention is a type of 'vital energy' used by their system and still not appreciated by conventional biomedical science.*
> Ted Kaptchuk [1]

SOME QUESTIONS AND RESULTS

Qi is not just one thing, and in fact is not a 'thing' at all. Rather like a Rorschach inkblot, it is interpretable in many ways. Is there in fact a core of such interpretations that unites the chapters in this book? Do the authors share a consensus view of *qi*, or only major differences of opinion? Have some aspects of energy medicine not been addressed, or even been missed or avoided? How does this book indicate possible areas for further investigation?

To make a start in answering these questions, one of the editors (David Mayor, DM) compiled a wide-ranging checklist of 98 keywords used by contributors as in some way potentially relevant to *qi*, and counted in how many chapters out of a possible 23 these words appeared (Table 25.1). Ideally, at least two readers should have reviewed the material independently and then created a consolidated checklist [2], but time constraints did not permit this.

Table 25.1   *Keywords appearing in six or more chapters (scores 6–7, 8–9, 10–22)*

Top 10 (score 10–22)	Score	Next 12 (score 8–9)	Score	Next 9 (score 6–7)	Score
Flow	22	Electric or other measurement	9	Heat	7
Energy	19	Life	9	Quantum	7
Life force/vital force	19	Emotional state	8	Resonance	7
Balance/ homeosta*	18	Information	8	Biophotons	6
Breath	13	Spine/*kundalini*	8	Circulation	6
Pathways	13	*Chakras*/centers	8	Electromagnetic	6
Block	13	Dynamic	8	Frequency	6
Yinyang	13	Emptiness	8	Spirit	6
Hands	11	Energy field	8	(W)hole	6
Movement	10	Interaction	8		
		Transforming *qi*	8		
		Awareness	8		

The search term 'homeosta' was used to include both 'homeostatic' and 'homeostasis'

Keywords scoring 1 to 5

   5. bioenergy; food; intention; matrix; network; pattern; process (vs. structure); self-organization; substance; subtle energy; wind
   4. coherence; connective tissue; feedback; force; holography; inscape; nonlocal; particle vs. wave; all-permeating; terrestrial (vs. celestial); transformative
   3. bridge (e.g. between physical/nonphysical); celestial (vs. terrestrial); cloud/vapor; consciousness; crystal; force field; *li* vs./& *qi*; pathogenic factor *qi*; structure (vs. process); synchronicity; universal; vibration
   2. chaos; complex systems; constant flux [flow]; correspondence between body/state/cosmos; electric metaphor; embodied; HRV; innate intelligence; microcurrent; pervades body; sexuality; shapes body; vitality; water; X-signal

1. atmosphere; biofield; embryogenesis; fertility; finest matter; fractal; influence; liminal; root/branch; shapes universe; synergy; vibe.

Notes: Numbers may not be precise, for several reasons: (1) searching was conducted manually rather than electronically and some keywords may have been missed, (2) sometimes different words were interpreted as synonyms, (3) some terms were used with different meanings in different contexts, and (4) scores were not verified by a second person. In addition, no account was taken consciously of how often a keyword occurs in each individual chapter.

Chapter 3 was excluded from this analysis, as it was written after these data were gathered and already includes some discussion of the incidence of terms used.

DISCUSSION

AREAS OF RELATIVE CONSENSUS – THE 'TOP TEN' AND RELATED TERMS

(Scores are shown in parentheses)

'Flow' (22), 'pathways (13), 'circulation' (6) and 'block' (13)

❝ *The blockage or impeded flow of* qi *is fundamental to every disease.*
Kevin V Ergil 2009 [3]

❝ *Those who are used to taking note of their own bodily sensations will certainly be able to sense the streamings which go through the whole body. With a full and deep breathing these wave-like movements give a feeling of being alive through and through. Those who have relaxed bodies and unclouded minds have these sensations as the regular and permanent background to all that they experience, and it is this which gives colour, taste, and freshness to their whole life.*
Ola Raknes (1887–1975) [4]

Not surprisingly, given that it was DM's interest in 'flow' that led him to coedit this book, this term appeared in nearly all chapters, so gave the highest score. However, this finding is not just a matter of editor bias: as mentioned in Chapters 3 and 13, 'flow' is definitely associated with the holistic, New Age (NA), feminist, processual and other discourses in which *qi* has found a place. (Incidentally, DM did not recruit the author of Ch. 13, and neither editor knew the content of her chapter prior to submission.)

Very much in keeping with the reductionist/processual polarity described in some detail in Chapter 13 and mentioned in Chapters 4 and 8 [5], the French philosopher Henri Bergson (1859–1841) noted that movement is inwardly experienced as continuous flow but mentally divisible into a juxtaposition of successive points, and so distinguished between 'intuition' (for which movement is reality) and 'intelligence' (based on immobility) [6]. Even our concept of *time* as flowing may arise from the 'nonlinguistic eidetic intuition' of spontaneous bodily self-movement [7] (the 'flow of kinesthesis' of the philosopher Edmund Husserl (1859–1938) [8]).

It is interesting that 'flow' occurs more frequently than its hypothesized 'pathways' and similar terms, while the even more sophisticated concept 'circulation' (Ch. 3) was used much less frequently, as was the more philosophical 'constant flux' (2). 'Block' and other terms indicating a disturbance of flow are still in the top ten, but not as common as 'flow'. This could be due partly to fewer chapters that were focused on disease and the pathologies of *qi* (in which context 'keeping the channels open' is important even from a biomedical perspective [9] – a high proportion of the causes of death involve a blockage and lack of flow of some sort).

Chapter 2 provides a stark reminder that pathological blocks to flow can have devastating and wide-ranging repercussions, not just in individual patients but throughout a community or nation. (Somewhat similar if less violently politicized accounts of flow and blockage occur in Papua New Guinea [10], while the image of flow and blockage in pathways within the body is commonly used by other African peoples, such as the Songhay of Niger [11] and the Yaka of Zaire [12].) A very African image of flow (of rain, of 'potency') occurs frequently in the rock art of the indigenous San people (Fig. 25.1).

'Energy' (19)

❝ *It is generally believed that* ki *itself is a form of energy.*
Kouzo Kaku [19, p 5]

❝ *The significance of energy comes close to being* hard orthodoxy *within the holistic milieu.*
Christopher Partridge [20]

Again, given the title of this book, it was to be expected that 'energy' would score highly, and many of the practitioner–contributors would happily consider *qi* and energy in the same breath, just as the character for *qi* is used in the terms for energy ('*qi* force', 氣力) in modern Chinese (*qili*) and Japanese (*kiryoku*). It is salutory though that some of the more academic authors (e.g. Chs 8, 12) warn about too glibly equating *qi* and energy.

Thus, although 'energy' is a frequently used (and now probably inescapable) word in any discussion of *qi*-related practices (and so will, in a perverse sense, always be 'conserved'), it is problematic. As with *qi* itself, its use by no means implies agreement as to what it actually means.

CONCLUSION

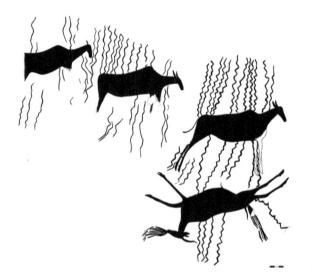

FIG 25.1 San rock art painting of eland, Bethlehem, South Africa. Zigzag pattern represents flow, and has been interpreted as rain [13] or as an entoptic phenomenon, the 'potency' that can be seen only by people in trance [14], specifically by shamans [15]. Such wavy power lines are also found in North American rock paintings [16] and shamanic artifacts [17]. They may mark 'events of tension' or liminality [18]. One San informant said 'if a "good" person placed his or her hand on a painting of an eland, power would flow from the image into the person' [15, p 105]. *(Reprinted with kind permission of the Rock Art Research Institute/SARADA, University of the Witwatersrand.)*

Qi is not 'energy'

Aristotle (384–322 BCE) first used the term 'energy' (*energeia*, ενεργεια) in the sense of 'being-at-work' [21]. In Newtonian mechanics, such a concept would relate more closely to 'force', or even 'work' itself (defined as 'force × distance'). The chemist-cum-physician Georg Ernst Stahl (1660–1734), a key figure in the history of scientific vitalism, used *energia*, but 'energy' in its modern sense came into general use in science only in the mid nineteenth century, as a more precise yet also more abstract substitute for the ambiguous term 'force' [22,23]. Energy so considered became 'the philosophical core of scientific materialism' [24], although in popular usage it has many other meanings [25].

In the late 1920s, despite the qualms of colleagues [26], George Soulié de Morant (1878–1955) translated '*qi*' as 'energy' 'for want of anything better' [27], influenced by the WW I era *élan vital* propounded by Henri Bergson [28]. Although many contemporary acupuncturists often use the word 'energy' and talk of 'vital energy' [29] or of 'energy circulating' through meridians [30], *qi* itself is neither 'substance'/'matter' nor 'energy' [31,32]. '*Qi* = energy is an equation that does not compute' [33, p 105]. The translation of *qi* as 'matter-energy' is also inexact [34], except for a handful of texts written since the eleventh century [35].

'Balance'/'homeostasis'/'homeodynamis' (18), and *yinyang* (13)

A score of 18 was higher than expected although, given the similarities between some interpretations of *qi* and humoral medicine [36] (see Chs 1 and 2), it is not altogether surprising. Homeostatic balance is emphasized in Chapter 22, for example. An association of 'balance' with *qi* would in part explain the score of 13 for *yinyang* (see Fig. 20.1).

'Life force'/'vital force' (19) or 'life' (9)

It is self-evident that terms such as 'life force' or 'vital force' would appear frequently – even if, to be accurate, only *sheng qi* ('living *qi*', 生氣) corresponds to 'life force', and then only loosely [37].

'Breath' (13), 'wind' (5), ['cloud'/'vapor' (3)], and 'heat' (7)

Worldwide, in prehistoric art and also more recent indigenous rock art, it has been suggested that the life-breath is the most frequently depicted form of the life-force [38]. It is well known that *qi* is traditionally associated with breath and wind, with a possible progression from 'wind' as a spirit entity to *qi* as 'vapors' by the time of the *Nanjing* [39] (see too the discussion of the breath-soul in Ch. 3). More startling – even breathtaking – is the biomedical interpretation of *qi* as 'homologous to oxygen' in Chapter 11. The association of warmth with life and its distillation/respiration processes [40] is also common. In acupuncture, a central role is played by the Fire of the Gate of Life (*mingmen*, 命門) in the lower abdomen [41], which is also closely related to the Kidney *zang* (associated with Water). Thus *mingmen* is where Fire and Water interact to produce the 'steam' or 'vapor' of *qi*; it is also where *jing* is stored within the body [35] (the storage of vital principle within the kidneys is found in Australia as well [42]). There are also many references in the subtle physiology literature of *daoyin*/*neigong* and yoga to methods of generating or conserving internal heat [43,44]. On another level, the warmth of close contact with others may be important for both life and health [45].

However, in terms of the 'elemental' associations of Air, Fire and Water (flow), hydraulic descriptions of qi in this book are well ahead of the pneumatic or thermal, while Earth, in the shape of 'substance' (5), or the physical body, trails even further behind. This finding relates to the terms next listed.

'Movement' (10), 'dynamic' (8)

> If we exclude the motion of the universe, living creatures are responsible for the motion of everything else, except such things as are moved by each other through striking against each other.
>
> Aristotle [46]

> Names *cannot do justice to dynamics.*
>
> Maxine Sheets-Johnstone [47]

It goes without saying that qi is dynamic, moving [48], as indeed is everything in the universe of modern science. In particular, the Heisenberg uncertainty principle states that one cannot precisely determine position and momentum of subatomic particles at the same time, giving an evanescent quality to the entire nature of reality and the universe in the quantum mechanical world. Like his fellow British physicist James Jeans (see Ch. 12), Arthur Eddington (1882–1944), who provided the first experimental observations confirming Einstein's general theory of relativity in 1919, stated that ultimately 'the stuff of the world is mind-stuff' and 'we live in an idea-like world, not a matter-like world' [49]. Thus, according to these eminent scientists, we live in a field of consciousness rather than a material universe – an idea espoused by an increasing number of leading-edge physicists [50] and philosophers [51]. Coeditor Marc Micozzi has pursued the relations among the ideas of qi, *prana* and spirit in traditional Indian, Tibetan, and Middle Eastern (Middle Asian) medicine and finds connections to twentieth-century views of the universe (relativity, quantum mechanics and superstring theories) under the 'Copenhagen interpretation' (encompassing wave–particle complementarity and the uncertainty principle). According to this view, the reality of the 'vital forces' or 'energies' of these ancient Asian healing traditions ultimately appears to lie in a mind–body–spirit connection to what can be considered as a 'universal consciousness' [52].

'Hands' (11)

Although the hands are inevitably the main parts of the body used in most forms of energy medicine, this high score was not foreseen. Yet 'the hands feel it' [53] in healing, 'it' usually being sensations of warmth or tingling [54–56] (A Morris, unpublished study, 2007) that are then interpreted as indicating the presence of qi or energy (as in *qigong*, for example [57]), though sometimes as denoting a 'blockage' [58]. So, for example, in contactful acupuncture such as *tōyōhari* (東洋鍼), 'our touch must be soft, water-like and most of all, receptive. Our hands must soften and melt to receive the qi' [59]. Handprints are indeed possibly the earliest and one of the most common motifs in indigenous rock art, whether in North America, Europe [16], Africa or Australia, where they have been interpreted as images (or even reservoirs) of potency [13], places where other hands can 'reach into the spiritual realm behind the membrane of rock' [60] (Fig. 25.2).

In this context, it is interesting to note that in the homunculus representation of the sensory cortex, the neurological mapping of the hand (i.e. representing conscious sensation) occupies an area second only in its size to that of the face. It is through both that we connect and communicate with the world about us.

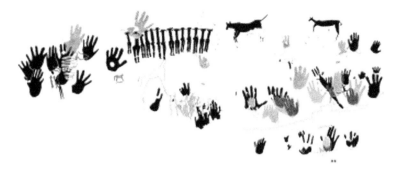

FIG 25.2 San rock art handprints, Waterberg district, South Africa. Handprints have been interpreted as images, or even reservoirs, of potency (as in the 'negative' Upper Paleolithic handprints created by blowing paint around the hand onto the rock, breathing life into it) [61], or simply the exuberant slap-dash of adolescent hunters. Compare Figures 5.1, 12.2 and 17.5. *(Reprinted with kind permission of the Rock Art Research Institute/SARADA, University of the Witwatersrand.)*

THE MIDDLE GROUND: SOME SELECTED TOPICS

'Emotional state' (8)

Emotions ('e-motions') are often described in terms of movement [47,62], the expression of an embodied 'flow of feeling', 'flow of energy' ('bodily energy can be envisioned as a stream of feeling' [63, p 440]), or even 'as the flow of *ki*' [64, p 111]. Thus, in both Chinese and Japanese, *qi* (or *ki*) is frequently a component of words describing states of emotion [32]. For William James writing in 1884, 'the perception of bodily changes as they occur' *was* the emotion itself [65]. More recently, for Christian de Quincey, emotion is 'a form of knowing that arises from paying deeper and more sensitive attention to messages from my body as it interacts with the world around me' [66, p 145]. Even from this single perspective, there seem to be associations among energy, flow, feeling, emotion and awareness (see below). In the words of one body psychotherapist: 'Flow is related to the freedom or restriction of breath, energy and the life force. (If you close your eyes and become receptive to the felt sense of emotion in the body, you will experience the quality of flow.)' [67]

'Spine'/'*kundalini*' (8) and '*chakras*'/'centers' (8)

❝ *Energy may be experienced as originating from below and moving up the body axis, originating above and moving down the axis, or both.*
Charles D Laughlin, Jr [43, p 113]

The experience of *kundalini* involves 'energy-like sensations usually starting at the base of the spine and then progressing rapidly with a powerful surge upwards through the body to the crown of the head', with other sensations (heat, tingling, pain, electric shock) that are similar to those experienced during panic attacks [68] and also during some forms of healing. These sensations are comparable to those experienced by participants in the San *!kia* (trance) dance (see Fig. 3.1B).

The term *kundalini* dates back to the tenth century CE, whereas the *chakras* were first discussed in the eighth century CE, when only four were considered, corresponding to different geographical sites. Since then, the system has continued to evolve, with each school of yoga creating its own [69]. The cosmophysiology of the seventeenth century Vaiṣṇava Sahajiyā' school, for example, was primarily based on metaphors of fluid and substance, in contrast to the more usual yoga metaphors of energy, sound and light [70]. One modern encyclopedia even defines *chakras* crudely as 'flywheels controlling the body's machinery' [71]. In a more sensitive interpretation, in keeping with the distinction between the transcendent/transfigurational aspirations of yoga and the Daoist preoccupation with prolonging the life of the material body (both based to a great extent on subtle physiologies derived from contemplative and embodied experience [72]), Richard Gerber has written about the *chakras* as 'emotional- and spiritual-energy transformers' (and so distinct from the 'life-energy' meridian system) [73]. C G Jung, for whom energy (as opposed to force) 'does not exist' except as an abstraction, considered the *chakras* as symbolic of psychic facts [74] – an approach also taken by some more recent commentators [75,76].

Others have taken a more embodied approach and noted the correspondence between the central axis of the body with its *chakras* and the seven 'segments' in which Wilhelm Reich observed chronic muscular armoring ('blocks') that could develop as a result of trauma – acting as a defense against the breakthrough of emotion and the upward movement of energy from the pelvis and belly (see Table 4.1) [77,78]. The loosening of such armor allowed the flow of what Reich called 'vegetative currents', with 'peculiar body sensations ... [such as] involuntary trembling and twitching of the muscles, sensations of cold and hot. Itching, the feeling of sitting on pins and needles, prickling sensations, the feeling of having the jitters, and somatic perceptions of anxiety, anger, and pleasure' [62, p 111]. Although it is arguable whether such sensations and emotions are a concomitant of the free flow of energy or arise from the conflict between flow and block, the parallels with *kundalini* are striking.

'Interaction' (8) [and 'feedback' (4)]

Practitioner–patient interaction and feedback can be important. Repeated feedback loops (for instance, as with pulse taking in acupuncture, Ch. 13) can reinforce inner awareness for both patient and practitioner. Interaction is a particular theme in Chapters 10 and 16.

A related term (not scored) is 'connection', another key to understanding energy medicine and *qi* in the sense of connecting different parts within the body, and the individual to others in the community, as well as more widely to nature and the cosmos (Chs 3 and 4).

'Awareness' (8)

❝ *Do not listen outwardly with your ears, nor even with your heart or mind, but with your essential qi and its open receptivity to all things.*
Zhuangzi Chapter 4 Pt II [79]

Such a primordial awareness of permeability is basic to an appreciation of *qi*, and very different from the reasoning, analytical focus of mind and words, which can in fact obscure it [80]. In some ways it is similar to the pleasurable esthetic experience of just allowing what appears to appear [81]. *Yi* (意), a word with many meanings, usually translated in acupuncture texts as 'intention', has also been defined as the 'power of awareness' [82], and *qi* itself as 'nothing else than my bodily awareness of being alive' [83]. The 'subjective turn' ('subjective-life', Ch. 3), interiority, or inner ('autocentric' [84], or even better 'interoceptive' [43]) awareness of *qi* is emphasized in many energy medicine trainings, and is important in practices ranging from *qigong* [85] and meditation [86] to Zero Balancing (Ch. 14), acupuncture (Chs 13, 15) and homeopathy [87]. Such awareness can therefore presumably be *increased* through careful training. It also clearly differentiates these CAM practices from the objectivizing perspective of conventional medicine, or even 'integrative' medicine when this approach incorporates/appropriates the outward forms (techniques) of CAM without its 'soul' (traditional theory and spirit).

A related term (not frequently used in this book) would be 'mindfulness' [88], or even 'bodyfulness' [89]. Practices such as quiet meditation increase awareness of body sensations [90], and as one writer on the Tibetan practice of *dumo* (*gTummo*) has put it in describing the healing or untangling of 'energy blocks': 'The experience of a greater flow of energy in the body/sensorium seems to be an inevitable consequence of the exercise of sustained concentration' [43, p 111]). This perspective is echoed in the 'breath work' of Ilse Middendorf (1910–2009), who found that simply by being present, aware of, and connecting with her breath, she could feel a sense of wellbeing 'streaming' throughout her body and her whole being, so that through the breath a source of healing and balance might be accessed (J Roffler, unpublished work, 2009).

More metaphorically, 'like the ice breaking free in a spring thaw, cumulative stresses seem to melt under this paradoxical attention, restoring natural flow to the bodymind whirlpool' [91]. Such an unthawing, associated with the freeing up of emotion (as described above), was for Reich an expression of the attempt by the orgone energy within the living organism to 'comprehend itself … [in] self-awareness'. For him, the function of this self-awareness was 'the greatest riddle of life' [62, p 517].

'Resonance' (7), 'frequency' (6), ['vibration' (3)]

❝ *Nature herself is perpetually rhythmic.*
Owen Barfield (1898–1997) [92]

❝ *If* ki *is a function of life, then rhythm may be an important element of* ki.
S Tsuyoshi Ohnishi and Tomoko Ohnishi [93]

It is indeed fascinating how often writers on 'subtle energy' use the above terms, even if only metaphorically (as in 'emotional resonance' or 'on the same wavelength'). Frequency in a more measurable sense is the topic of Chapter 9.

Oscillation and frequency are also implicit in the close association of *qi* with *yin-yang* (see Fig. 4.1). 'Pulsation' has been emphasized in the writings of Reich ('it is the task of orgone therapy to reestablish the full capacity for pulsation' [62, p 147]) and Stanley Keleman ('the whole organism is … a series of peristaltic tubes, pulsating with different intensities and amplitudes' [94]). In one survey of the phenomena of *qi* experienced by five practitioners of different forms of energy medicine (A Morris, unpublished study, 2007), all used the word 'vibration' to describe something of what they felt (compare the shivers, shudders and tinglings of Table 3.6).

AREAS OF RELATIVE DISAGREEMENT

The 98 keywords with which we began can be categorized as in Table 25.2. Here 'embodied experience' refers to experience *within*, or while being aware of, the body (rather than, for example, thinking *about* the body), whereas terms of 'objectivity or physical theory' will be those more familiar to those accustomed to the language of scientific discussion. 'Philosophical' terms are those that would be used in a more general, even metaphysical discourse, while 'contemporary terms about the body' are those used in contrast by writers such as James L Oschman in his books on energy medicine [95,96]. 'Polarities and boundaries' is a catch-all category to include a number of suggested dichotomies within this book, together with the image of bridging or moving between levels or states of awareness or experience.

Table 25.2 *Keywords analyzed by type*

A. Terms of embodied experience	B. Terms of objectivity or physical theory	C. General terms applicable to A or B
Breath (13)	Energy (19)	Flow (22) & block (13)
Pathways (13)	Electric or other measurement (9)	Life force (19)
Hands (11)	Information (8)	Balance (18)
Emotional state (8)	Energy field (8)	*Yinyang* (13)
Spine/kundalini (8)	Quantum (7)	Movement (10)
Chakras/centers (8)	Biophotons (6)	Life (9)
Transforming *qi* (8)	Electromagnetic (6)	Dynamic (8)
Awareness (8)	Frequency (6)	Interaction (8)
Heat (7)	Self-organization (5)	Resonance (7)
Circulation (6)	Substance (5)	(W)hole (6)
Spirit (6)	Coherence (4)	Food (5)
Intention (5)	Force (4)	Subtle energy (5)
Inscape (4)	Holography (4)	Pattern (5)
Transformative (4)	Nonlocal (4)	Wind (5)
Consciousness (3)	Force field (3)	Feedback (4)
Embodied (2)	Vibration (3)	Cloud/vapor (3)
Pervades body (2)	Chaos (2)	Pathogenic factor *qi* (3)
Sexuality (2)	Electric metaphor (2)	Vitality (2)
Fertility (1)	Microcurrent (2)	Water (2)
	Fractal (1)	Atmosphere (1)
		Influence (1)
		Vibe (1)
Total: 119	Total: 108	Total: 170
Mean: 6.3	Mean: 5.4	Mean: 7.4

D. Philosophical terms	E. Contemporary terms about the body	F. Polarities and boundaries
Emptiness (8)	Bioenergy (5)	Process vs. structure (5+3)
All-permeating (4)	Matrix (5)	Particle vs. wave (4)
Terrestrial/celest'l (4+3)	Network (5)	*li* vs. *l*& *qi* (3)
Synchronicity (3)	Connective tissue (4)	Liminality (1)
Universal (3)	Crystal (3)	Bridging (e.g. physical/ nonphysical) (3)
Constant flux (2)	Complex systems (2)	
Correspondence between body/state/ cosmos (2)	Embryogenesis (1)	
Shapes body (2)	HRV (2)	
Shapes universe (1)	X-signal (2)	
Finest matter (1)	Biofield (1)	
Root/branch (1)		
Synergy (1)		
Total: 35	Total: 30	Total: 19
Mean: 2.7	Mean: 3.0	Mean: 3.8

Note: A number of these keywords will mean different things to different people and, as with the terms in Table 25.1, ideally they should have been reviewed by several readers independently before forming a consensus categorization. Some terms could be included in more than one category (for example, 'heat 'may be objective and quantifiable as well as felt, 'spirit' might be considered as philosophical, and so on), and other methods of categorization are of course also feasible (for instance, based on a more precise analysis of clusters of terms in different chapters).

As a generalization, *qi* tends to be considered either as a universal ('the basis of existence … which permeates the entire universe'), or as associated with the individual person ('the basis of the life-force … made manifest by subtle breath control' [19, p 144]). Correspondingly, for some the search for understanding/meaning is externally directed, to measurement, to concepts in published papers (**B** in Table 25.2), but to others it is more an interior process, subjectivized, embodied (**A**). Others again prefer a more philosophical approach (**D**), try to understand the body in terms of contemporary science (**E**), or look for *yinyang* patterns of polarity, what happens at the 'edges' of experience and knowledge and in transitions between 'levels', and ways of bridging these (**F**).

However, these types are not mutually exclusive, and at least according to this rather basic method of analysis, in this book most contributors appear happy to mix their type **A** and type **B** (or type **D** and type **E**) metaphors, rather than gravitating to one extreme or the other. In particular, Chapter 4 scored high for all five types, and Chapter 16 for three types, while low scorers included Chapter 21 (for four types), and Chapters 20 and 23.1 (three types). Only Chapters 6 and 13 showed a marked preference (7-point difference) for type **A** over type **B** terms, Chapters 1 and 7 for **D** over **E** terms (4-point difference), and Chapter 12 for **B** over **A** (again, 4-point difference). Some type **A**/type **B** issues are now examined.

'Electrical or other measurement' (9)

This score is a reasonable outcome, given the assumed need for the evidence of objective verification in our scientized culture. Several chapters have taken this approach (e.g. Chs 9, 10 and 25). However, that any form of measurement has been attempted of the effects of what in itself is by some definitions unmeasurable (Ch. 3) might well be construed by the skeptical as misguided rather than admirable.

'Embodiment' (2), 'quantum' (7) and 'information' (8)

❝ As soon as I treat my body as a thing, I exile myself in infinite degree.
Gabriel Marcel (1889–1973) [97]

❝ In a very real sense, … the practice of Chinese medicine – working with qi – is an embodied undertaking.
Diane Dutton [98]

❝ The unconscious, bodily based, vital force, which connects the physical body with the deeper consciousness in which it has its source, is the central agent within the healing process.
Anne Scott [99, p 12]

In contrast to the previous item ('measurement'), the score for the seemingly rather abstract term 'embodiment' was unexpectedly very low. This may highlight the difficulty of writing from the perspective of feeling (*sentio, ergo sum* [100]) rather than thinking (*cogito, ergo sum*), but also reflects the very different approaches to *qi* taken by contributors to this volume.

Traditionally, *qi* has been discussed using keywords of type **A**, **C** or **D**. Another interpretation is that of Fritjof Capra, who in 1975 published his influential book *The Tao of Physics*, comparing *qi* with the quantum field of modern physics [101]. Partly as a result, in addition to 'subtle energy', a particularly tenacious label in recent decades has been the term 'quantum', popularized by Deepak Chopra [102], albeit admittedly as a metaphor. Proponents of a quantum model often consider that their work is at the cutting edge of an 'emerging paradigm' and so 'in advance of, rather than in opposition to, mainstream scientific research' [99, p 109]. Others might describe such a dematerializing, 'superorganic' approach as simply an outgrowth of bourgeois science, with its denial of the sensual body [103]. Others again, critical of CAM in general, believe the term 'quantum' is overused or employed so vaguely in this context as to be meaningless ('quantum silliness') [104].

A more recent view is that *qi* is not a form of electricity, energy or field, but rather of *information*, more precisely 'the information needed to maintain a complex system' [33, p 108], or 'the free flow of information carried by biochemicals of emotions, the neuropeptides and their receptors' [105]. While a fascination with energy in most modalities of CAM, like the fascination with contrasting mechanist views of the body as a machine, has been attributed to industrialisation [106] (even dubbed 'Fordist' by one sociologist [107]), reinterpretations as something more 'subtle' have been described as in keeping with an increasingly common postmodern dematerialization of the body [108,109] In fact, Birch's view of *qi* is quite appropriate in an age of cybernetics, information flow and global interconnection – even universal consciousness.

Overall, there is a fairly even balance in this book between a body-centered (if not always 'embodied') approach to *qi* and what might be called the electrical–quantum–informational one (emphasized in Chs 8, 12 and 23.1, for example), with the former having possibly a slight advantage. There is a similar balance between the philosophers and the biologists, but those with more of a *yinyang* or emphasized bridging perspective are surprisingly few (Chs 10, 15).

To try to determine whether there is really any serious divide between the quantum theorists with their abstract mind fields, the bodyworkers (and some homeopaths [87]) with their flows and feelings, and the information biologists, would probably not be either helpful or meaningful, and would require a more sensitive method of analysis than is possible here (although it is always tempting to impose a left/right brain dichotomy on such polarities [110]).

LACUNAE

Also of note are the topics that are *not* well covered in this book.

Sexuality

❝ *The healer becomes aware of a feeling of intense pleasure, as he knows inwardly that the healing has been successful. A feeling of ecstasy pervades his whole being.*
Harry Edwards (1893–1976) [54, p 55]

In early Greek physiology [111], as in traditional Chinese, Indian and many other cultures (e.g. in ancient Sumer and Egypt [112], or in modern times for the Samo in Burkina Faso [113], the Yukanoa in Colombia [114], the Hua in New Guinea [115], and elsewhere [116]), semen and marrow as the body's store of *jing* (精), essence or potency are virtually interchangeable. (An intriguing modern connection might be the carrying of 'information' in the DNA of the sperm (see Ch. 23.2).) Possibly from his own experience of orgasm [117], but also from the Homeric equivalence of life-force or life-fluid (*aion*, αἰών) with the cerebrospinal fluid [118], the philosopher Plato hypothesized that a universal 'panspermia' (closely bonded with 'soul') is present in the brain, spine and sex organs. (The spine was still suggested as a potential site for the body–soul relation in the late eighteenth century by the prominent Montpellier vitalist Paul Joseph Barthez (1734–1806), one of Napoleon's physicians [119].) In classical Rome, authors took this association metaphorically: love became a sexual fire of the spinal marrow [111], the 'sap' of Zola or D H Lawrence two millennia later (Ch. 3).

The close association of the movement of something through the spine (or other central pathways in the body) – as in orgasm (ecstasy) or even internally with visualization (enstasy) – occurs in much Chinese internal alchemy (see Ch. 3 and Fig. 7.2), in Indian *kundalini* and tantra and in modern methods of body psychotherapy based on the work of Wilhelm Reich, for whom 'every psychic illness has a core of dammed-up sexual excitation' and 'orgastic potency is the capacity to surrender to the streaming of biological energy, free of any inhibitions' [62, p 29, 37]. The laying on of hands in the intimate ritual of healing may have erotic overtones for both those involved [54,120,121], as may even *imaginal* encounter in a therapeutic setting [122]. Yet sexuality (and indeed fertility and reproduction) are barely mentioned in this book, even though they are important components of the traditional Chinese, Indian and Tibetan formulation of vital essence and health.

The work of Wilhelm Reich (1897–1957)

Reich, with his emphasis on the psychosexual energy he termed 'orgone', remains a controversial figure. The Reichian and post-Reichian tradition has been described as 'the central element in body psychotherapy' [123]. Yet, despite the editors' best efforts, no one was found to contribute a chapter on the current state of neo-Reichian body psychotherapies. Thus, although his work has been touched on several times in the present chapter, it barely receives a mention elsewhere in this book (Chs 3, 14).

Yet there are important parallels between *qi* and orgone, and indeed 'orgone-acupuncture' has been practiced since the 1970s [55,124]. Leon Southgate has listed 50 such parallels (and two important differences) [55]. For example, in both Chinese medicine (CM) and Reichian theory, 'a singular, universal, cosmic and biological energy ... is thought to give rise to form and to animate organisms', with the *yinyang* antithesis of CM echoed in Reich's contraction/expansion of the pulsating orgone. In particular, 'expansion of orgone ... corresponds to the free flow of *qi*' (and health), and is functionally equivalent to parasympathetic activation, while 'contraction of orgone ... corresponds to stagnation of *qi*' (and disease), and to sympathetic dominance. Reich observed that parasympathetic activation (orgone expansion, free flow of *qi*) was associated with pleasure, joy, and relaxation [62]. A state of relaxation often follows energy medicine treatments (A Morris, unpublished study, 2007), sometimes being a primary objective.

According to Reich's close student Ola Raknes (above) and Raknes's own former trainee David Boadella (cited in Ch. 3), streaming sensations will most easily be felt within the body when in a state of relaxation (in *qigong* similarly, *qi* flows optimally through the channels when relaxation is greatest [125]). Given the equivalence between 'free flow' and 'expansion' posited by Southgate, this now appears self-evident, and is supported by studies demonstrating that decreased muscle tone is correlated with increased body-perception scores [126,127], although it has also been suggested that what is felt when attending to a body part is perhaps the result of a slight muscle contraction [128].

Breathing (along with the production of heat [62] – see Ch. 3) is also a key element in both CM and post-Reichian bodywork (as well as in methods such as Middendorf's breathwork). More explicitly, the erotic arts have always played an important role in Indian and Chinese culture, particularly in Daoist practices, while the sexual nature of reality is fundamental to Reich's theory of the orgone. However, sexuality is mostly played down in Chinese and other forms of energy medicine, as we have already seen. (Other parallels between *qi* and orgone are discussed in Southgate's work [55].)

Shamanism – some parallels and contrasts

The concept of 'vital energy' is shared by many ethnomedical healing and shamanic traditions (Ch. 7). There are notable parallels between *qi* and the 'something' that flows between the shaman and all living things, and as vitality through the shaman into the community [17], as well as between *qi* and the various vaporous 'souls' that only trained shamans can see (Ch. 3). 'Energy flows' are explicitly described in some shamanistic writing [129,130]. There are also parallels between acupuncture techniques and those of shamanic healing (e.g. mastery of fire/moxibustion, sucking/cupping, bleeding/needling). Indeed, one possible shamanic origin of acupuncture may even have been the hallucinations of piercing that can accompany the prickling sensations triggered in altered states of consciousness (ASCs) [131]. However, the importance of shamanism in Chinese culture may well have diminished (at least in official circles) by the time the Chinese medicine we know developed [32], and no contributors have paid more than passing attention to possible links and influences. Again, the topics of ecstasy, or even ASCs in general, are avoided.

This anomaly has an intriguing parallel in one US study, where ASC in Christian (Pentecostal or charismatic) healing groups frequently involved somesthesia (reports of tingling, warmth, buzzing in ears, or 'electric shocks'), whereas those in metaphysical (NA) healing groups were more likely to report feelings of harmony and calm [132]. (However, other authors have noted that feelings of calm, floating, or waves of love occur more frequently than heat or tingling in charismatic healing [133].) This difference is echoed in one analysis of bodily sensations in Tibetan *dumo*: feelings of warmth and relaxation may indicate greater parasympathetic (trophotropic) than sympathetic (ergotropic) activity, 'energy rushes' a state of 'hyper-trophotropic tuning with ergotropic eruption', and the contrary ('hyper-ergotropic tuning with trophotropic eruption' or rebound) a state of ecstasy or 'a generalized sense of flow' [43, p 126].

Indigenous shamanism often makes use of natural hallucinogens, as in the ayahuasca ceremony of the Amazon, or the peyote religion of the American Southwest [134]. Descriptions of drug-induced ASC not infrequently include words such as 'energy', 'current', vitality' [135], with feelings of melting and fluidity, shimmering electricity [136], tingling [137], oneness, or wavelike movements of the body [138].

It would seem that most of the energy medicine modalities described in this book are more concerned with parasympathetic than sympathetic activation, with 'de-tensionality' and 'attunement' [139], quite appropriately in our age of technological acceleration and autonomic overload. However, there is conflicting evidence on the autonomic effects of acupuncture (stimulation at one and the same point can exert both sympathetic and parasympathetic actions, for example, depending on depth of needling, stimulation intensity, and other factors). Given the importance of the goal of *yinyang* balance in Chinese medicine, and the frequent interpretation of this polarity in terms of autonomic balance, as for example in the Japanese *ryodoraku* (良導絡) system [140], it would be most interesting to analyze a broader spectrum of interventions and methods in this manner.

The philosophy of *qi*: a third way of knowing?

❝ The number 2 is a very dangerous number: that is why the dialectic is a dangerous process. Attempts to divide anything into two ought to be regarded with much suspicion.
C P Snow (1905–1980) [141]

There are a number of apparent dichotomies in the above discussion (and also in the final sections of Ch. 3), such as those between intuition (movement/flow/

process) and intelligence/reason (immobility/block/reductionism), experience/ feeling and theory/thinking, embodiment and dematerialization. To oversimplify, from one angle these can be seen to boil down to the Cartesian philosophical dualism of matter and mind. Yet even Descartes retained the traditional concept of something that moved between the two, the 'animal spirits' (*anima*), seated in the pineal gland [142].

Elsewhere DM has argued that there are parallels between *qi* and the animal spirits [5], themselves heir to the *pneuma* that from our perspective can be seen as a 'third potency' mediating between *hyle* (ύλη, matter) and *psyche* (ψυχή) [143]. One philosopher who has very sensitively explored how *qi* and the acupuncture channels can bring body and mind together in a worldview of 'correlative dualism' rather than separation [144], is the Japanese Yuasa Yasuo (at one time a close associate of Motoyama Hiroshi [145]). For Yuasa, whose work has not been mentioned elsewhere in this book, the 'third term' of the channel system forms an 'unconscious quasi-body [mediating] between the mind and body' [64, p 220], a potential circuit below consciousness which engenders the living human body 'with vigor and life force' [146, p 138]. Further, the interfusion of *qi* through the acupuncture points at the skin boundary mediates the (felt) interior and the (observed) exterior [147]. He even suggests that 'this unique energy system, or the unconscious quasi-body, is basically a network of functions, and the "mind" and the "body" are two Cartesian substances that appear to consciousness out of this indivisible system' [148, p 274].

If we *think* about the body as object, or even the body-mind posited by John Dewey (1852–1952), it eludes us in some way. What we cannot grasp is its life [149] – rather as with Heisenberg's Uncertainty Principle, according to which movement at the quantum level cannot be measured when location is accurately determined. In actual interaction, we realize that 'mind' and 'body' are just convenient abstractions [150]. Conversely, if we wallow in the flow of our *feelings* we may end up drowning. Yuasa's very Japanese solution is to unify the mind with *qi* by using the intermediary being of one's own body [147].

Others have suggested that the 'flow of feeling' (which Yuasa allots to a different, if related, 'circuit' in his body-mind schema to that of the circulation of *qi*) may be both substantive and spiritual [63] or, like Susanne K Langer (1895–1985), that the felt process anyway shifts all the time between objective and subjective [151]. A different approach was taken by the philosopher Alfred North Whitehead (1861–1947), who proposed – rather like William James before him with his 'pure experience' [152] – that 'nature is nothing else than the deliverance of sense-awareness', so avoiding its bifurcation into the sensed and the conceived [153]. More recently, Christian de Quincey has suggested that 'consciousness is the process of matter-energy informing itself' [66, p 61], and that matter itself 'tingles with interiority' [66, p xx].

It has been stated (often disparagingly) that the tingling of *qi* is just a metaphor, and so has no place in scientific discourse (although it certainly does in literature, as shown in Ch. 3). However, metaphor is powerful, and itself 'unites reason and imagination' [154], so can be widely appealing. Indeed, perhaps it would be more accurate to say that we live in a field of metaphor rather than a field of consciousness. As a virtually universal metaphor (Ch. 3), *qi* in fact provides a fascinating way of exploring the multidimensional nature of reality [155], and could perhaps be a factor in a future democratization of medicine based more on common knowledge than on specialist jargons [103].

Qi in itself offers us a third way, leading us out of the potential conflicts that beset discussions of what it may or may not be.

Risks and side effects

Adverse effects are not mentioned in this book. They are usually associated with strong medication or invasive procedures. However, some people are more susceptible to side effects than others, and those who use the usually gentler methods of energy medicine (e.g. Ch. 17) may do so precisely because they are particularly sensitive. This sensitivity (Ch. 3) may also affect their responses to more subtle methods. Indeed, for some patients in certain situations there is a distinct possibility of energy 'overdose'. Dependency (even sexual involvement) can also become an issue, and there may be particular problems in those with a prior history of abuse (for instance, if therapy involves body contact), posttraumatic stress disorder (PTSD), or a borderline personality [156]. As Babette Rothschild has pointed out, 'those with PTSD become overly attentive to interoceptive reminders of the past danger, whilst losing their connection to extroceptive cues (the five 'senses') that appraise the present environment' [157]. The interoceptive vocabulary easily becomes fixated on pain or discomfort [158].

This view is echoed by David Boadella, who has written of the need in somatic psychotherapy to work with great respect for the pace and energetic level of the person. Encouraging too much 'flow' of ideas and feelings from one level of the body-mind to another without providing adequate structure and boundary can lead to psychological disturbance [159]. Bodily sensations may become threatening and, for example, be experienced as persecutory forces: 'the world of uncontained de-personalised streamings is the world of the schizophrenic who is deeply alive and sensitive underneath his contactlessness. He or she senses the tremor of life, but does not recognise it as coming from their own body. In extreme forms the streamings may be experienced as persecutory electric currents … [or] mystified into "Christ sensations" with the conviction that one has been specially chosen or is in touch with some special force' [78, p 89]. Reich wrote similarly about 'a dividing wall between excitation and sensation … at the root of the mystical experience' [62, p 293]. (See Ch. 3 for some examples of this.)

Although rare, such frankly psychotic episodes have been reported as a result of *qigong*, *kundalini* and *subud* practice [57,160,161]. Gopi Krishna, for example, described his dramatic experiences of 'energy-sensation' or 'currents' when 'blocks' in the *susumna* or other *nadi* were encountered [162]. In China, '*qigong*-induced psychosis' or '*qigong* deviation syndrome' (*zouhuo lümo*, 作火鲁莫) was found to occur particularly in practitioners who followed methods involving spontaneous movement [163,164] or without proper guidance [165]. On the other hand, *taiji* has been used to help those experiencing psychotic fragmentation [166]. Psychosis is probably far more likely to result from drug abuse or dabbling unsupervised in shamanic or magical practices than from receiving energy medicine treatment from a properly trained practitioner, although research to prove this would be problematic for many reasons.

Who is a strong responder?

From much of the above it also seems likely that being relatively 'sensitive' and able to 'tune in' to internal states would be associated with a greater responsiveness to subtle energy, as originally adumbrated by Reich [62], and observed in the practice of orgone-acupuncture by Southgate [55]. Such sensitivity is in fact mentioned in Chapter 14, and in the context of treating children in Chapter 20 (similarly, Southgate has observed that young people may be more responsive to orgone-acupuncture). Michael Jawer has reiterated that responders may be those who 'aren't just extraordinarily sensitive to their surroundings, they're also extra sensitive to their own, *internal landscape of feeling*' [63, p 307]; in other words, such 'thin-boundary people ... have a greater connectedness among their bodies' various systems', the result being 'a more rapid and direct flow of feeling' [63, p 330]. However, at least one study on conventional acupuncture has shown an opposite association [167], and whether an individual's responsiveness to one form of energy medicine indicates that other forms may be helpful is a complete unknown. Other factors such as an openness to change (Ch. 16), the ability to suspend doubt and judgment (which may stop 'the harmonious flow of experience' [150]), suggestibility, and trust in the practitioner and the healing process, the therapeutic relationship in general, and of course the practitioner's own sensitivity and abilities, may clearly be important.

This question may also relate to the brief discussions of parasympathetic/sympathetic activation above, to studies of synesthesia (D F Mayor, unpublished work, 1998) [168], and also to some forms of repetitive self-harm such as cutting and burning, which is more prevalent in women than in men, and which may be a way for some sufferers to 'feel alive' [169,170] – as may deliberate self-injury in some religious contexts, sometimes followed by remarkably rapid healing [171].

FUTURE POSSIBILITIES

❝ To those of you who may be vitalists, I would make this prophecy:
... what everyone believed yesterday, and you believe today, only cranks will believe tomorrow.
Francis Crick [172]

❝ There are serious limitations in attempting to embrace the indigenous knowledge system of the East, one of the oldest systems of empirical knowledge, by a 300-year-old science of the West.
Beverly Rubik [173]

Clearly, there is much scope for research in this area – and for improving research methodology (see Ch. 7), especially the adoption of paradigms appropriate to what is being investigated (Ch. 13). In particular, we would like to see more experiential research on *qi*, along the lines of that described in Chapter 13 or a recent UK undergraduate dissertation on the phenomenon of *qi* (A Morris, unpublished study, 2007). It is important that we do not lose the 'felt sense' that is so vital to energy medicine, but at the same time that we work respectfully to bring together aspects of *both* patient-centered (subjective/qualitative) *and* evidence-based (objective/quantitative) medicine, rather than focusing exclusively on one or the other [174]. We need also to continue to develop ideas about what we are doing rather than, on the one hand, becoming entrenched in positions hedged about with hubris and competitive denigration or, on the other, attempting to 'synthesize all variations into one gigantic, panhuman hodgepodge' [175]. Times change in our accelerating world, and what may be orthodoxy today may be considered best forgotten tomorrow. Only time will tell, for example, whether attempts to create life from computer-generated sequences of nucleotides ('information') activated by ATP ('energy') are realistic, or overly simplistic and soulless.

On the other hand, questions that may well remain unanswerable are those about whether *qi* 'exists' substantively, or (as orthodox science concluded about Mesmer's *fluidum* – see Ch. 22) is a matter of the imagination (Bergsonian 'intuition'), or even 'magical ideation' [176], merely a conceptualization of process underlying placebo effects. No doubt there will always be proponents of both views, and hopefully each will remain open minded enough at least to acknowledge the other and that in this field no single truth is final.

CONCLUSION

❝ Qi has as many definitions as authors who have written about it.

Lisa Swartz [177]

We hope that this book will contribute to the theory and practices of energy medicine, both in broadening how we think about what we are doing as practitioners or patients, and in deepening our awareness of what it is to experience *qi* in therapy and in life. We would not ask you to accept it all at face value, but to use it selectively, and critically, as a tool in your own further development.

As our authors have made abundantly clear, *qi* is polysemous and reinterpretable according to the *Zeitgeist* or the worldview of the interpreter, as against the monoparadigmatic and hegemonic tendencies of Western science and medicine. Pluralism (Ch. 1), variety (Ch. 6), multidimensionality (Ch. 22), synergy (Ch. 18) and even integration (Ch. 23.1) are implicit in working with *qi*. *Qi* itself remains unexplainable (Ch. 4), and life a mystery (Ch. 12) that will always beckon us to further exploration.

Despite the somewhat limited methodology of the content analysis undertaken here, it is clear that there is at least some agreement among contributors to this book on the topics associated with *qi* that warrant discussion, but also that there are areas where views diverge widely and some topics about which writers feel uncomfortable or which they consider as irrelevant. The dozen or so definitions of *qi* presented here are in many ways consistent with Chinese medicine itself as a multivalent, diverse system of healing philosophies, schools and techniques (which can also be said of the formulaic approaches adapted and practiced in the West today). In practical terms, this ambiguity leaves room for both practitioner and patient and preserves the possibility for as many successful *qi* practices as there are practitioners, and as many *qi* treatments as there are patients.

ACKNOWLEDGMENTS

To Leon Southgate, for his last-minute assistance with information about the relationship between *qi* and orgone, and Mark Bovey and Charles Buck for their helpful critiques of preliminary versions of this chapter.

References and Further Reading

1. *QI* IN ASIAN MEDICINE

[1] Kohn L. Taoist Meditation and Longevity Techniques. Ann Arbor, MI: University of Michigan Center for Chinese Studies; 1989. p. 135.

[2] Leslie C. Asian Medical Systems: A comparative study. Berkeley, CA: University of California Press; 1977.

[3] Leslie C, Young A. Paths to Asian Medical Knowledge. Berkeley, CA: University of California Press; 1992.

[4] Herfel W, Rodrigues H, Gao Y. Chinese medicine and the dynamic conceptions of health and disease. Journal of Chinese Philosophy 2007;34(Suppl. 1): 57–79.

[5] Kuriyama S. The Expressiveness of the Body and the Divergence of Greek and Chinese Medicine. New York: Zone Books; 1999.

[6] Hsü E. The Transmission of Chinese Medicine. Cambridge, UK: Cambridge University Press; 1999.

[7] Scheid V. Chinese Medicine in Contemporary China: Plurality and synthesis. Durham, NC: Duke University Press; 2002. p. 9.

[8] Farquhar J. Knowing Practice: The clinical encounter with Chinese medicine. Boulder, CO: Westview Press; 1996.

[9] Sivin N. Huang ti nei ching Suwen. Loewe M, editor. Early Chinese Texts: A bibliographical guide. Berkeley, CA: University of California Press; 1993. p. 196–215.

[10] Yang SZ, editor and translator. The Divine Farmer's Materia Medica: A translation of the Shen Nong Ben Cao Jing. Boulder, CO: Blue Poppy Press; 1998.

[11] Harper D. Early Chinese Medical Literature: The Mawangdui medical manuscripts. London: Kegan Paul International; 1998.

[12] Lo V. The influence of yangsheng culture on early Chinese medical theory. Hsü E, editor. Innovation in Chinese Medicine. Cambridge, UK: Cambridge University Press; 2001. p. 22–48.

[13] Furth C. A Flourishing Yin: Gender in China's medical history. Berkeley, CA: University of California Press; 1999.

[14] Chen NN. Embodying qi and masculinities in post-Mao China. Brownell S, Wasserstrom JN, editors. Chinese Femininities/Chinese Masculinities: A reader. Berkeley, CA: University of California Press; 2002. p. 315–29.

[15] Unschuld PU. Huang Di Nei Jing Su Wen: Nature, knowledge, and imagery in an ancient Chinese medical text. Berkeley, CA: University of California Press; 2003. p. 161, 164.

[16] Sivin N. State, cosmos, and body in the last three centuries B.C. Harvard Journal of Asiatic Studies 1995;55(1):5–37.

[17] Goldschmidt AM. The Evolution of Chinese Medicine: Northern Song dynasty 960–1200. New York: Routledge; 2008.

[18] Jeon SW. Science and Technology in Korea: Traditional instruments and techniques. Cambridge, MA: MIT Press; 1974.

[19] Kosoto H. Kajiwara Shozen (1265–1337) and the medical silk road. In: Goble AE, Robinson KR, Wakabayashi HN, editors. Tools of Culture: Japan's cultural, intellectual, medical, and technological contacts in East Asia, 1000–1500s. Ann Arbor, MI: Association for Asian Studies; 2009. p. 211–30.

[20] Deal WE. Handbook to Life in Medieval and Early Modern Japan. Oxford: Oxford University Press; 2007.

[21] Goble AE, Robinson KR, Wakabayashi HN, editors. Tools of Culture: Japan's cultural, intellectual, medical, and technological contacts in East Asia, 1000–1500s. Ann Arbor, MI: Association for Asian Studies; 2009.

[22] Oka T. The role of Kampo (Japanese traditional herbal) medicine in psychosomatic medicine practice in Japan. In:Psychosomatic Medicine: Proceedings of the 18th World Congress on Psychosomatic Medicine,

339

Kobe, Japan, 21–26 August 2005. International Congress Series 1287; 2006. p. 304–8.

[23] Alter J. Yoga in Modern India: The body between science and philosophy. Princeton, NJ: Princeton University Press; 2004.

[24] Chopra A. Ayurvedic medicine: core concept, therapeutic principles, and current relevance. Med Clin North Am 2002;86(1):75–89.

[25] Alter J. Yoga in Asia – mimetic history: problems in the location of secret knowledge. Comparative Studies of South Asia, Africa, and the Middle East 2009;29(2):213–29.

[26] Sheehan HE, Hussain SJ. Unani Tibb: History, theory, and contemporary practice in South Asia. Ann Am Acad Pol Soc Sci 2002;583(1):122–35.

[27] Leslie C. The professionalization of Ayurvedic and Unani medicine. Trans N Y Acad Sci 1968;30(4):559–72.

[28] Liebeskind C. Unani medicine of the subcontinent. Van Alphen J, Aris A, editors. Oriental Medicine: An illustrated guide to the Asian arts of healing. London: Serindia Publications; 1995. p. 39–65.

[29] Dönden Y. Health Through Balance: An introduction to Tibetan medicine. Ithaca, NY: Snow Lion Publications; 2003.

[30] Schrempf M. Soundings in Tibetan Medicine: Anthropological and historical perspectives. Leiden: Brill; 2007.

[31] Kunzang JP. Tibetan Medicine, Illustrated in Original Texts. London: Wellcome Institute of the History of Medicine; 1973.

[32] Meyer F. Theory and practice of Tibetan medicine. Van Alpen J, Aris A, editors. Oriental Medicine: An illustrated guide to the Asian arts of healing. London: Serindia Publications; 1995. p. 109–41.

[33] Adams V. The sacred in the scientific: ambiguous practices of science in Tibetan medicine. Cultural Anthropology 16(4):542–75.

[34] Janes CR. The transformations of Tibetan medicine. Med Anthropol Q 1995;9(1):6–39.

[35] Chen NN. Breathing Spaces: Qigong, psychiatry, and healing in China. New York: Columbia University Press; 2003.

[36] Alter J, editor. Asian Medicine and Globalization: Encounters with Asia. Philadelphia, PA: University of Pennsylvania Press; 2005.

2. FLOWS AND BLOCKAGES IN RWANDAN RITUAL AND NOTIONS OF THE BODY

[1] Janzen JM, Green EC. Continuity, change, and challenge in African medicine. Selin H, editor. Medicine across Cultures: The history of non-Western medicine. Dordrecht, Netherlands: Kluwer Academic; 2003. p. 1–26.

[2] Taylor C. Milk, Honey, and Money: Changing concepts in Rwandan healing. Washington, DC: Smithsonian Institution Press; 1992.

[3] Zhang YH. Transforming Emotions with Chinese Medicine. Albany, NY: State University of New York Press; 2007.

[4] Farquhar J. Knowing Practice: The clinical encounter of Chinese medicine. Boulder, CO: Westview Press; 1994.

[5] Kakar S. Shamans, Mystics and Doctors: A psychological inquiry into India and its healing. New York: Knopf; 1982. p. 187.

[6] de Mahieu W. Qui a Obstrué la Cascade? Analyse sémantique du rituel de la circoncision chez les Komo du Zaïre. Cambridge, Cambs: Cambridge University Press; 1985.

[7] Bekaert S. System and Repertoire in Sakata Medicine. PhD dissertation. Belgium: Department of Social and Cultural Anthropology, Katholieke Universiteit Leuven; 1997. p. 351.

[8] d'Hertefelt M, Coupez A. La Royauté Sacrée de l'Ancien Rwanda. Tervuren, Belgium: Musée Royal de l'Afrique Centrale; 1964. p. 17, 20, 27–31, 286, 460.

[9] Kagame A. La Philosophie Bantu-Rwandaise de l'Être. Bruxelles: Académie Royale des Sciences Coloniales; 1956. p. 15.

[10] Beattie J. Bunyoro: An African kingdom. New York: Holt, Rinehart & Winston; 1960. p. 28.

[11] Rodegem F. Dictionnaire Rundi–Français. Tervuren, Belgium: Musée Royal de l'Afrique Centrale; 1970. p. 209.

[12] Origine de la mort. In: Smith P, editor. Le Récit Populaire au Rwanda. Paris: Armand Colin; p.129–33.

[13] Smith P, editor. Le Récit Populaire au Rwanda. Paris: Armand Colin; p. 39.

[14] Jacob I. Dictionnaire Rwandais–Français, Extrait du Dictionnaire de l'Institut National de Recherche Scientifique. vol. 1. Kigali, Rwanda: l'Institut National de Recherche Scientifique; 1985. p. 456.

3. ELEMENTAL SOULS AND VERNACULAR *QI*: SOME ATTRIBUTES OF WHAT MOVES US

[1] Neijing Ling Shu, Ch. 6, cited in Sivin N. State, cosmos, and body in the last three centuries BC. Harvard Journal of Asiatic Studies 1995;55(1): 5–37. p. 14.

[2] Boadella D. Lifestreams: An introduction to biosynthesis. London: Routledge & Kegan Paul; 1987. p. 87.

[3] Liu CL. The life philosophy of ancient China and qi. Kawakita Y, Sakai S, Otsuka Y, editors. The comparison between concepts of life-breath in East and West: Proceedings of the 15th international syposium on the comparative history of medicine, East and West. St. Louis, MO: Ishiyaku EuroAmerica; 1995. p. 121–37.

[4] Robinet I. Taoism: Growth of a religion. Stanford, CA: Stanford University Press; 1997. p. 8.

[5] de Bary T, Chan WT, Watson B. Sources of Chinese Tradition. I. New York: Columbia University Press; 1960. p. 193n.

[6] Unschuld PU. Medicine in China: A history of ideas, comparative studies of health systems and medical care. Berkeley, CA: University of California Press; 1985. p. 67.

[7] Lloyd G, Sivin N. The Way and the Word: Science and medicine in early China and Greece. New Haven, CT: Yale University Press; 2002.

[8] Rochat de la Vallée E. A Study of Qi in Classical Texts. Cambridge, Cambs: Monkey Press; 2006. p. 5, 10.

[9] Lo V. The Influence of Yangsheng Culture on Early Chinese Medical Theory. 1998 Thesis submitted for the degree of Doctor of Philosophy of the University of London.

[10] Sivin N. Traditional Medicine in Contemporary China. A partial translation of Revised Outline of Chinese Medicine (1972) with an introductory study on change in present-day and early medicine. Ann Arbor, MI: Center for Chinese Studies, University of Michigan; 1987.

[11] Chu CY. Discussion of the sages with one single qi. In: Zhang YH, Rose K 2001 A Brief History of Qi. Brookline, MA: Paradigm; 2000. p. vi–xiv.

[12] Graham AC. Disputers of the Tao: Philosophical argument in ancient China. La Salle, IL: Open Court; 1989. p. 101,158.

[13] Birrell A, translator. The Classic of Mountains and Seas. London: Penguin; 1999.

[14] Ergil MC. History. Ergil MC, Ergil KV, editors. Pocket Atlas of Chinese Medicine. New York: Thieme; 2009. p. 1–51.

[15] Allan S. The Way of Water and Sprouts of Virtue. Albany, NY: State University of New York Press; 1997.

[16] Needham J, Wang L. History of Scientific Thought. Science and Civilisation in China. II. Cambridge, Cambs: Cambridge University Press; 1956.

[17] Rickett WA. Guanzi. Political, economic, and philosophical essays from early China. A study and translation. vol. 2. Princeton, NJ: Princeton University Press; 1998. p. 100.

[18] Hsu E. The experience of wind in early and medieval Chinese medicine. Journal of the Royal Anthropological Institute (NS) 2007;13(S1):S117–34.

[19] Unschuld PU. Huang Di Nei Jing Su Wen: Nature, knowledge, and imagery in an ancient Chinese medical text. Berkeley, CA: University of California Press; 2003. p. 163.

[20] Beinfield H, Korngold E. Between Heaven and Earth: A guide to Chinese medicine. New York: Ballantine; 1991. p. 32.

[21] Scheid V. Currents of Tradition in Chinese Medicine 1626–2006. Seattle, WA: Eastland Press; 2007.

[22] Ekken K. The Philosophy of Qi: The record of great doubts. New York: Columbia University Press; 2007. p. 66–143.

[23] Birch SJ, Felt RL. Understanding Acupuncture. Edinburgh: Churchill Livingstone; 1999. p. 52, 97.

[24] Ni MS. The Yellow Emperor's Classic of Medicine. A new translation of the Neijing Suwen. Boston, MA: Shambhala; 1995. p. 148.

[25] Lo V. Tracking the Pain. Jue[a,b,c] and the formation of a theory of circulating qi through the channels. Sudhoffs Archiv für Geschichte der Medizin und der Naturwissenschaften 1999;83(2):191–211.

[26] Hsü E. Mai and qi in the Western Han: introduction. Hsü E, editor. Innovation in Chinese Medicine. Cambridge,

Cambs: Cambridge University Press; 2001. p. 13–7.

[27] Lo V. Healing and medicine. Shaughnessy EL, editor. China: The land of the heavenly dragon. London: Duncan Baird; 2000. p. 148–65.

[28] Lo V. Huangdi Hama jing (Yellow Emperor's Toad Canon). Asia Major 2001;14(2):61–99.

[29] Unschuld PU, translator. Nan-Ching: The classic of difficult issues. With commentaries by Chinese and Japanese authors from the third through the twentieth century. Berkeley, CA: University of California Press; 1986.

[30] Harper D. Dunhuang iatromantic manuscripts: P. 2856 R and P. 2675 V. Lo V, Cullen C, editors. Medieval Chinese Medicine: The Dunhuang medical manuscripts. London: RoutledgeCurzon; 2005. p. 134–64.

[31] Hall TS. History of General Physiology, 600 BC to AD 1900. II. From the Enlightenment to the end of the nineteenth century. Chicago, IL: University of Chicago Press; 1975.

[32] Ots T. The silenced body – the expressive Leib: on the dialectic of mind and life in Chinese cathartic healing. Csordas TJ, editor. Embodiment and Experience: The existential ground of culture and self. Cambridge, Cambs: Cambridge University Press; 1994. p. 116–36.

[33] Eisenberg L. Disease and illness: distinctions between professional and popular ideas of sickness. Cult Med Psychiatry 1977;1(1):9–23.

[34] Chen NN. Embodying qi and masculinities in post-Mao China. Brownell S, Wasserstrom JN, editors. Chinese Femininities/Chinese Masculinities: A reader. Berkeley, CA: University of California Press; 2002. p. 315–29.

[35] Messner AC. Translations and transformations: toward creating new men in early twentieth-century China. Bala P, editor. Biomedicine as a Contested Site: Some revelations in imperical contexts. Lanham, MD: Lexington Books; 2009. p. 99–114.

[36] Ho EY. Behold the power of qi: the importance of qi in the discourse of acupuncture. Research on Language and Social Interaction 2006;39(4):411–40.

[37] Yuasa Y. The Body, Self-cultivation, and Ki-energy. Albany, NY: State University of New York Press; 1993. p. 78.

[38] Hall DL, Ames RT. Anticipating China: Thinking through the narratives of Chinese and Western culture. Albany, NY: State University of New York Press; 1995. p. 188.

[39] Hufford DJ. Contemporary folk medicine. Gevitz N, editor. Other Healers: Unorthodox medicine in America. Baltimore, MD: Johns Hopkins University Press; 1988. p. 240.

[40] Crawley AE. The Idea of the Soul 1909. London: Adam and Charles Black; p. 222, 254.

[41] van der Leeuw G. Religion in Essence and Manifestation. Gloucester, MA: P Smith; 1967. p. 276.

[42] Lewis-Williams JD, Pearce DG. San Spirituality: Roots, expression, and social consequences. Walnut Creek, CA: AltaMira Press; 2004.

[43] Grim JA. The Shaman: Patterns of Siberian and Ojibway healing. Norman, OK: University of Oklahoma Press; 1983.

[44] Alexander HB. SOUL (Primitive). Hastings J, editor. Encyclopaedia of Religion and Ethics, vol. 11. Edinburgh: T and T Clark; 1920. p. 725–31.

[45] Hultkrantz Å. Conceptions of the Soul among North American Indians. Stockholm: Ethnographical Museum of Sweden; 1953.

[46] Hultkrantz Å. Shamanism and soul ideology. Hoppál M, editor. Shamanism in Eurasia. Göttingen, Germany: Edition Herodot; 1984. p. 28–36.

[47] VanStone JW. Athapascan Adaptations: Hunters and fishermen of the sub-arctic forests. Chicago, IL: Aldine; 1974.

[48] Wundt W. Elements of folk psychology: outlines of a psychological history of the development of mankind. London: George Allen & Unwin; 1916.

[49] Tu WM. Soul: Chinese concepts. Eliade M, editor. The Encyclopedia of Religion, vol. 13. New York: Macmillan; 1987. p. 447–50.

[50] Maciocia G. The Psyche in Chinese Medicine. Treatment of mental and emotional disharmonies with

acupuncture and Chinese herbs. Edinburgh: Churchill Livingstone; 2009.

[51] Eliade M. The Two and the One. London: Harvill Press; 1965.

[52] Wile D. Tai ji quan. Ergil MC, Ergil KV, editors. Pocket Atlas of Chinese Medicine. New York: Thieme; 2009. p. 345–65.

[53] Connolly P. Vitalistic Thought in India: A study of the prana concept in Vedic literature and its development in the Vedanta, Samkhya and Pancaratra traditions. Delhi: Sri Satguru Publications; 1992.

[54] Mbiti JS. African Religions and Philosophy. Oxford: Heinemann International; 1989.

[55] Tempels P. Bantu Philosophy. Paris: Présence Africaine; 1969.

[56] Keesing RM. Solomon Islands religions. Eliade M, editor. The Encyclopedia of Religion, vol. 13. New York: Macmillan; 1987. p. 410–2.

[57] Arbman E. Seele und Mana. Archiv für Religionswissenschaft 1931;29(2):293–394.

[58] Lévy-Bruhl L. The 'Soul' of the Primitive. London: Allen & Unwin; 1965.

[59] Matthews C, Matthews J. Encyclopaedia of Celtic Wisdom: The Celtic shaman's sourcebook. London: Rider; 2001.

[60] McKenzie D. The Infancy of Medicine: An enquiry into the influence of folklore upon the evolution of scientific medicine. London: Macmillan; 1927.

[61] McCarthy Brown K. Healing relationships in the African Caribbean. Selin H, editor. Medicine across Cultures: The history of non-Western medicine. Dordrecht, Netherlands: Kluwer Academic; 2003. p. 285–303.

[62] Devisch R. Weaving the Threads of Life: The Khita gyn-eco-logical healing cult among the Yaka. Chicago, IL: University of Chicago Press; 1993.

[63] Reinard A, Réquéna Y. Qi gong. Ergil MC, Ergil KV, editors. Pocket Atlas of Chinese Medicine. New York: Thieme; 2009. p. 319–43.

[64] Vinnicombe P. People of the Eland: Rock paintings of the Drakensberg Bushmen as a reflection of their life and thought. Pietermaritzburg, KwaZulu-Natal: University of Natal Press; 1976.

[65] Heinze RI. Tham Khwan: How to contain the essence of life. A socio-psychological comparison of a Thai custom. Singapore: Singapore University Press; 1982.

[66] Darnton R. Mesmerism and the End of the Enlightenment in France. Cambridge, MA: Harvard University Press; 1968.

[67] James W. Does 'consciousness' exist? Journal of Philosophy, Psychology and Scientific Method 1904;1(18):477–91.

[68] Spicker SF. Introduction. Spicker SF, editor. The Philosophy of the Body: Rejections of Cartesian dualism. Chicago, IL: Quadrangle Books; 1970. p. 21.

[69] Siegfried Benignus S. German. The Course of Study 1900;1(4):312.

[70] Currier RL. The hot-cold syndrome and symbolic balance in Mexican and Spanish-American folk medicine. Ethnology 1966;5(3):251–63.

[71] de Heusch L. Heat, physiology, and cosmogony: rites de passage among the Thonga. Karp I, Bird CS, editors. Explorations in African Systems of Thought. Bloomington, IN: Indiana University Press; 1980. p. 27–43.

[72] Turner VW. The Ritual Process: Structure and anti-structure. London: Routledge & Kegan Paul; 1969.

[73] Beidelman TO. Moral Imagination in Kaguru Modes of Thought. Bloomington, IN: Indiana University Press; 1986.

[74] Bardinet T. Les Papyrus Médicaux de l'Égypte Pharaonique. Paris: Fayard; 1995.

[75] Comaroff J. Body of Power, Spirit of Resistance: The culture and history of a South African people. Chicago: University of Chicago Press; 1985.

[76] Whitehead AN. Process and Reality. New York: Free Press; 1978. p. 208.

[77] Precope J. Hippocrates on Diet and Hygiene. London: Zeno; 1952. p. 174.

[78] Ghalioungui P. Magic and Medical Science in Ancient Egypt. London: Hodder & Stoughton; 1963.

[79] Ghalioungui P. The House of Life: Per ankh. Magic and medical science in ancient Egypt. Amsterdam: B M Israël; 1973.

[80] Onions CT, editor. The Shorter Oxford English Dictionary on Historical Principles, vol. 2. Oxford: Clarendon Press; 1933. p. 2364.

[81] Mayor DF. Vitalism: flow, connection, and the awareness of being alive. Micozzi MS, editor. Fundamentals of Complementary and Alternative Medicine. 4th ed. St Louis, MO: Saunders; 2011. p. 61–80.

[82] Coulter ID, Willis EM. The rise and rise of complementary and alternative medicine: a sociological perspective. Med J Aust 2004;180(11):587–9.

[83] Synnott A. Tomb, temple, machine and self: the social construction of the body. Br J Sociol 1992;43(1):79–110.

[84] Hall TS. History of General Physiology, 600 BC to AD 1900. I. From Pre-Socratic times to the Enlightenment. Chicago: University of Chicago Press; 1975.

[85] Lewis CT. An Elementary Latin Dictionary. Oxford: Clarendon Press; 1904.

[86] Wheeler LR. Vitalism: Its history and validity. London: HF & G Witherby; 1939.

[87] Bishop LM. Words, Stones, and Herbs: The healing word in medieval and early modern England. Syracuse, NY: Syracuse University Press; 2007.

[88] French RK. Ether and physiology. Cantor GN, Hodge MJS, editors. Conceptions of Ether: Studies in the history of ether theories 1740–1900. Cambridge, Cambs: Cambridge University Press; 1981. p. 111–34.

[89] Duffin J. History of Medicine: A scandalously short introduction. London: Macmillan; 2000.

[90] Mendelsohn E. Heat and Life: The development of the theory of animal heat. Cambridge, MA: Harvard University Press; 1964.

[91] Sheets-Johnstone M. The Primacy of Movement. Amsterdam: John Benjamins; 1999.

[92] Porter R. Flesh in the Age of Reason. London: Allen Lane; 2003.

[93] Jung CJ. Psychology and Alchemy. London: Routledge & Kegan Paul; 1968.

[94] Raff J. Jung and the Alchemical Imagination. Berwick, ME: Nicholas-Hays; 2000.

[95] Noll R. The Jung Cult: Origins of a charismatic movement. Princeton, NJ: Princeton University Press; 1994.

[96] Hillman J. Emotion: A comprehensive phenomenology of theories and their meanings for therapy. London: Routledge; 1999.

[97] Benz E. The Theology of Electricity: On the encounter and explanation of theology and science in the 17th and 18th centuries. Princeton Theological Monograph Series 19. Allison Park, PA: Pickwick; 1989.

[98] Wilson B. A Treatise on Electricity. London: C Davis, R Dodsley, E Comyns, C Corbet; 1750.

[99] Molenier J. Essai sur le Méchanisme de l'Électricité, et l'Utilité que l'on Peut en Tirer pour la Guérison de quelques Maladies. Bordeaux, France: Veuve de F Sejourne; 1768.

[100] Philip APW. An Experimental Inquiry into the laws of the Vital Functions, with some observations on the nature and treatment of internal diseases. London: Thomas & George Underwood; 1817.

[101] Cloquet J. Traité de l'Acupuncture d'après les Observations de M J Cloquet, publié sous ses yeux par M Dantu. Paris: Bichet; 1826.

[102] Tatar MM. Spellbound: Studies on mesmerism and literature. Princeton, NJ: Princeton University Press; 1978.

[103] Cheung. Regulating agents, functional interactions, and stimulus-reaction-schemes: the concept of 'organism' in the organic system theories of Stahl, Bordeu, and Barthez. Sci Context 2008;21(4):495–519.

[104] Benton E. Vitalism in nineteenth-century scientific thought: a typology and reassessment. Studies in History of Philosophy and Science 1974;5(1):17–48.

[105] Kaptchuk T. Vitalism. Micozzi M, editor. Fundamentals of Complementary and Integrative Medicine. 3rd ed. St Louis, MO: Saunders; 2006. p. 53–66.

[106] Mesmer FA. Dissertation on the Discovery of Animal Magnetism. Bloch GJ, editor. Mesmerism: A translation of the original medical and scientific writings of FA Mesmer, MD. Los Altos, CA: William Kaufmann; 1980.

[107] Fara P. Fatal Attraction. Magnetic mysteries of the enlightenment. Revolutions in Science. Thriplow, Cambs: Icon; 2005.

[108] Rzepka CJ. Re-collecting spontaneous overflows: Romantic passions, the sublime, and Mesmerism. Romantic Circles; 1998. Online. Available: http://www.rc.umd .edu/praxis/passions/rzepka/rzp .html 20 Mar 2010.

[109] Breuer J, Freud S. Studies on Hysteria. Harmondsworth, Middx: Penguin; 1974.

[110] Zweig S. Mental healers: Franz Anton Mesmer, Mary Baker Eddy, Sigmund Freud. London: Cassell; 1933.

[111] Wolff W, Bateman A, Sturgeon D, editors. UCH Textbook of Psychiatry. London: Gerald Duckworth; 1990.

[112] Hall CS. A Primer of Freudian Psychology. New York: World Publishing Company; 1954.

[113] Kelley CR. What is orgone energy? n.d. Online. Available: Public Orgonomic Research Exchange website http://www.orgone.org/ articles/ax9kelley1a.htm 28 Nov 2004.

[114] Conger JP. Jung and Reich: The body as shadow. Berkeley, CA: North Atlantic; 1988.

[115] DeMeo J. A brief history of Wilhelm Reich's discoveries, and the developing science of orgonomy. 1998. Online. Available: Orgone Biophysical Research Lab website www.orgonelab.org/wrhistory.htm 28 Nov 2004.

[116] Trettin J. Wilhelm Reich and Orgonomy: a science-biography. 1997. Online. Available: Public Orgonomic Research Exchange website http:// www.orgone.org/IOOeng/historie. htm 28 Nov 2004.

[117] Reich W. Character Analysis. 3rd ed. New York: Farrar, Straus and Giroux; 1972.

[118] Peers EA, editor. The Complete Works of Saint John of the Cross, Doctor of the Church, London: Burns Oates and Washbourne; 1953. vol. 2, p. 258, 276, 448, vol. 3, p. 36, 57.

[119] Menzies L. The Revelations of Mechthild of Magdeburg (1210–1297) The flowing light of the Godhead. London: Longmans Green; 1953. p. 9 110, 129, 152, 254.

[120] Feild R. Breathing Alive. A guide to conscious living. Shaftesbury, Dorset: Element; 1988. p. 3.

[121] Madden D. 'A Cheap, Safe and Natural Medicine': Religion, medicine and culture in John Wesley's Primitive Physic. Amsterdam: Rodopi; 2007.

[122] King U. Christ in All Things: Exploring spirituality with Teilhard de Chardin. London: SCM Press; 1997.

[123] de St R, Victor. The Twelve Patriarchs, The Mystical Ark, Book Three of the Trinity. London: SPCK; 1979.

[124] Heiler F. Erscheinungsformen und Wesen der Religion. Stuttgart, Germany: Kohlhammer; 1961. p. 49 (trans DM).

[125] Thurston H. The Physical Phenomena of Mysticism. London: Burns Oates; 1952.

[126] Schimmel A. As Through a Veil: Mystical poetry in Islam. New York: Columbia University Press; 1982.

[127] Happold FC. Mysticism. A study and an anthology. Harmondsworth, Middx: Penguin Books; 1970.

[128] Lewis D translator. The Life of St Teresa of Avila. Including the relations of her spiritual state. London: Burns and Oates; 1962. p. 238, 144.

[129] Erickson C. The Medieval Vision: Essays in history and perception. New York: Oxford University Press; 1976.

[130] Zum Brunn E, Epiney-Burgard G. Women Mystics in Medieval Europe. New York: Paragon House; 1989. p. 8–87.

[131] Merrell-Wolff F. Franklin Merrell-Wolff's Experience and Philosophy. A personal record of transformation and a discussion of transcendental consciousness. Containing his Philosophy of Consciousness Without an Object and his Pathways Through to Space. NY: State University of New York; 1994. p. 37, 270.

[132] Minkin JS. The Romance of Hassidism. London: Thomas Yoseloff; 1955.

[133] Dwyer WJ. Bhakti in Kabir. Patna, India: Associated Book Agency; 1981.

[134] Franklin JC. Mystical Transformations: The imagery of liquids in the work of Mechthild von Magdeburg. Rutherford, NJ: Fairleigh Dickinson University Press; 1978. p. 161–62.

[135] Bynum CW. The female body and religious practice in the later Middle

Ages. Feher M, with Naddaff R, Tazi N, editors. Fragments for a History of the Human Body. Part One. New York: Zone; 1989. p. 160–219.

[136] Armstrong K, editor. The English Mystics of the Fourteenth Century. London: Kyle Cathie; 1991.

[137] Rolle R. The Fire of Love. Harmondsworth, Middx: Penguin Books; 1972.

[138] Mali A. Mystic in the New World: Marie de L'Incarnation (1599–1672). Leiden: E J Brill; 1996. p. 70.

[139] Flinders CL. Enduring Grace: Living portraits of seven women mystics. San Francisco, CA: HarperSanFrancisco; 1993.

[140] Nygren A. Agape and Eros. London: SPCK; 1982. p. 735.

[141] Matthew. Ch. 11, v. 25 Catholic Online Bible. Online. Available: www.catholic .org/bible/book.php?id=47&bible_ chapter=11 20 Mar 2010.

[142] McDonald ED, editor. Phoenix. The posthumous papers of D H Lawrence. London: William Heinemann; 1936. p. 769.

[143] Sheets-Johnstone M. The Corporeal Turn: An interdisciplinary reader. Exeter: Imprint Academic; 2009.

[144] Thompson PA. Subversive Bodies: Embodiment as discursive strategy in women's popular literature in the long eighteenth century. PhD Dissertation. Baton Rouge, LA: Department of English, Louisiana State University; 2003.

[145] Grabo C. A Newton among Poets: Shelley's use of science in Prometheus Unbound. Chapel Hill, NC: University of North Carolina Press; 1930.

[146] Balzac H. La Peau de Chagrin (The Magic Skin). 1831. Online. Available: Nalanda Institute of Technology Calicut website http:// www.nalanda.nitc.ac.in/resources/ english/etext-project/balzac/ TheMagicSkin.pdf 18 Jun 2005.

[147] Meyrink G. Der Golem. Ein Roman. Munich, Germany: Kurt Wolff; 1915.

[148] Lawrence DH. Women in Love. Ware, Herts: Wordsworth Classics; 1999.

[149] Okri B. Infinite Riches. London: Phoenix; 1999.

[150] Costantini M. Behind the mask: A study of Ben Okri's fiction. Rome: Carocci; 2002.

[151] Lorca FG. The Duende: Theory and divertissement. 1930. Online. Available: Athenaeum Reading Room website http://evans-experientialism.freewebspace .com/lorca_duende.htm 16 Apr 2010.

[152] Wan MB. Green Peony and the Rise of the Chinese Martial Arts Novel. Albany, NY: State University of New York Press; 2009.

[153] Barfield O. Poetic Diction: A study in meaning. London: Faber & Gwyer; 1928.

[154] Higginson TW. Letter 342a. Johnson TH, editor. 1958 The Letters of Emily Dickinson. Cambridge, MA: Belknap Press of Harvard University Press; 1870. p. 472–4.

[155] Sheets-Johnstone M. The Roots of Thinking. Philadelphia, PA: Temple University Press; 1990. p. 241.

[156] Carroll R. Neuroscience and the 'law of the self': the autonomic nervous system updated, re-mapped and in relationship. Totton N, editor. New Dimensions in Body Psychotherapy. Maidenhead, Berks: Open University Press; 2005. p. 13–29.

[157] Greyson B. Near-death experiences and the physio-kundalini syndrome. J Relig Health 1993;32(4):277–90.

[158] Eliade M. Yoga: Immortality and freedom. London: Routledge & Kegan Paul; 1958.

[159] Onians RB. The Origins of European Thought about the Body, the Mind, the Soul, the World, Time, and Fate. New interpretations of Greek, Roman and kindred evidence also of some basic Jewish and Christian beliefs. New York: Arno Press; 1973.

[160] Euripides. The Bacchae and Other Plays. Harmondsworth, Middx: Penguin; 1973.

[161] Fraser VM, translator. The Songs of Peire Vidal. New York: Peter Lang; 2006.

[162] Wilhelm JJ. translator. The poetry of Arnaut Daniel. New York: Garland; 1981.

[163] Fraser V. The goddess natura in the Occitan lyric. Salisbury JE, editor. The Medieval World of Nature: A book of essays. London: Garland; 1993. p. 129–44.

[164] Lakoff G, Johnson M. Metaphors We Live By. Chicago, IL: University of Chicago Press; 1980.

[165] Lakoff G, Turner M. More than Cool Reason: A field guide to poetic metaphor. Chicago, IL: University of Chicago Press; 1989. p. 52.

[166] Johnson M. The Meaning of the Body: Aesthetics of human understanding. Chicago, IL: University of Chicago Press; 2007.

[167] Johnson M. The Body in the Mind: The bodily basis of meaning, imagination, and reason. Chicago, IL: University of Chicago Press; 1987.

[168] Lakoff G, Johnson M. Philosophy in the Flesh: The embodied mind and its challenge to Western thought. New York: Basic Books; 1999.

[169] Katz R. The Straight Path of the Spirit: Ancestral wisdom and healing traditions in Fiji. Rochester, VT: Park Street Press; 1999.

[170] Jackson M. Paths Toward a Clearing: Radical empiricism and ethnographical inquiry. Bloomington, IN: Indiana University Press; 1989. p. 141, 147.

[171] Fox A. Guarding what is essential: critiques of material culture in Thoreau and Yang Zhu. Philosophy East & West 2008;58(3):358–71.

[172] Stern DN. The Interpersonal World of the Infant. A view from psychoanalysis and developmental psychology. New York: Basic Books; 1985.

[173] Leder D. The Absent Body. Chicago, IL: University of Chicago Press; 1990.

[174] Yuasa Y. The Body: Toward an Eastern mind-body theory. Albany, NY: State University of New York Press; 1987.

[175] Staal F. Indian bodies. Kasulis TP, with Ames RT, Dissanayake W, editors. Self as Body in Asian Theory and Practice. Albany, NY: State University of New York Press; 1993. p. 59–102.

[176] Shamdasani S, editor. The Psychology of Kundalini Yoga: Notes of the seminar given in 1932 by C G Jung. London: Routledge; 1996.

[177] Freud S. The Ego and the Id. 4th ed. London: Hogarth Press; 1947. p. 31.

[178] Berleant A. The sensuous and the sensual in aesthetics. Journal of Aesthetics and Art Criticism 1964;23(2):185–92.

[179] Langer SK. Mind: An essay on human feeling. Abridged edn. Baltimore, MD: Johns Hopkins University Press; 1988

[180] Langer SK. Problems of Art: Ten philosophical lectures. New York: Charles Scribner's Sons; 1957. p. 25.

[181] Graham H. Time, Energy and the Psychology of Healing. London: Jessica Kingsley; 1990.

[182] Hay J. The human body as a microcosmic source of macrocosmic values in calligraphy. Kasulis TP, with Ames RT, Dissanayake W, editors. Self as Body in Asian Theory and Practice. Albany, NY: State University of New York Press; 1993. p. 179–211.

[183] Tu WM. Confucian Thought: Selfhood as creative transformation. Albany, NY: State University of New York Press; 1985. p. 43.

[184] Kaku K. The Mysterious Power of Ki – the force within. Folkestone, Kent: Global Oriental; 2000. p. 10, 318,327.

[185] Barnes LL. Multiple meanings of Chinese healing in the United States. Barnes LL, Sered SS, editors. Religion and Healing in America. Oxford: Oxford University Press; 2005. p. 318.

[186] Lawrence DH. Fantasia of the Unconscious. Harmondsworth, Middx: Penguin; 1971.

[187] Hanegraaff WJ. New Age Religion and Western Culture: Esotericism in the mirror of secular thought. Leiden: E J Brill; 1996.

[188] Krus DJ, Blackman HS. Contributions to psychohistory: V. East-West dimensions of ideology measured by transtemporal cognitive matching. Psychol Rep 1980;47:947–55.

[189] Moore RL. In Search of White Crows: Spiritualism, parapsychology, and American culture. New York: Oxford University Press; 1977.

[190] Turner E. Taking seriously the nature of religious healing in America. Barnes LL, Sered SS, editors. Religion and Healing in America. Oxford: Oxford University Press; 2005. p. 390.

[191] Lewis-Williams D. The Mind in the Cave: Consciousness and the origins of art. London: Thames & Hudson; 2002. p. 121.

[192] Partridge CH. The Re-enchantment Of The West: Alternative spiritualities, sacralization, popular culture, and occulture. vol. 2. London: T & T Clark; 2005. p. 2.

[193] Heelas P, Woodhead L, with Seel B, et al. The Spiritual Revolution: Why

religion is giving way to spirituality. Oxford: Blackwell; 2005. p. 26 27.

[194] Sutcliffe S, Bowman M. Introduction. Sutcliffe S, Bowman M, editors. Beyond New Age: Exploring alternative spirituality. Edinburgh: Edinburgh University Press; 2000. p. 1–13.

[195] Green M. New centres of life. Sutcliffe S, Bowman M, editors. Beyond New Age: Exploring alternative spirituality. Edinburgh: Edinburgh University Press; 2000. p. 63–4.

[196] Otto H, Knight J, editors. Dimensions in Wholistic Healing. Chicago: Nelson-Hall; 1979.

[197] English-Lueck JA. Health in the New Age: A study in Californian holistic practices. Albuquerque, NM: University of New Mexico Press; 1990.

[198] Ferguson M. The Aquarian Conspiracy: Personal and social transformation in the 1980s. London: Granada; 1982.

[199] Fuller R. Alternative Medicine and American Religious Life. New York: Oxford University Press; 1989.

[200] Albanese CL. The subtle energies of spirit: explorations in metaphysical and New Age spirituality. Journal of the American Academy of Religion 1999;67(2):305–25.

[201] Gulmen FM. Energy medicine. Am J Chin Med 2004;32(5):651–8.

[202] Albanese CL. Nature Religion in America: From the Algonkian Indians to the New Age. Chicago, IL: University of Chicago Press; 1990.

[203] Starhawk. The Spiral Dance: A rebirth of the ancient religion of the Great Goddess. San Francisco: Harper and Row; 1979. p. 13, 129.

[204] Scott A. The knowledge in our bones: standpoint theory, alternative health and the quantum model of the body. Maynard M, editor. Science and the Construction of Women. London: UCL Press; 1997. p. 14.

[205] Dutton D. The lived body: changing conceptions of embodiment and their challenge to modern Chinese medicine. European Journal of Oriental Medicine 2009;6(4):43–51.

[206] Johnston J, Barcan R. Subtle transformations: imagining the body in alternative health practices. International Journal of Cultural Studies 2006;9(1):25–44.

[207] European Commission Directorate General Press and Communication. Social Values, Science and Technology. 2005. Special Eurobarometer 225(wave 63.1) Online. Available: http:// ec.europa.eu/public_opinion/ archives/ebs/ebs_225_report_ en.pdf 1 Apr 2010.

[208] McCarthy Brown K. Mama Lola: A Vodou priestess in Brooklyn. Berkeley, CA: University of California Press; 2001.

[209] Taylor C. Milk, Honey, and Money: Changing concepts in Rwandan healing. Washington, DC: Smithsonian Institution Press; 1992.

[210] Heelas P. Introduction: detraditionalization and its rivals. Heelas P, Lash S, Morris P, editors. Detraditionalization: Critical reflections on authority and identity. Oxford: Blackwell; 1996. p. 1–20.

[211] Nüchtern E. Was Alternativmedizin populär macht. Berlin: Evangelische Zentralstelle für Weltanschauungsfragen; 1998.

[212] Nader L. The three-cornered constellation: magic, science, and religion revisited. Nader L, editor. Naked Science: Anthropological inquiry into boundaries, power, and knowledge. London: Routledge; 1996. p. 259–75.

[213] Salk J. The Anatomy of Reality: Merging of intuition and reason. New York: Columbia University Press; 1983.

[214] Puttick E. Personal development: the spiritualisation and secularisation of the human potential movement. Sutcliffe S, Bowman M, editors. Beyond New Age: Exploring alternative spirituality. Edinburgh: Edinburgh University Press; 2000. p. 201–19.

[215] Kenyon J 2004 Subtle energies: a lifetime's scientific quest. Online. Available: Dove Clinic for Integrated Medicine website http://www. doveclinic.com/downloads/Papers/ Subtle%20Energies_lifetime.pdf; 24 Mar 2010.

[216] Scheler M. Lived body, environment, and ego. Spicker SF, editor. The Philosophy of the Body: Rejections of Cartesian dualism. Chicago, IL: Quadrangle Books; 1970. p. 159–86.

[217] Macy J. Working through environmental despair. Roszak T, Gomes ME, Kanner AD, editors. Ecopsychology: Restoring the earth, healing the mind. San Francisco, CA: Sierra Club; 1995. p. 253.

[218] Drengson A, Devall B, editors. Ecology of Wisdom: Writings by Arne Næss. Berkeley, CA: Counterpoint; 2008.

[219] Turner E. The Hands Feel It: Healing and spirit presence among a northern Alaskan people. DeKalb, IL: Northern Illinois University Press; 1996.

[220] Desjarlais RR. Body and Emotion: The aesthetics of illness and healing in the Nepal Himalayas. Philadelphia, PA: University of Pennsylvania Press; 1992.

[221] Aizenstat S. Jungian psychology and the world unconscious. Roszak T, Gomes ME, Kanner AD, editors. Ecopsychology: Restoring the earth, healing the mind. San Francisco, CA: Sierra Club; 1995. p. 96.

[222] McVay S. Prelude: 'A Siamese connexion with a plurality of other mortals'. Kellert SR, Wilson EO, editors. The Biophilia Hypothesis. Washington DC: Shearwater Books; 1993. p. 4.

[223] Harding S. Animate Earth. Science, intuition and Gaia. Dartington, Devon: Green Books; 2006. p. 21.

[224] Glendinning C. Technology, trauma, and the wild. Roszak T, Gomes ME, Kanner AD, editors. Ecopsychology: Restoring the earth, healing the mind. San Francisco, CA: Sierra Club; 1995. p. 41–54.

[225] Macy J. The ecological self: postmodern ground for right action. Griffin DR, editor. Sacred Interconnections: Postmodern spirituality, political economy, and art. Albany, NY: State University of New York Press; 1990. p. 35–48.

[226] Orr DW. Love it or lose it: the coming biophilia revolution. Kellert SR, Wilson EO, editors. The Biophilia Hypothesis. Washington, DC: Shearwater Books; 1993. p. 415–40.

[227] Lovelock JE. Gaia: A new look at life on earth. Oxford: Oxford University Press; 1979.

[228] Graves T. Needles of Stone. London: Turnstone; 1978.

[229] Skinner S. The Living Earth Manual of Feng-shui: Chinese geomancy. London: Routledge & Kegan Paul; 1982.

[230] Gomes ME, Kanner AD. The rape of the well-maidens. Roszak T, Gomes ME, Kanner AD, editors. Ecopsychology: Restoring the earth, healing the mind. San Francisco, CA: Sierra Club; 1995. p. 111–21.

[231] Weiss G. Body Images: Embodiment as intercorporeality. London: Routledge; 1999.

[232] Bynum CW. The Resurrection of the Body in Western Christianity, 200–1336. New York: Columbia University Press; 1995. p. 113.

[233] Grosz E. Volatile Bodies: Toward a Corporeal Feminism. Bloomington IN: Indiana University Press; 1994. p. 203.

[234] Shilling C. The Body and Social Theory. London: Sage; 1993.

[235] Keller C. Warriors, women, and the nuclear complex: toward a postnuclear postmodernity. Griffin DR, editor. Sacred Interconnections: Postmodern spirituality, political economy, and art. Albany, NY: State University of New York Press; 1990. p. 63–82.

[236] Daly M. Pure Lust: Elemental feminist philosophy. London: Women's Press; 1984.

[237] Nelson LA, Schwartz GE. Human biofield and intention detection: individual differences. J Altern Complement Med 2005;11(1):93–101.

[238] Thalbourne MA, Fox B. Paranormal and mystical experience: the role of panic attacks and kundalini. Journal of the American Society for Psychical Research 1999;93(1):99–115.

[239] Klosterhalfen S, Enck P. Neurophysiology and psychobiology of the placebo response. Curr Opin Psychiatry 2008;21(2):189–95.

[240] Canter PH, Brown LB, Greaves C, et al. Johrei family healing: a pilot study. Evidence-based Complementary and Alternative Medicine 2006;3(4):533–40.

[241] Winter A. Mesmerized: Powers of mind in Victorian Britain. Chicago, IL: University of Chicago Press; 1998.

[242] Barnes PM, Powell-Griner E, McFann K, et al. Complementary and alternative medicine use among

adults: United States, 2002. Advance Data from Vital and Health Statistics (343). Hyattsville, MD: National Center for Health Statistics; 2004. Online. Available: http://nccam.nih.gov/news/camstats/2002/report.pdf 24 Mar 2010.

[243] Walker K. Nursing, gender, aporia. Contem Nurse 2009;33(2):163–5.

[244] Gevitz N, editor. Other Healers: Unorthodox medicine in America. Baltimore, MD: Johns Hopkins University Press; 1988.

[245] Palmer DA. La fièvre du Qigong: Guérison, religion et politique en Chine, 1949–1999. Paris: École des Hautes Études en Sciences Sociales; 2005.

[246] Cooke PA, Klopf D, Ishii S. Perceptions of world view among Japanese and American university students: a cross-cultural comparison. Communication Research Reports 1991;8(2):81–8.

[247] Dean K. Lord of the Three in One: The spread of a cult in Southeast China. Princeton, NJ: Princeton University Press; 1989. p. 7.

[248] Conrad E. Continuum movement. Totton N, editor. New Dimensions in Body Psychotherapy. Maidenhead, Berkshire: Open University Press; 2005. p. 144.

[249] White DG. The Alchemical Body: Siddha traditions in medieval India. Chicago IL: University of Chicago Press; 1996.

[250] Taylor CC. Sacrifice as Terror: The Rwandan genocide of 1994. Oxford: Berg; 1999.

[251] Bastien JW. Qollahuaya-Andean body concepts: a topographical-hydraulic model of physiology. American Anthropologist NS 1985;87(3):595–611.

[252] Crisp T. Relax with Yoga. London: Sphere; 1978.

[253] Jonas WB. Magic and methodology: when paradigms clash. Guest editorial. J Altern Complement Med 1999;5(4):319–21.

[254] Chen NN. Breathing Spaces: Qigong, psychiatry, and healing in China. New York: Columbia University Press; 2003.

[255] Xu J. Body, discourse, and the cultural politics of contemporary Chinese qigong. Journal of Asian Studies 1999;58(4):961–91.

[256] Zhang HH, Baker G. Think Like Chinese. Leichhardt, New South Wales: Federation Press; 2008.

[257] Weller RP. Resistance, Chaos and Control in China: Taiping rebels, Taiwanese ghosts and Tiananmen. Basingstoke, Hants: Macmillan; 1994.

[258] Farquhar J, Zhang QC. Biopolitical Beijing: pleasure, sovereignty, and self-cultivation in China's capital. Cultural Anthropology 2005;20(3):303–27.

[259] Grosz E. Space, Time, and Perversion. London: Routledge; 1995.

[260] Coward R. The Whole Truth: The myth of alternative health. London: Faber & Faber; 1989.

[261] Hahn RA. Sickness and Healing: An anthropological perspective. New Haven, CT: Yale University Press; 1995.

4. THE ANATOMICAL FOUNDATIONS OF QI

[1] Keleman S. Emotional Anatomy. Berkeley, CA: Center Press; 1985.

[2] Kaptchuk T. The Web That Has No Weaver. New York: Congdon & Weed; 1992.

[3] Beinfield H, Korngold E. Between Heaven and Earth. New York: Ballantine Books; 1991.

[4] Sheldon H. Boyd's Introduction to the Study of Disease. Philadelphia: Lea & Febiger; 1984.

[5] Brennan B. Hands of Light. New York: Bantam Books; 1987.

[6] Targ R, Katra J. Miracles of Mind. Novato, CA: New World Library; 1998.

[7] Maxwell JC. A dynamical theory of the electromagnetic field. Philos Trans R Soc Lond B Biol Sci 1865;155:459–512.

[8] Gerber R. Vibrational Medicine for the 21st Century: A complete guide to energy healing and spiritual transformation. New York: Eagle Brook; 2000.

[9] Gerber R. Vibrational Medicine: New choices for healing ourselves. Santa Fe, NM: Bear; 1988.

[10] Dobrin R, Conway B, Pierrakos J. Instrumental Measurements of the Human Energy Field. New York: Institute for New Age; 1978.

[11] Eddington A. The Philosophy of Physical Science. Ann Arbor, MI: University of Michigan Press; 1958.

[12] Barrow JD. New Theories of Everything: The quest for ultimate

explanation. New York: Oxford University Press; 2007.

[13] Capra F. Tao of Physics. Boston, MA: Shambhala; 1991.

[14] Cohen MR, Doner K. The Chinese Way of Healing. New York: Berkley; 1996.

[15] Hanegraaff WJ. New Age Religion and Western Culture: Esotericism in the mirror of secular thought. Leiden, Netherlands: E J Brill; 1996.

[16] Bohm D. Wholeness and the Implicate Order. London: Routledge Classics; 1980.

[17] Hall DL, Ames RT. Anticipating China: Thinking through the narratives of Chinese and Western culture. Albany, NY: State University of New York Press; 1995.

[18] Manning CA, Vanrenen LJ. Bioenergetic Medicine. Berkeley, CA: North Atlantic Books; 1988.

[19] Maciocia G. The Foundations of Chinese Medicine: A comprehensive text for acupuncturists and herbalists. 2nd ed. Edinburgh: Churchill Livingstone; 2005.

[20] Leskowitz R. Energy medicine 101: subtle anatomy and physiology. Integrative Medicine 2006;5(4):30–4.

[21] Manaka Y, Itaya K, Birch S. Chasing The Dragon's Tail: The theory and practice of acupuncture in the work of Yoshio Manaka. Brookline, MA: Paradigm; 1995.

[22] Oschman JL. Energy Medicine: The scientific basis. Edinburgh: Churchill Livingstone; 2000.

[23] Palmer DD. The Science, Art, and Philosophy of Chiropractic. Portland, OR: Portland Printing House Company; 1910.

[24] Baldwin D. Odic Energy. Lyons, CO: Odic Energy Research Institute; 2007.

[25] Stump J. The Theory and Philosophy of Acupuncture. Teaching Manual, vol. 1. Delmar, DE: Sportec International; 1975. p. 71.

[26] Harpur T. The Uncommon Touch: An investigation of spiritual healing. Toronto: McCelland & Stewart; 1994.

[27] Moyers B. Healing and the Mind. New York: Doubleday; 2001. p. 45.

[28] Eden D, Feinstein D. Energy Medicine: Balancing your body's energy for optimal health, joy, and vitality. New York: Penguin Group; 2008.

[29] Hunt V. Electronic evidence of auras, chakras in UCLA study. Brain/Mind Bulletin 1978;3(9):1–2.

[30] Leadbeater CW. The Chakras: A monograph. Wheaton, IL: Theosophical Publishing House; 1927 (1973).

[31] Karagulla S, van Gelder Kunz D. The Chakras and the Human Energy Fields. Wheaton, IL: Theosophical Publishing House; 1989.

[32] Myss C. Anatomy of the Spirit: The seven stages of power and healing. New York: Three Rivers Press; 1996.

[33] Judith A. Eastern Body, Western Mind: Psychology and the chakra system as a path to the self. Berkeley, CA: Celestial Arts; 2004.

[34] Cross J. The Chakra energy system. Charman RA, editor. Complementary Therapies for Physical Therapists. Oxford: Butterworth-Heinemann; 2000. p. 78–93.

[35] Greenwood M. Acupuncture and the chakras. Medical Acupuncture 2006;17(3):27–32.

[36] Boadella D. Lifestreams: An introduction to Biosynthesis. London: Routledge & Kegan Paul; 1987.

[37] Motoyama H. Karma and Reincarnation: The key to spiritual evolution and enlightenment. London: Judy Piatkus; 1992.

[38] Motoyama H. Theories of the Chakras: Bridge to higher consciousness. Wheaton, IL: Theosophical Publishing House; 1981.

[39] Majumdar B. History of Indian Social and Political ideas, from Rammohan to Dayananda. Calcutta: Bookland; 1967.

[40] Deadman P, Al-Khafaji M, Baker K. A Manual of Acupuncture. Hove: Journal of Chinese Medicine Publications; 2001.

[41] Ross J. Zang Fu. Edinburgh: Churchill Livingstone; 1985.

[42] Rothfeld GS, Levert S. The Acupuncture Response. New York: Contemporary Books; 2002.

[43] Ellis A, Wiseman N, Boss K. Fundamentals of Chinese Acupuncture. Brookline, MA: Paradigm Publications; 1991.

[44] Cassidy CM, editor. Contemporary Acupuncture. New York: Churchill Livingstone; 2002.

[45] Matsumoto K, Birch S. Extraordinary Vessels. Brookline, MA: Paradigm; 1986.

[46] Mei JH. The extraordinary channel chong mai and its clinical applications. Journal of Chinese Medicine 1993;(43)27–31.

[47] Stump J. The Theory and Philosophy of Acupuncture. Teaching Manual, vol. 3. Delmar, DE: Sportec International; 1985.

[48] Soh KS, Choi SM. Recent progress in Bonghan system research. Journal of the International Society of Life Information Science 2005;23(2):280–5.

[49] Wei HF, Hung LCL, Kong J. The substrate and properties of meridians: a review of modern research. Acupunct Med 1999;17(2):134–9.

[50] Myers TW. Anatomy Trains: Myofascial meridians for manual and movement therapists. 2nd ed. New York: Churchill Livingstone; 2009.

[51] Langevin HM, Yandow JA. Relationship of acupuncture points and meridians to connective tissue planes. Anat Rec 2002;269(6):257–65.

[52] Lee JK, Bae SK. Acupuncture. Seoul: Sam Wha Publishing; 1978.

[53] Stump J. The Theory and Philosophy of Acupuncture. Teaching Manual, vol. 2. Delmar, DE: Sportec International; 1981.

[54] Gerwin R. Differential diagnosis of trigger points. Journal of Musculoskeletal Pain 2005;12(3–4):23–8.

[55] Yan ZG. Anatomical Atlas of Acupuncture Points: A photo location guide. St Albans, Herts: Donica Publishing; 2003.

[56] Chen E. Cross-Sectional Anatomy of Acupoints. Edinburgh: Churchill Livingstone; 1995.

[57] Heine H. Anatomical structure of acupoints. J Tradit Chin Med 1988;8(3):207–12.

[58] Mayor DF. The Chinese back shu and front mu points and their segmental innervation. Deutsche Zeitschrift für Akupunktur/German Journal of Acupuncture and Related Techniques 2008;51(2):26–36.

[59] Shang C. Prospective tests on biological models of acupuncture. Evidence-based Complementary and Alternative Medicine 2009;6(1):31–9.

[60] Lo V. The Influence of Yangsheng Culture on Early Chinese Medical Theory. Thesis submitted for the degree of Doctor of Philosophy of the University of London. 1998.

[61] Epler Jr DC. Bloodletting in early Chinese medicine and its relation to the origin of acupuncture. Bull Hist Med 1980;54(3):337–67.

5. *QI* IN CHINA'S TRADITIONAL MEDICINE: THE EXAMPLE OF *TUINA*

[1] Kleinman A. Social Origins of Distress and Disease: Depression, neurasthenia, and pain in modern China. New Haven, CT: Yale University Press; 1986.

[2] Wiseman N, Boss K. Glossary of Chinese Medical Terms and Acupuncture Points. Brookline, MA: Paradigm Publications; 1990.

[3] Wiseman N, Ellis A. Fundamentals of Chinese Medicine. Brookline, MA: Paradigm Publications; 1995.

[4] Wong CK, Wu TL. History of Chinese Medicine: Being a chronicle of medical happenings in China from ancient times to the present period. Taipei, Taiwan: Southern Materials Center; 1985.

[5] Sivin N. Huang ti nei ching 黃帝內經. Loewe M, editor. Early Chinese Texts: A bibliographical guide. Berkeley, CA: University of California Press; 1993. p. 196–215.

[6] Unschuld PU. Medicine in China: A history of ideas. Berkeley, CA: University of California Press; 1985.

[7] Chuang YM. The Historical Development of Acupuncture. Los Angeles, CA: Oriental Healing Arts Institute; 1982.

[8] Wang XT. A research on the origin and development of Chinese acupuncture and moxibustion. In: National Symposia of Acupuncture and Moxibustion and Acupuncture Anaesthesia. Beijing, 1–5 June 1979. p. 121–3.

[9] Lloyd G, Sivin N. The Way and the Word: Science and medicine in early China and Greece. New Haven, CT: Yale University Press; 2002.

[10] Maciocia G. The Foundations of Chinese Medicine: A comprehensive text for acupuncturists and herbalists. 2nd ed. Edinburgh: Churchill Livingstone; 2005.

[11] Wang GC, Fan YL, Guan Z. Chinese Massage. Shanghai: Shanghai College of Traditional Chinese Medicine; 1990.

[12] Engelhardt U. Qi for life: longevity in the Tang. Kohn L, editor. Taoist Meditation and Longevity Techniques. Ann Arbor, MI: Center for Chinese Studies, University of Michigan; 1989. p. 263–96.

[13] Zhang EQ. Clinic of Traditional Chinese Medicine. Shanghai: Shanghai

College of Traditional Chinese Medicine; 1990.

[14] Despeux C. Gymnastics: the ancient tradition. Kohn L, editor. Taoist Meditation and Longevity Techniques. Ann Arbor, MI: Center for Chinese Studies, University of Michigan; 1989. p. 225–61.

[15] Watson B. The Complete Works of Chuang Tzu. New York: Columbia University Press; 1968.

[16] Eckman P. In the Footsteps of the Yellow Emperor: Tracing the history of traditional acupuncture. San Francisco, CA: Cypress Books; 1996.

[17] Ergil KV, Micozzi MS. Qi gong and tui na. Coughlin P, editor. Principles and Practice of Manual Therapies. Edinburgh: Churchill Livingstone; 2002. p. 165–72.

6. *QI* CULTIVATION IN *QIGONG* AND *TAIJI QUAN*

[1] Li DC. The Book of Balance and Harmony [Cleary T, Trans.]. Boston, MA: Shambhala; 1989.

[2] Maciocia G. The Psyche in Chinese Medicine: Treatment of emotional and mental disharmonies with acupuncture and Chinese herbs. Edinburgh: Churchill Livingstone; 2009.

[3] Johnson JA. Chinese Medical Qigong Therapy. vol. 4. Pacific Grove, CA: International Institute of Medical Qigong; 2002. p. 99–100, 441, 442, 437.

[4] van Lysebeth A. Tantra: The cult of the feminine. York Beach, ME: Samuel Weiser; 1995.

[5] Hsu A. The Sword Polisher's Record: The way of kung-fu. Boston, MA: Tuttle Martial Arts; 1998.

[6] Lü TP. The Secret of the Golden Flower: The classic Chinese book of life [Cleary T, Trans.]. San Francisco, CA: HarperSanFrancisco; 1991. p. 10.

[7] Chuen LK. The Way of Healing: Chi Kung. New York: Broadway Books; 1999.

[8] Sim DSV, Gaffney D. Chen Style Taijiquan: The source of taiji boxing. Berkeley, CA: North Atlantic Books; 2002. p. 29, 101.

[9] Li DC. The Book of Balance and Harmony [Cleary T, Trans.] Boston, MA: Shambhala; 1989.

[10] Johnson JA. Chinese Medical Qigong Therapy. vol. 1. Pacific Grove, CA:

International Institute of Medical Qigong; 2002. p. 207.

[11] Lu KY. Taoist Yoga: Alchemy and immortality. New York: Samuel Weiser; 1980.

[12] Yang JM. Tai Chi Chuan Martial Applications. Wolfeboro, NH: YMAA Publication Center; 1996. p. 326.

[13] Jou TH. The Dao of Taijiquan: Way to rejuvenation. Warwick, NY: Tai Chi Foundation; 1998. p. 177.

[14] Liao WS, translator. The Tai Chi Classics. New York: Shambhala; 1990.

[15] Wong E, translator. Harmonizing Yin and Yang: The dragon-tiger classic. A manual of Taoist yoga: Internal, external, and sexual. Boston, MA: Shambhala; 1997.

7. *QIGONG* THEORY AND RESEARCH

[1] Ai AL, Peterson C, Gillespie B, et al. Designing clinical trials on energy healing: ancient art encounters medical science. Altern Ther Health Med 2001;7(4):83–90.

[2] Ai AL. Assessing mental health in clinical study on qigong: between scientific investigation and holistic perspectives. Seminars in Integrative Medicine 2003;1(2):112–21.

[3] Ai AL. Qi gong. Micozzi MS, editor. Fundamentals of Complementary and Alternative Medicine. 4th ed. St Louis, MO: Saunders; 2011. p. 438–54.

[4] Ai AL. Psychosocial adjustment and health care practices following coronary artery bypass surgery (CABG). PhD Dissertation, University of Michigan; 1996.

[5] Capra F. The Tao of Physics: An exploration of the parallels between modern physics and Eastern mysticism. 3rd ed. Boston, MA: Shambhala; 1991. p. 281.

[6] Rosenthal S, translator. Tao Te Ching. Feb 2006. Online. Available: Taoism Virtual Library website http://www.vl-site.org/taoism/ttcstan3.html. 17 Nov 2010.

[7] Peng K, Nisbett EN. Culture, dialectics, and reasoning about contradiction. Am Psychol 1999;54:741–54.

[8] Plato. A Bloom, translator. The Republic of Plato: Translated with notes and an interpretive essay. New York: Basic Books; 1968.

[9] Crosby DA. A Religion of Nature. Albany, NY: State University of New York Press; 2002.

[10] Maciocia G. The Psyche in Chinese Medicine: Treatment of emotional and mental disharmonies with acupuncture and Chinese herbs. Edinburgh: Churchill Livingstone; 2009.

[11] Yuan CH. Chinese medicine is not the abbreviation of the medicine of China: I-Ching expert Lui Dajun's definition of Chinese medicine. Chinese News [Zhongguo Xin Wen] 1997;28:23.

[12] Garrison FH. History of Medicine. Philadelphia, PA: W B Saunders; 1966.

[13] Ng BH, Tsang HW. Psychophysiological outcomes of health qigong for chronic conditions: a systematic review. Psychophysiology 2009;46(2):257–69.

[14] Rogers CE, Larkey LK, Keller C. A review of clinical trials of tai chi and qigong in older adults. West J Nurs Res 2009;31(2):245–79.

[15] Lee MS, Lee MS, Kim HJ, et al. Effects of qigong on blood pressure, high-density lipoprotein cholesterol and other lipid levels in essential hypertension patients. Int J Neurosci 2004;114(7):777–86.

[16] Lee MS, Lim HJ, Lee MS. Impact of qigong exercise on self efficacy and other cognitive perceptual variables in patients with essential hypertension. J Altern Complement Med 2004;10(4):675–80.

[17] Lee MS, Lee MS, Choi ES, et al. Effects of qigong on blood pressure determinants and ventilatory function in middle-aged patients with essential hypertension. Am J Chin Med 2003;31(3):489–97.

[18] Lee MS, Lee MS, Kim HJ, et al. Qigong reduced blood pressure and catecholamine levels of patients with essential hypertension. Int J Neurosci 2003;113(12):1691–701.

[19] Cheung BM, Lo JL, Fong DY, et al. Randomised controlled trial of qigong in the treatment of mild essential hypertension. J Hum Hypertens 2005;19(9):697–704.

[20] Liu X, Miller YD, Burton NW, et al. A preliminary study of the effects of Tai Chi and Qigong medical exercise on indicators of metabolic syndrome, glycaemic control, health related quality of life, and psychological health in adults with elevated blood glucose. Br J Sports Med 2009;43(11):840–94.

[21] Liu JR, Jiang XJ, Xia XW, et al. Influences of badua njin on the metabolism of high-density lipoprotein, low-density lipoprotein, total cholesterol and triglyceride. Chinese Journal of Gerontology [Zhongguo Laonian Xue Zazhi] 2006;26(3):317–9.

[22] Iwao M, Kajiyama S, Mori H, et al. Effects of qigong walking on diabetic patients: a pilot study. J Altern Complement Med 1999;5(4):353–8.

[23] Tsujiuchi T, Kumano H, Yoshiuchi K, et al. The effect of qi-gong relaxation exercise on the control of type 2 diabetes mellitus: a randomized controlled trial. Diabetes Care 2002;25(1):241–2.

[24] Pippa L, Manzoli L, Corti I, et al. Functional capacity after traditional Chinese medicine (qi gong) training in patients with chronic atrial fibrillation: a randomized controlled trial. Prev Cardiol 2007;10(1):22–5.

[25] Stenlund T, Ahlgren C, Lindahl B, et al. Cognitively oriented behavioral rehabilitation in combination with qigong for patients on long-term sick leave because of burnout: REST – a randomized clinical trial. Int J Behav Med 2009;16(3):294–303.

[26] Du SW, Cheng QL, Wang H, et al. The effects of health qigong yi jin jing on cardiac function of the elderly. Chinese Journal of Sports Medicine [Zhongguo Yundong Yixue Zazhi] 2006;25(6):721–2.

[27] Wang YN, Shi JF, Tan P, et al. Ultrasound evaluation of cardiac function of the elderly upon the practice of health qigong yi jin jing. Chinese Journal of Ultrasound Diagnosis [Zhongguo Chaosheng Zhenduan Zazhi] 2006;7(10):762–83.

[28] Xu GH. Study on the rehabilitating effects of respiration qigong on the COPD patients. Nanfang Journal of Nursing [Nanfang Huli Zazhi] 2000;7(6):2–4.

[29] Mannerkorpi K, Arndorw M. Efficacy and feasibility of a combination of body awareness therapy and qigong in patients with fibromyalgia: a pilot study. J Rehabil Med 2004;36(6):279–81.

[30] Astin JA, Berman BM, Bausell B, et al. The efficacy of mindfulness meditation plus Qigong movement therapy in the treatment of fibromyalgia: a

randomized controlled trial.
J Rheumatol 2003;30(10):2257–62.

[31] Tsang HWH, Mok CK, Au Yeung YT, et al. The effect of qigong on general and psychosocial health of elderly with chronic physical illnesses: a randomized clinical trial. Int J Geriatr Psychiatry 2003;18(5):441–9.

[32] Tsai YK, Chen HH, Lin IH, et al. Qigong improving physical status in middle-aged women. West J Nurs Res 2008;30(8):915–27.

[33] Wenneberg S, Gunnarsson LG, Ahlstrom G. Using a novel exercise programme for patients with muscular dystrophy. Part II: A quantitative study. Disabil Rehabil 2004;26(10):595–602.

[34] Yang Y, Verkuilen J, Rosengren KS, et al. Effect of combined taiji and qigong training on balance mechanisms: A randomized controlled trial of older adults. Med Sci Monit 2007;13(8):CR339–48.

[35] Schmitz-Hübsch T, Pyfer D, Kielwein K, et al. Qigong exercise for the symptoms of Parkinson's disease: A randomized, controlled pilot study. Mov Disord 2006;21(4):543–8.

[36] Chen HH, Yeh ML, Lee F. The effects of baduanjin qigong in the prevention of bone loss for middle-aged women. Am J Chin Med 2006;34(5):741–7.

[37] Manzaneque JM, Vera FM, Maldonado EF, et al. Assessment of immunological parameters following a qigong training program. Med Sci Monit 2004;10(6):264–70.

[38] Lee MS, Huh HJ, Jeong SM, et al. Effects of qigong on immune cells. Am J Chin Med 2003;31(2):327–35.

[39] Lee MS, Kang CW, Ryu H. Acute effect of qi-training on natural killer cell subsets and cytotoxic activity. Int J Neurosci 2005;115(2):285–97.

[40] Yang Y, Verkuilen J, Rosengren KS, et al. Effects of a taiji and qigong intervention on the antibody response to influenza vaccine in older adults. Am J Chin Med 2007;35(4):597–607.

[41] Tsang HWH, Fung KMT, Chan ASM, et al. Effect of a qigong exercise program on elderly with depression. Int J Geriatr Psychiatry 2006;21(9):890–7.

[42] Zhang WC, Zhong ZB, Wu QH. A research on health qigong yi jin jing for slowing down intelligence decline of the aged. Chinese Journal of Behavioral Medical Science [Zhongguo Xingwei Yixue Kexue] 2006;15(9):827–8.

[43] Li M, Chen K, Mo ZX. Use of qigong therapy in the detoxification of heroin addicts. Altern Ther Health Med 2002;8(1):50–4, 56, 59.

[44] Chen K, Perlman A, Liao J, et al. Effects of external qigong therapy on osteoarthritis of the knee. Clin Rheumatol 2008;27(12):1497–505.

[45] Wu WH, Bandilla E, Ciccone DS, et al. Effects of qigong on late-stage complex regional pain syndrome. Altern Ther Health Med 1999;5(1):45–54.

[46] Jang HS, Lee MS. Effects of qi therapy (external qigong) on premenstrual syndrome: a randomized placebo-controlled study. J Altern Complement Med 2004;10(3):456–62.

SECTION 3 INTRODUCTION

[1] Albanese CL. Nature Religion in America: From the Algonkian Indians to the New Age. Chicago, IL: University of Chicago Press; 1990.

8. THE LANGUAGE OF *QI*, QUANTUM PHYSICS AND THE SUPERIMPLICATE BODY

[1] Whorf BL. Language, Thought and Reality. Cambridge, MA: MIT Press; 1956.

[2] Sabbadini SA. Tao Te Ching: Una guida all'interpretazione del libro fondamentale del taoismo. Milan: Urra; 2009.

[3] Tsu Lao. Tao Te Ching: A new translation by Gia-Fu Feng and Jane English. London: Wildwood House; 1973.

[4] Leibniz's Philosophy of Mind. Stanford Encyclopedia of Philosophy. 2007. Online. Available: http://plato.stanford.edu/entries/leibniz-mind 13 Oct 2009.

[5] Slater JG, editor. Collected Papers of Bertrand Russell, vol. 8. The Philosophy of Logical Atomism and Other Essays (1914–1919). London: Allen & Unwin; 1986.

[6] Wittgenstein L. Tractatus Logico-philosophicus. London: Routledge; 2001.

[7] Wittgenstein L. Philosophical Investigations. Hoboken, NJ: Wiley Blackwell; 2009.

[8] Wheeler JA, Zurek WH. Quantum Theory and Measurement. Princeton, NJ: Princeton University Press; 1983.

[9] Bohm D. Wholeness and the Implicate Order. London: Routledge; 2002.

[10] David Peat FD. Blackfoot Physics: A journey into the Native American universe. Newberryport, MI: Red Wheel/Weiser; 2005.

[11] Bohm D, Peat FD. Science, Order and Creativity. London: Routledge; 2000.

[12] Peat FD. Pathways of Chance. Pari, Tuscany: Pari Publishing; 2007.

[13] Bohm D. A new theory of the relationship of mind and matter. Philosophical Psychology 1990;3(2):271–86.

[14] Peat FD. Gentle Action: Bringing creative change to a turbulent world. Pari, Tuscany: Pari Publishing; 2008.

[15] Bohm D, Hiley BJ. The Undivided Universe. London: Routledge; 1993.

9. *QI* AND THE FREQUENCIES OF BIOELECTRICITY

[1] Fröhlich H. Coherence in biology. Fröhlich H, Kremer F, editors. Coherent Excitations in Biological Systems. BerlSpringer; 1983. p. 1–5.

[2] Fröhlich H. Theoretical physics and biology. Fröhlich H, editor. Biological Coherence and Response to External Stimuli. BerlSpringer; 1988. p. 1–24.

[3] Smith CW. Fröhlich's interpretation of biology through theoretical physics. Hyland GJ, Rowlands P, editors. Herbert Fröhlich FRS: A physicist ahead of his time. 2nd ed. Liverpool: University of Liverpool; 2008. p. 107–54.

[4] Smith CW, Best S. Electromagnetic Man: Health and hazard in the electrical environment. Dent, London: 1989.

[5] Arani R, Bono I, del Giudice E, et al. QED coherence and the thermodynamics of water. International Journal of Modern Physics B 1995;9(15):1813–41.

[6] Smith CW. Coherent frequencies, consciousness and the laws of life. In: Proceedings of the 9th International Conference on Computing Anticipatory Systems. HEC-ULg, Liège, Belgium, 3–8 August 2009. Abstract: CASYS '09 Symposium 10, 2009. p. 17.

[7] Milani M, del Giudice E, Doglia S, et al. Superconductive and Josephson-like behaviour of cells. Radiologica Medica 1991;81(4 Suppl. 1):51–5.

[8] Smith CW. Electromagnetic and magnetic vector potential bio-information and water. Endler PC, Schulte J, editors. Ultra High Dilution: Physiology and physics. Dordrecht, Netherlands: Kluwer Academic; 1994. p. 187–202.

[9] Marcer P, Schempp W. The brain as a conscious system. International Journal of General Systems 1998;27(1–3):231–48.

[10] Smith CW. Homeopathy – How It Works and How It Is Done, chs 1–7. Homeopathic Research (Hpathy Ezine). Jan–July. 2008. Online. Available: www.hpathy.com/ezine 17 Nov 2010.

[11] Jafary-Asl AH, Solanki SN, Aarholt E, et al. Dielectric measurements on live biological materials under magnetic resonance conditions. Journal of Biological Physics 1983;11(1):15–22.

[12] Aarholt E, Jaberansari J, Jafary-Asl AH, et al. NMR conditions and biological systems. Marino AA, editor. Modern Bioelectricity. New York: Marcel Dekker; 1990. p. 75–104.

[13] Smith CW. Water – its clinical and scientific depths. Emoto M, editor. The Healing Power of Water. London: Hay House; 2007. p. 77–88.

[14] Smith CW. Correspondence: dowsing as a quantum phenomenon. Frontier Perspectives 2004;13(1):4–6.

[15] Smith CW. Can homeopathy ameliorate ongoing sickness? J Altern Complement Med 2009;15(5):465–7.

[16] Smith CW. Bioluminescence, coherence and biocommunication. Jezowska-Trzebiatowska B, Kochel B, Slawinski J, et al., editors. Biological Luminescence. Singapore: World Scientific; 1990. p. 3–18.

[17] Kenyon JN. Modern Techniques of Acupuncture, vol 3. A critical review of the latest developments in European and Japanese acupuncture. London: Thorsons; 1985.

[18] Bechtloff F. Elektroakupunktur nach Voll – Eine Darstellung in Bereichen. Uelzen: Medizinisch Literarische Verlag; 1991.

[19] Tiller WA. Psychoenergetic Science: A second Copernican revolution. Walnut Creek, CA: Pavior; 2007.

[20] Jahn RG, Dunne B. Sensors, filters, and the source of reality. Journal of Scientific Exploration 2004;18(4):547–70.

[21] Smith CW. Effects of electromagnetic fields in the living environment. Proceedings of the International Conference on Electromagnetic Environments and Health in Buildings, Royal College of Physicians, London, England, 16–17 May 2002. Clements-Croome D, editor. Electromagnetic Environments and Health in Buildings. London: Taylor & Francis; 2003. p. 53–118.

[22] Rowlands P. Zero to Infinity. Singapore: World Scientific; 2007.

[23] Hicks J, Hicks A, Mole P. Five Element Constitutional Acupuncture. Edinburgh: Churchill Livingstone; 2004.

[24] Qigong master projecting his chi energy. Online. Available: YouTube website http://www.youtube.com/watch?v=nu99GRUUN6Y 17 Nov 2010.

10. SYSTEMS THEORY: TRAPPING AND MAPPING HEALING WITH *QI*

[1] Turner JA, Deyo RA, Loeser JD, et al. The importance of placebo effects in pain treatment and research. J Am Med Assoc 1994;271(20):1609–14.

[2] Latey P. Placebo responses in bodywork. Peters D, editor. Understanding the Placebo Effect in Complementary Medicine: Theory, practice and research. 1st ed. Edinburgh: Churchill Livingstone; 2001. p. 147–63.

[3] Radin D. The Conscious Universe: The scientific truth of psychic phenomena. 1st ed. New York: HarperEdge; 1997.

[4] Targ R, Puthoff HE. Information transmission under conditions of sensory shielding. Nature 1974;251(5476):602–7.

[5] Seto A, Kusaka C, Nakazato S, et al. Detection of extraordinary large bio-magnetic field strength from human hand during external Qi emission. Acupunct Electrother Res 1992;17(2):75–94.

[6] Larre C, Schatz J, Rochat de la Vallée E Survey of Traditional Chinese Medicine. 1st ed. Columbia, MD: Institut Ricci and Traditional Acupuncture Foundation; 1986.

[7] Low C. Perfectly organised chaos: acupuncture as the model for a mediating function in therapeutics. European Journal of Oriental Medicine 1996;2(1):18–25.

[8] Miura K. The revival of qi: qigong in contemporary China. Kohn L, editor. Taoist Meditation and Longevity Techniques. 1st ed. Ann Arbor, MI: University of Michigan Press; 1989. p. 331–62.

[9] Schipper K. The Taoist Body. Berkeley, CA: University of California Press; 1993.

[10] Despeux C. Gymnastics: the ancient tradition. Kohn L, editor. Taoist Meditation and Longevity Techniques. 3rd ed. Ann Arbor, MI: University of Michigan Press; 1989. p. 225–61.

[11] Kohn L. Taoist Mystical Philosophy. 1st ed. Albany, NY: State University of New York Press; 1991.

[12] Kohn L. Physical practices: gymnastics. Kohn L, editor. The Daoist Experience: An anthology. 1st ed. Albany, NY: State University of New York Press; 1993. p. 142–8.

[13] Jiao GR. Qigong Essential for Health Promotion. Beijing: China Reconstructs; 1990.

[14] Cohen KS. Qigong: The art and science of Chinese energy healing. New York: Ballantine Books; 1997.

[15] Glass L, Mackey MC. Pathological conditions resulting from instabilities in physiological control systems. Ann N Y Acad Sci 1979;316:214–35.

[16] Goldberger AL. Fractals and the birth of Gothic: reflections on the biologic basis of creativity. Mol Psychiatry 1996;1(2):99–104.

[17] Ivanov PC, Amaral LA, Goldberger AL, et al. Multifractality in human heartbeat dynamics. Nature 1999;399(6735):461–5.

[18] West GB, Brown JH, Enquist BJ. The fourth dimension of life: fractal geometry and allometric scaling of organisms. Science 1999;284(5420):1677–9.

[19] Peng CK, Mietus J, Hausdorff JM, et al. Long-range anticorrelations and non-Gaussian behavior of the heartbeat. Phys Rev Lett 1993;70(9):1343–6.

[20] Iyengar N, Peng CK, Morin R, et al. Age-related alterations in the fractal scaling of cardiac interbeat interval dynamics. Am J Physiol 1996;271 (4 Pt 2):R1078–84.

[21] Goldberger AL, Amaral LAN, Hausdorff JM, et al. Fractal dynamics in physiology: alterations with disease and aging. Proc Natl Acad Sci U S A 2002;99(1):2466–72.

[22] Low CJ. Therapeutic Agency: An investigation using daoyin healing with single and concurrent ECG data. Thesis for the degree of Doctor of Philosophy in Complementary Heatlh Studies, University of Exeter; 2005.

[23] Peng CK, Havlin S, Stanley HE, et al. Quantification of scaling exponents and crossover phenomena in nonstationary heartbeat time series. Chaos 1995;5(1):82–7.

[24] Ho KKL, Moody GB, Peng CK, et al. Predicting survival in heart failure case and control subjects by use of fully automated methods for deriving nonlinear and conventional indices of heart rate dynamics. Circulation 1997;96(3):842–8.

[25] Goldberger AL. Fractal variability versus pathologic periodicity: complexity loss and stereotypy in disease. Perspect Biol Med 1997;40(4):543–61.

[26] Goldberger AL. Complex systems. Proc Am Thorac Soc 2006;3:467–71.

[27] Poon CS, Merrill CK. Decrease of cardiac chaos in congestive heart failure. Nature 1997;389(6650):492–5.

[28] Costa M, Goldberger AL, Peng CK. Multiscale entropy analysis of complex physiologic time series. Phys Rev Lett 2002;89(6):068102 (4 pp).

[29] Altman DG, Bland JM. How to randomise. Br Med J 1999;319(7211):703–4.

[30] Task Force of the European Society of Cardiology and the North American Society of Pacing and Electrophysiology. Heart rate variability: standards of measurement, physiological interpretation and clinical use. Circulation 1996;93(5):1043–65.

[31] Maturana HR, Varela FJ. Autopoiesis and Cognition: The realization of the living. Dordrecht: D Reidel; 1979.

[32] Goodwin BC. How the Leopard Changed its Spots: The evolution of complexity. London: Wiedenfeld & Nicolson; 1994.

[33] Buchanan M. Ubiquity: The Science of History … Or why the world is simpler than we think. London: Wiedenfeld & Nicolson; 2000.

[34] West BJ, Goldberger AL. Physiology in fractal dimensions. Am Sci 1987;75(4):354–65.

[35] West GB, Brown JH, Enquist BJ. A general model for the origin of allometric scaling laws in biology. Science 1997;276:122–6.

[36] Rössler OE. Continuous chaos: four prototype equations. Ann N Y Acad Sci 1979;316:376–92.

[37] Goldberger AL. Non-linear dynamics for clinicians: chaos theory, fractals, and complexity at the bedside. Lancet 1996;347(9011):1312–4.

[38] Goldberger AL, Rigney DR, Mietus J, et al. Nonlinear dynamics in sudden cardiac death syndrome: heart rate oscillations and bifurcations. Experientia 1988;44(11–12):983–7.

[39] Zweiner U, Hoyer D, Luthke B, et al. Relations between parameters of spectral power densities and deterministic chaos of heart-rate variability. J Auton Nerv Syst 1996;57(3):132–5.

[40] Glass L, Mackey MC. From Clocks to Chaos: The rhythms of life. 1st ed. Princeton, NJ: Princeton University Press; 1988.

[41] Skinner JE, Goldberger AL, Gottfried Mayer-Kress G, et al. Chaos in the heart: implications for clinical cardiology. Nat Biotechnol 1990;8(11):1018–24.

[42] Griffith TM, Edwards DH. Complexity of chaotic vasomotion is insensitive to flow and pressure but can be regulated by external control. Am J Physiol Heart Circ Physiol 1995;269(2):H656–68.

[43] Achterberg J, Cooke K, Richards T, et al. Evidence for correlations between distant intentionality and brain function in recipients: a functional magnetic imaging analysis. J Altern Complement Med 2005;11(6):965–71.

[44] Richards TL, Kozak L, Johnson C, et al. Replicable functional magnetic resonance imaging evidence of correlated brain signals between physically and sensory isolated subjects. J Altern Complement Med 2005;11(6):955–63.

[45] Pizzi R, Fantasia A, Gelain F, et al. Non-local correlation between human neural networks. Donker E, Pirick AR, Brandt HE, editors. Quantum Information and Computation 11, SPIE Conference Proceeding vol. 436. 2004. p. 107–17.

11. THE PHYSIOLOGY OF QI

[1] Lane N. Power, Sex, Suicide: Mitochondria and the meaning of life. Oxford: Oxford University Press; 2006.

[2] De Bary WT, Chan WT, Watson B. Sources of Chinese Tradition. New York: Columbia University Press; 1960.

[3] Kuriyama S. Pneuma, qi, and the problematic of breath. Kawakita Y, Sakai S, Otsuka Y, editors. The Comparison between Concepts of Life-Breath in East and West: Proceedings of the 15th International Syposium on the Comparative History of Medicine, East and West. St Louis, MO: Ishiyaku EuroAmerica; 1995. p. 1–31.

[4] Kendall DE. Dao of Chinese Medicine: Understanding an ancient healing art. Oxford: Oxford University Press; 2002.

[5] Amri H, Abu-Asab MS. Unani Medicine. Micozzi M, editor. Fundamentals of Complementary and Alternative Medicine. 4th ed. St Louis, MO: Saunders; 2011. p. 468–81.

[6] Zysk KG. Vital breath (prana) in ancient Indian medicine and religion. Kawakita Y, Sakai S, Otsuka Y, editors. The Comparison between Concepts of Life-Breath in East and West: Proceedings of the 15th International Syposium on the Comparative History of Medicine, East and West. St Louis, MO: Ishiyaku EuroAmerica; 1995. p. 33–65.

[7] Hanawa T. The interpretation of qi according to Japanese herbalists: two theories of etiology in eighteenth century Japan. Kawakita Y, Sakai S, Otsuka Y, editors. The Comparison between Concepts of Life-Breath in East and West: Proceedings of the 15th International Syposium on the Comparative History of Medicine, East and West. St Louis, MO: Ishiyaku EuroAmerica; 1995. p. 199–228.

[8] Ebrey PB, Walthall A, Palais JB. East Asia: A cultural, social, and political history. Boston, MA: Houghton Mifflin; 2006.

[9] WHO. Traditional Medicine. 2010. Online. Available: World Health Organization website http://www.who.int/mediacentre/factsheets/fs134/en 17 Nov 2010.

[10] Elstein D. Zhang Zai (Chang Tsai, 1020–1077 CE). 2004. Online. Available: Internet Encyclopedia of Philosophy website http://www.iep.utm.edu/zhangzai 17 Nov 2010.

[11] Tavassoli M. The cell theory: a foundation to the edifice of biology. Am J Pathol 1980;98(1):44.

[12] Tuch BE. Stem cells: a clinical update. Aust Fam Physician 2006;35(9):719–21.

[13] Yang Y, Valera VA, Padilla-Nash HM, et al. UOK 262 cell line, fumarate hydratase deficient (FH-/FH-) hereditary leiomyomatosis renal cell carcinoma: in vitro and in vivo model of an aberrant energy metabolic pathway in human cancer. Cancer Genet Cytogenet 2010;196(1):45–55.

[14] Voet D, Voet JG. Biochemistry. 3rd ed. New York: John Wiley; 2004.

[15] Tornroth-Horsefield S, Neutze R. Opening and closing the metabolite gate. Proc Natl Acad Sci U S A 2008;105(50):19565–6.

[16] Dykens JA, Will Y. Drug-induced Mitochondrial Dysfunction. Hoboken, NJ: John Wiley; 2008.

[17] Reed JC. Apoptosis and cell death. Foreword. Oncogene 2008;27(48):6192–3.

[18] Lane N. Oxygen: The molecule that made the world. Oxford: Oxford University Press; 2002.

[19] Avicenna. al-Qanoon fi tibb. New Delhi: Department of Islamic Studies, Jamia Hamdard; 1993.

[20] Ko KM, Leon TY, Mak DH, et al. A characteristic pharmacological action of 'Yang-invigorating' Chinese tonifying herbs: enhancement of myocardial ATP-generation capacity. Phytomedicine 2006;13(9–10):636–42.

[21] Li XT, Chen R, Jin LM, Chen HY. Regulation on energy metabolism and protection on mitochondria of *Panax ginseng* polysaccharide. Am J Chin Med 2009;37(6):1139–52.

[22] Cheng JH. Effect of preventive and therapeutical function of jian-pi yi-qi li-shui decoction on cisplatin nephrotoxicity in rats. Zhongguo Zhongxiyi jiehe zazhi (Chinese Journal of Integrated Traditional and Western Medicine) 1992;12(10):581–2, 614, 616.

[23] Cheng N, Van Hoof H, Bockx E, et al. The effects of electric currents on ATP generation, protein synthesis, and membrane transport of rat skin. Clin Orthop Relat Res 1982;(171):264–72.

12. ENERGY AND MEDICINE

[1] Ohnishi ST, Ohnishi T. Philosophy, psychology, physics and practice of ki. Evidence-based Complementary and Alternative Medicine 2008;6(2):175–83.

[2] Jonas WB, Crawford CC, editors. Healing, Intention and Energy

Medicine: Science, research methods and clinical implications. Edinburgh: Churchill Livingstone; 2003.

[3] Benor DJ. Consciousness, Bioenergy, and Healing: Self-healing and energy medicine for the 21st Century. Healing Research, vol. 2. Medford, NJ: Wholistic Healing Publications; 2004.

[4] Lu Z. Scientific Qigong Exploration: The wonders and mysteries of qi. Malvern, PA: Amber Leaf Press; 1997.

[5] Zha LP. Review of history, findings and implications of research on exceptional functions of the human body in China. Bridging Worlds and Filling Gaps in the Science of Spiritual Healing. Proceedings. Kona, Hawaii: Samueli Institute Meeting; 2001. p. 177–202, 29 Nov-4 Dec 2001.

[6] Hintz KJ, Yount GL, Kadar I, et al. Bioenergy definitions and research guidelines. Altern Ther Health Med 2003;9(Suppl. 3):A13–30.

[7] Yan X, Shen H, Jiang H, et al. External qi of yan xin qigong induces G2/M arrest and apoptosis of androgen-independent prostate cancer cells by inhibiting Akt and Nf-Kappa B pathways. Mol Cell Biochem 2008;310(1–2):227–34.

[8] Tsang HW, Fung KM. A review on neurobiological and psychological mechanisms underlying the anti-depressive effect of qigong exercise. J Health Psychol 2008;13(7):857–63.

[9] Mayor DF. Vitalism: flow, connection, and the awareness of being alive. In: Micozzi MS, editor. Fundamentals of Complementary and Alternative Medicine. 4th ed. St Louis, MO: Saunders; 2011. p. 61–80.

[10] Gordon JS. (Chairman) White House Commission on Complementary and Alternative Medicine Policy: Final Report. 2002. Online. Available: http://www.whccamp.hhs.gov 17 Nov 2010.

[11] Yount G, Solfvin J, Moore D, et al. In vitro test of external qigong. BMC Complement Altern Med 2004;4:5.

[12] Jonas WB, Crawford CC. Science and spiritual healing: a critical review of spiritual healing, 'energy' medicine, and intentionality. Altern Ther Health Med 2003;9(2):56–61.

[13] Sparber AG, Crawford CC, Jonas WB. Laboratory research on bioenergy healing. Jonas WB, Crawford CC, editors. Healing, Intention and Energy

Medicine: Science, research methods and clinical implications. Edinburgh: Churchill Livingstone; 2003. p. 139–50.

[14] Yu T, Tsai HL, Hwang ML. Suppressing tumor progression of in vitro prostate cancer cells by emitted psychosomatic power through Zen meditation. Am J Chin Med 2003;31(3):499–507.

[15] Ventura C. CAM and cell fate targeting: molecular and energetic insights into cell growth and differentiation. Evidence-based Complementary and Alternative Medicine 2005;2(3):277–83.

[16] Tiller WA. Science and Human Transformation: Subtle energies, intentionality and consciousness. Walnut Creek, CA: Pavior Publishing; 1997.

[17] Vickers AJ, Fisher P, Smith C, et al. Homeopathic arnica 30x is ineffective for muscle soreness after long-distance running: a randomized, double-blind, placebo controlled trial. Clin J Pain 1998;14(3):227–31.

[18] Bell IR, Lewis DAII, Schwartz GE, et al. Electroencephalographic cordance patterns distinguish exceptional clinical responders with fibromyalgia to individualized homeopathic medicines. J Altern Complement Med 2004;10(2):285–300.

[19] Moerman DE, Jonas WB. Deconstructing the placebo effect and finding the meaning response. Ann Intern Med 2002;136(6):471–6.

[20] Kiang JG, Ives JA, Jonas WB. External bioenergy-induced increases in intracellular free calcium concentrations are mediated by Na^+/Ca^{2+} exchanger and L-type calcium channel. Mol Cell Biochem 2005;271(1–2):51–9.

[21] Cassidy CM. Social science theory and methods in the study of alternative and complementary medicine. J Altern Complement Med 1995;1(1):19–40.

[22] Engebretson J, Wardell DW. Energy-based modalities. Nurs Clin North Am 2007;42(2):243–59 vi.

[23] Krieger D. Accepting Your Power to Heal. Santa Fe, NM: Bear & Company; 1993.

[24] Mentgen JL. Healing touch. Nurs Clin North Am 2001;36(1):143–58.

[25] North American Nursing Diagnosis Association. Nursing Diagnoses: Definitions and classifications, 2007–2008. Philadelphia, PA: NANDA; 2008.

[26] Peters RM. The effectiveness of Therapeutic Touch: a meta-analytic review. Nurs Sci Q 1999;12(1):52–61.

[27] Winstead-Fry P, Kijek J. An integrative review and meta-analysis of Therapeutic Touch research. Altern Ther Health Med 1999;5(6):58–67.

[28] Astin JA, Harkness E, Ernst E. The efficacy of 'distant healing': a systematic review of randomized trials. Ann Intern Med 2000;132(11):903–10.

[29] O'Mathuna DP, Ashford RL. Therapeutic touch for healing acute wounds. Cochrane Database Syst Rev 2009;(4) CD002766.

[30] Warber SL, Gordon A, Gillespie BW, et al. Standards for conducting clinical biofield energy healing research. Altern Ther Health Med 2003;9(Suppl. 3):A54–64.

[31] Leskowitz E. Energy-based therapies for chronic pain. Audette JF, Bailey A, editors. Integrative Pain Medicine: The science and practice of complementary and alternative medicine in pain management. New York: Springer; 2008. p. 225–41.

[32] Engebretson J, Wardell DW. Experience of a Reiki session. Altern Ther Health Med 2002;8(2):48–53.

[33] Miles P, True G. Reiki – a review of a biofield therapy history, theory, practice and research. Altern Ther Health Med 2003;9(2):62–72.

[34] So PS, Jiang Y, Qin Y. Touch therapies for pain relief in adults. Cochrane Database Syst Rev 2008;(4) CD006535.

[35] Van Wijk R, Van Wijk EP, Wiegant FA, et al. Free radicals and low-level photon emission in human pathogenesis: state of the art. Indian J Exp Biol 2008;46(5):273–309.

[36] Einstein A. Letter to Max Born. 1971 Born I, editor. The Born–Einstein Letters: Correspondence between Albert Einstein and Max and Hedwig Born from 1916 to 1955, with commentaries by Max Born. New York: Walker; 1947. p. 158.

[37] Jeans JH. The Mysterious Universe. Cambridge: Cambridge University Press; 1930. p. 148.

[38] Julsgaard B, Kozhekin A, Polzik ES. Experimental long-lived entanglement of two macroscopic objects. Nature 2001;413(6854):400–3.

[39] Bennett CH, DiVincenzo DP. Quantum information and computation. Nature 2000;404(6775):247–55.

[40] Smith CW. Is a living system a macroscopic quantum system? Frontier Perspectives 1998;7(1):9–15.

[41] Smith CW. Straws in the wind. J Altern Complement Med 2003;9(1):1–6.

[42] Jahn RG, Dunne BJ. On the quantum mechanics of consciousness, with application to anomalous phenomena. Found Phys 1986;16(8):721–72.

[43] Energy Medicine: An Overview from the National Center for Complementary and Alternative Medicine. Online. Available: Healthy. Net website http://healthy.net/scr/article.aspx?Id=2407; Mar 2010.

[44] Atmanspacher H, Romer H, Walach H. Weak quantum theory: complementarity and entanglement in physics and beyond. Found Phys 2002;32(3):379–406.

[45] Walach H. Entanglement model of homeopathy as an example of generalized entanglement predicted by weak quantum theory. Forschende Komplementärmedizin und Klassische Naturheilkunde 2003;10(4):192–200.

[46] Milgrom LR. A new geometrical description of entanglement and the curative homeopathic process. J Altern Complement Med 2008;14(3):329–39.

[47] Milgrom LR. Treating Leick with like: response to criticisms of the use of entanglement to illustrate homeopathy. Homeopathy 2008;97(2):96–9.

[48] Milgrom LR. Towards a new model of the homeopathic process based on quantum field theory. Forschende Komplementärmedizin 2006;13(3):174–83.

[49] Walach H. Generalized entanglement: a new theoretical model for understanding the effects of complementary and alternative medicine. J Altern Complement Med 2005;11(3):549–59.

[50] Bergson H. Creative Evolution. New York: Henry Holt; 1911.

[51] Rubik B. The biofield hypothesis: its biophysical basis and role in medicine. J Altern Complement Med 2002;8(6):703–17.

[52] Walach H, Jonas WB, Ives J, et al. Research on homeopathy: state of the art. J Altern Complement Med 2005;11(5):813–29.

[53] May E. Challenges for healing and intentionality research: causation and information. Jonas WB, Crawford CC, editors. Healing, Intention and Energy Medicine: Science, research methods

and clinical Iimplications. Edinburgh: Churchill Livingstone; 2003. p. 283–92.

[54] Dossey L. Signal versus information in DMILS research protocols (response to Kevin Chen). Journal of Non-Locality and Remote Mental Interactions 2003;2(1). Online. Available: http://www.emergentmind.org/letters1.htm#6 Signal versus information in DMILS research protocols (Response to Kevin Chen) 17 Nov 2010.

[55] Rein G. Bioinformation within the biofield: beyond bioelectromagnetics. J Altern Complement Med 2004;10(1):59–68.

13. WHAT DOES IT MEAN TO PRACTICE AN ENERGY MEDICINE?

[1] Cassidy CM. Social and cultural factors in medicine. Micozzi MS, editor. Fundamentals of Complementary and Integrative Medicine. 4th ed. St Louis, MO: Saunders; 2011. p. 42–60.

[2] Schulman D. Editorial: Is 'energy medicine' a good label for acupuncture? J Altern Complement Med 2004;10(3):419–21.

[3] Helms JM. Acupuncture Energetics: A clinical approach for physicians. New York: Thieme; 1995.

[4] MacPherson H, Kaptchuk TJ. Acupuncture in Practice: Case history insights from the West. Edinburgh: Churchill Livingstone; 1997.

[5] Cassidy CM. Chinese medicine users in the United States, art I: Utilization, satisfaction, medical plurality. J Altern Complement Med 1998;4(1):17–27.

[6] Maciocia G. The Practice of Chinese Medicine: The treatment of diseases with acupuncture and Chinese herbs. Edinburgh: Churchill Livingstone; 1994.

[7] Ross J. Acupuncture Point Combinations: The key to clinical success. Edinburgh: Churchill Livingstone; 1995.

[8] Matsumoto K, Euler D. Kiiko Matsumoto's Clinical Strategies, in the Spirit of Master Nagano. vol. 1. Natick, MA: Kiiko Matsumoto International; 2005.

[9] Zhang ZJ, Ye F, Wiseman N, et al. Shang Han Lun: On cold damage. Translation and commentaries. Taos, NM: Paradigm; 1999.

[10] Matsumoto K, Euler D. Kiiko Matsumoto's Clinical Strategies, in the Spirit of Master Nagano, vol. 2. Natick, MA: Kiiko Matsumoto International; 2008.

[11] Worsley JR. Traditional Acupuncture, vol 2: Traditional Diagnosis. Royal Leamington Spa, Warwickshire: College of Traditional Acupuncture; 1990.

[12] Cassidy CM. Chinese medicine users in the United States, Part I: Utilization, satisfaction, medical plurality. J Altern Complement Med 1998;4(1):17–27.

[13] Cassidy CM. Chinese medicine users in the United States, Part II: Preferred aspects of care. J Altern Complement Med 1998;4(2):189–202.

[14] Gould A, MacPherson H. Patient perspectives on outcomes after treatment with acupuncture. J Altern Complement Med 2001;7(3):261–8.

[15] MacPherson H, Thorpe L, Thomas K. Beyond needling – therapeutic processes in acupuncture care; a qualitative study nested within a low back pain trial. J Altern Complement Med 2006;12(9):873–80.

[16] Mulkins AL, Verhoef MJ. Supporting the transformative process: experiences of cancer patients receiving integrative care. Integr Cancer Ther 2004;3(3):230–7.

[17] Price S, Mercer S, MacPherson H. Practitioner empathy, patient enablement and health outcomes: a prospective study of acupuncture patients. Patient Educ Couns 2006;63(1–2):239–45.

[18] Cassidy CM, Thomas K. Patient patterns of use and experience of acupuncture. MacPherson H, Hammerschlag R, Lewith G, et al., editors. Acupuncture Research: Strategies for establishing an evidence base. Edinburgh: Churchill Livingstone; 2007. p. 37–56.

[19] Paterson C, Schnyer R. Measuring patient-centered outcomes. MacPherson H, Hammerschlag R, Lewith G, et al., editors. Acupuncture Research: Strategies for establishing an evidence base. Edinburgh: Churchill Livingstone; 2007. p. 77–93.

[20] Paterson C, Britten N. Acupuncture as a complex intervention: a holistic model. J Altern Complement Med 2004;10(5):791–801.

[21] Paterson C, Britten N. Acupuncture for people with chronic illness: combining qualitative and quantitative outcome

assessment. J Altern Complement Med 2003;5(9):671–81.

[22] Frank R, Stollberg G. Medical acupuncture in Germany: patterns of consumerism among physicians and patients. Sociol Health Illn 2004;26(3):351–72.

[23] Kaufman K, Salkeld EJ. Home hospice acupuncture: a preliminary report of treatment delivery and outcomes. Permanente Journal 2008;12(1):23–6.

[24] Emad M. Feeling the qi: emergent bodies and disclosive fields in American appropriations of acupuncture. PhD Dissertation, Houston, TX: Rice University; 1998.

[25] Ryan JD. The use of evidence in acupuncture clinical practice. Australian Journal of Acupuncture and Chinese Medicine 2006;1(1):19–23.

[26] Cassidy CM. Unraveling the ball of string: reality, paradigms, and alternative medicine. Advances: The Journal of Mind-Body Health 1994;10(1):5–31.

[27] Goozner M. The $800 Million Pill. Berkeley, CA: University of California Press; 2004.

[28] Schnyer RN, Allen JJB. Acupuncture in the Treatment of Depression: A manual for practice and research. Edinburgh: Churchill Livingstone; 2001.

[29] Cassidy CM. Social science theory and methods in the study of alternative and complementary medicine. J Altern Complement Med 1995;1(1):19–40.

[30] Verhoef MJ, Lewith G, Ritenbaugh C, et al. Whole systems research: moving forward. FACT: Focus on Alternative and Complementary Therapies 2005;9(2):87–90.

[31] Walach H, Falkenberg T, Fonnebø V, et al. Circular instead of hierarchical: methodological principles for the evaluation of complex interventions. BMC Med Res Methodol 2006;6:29.

[32] Campbell NC, Murray E, Darbyshire J, et al. Designing and evaluating complex interventions to improve health care. Br Med J 2007;334(7591):455–9.

14. EVIDENCING ENERGY: EXPERIENCES IN ACUPUNCTURE AND THERAPEUTIC BODYWORK (ZERO BALANCING)

[1] Berleant A. The Aesthetics of Environment. Philadelphia, PA: Temple University Press; 1992.

[2] Murcott T. The Whole Story: Alternative medicine on trial? Basingstoke, Hants: Macmillan; 2005.

[3] Tzu Lao. Tao Te Ching. Harmondsworth, Middx: Penguin; 1963.

[4] Copeland M, Phillpot C, Armleder J, et al. Voids: A retrospective. Zürich: JRP Ringier; 2009.

[5] Graham AC. Disputers of the Tao: Philosophical argument in ancient China. La Salle, IL: Open Court; 1989.

[6] Smith F. Inner Bridges: A guide to energy movement and body structure. Atlanta, GA: Humanics New Age; 1986.

[7] Smith F. Introduction. Hamwee J, editor. Zero Balancing: Touching the energy of bone. London: Frances Lincoln; 1999. p. 11–2.

[8] Smith F. Second International Zero Balancing Teacher Training Program. Mexico: Rio Caliente; 1996.

[9] Newman T. An introduction to Zero Balancing for Acupuncturists. British Acupuncture Council Conference. Egham, Surrey: Royal Holloway College; 2009. September 13.

[10] Hamwee J. Zero Balancing: Touching the energy of bone. London: Frances Lincoln; 1999.

[11] Mayor D, Newman T. Qi: The experience of flow and the origins of acupuncture. A historical/experiential workshop. British Acupuncture Council Conference; Egham, Surrey: Royal Holloway College; 2009 September 13.

[12] Reich W. The Cancer Biopathy. Isle of Arran, Scotland: Banton Press; 1998.

[13] Lipton B. The Biology of Belief: Unleashing the power of consciousness, matter, and miracles. Carlsbad, CA: Hay House; 2008.

[14] Lewis JM. Ooishi's Observation: viewed in the context of jet stream discovery. Bulletin of the American Meteorological Society 2003;84(3):357–69.

[15] Schwenk T. Sensitive Chaos: The creation of flowing forms in water and air. London: Rudolph Steiner Press; 1976.

[16] DeBlieu J. Wind: How the flow of air has shaped life, myth, and the land. Boston, MA: Houghton Mifflin; 1998.

[17] Tournier P. The Meaning of Persons. London: SCM Press; 1957.

[18] Schwartz GE, Russek LG. The Living Energy Universe: A fundamental

discovery that transforms science and medicine. Newburyport, MA: Hampton Roads; 1999.

15. EIGHT MODALITIES FOR WORKING WITH *QI*: *CHAKRA* ACUPUNCTURE, WITH *QIGONG*, MEDITATION AND THE FIVE SOURCES OF ENERGY (FURTHER READING)

[1] Jung CG. Über psychische Energie und das Wesen der Träume. Zürich: Rascher; 1948.

[2] Krieger D. Therapeutic Touch: How to use your hands to help or to heal. Englewood Cliffs, NJ: Prentice-Hall; 1979.

[3] Stux G. Was ist Energie-Medizin? Therapeutikon 1992;6(4):171–2.

[4] Stux G. Chakra acupuncture. Pacific Journal of Oriental Medicine 1994;(2):16–8.

[5] Stux G. Chakra flow meditation. Frontier Perspectives 1996;6(1):39–40.

[6] Stux G. Einführung in die Akupunktur. 7th ed. Berlin: Springer; 2008.

[7] Stux G. 12 lichtvolle Punkte entdeckt. 2009. Online. Available: http://akupunktur-aktuell.de/2009/beitrag/Lichtpunkte.htm 17 Nov 2010.

[8] Stux G. Spirituelle Anwendung der Akupunktur Eine zusammenfassende Darstellung. 2009. Online. Available: http://akupunktur-aktuell.de/2009/beitrag/Spirituelle_Akupunktur.htm 17 Nov 2010.

16. *KI* IN *SHIATSU*

[1] Maciocia G. I Fondamenti della Medicina Tradizionale Cinese. Milan, Italy: Editrice Ambrosiana; 1989.

[2] Beresford-Cooke C. Shiatsu Theory and Practice: A comprehensive text for the student and professional. Edinburgh: Churchill Livingstone; 1996.

[3] Masunaga S. Manuale di Diagnosi. Tokyo, Japan: Iokai Shiatsu Center; 1977.

[4] Szent-Györgyi A. Bioenergetics. New York: Academic Press; 1957.

[5] Tappan FM. Healing Massage Techniques. Norwalk, CT: Appleton-Lange; 1988.

[6] Masunaga S. Zen Imagery Exercises: Meridian exercises for wholesome living. Tokyo: Japan Publications; 1987.

[7] Stefanini P. Masunaga in quantumland. Shiatsu Society News 2001;(75):24–5.

[8] Stefanini P. Quantum physics and shiatsu. Shiatsu Society News 2000;(72):2–4.

[9] Smith CW. Is a living system a macroscopic quantum system? Frontier Perspectives 1998;7(1):9–15.

[10] Del Giudice E, Pulselli RM, Tiezzi E. Thermodynamics of irreversible processes and quantum field theory: an interplay for the understanding of ecosystem dynamics. Ecological Modelling 2009;220(16):1874–9.

[11] Brizhik LS, Del Giudice E, Popp FA, et al. On the dynamics of self-organization in living organisms. Electromagn Biol Med 2009;28(1):28–40.

[12] Brizhik LS, Popp FA, Schlebusch KP. Meridians as optical pathways. Abstracts, Acupuncture, Auriculo-Acupuncture, Sciences et Neurosciences: Des laboratoires à nos consultations médicales. Échanges Soulié de Morant. Paris: Les Invalides; 2008 8 March.

[13] Brizhik LS. Nonlinear charge transport and dynamics of self-organization in living organisms. Neuss, Germany: IIB Summer School; 2009.

[14] Hado.Net. Hado Life USA. 2006. Dr Emoto Online. Available: http://www.hado.net/dremoto/index.php 17 Nov 2010.

[15] Niggli H. Biophotons: the language of cells. Neuss, Germany: IIB Summer School; 2009.

[16] Popp FA, Klimek W, Marić-Oehler W, et al. Visualisierung von meridianähnlichen Ausbreitungspfaden nach optischer Reizung im infraroten Spektralbereich-Vorläufige Ergebnisse. Deutsche Zeitschrift für Akupunktur 2006;49(1):6–16.

[17] Oschman JL. Energy Medicine: The scientific basis. Edinburgh: Churchill Livingstone; 2000.

[18] Chien CH, Tsuei JJ, Lee SC, et al. Effect of emitted bioenergy on biochemical functions of cells. American Journal of Chinese Medicine 1991;19(3–4):285–92.

[19] Schwartz SA, De Mattei RJ, Brame Jr EG, et al. Infrared spectra alteration in water proximate to the palms of therapeutic practitioners. Subtle Energies 1990;1(1):43–72.

[20] Zimmerman J. Laying-on-of hands healing and therapeutic touch. A testable theory. BEMI Currents, Journal of the Bio-Electro-Magnetics Institute 1990;2:8–17.

[21] Popp FA, Yan Y, Popp A, et al. Electromagnetic man – biophoton emission is correlated to resistance values of the skin, but even to the distribution function of electric parameters of the skin. 2006. Online. Available: www.biophotonen-online .de/news/2006/electro.pdf 17 Nov 2010.

[22] Seto A, Kusaka C, Nagazato S, et al. Detection of extraordinary large bio-magnetic field strength from human hand during external qi emission. Acupunct Electrother Res 1992;17(2):75–94.

[23] International Institute of Biophysics. History of Biophotonik or biophotonics from the German point of view. 2003. Online. Available: www. lifescientists.de/history.htm 17 Nov 2010.

[24] Ho MW. The Rainbow and the Worm: The physics of organisms. 2nd ed. Singapore: World Scientific; 1998. p. 233.

17. BIOELECTRICITY AND *QI*: A MICROCURRENT APPROACH

[1] Sheldrake R. A New Science of Life: The hypothesis of formative causation. Los Angeles: J P Tarcher; 1981.

[2] Nordenström BEW. Biologically Closed Electric Circuits: Clinical, experimental and theoretical evidence for an additional circulatory system. Stockholm: Nordic Medical; 1983.

[3] Burr HS. Blueprint for Immortality: The electric patterns of life. London: Neville Spearman; 1972.

[4] Manning CA, Vanrenen LJ. Bioenergetic Medicines East and West: Acupuncture and homeopathy. Berkeley, CA: North Atlantic Books; 1988. p. 14–5.

[5] Pankratov S. Meridiane leiten Licht. Raum und Zeit 1991;7(35):16–8.

[6] Popp FA. Biophotons – background, experimental results, theoretical approach and applications. Frontier Perspectives 2002;11(1):16–28.

[7] Oschman JL. Energy Medicine: The scientific basis. Edinburgh: Churchill Livingstone; 2000. p. 48.

[8] Motoyama H. Measurements of Ki Energy, Diagnoses and Treatments: Treatment principles of Oriental medicine from an electrophysiological viewpoint. Tokyo: Human Science Press; 1997.

[9] Szent-Györgyi A. Introduction to a Submolecular Biology. New York: Academic Press; 1960.

[10] Becker RO, Selden G. The Body Electric: Electromagnetism and the foundation of life. New York: William Morrow; 1985.

[11] Bulkley D. Bio-Magnetics and Life. 2nd ed. Washington DC: Rogue Press; 1972.

[12] Buchanan GR. Sona: Healing with wave front bioresonance. Reno, NV: Gary Robert Buchanan and The Music Guild; 2008. p. 31–3.

[13] Manaka Y, Itaya K, Birch S. Chasing the Dragon's Tail: The theory and practice of acupuncture in the work of Yoshio Manaka. Brookline, MA: Paradigm; 1995.

[14] Matsumoto K, Birch S. Hara Diagnosis: Reflections on the sea. Brookline, MA: Paradigm; 1988.

[15] Oschman JL. Energy Medicine in Therapeutics and Human Performance. Philadelphia, PA: Butterworth-Heinemann; 2003. p. 282.

[16] Microcurrent's NewWave: Microlight therapy. Online. Available: East-West Seminars website http://www.east-westseminars.com/info.php.

[17] Nelson RM, Currier DP, editors. Clinical Electrotherapy. Norwalk, CT: Appleton & Lange; 1991.

[18] Greenlee C, Greenlee DL, Wing TW. Basic Microcurrent Therapy Acupoint and Body Work Manual. Kelseyville, CA: Earthen Vessel; 1999.

[19] Kaptchuk TJ. The Web that has no Weaver: Understanding Chinese medicine. 1st ed. New York: Congdon & Weed; 1983. p. 22.

[20] Online. Available: EastWestMed website: http://www.eastwestmed. com 17 Nov 2010.

[21] Kubiena G, Sommer B. Practice Handbook of Acupuncture. Edinburgh: Churchill Livingstone; 2010.

[22] Starwynn D. Microcurrent Electro-Acupuncture: Bio-electric principles, evaluation and treatment. Phoenix, AZ: Desert Heart Press; 2001.

[23] Tan RTF, Ruch S. Twelve and Twelve in Acupuncture: Unique point applications and case studies for effective pain treatment. San Diego, CA: Richard Tan; 1991.

18. ENERGY PSYCHOLOGY: WORKING WITH MIND–BODY SYNERGY

[1] Callahan RJ. Tapping the Healer Within. New York: Contemporary Books; 2001.

[2] Callahan RJ, Callahan J. Stop the Nightmares of Trauma. LaQuinta, CA: Callahan; 2000.

[3] Diepold JH, Britt V, Bender SS. Evolving Thought Field Therapy. The Clinician's Handbook of Diagnosis, Treatment, and Theory. New York: Norton; 2004.

[4] Frost R. Applied Kinesiology. Berkeley, CA: North Atlantic Books; 2002.

[5] Walther DS. Applied Kinesiology: Synopsis. Pueblo, CO: Systems DC; 1988.

[6] Monti D, Sinnot J, Marchese M, et al. Muscle test comparisons of congruent and incongruent self-referential statements. Percept Mot Skills 1999;88(3 part 1):1019–28.

[7] Diamond J. Your Body Doesn't Lie: An introduction to behavioural kinesiology. 1997 ed. Enfield, Middx: Eden Grove; 1979.

[8] Diamond J. Life Energy. St Paul, MN: Paragon House; 1985.

[9] Callahan R. TFT Diagnostics 'Step A' DVD Course. La Quinta, CA: Callahan Techniques; 1997. Online. Available: http://www.rogercallahan.com 17 Nov 2010.

[10] Callahan RJ. Self-acceptance and Thought Field Therapy: a recommendation for complex cases. The Thought Field 2001;7(2). Online. Available: http://www.rogercallahan.com 17 Nov 2010.

[11] Gruder D. The Energy Psychology Desktop Companion. Del Mar, CA: Willingness Works; 2003.

[12] ACEP. Association for Comprehensive Energy Psychology: Certification training manual. Haverford, PA: Association for Comprehensive Energy Psychology; 2007.

[13] Connolly SM. Thought Field Therapy: Clinical applications, integrating TFT in psychotherapy. Sedona, AZ: George Tyrrell Press; 2004.

[14] Callahan RJ, Callahan J. Sensitivities, Intolerances and Individual Energy Toxins: How to identify and neutralize them with TFT. DVD set. La Quinta, CA: Callahan Techniques; 2003. Online. Available: http://www.rogercallahan.com 17 Nov 2010.

[15] Callahan R. How Executives Overcome the Fear of Public Speaking and Other Phobias [previously titled The Five Minute Phobia Cure]. Wilmington, DE: Enterprise Publishing; 1985.

[16] Bray RL. Working through traumatic stress without the overwhelming responses. Journal of Aggression, Maltreatment and Trauma 2006;12(1):103–24.

[17] Durlacher JV. Freedom From Fear Forever: The Acu-Power way to overcoming your fears, phobias and inner problems. Mesa, AZ: Van Ness Publishing; 1994.

[18] Gallo FP. Energy Psychology: Explorations at the interface of energy, cognition, behavior, and health. Boca Raton, FL: CRC Press; 1999.

[19] Hartung JG, Galvin MD. Energy Psychology and EMDR: Combining forces to optimize treatment. New York: Norton; 2003.

[20] Gallo FP, editor. Energy Psychology in Psychotherapy: A comprehensive source book. New York: Norton; 2002.

[21] Mollon P. EMDR and Energy Therapies: Psychoanalytic perspectives. London: Karnac; 2005.

[22] Mollon P. Psychoanalytic Energy Psychotherapy: Inspired by Thought Field Therapy, EFT, TAT, and Seemorg Matrix. London: Karnac; 2008.

[23] Elder C, Ritenbaugh C, Mist S, et al. Randomised trial of two mind-body interventions for weight loss maintenance. J Altern Complement Med 2007;13(1):67–78.

[24] Baker AH, Siegel LS. Can a 45 minute session of EFT lead to reduction of intense fear of rats, spiders and water bugs? A replication and extension of the Wells et al (2003) laboratory study. Paper presented at the Seventh International Conference of the Association for Comprehensive Energy Psychology, Baltimore, MD, 27 April–4 May. 2005.

[25] Wells S, Polglase K, Andrews HB, et al. Evaluation of a meridian based intervention, emotional freedom techniques (EFT) for reducing specific phobias of small animals. J Clin Psychol 2003;59(9):943–66.

[26] Feinstein D. Energy psychology: a review of the preliminary evidence. Psychotherapy: Theory, Research, Practice, Training 2008;45(2):199–213.

[27] Johnson C, Shala M, Sejdijaj X, et al. Thought field therapy – soothing the bad moments of Kosovo. J Clin Psychol 2001;57(10):1241–4.

[28] Cho ZH, Chung SC, Jones JP, et al. New findings of the correlation between acupoints and corresponding brain cortices using functional MRI. Proc Natl Acad Sci U S A 1998;95(5):2670–3.

[29] Hui KKS, Liu J, Makris N, et al. Acupuncture modulates the limbic system and subcortical gray structures of the human brain: evidence from fMRI studies in normal subjects. Hum Brain Mapp 2000;9(1):13–25.

[30] Pignotti M, Steinberg M. Heart rate variability as an outcome measure for Thought Field Therapy in clinical practice. J Clin Psychol 2001;57(10):1193–206.

[31] Callahan R. The impact of Thought Field Therapy on heart rate variability (HRV). J Clin Psychol 2001;57(10):1153–70.

[32] Callahan R. Raising and lowering heart rate variability: some clinical findings of Thought Field Therapy. J Clin Psychol 2001;57(10):1175–86.

[33] Rowe JE. The effects of EFT on long-term psychological symptoms. Counseling and Clinical Psychology 2005;2(3):104–11.

[34] Sakai C, Paperny D, Mathews M, et al. Thought field therapy clinical applications: utilization in an HMO in behavioral medicine and behavioral health services. J Clin Psychol 2001;57(10):1215–27.

[35] Pert C. Molecules of Emotion: The science behind mind-body medicine. New York: Simon & Schuster; 1999.

[36] Oschman JL. Energy Medicine: The scientific basis. Edinburgh: Churchill Livingstone; 2000.

[37] Ruden RA. A model for disrupting an encoded traumatic memory. Traumatology 2007;13(1):71–5.

[38] Tiller WA. Science and Human Transformation: Subtle energies, intentionality and consciousness. Walnut Creek, CA: Pavior Publishing; 1997.

[39] Andrade J, Feinstein D. Energy psychology: theory, indications, evidence (appendix). Feinstein D, editor. Energy Psychology Interactive. Ashland, OR: Innersource; 2004. p. 199–214.

[40] Aalberse M. Sutherland C. The South American studies. Summary and discussion of the clinical data (n.d.) Online. Available: BMSA International website http://www.realhelpfordepression.com/south_american_studies.htm 17 Nov 2010.

[41] Waite WL, Holder MD. Assessment of the emotional freedom technique: an alternative treatment for fear. Scientific Review of Mental Health Practice 2003;2(1):20–6.

19. CRANIOSACRAL BIODYNAMICS

[1] Sutherland WG. Teachings in the Science of Osteopathy. Cambridge, MA: Rudra Press; 1990.

[2] Sutherland WG. 1998 Contributions of Thought. Cambridge, MA: Rudra Press; 1971.

[3] Bivins RE. Alternative Medicine? A history. Oxford: Oxford University Press; 2007.

[4] Becker R. The Stillness of Life. Portland, OR: Stillness Press; 2000.

[5] Cleary T. Translator. Kensho: The heart of Zen. Boston, MA: Shambala; 1997.

[6] Coats C. Living Energies: An exposition of concepts related to the theories of Viktor Schauberger. Dublin: Gateway; 2001.

[7] Ho MW. The Rainbow and the Worm: The physics of organisms. 2nd ed. Singapore: World Scientific; 1998.

[8] Becker R. Life In Motion. Cambridge, MA: Rudra Press; 1997.

[9] Stone R. Polarity Therapy. Summertown, TN: Book Publishing Company; 1999.

20. *QI* IN CHILDREN (FURTHER READING)

[1] Cao JM, Su XM, Cao JQ. Essentials of Traditional Chinese Pediatrics. Beijing: Foreign Language Press; 1990.

[2] Deadman P, Al-Khafaji M, Baker K. A Manual of Acupuncture. Hove, Sussex: Journal of Chinese Medicine Publications; 2001.

[3] Diagnosis and Treatment of Gynecology and Pediatrics. Wang DS, Yan ZG, editors. Chinese Zhenjiuology, Acupuncture & Moxibustion, vol. 13. Beijing: Chinese Medical Audio-Video Organization and Meditalent Meditalent Enterprises; 1990 (videotape).

[4] Diagnostic and Statistical Manual of Mental Disorders: DSM-IV. 4th ed. Washington, DC: American Psychiatric Association; 1994.

[5] Ellis E, Wiseman N, Boss K. Fundamentals of Chinese Acupuncture. Revised ed. Brookline, MA: Paradigm Publications; 1991.

[6] Flavel JH. The Developmental Psychology of Jean Piaget. Princeton, NJ: Van Nostrand; 1963.

[7] Flaws B. A Handbook of TCM Pediatrics: A practitioner's guide to the care and treatment of common childhood diseases. Boulder, CO: Blue Poppy Press; 1997.

[8] Freud S. Character and anal eroticism. Strachey J, editor. The Standard Edition of the Complete Psychological Works of Sigmund Freud, vol. 9. London: Hogarth Press; 1908. p. 167–75.

[9] Helms J. Acupuncture Energetics: A clinical approach for physicians. Berkeley, CA: Medical Acupuncture Publishers; 1995.

[10] Kline P. Facts and Fantasy in Freudian Theory. London: Methuen; 1972.

[11] Loo M. Select populations: children. Spencer JW, Jacobs JJ, editors. Complementary and Alternative Medicine: An evidence-based approach. St Louis, MO: Mosby; 2002. p. 409–57.

[12] Loo M. Integrative Medicine for Children. St Louis, MO: Saunders; 2009.

[13] Maciocia G. The Foundations of Chinese Medicine: A comprehensive text for acupuncturists and herbalists. Edinburgh: Churchill Livingstone; 1989.

[14] Maciocia G. The Practice of Chinese Medicine: The treatment of diseases with acupuncture and Chinese herbs. Edinburgh: Churchill Livingstone; 1994.

[15] Maciocia G. The Psyche in Chinese Medicine: Treatment of emotional and mental disharmonies with acupuncture and Chinese herbs. Edinburgh: Churchill Livingstone; 2009.

[16] Mahler MS. On Human Symbiosis and the Vicissitudes of Individuation. I. Infantile psychosis. New York: International Universities Press; 1968.

[17] Menninger WC. Characterologic and symptomatic expressions related to the anal phase of psychosexual development. Psychoanal Q 1943;12:161–93.

[18] O'Connor J, Bensky D, editors. Acupuncture: A comprehensive text. Seattle, WA: Eastland Press; 1981.

[19] Oschman JL. Energy Medicine: The scientific basis. Edinburgh: Churchill Livingstone; 2000.

[20] Piaget J. The Child's Conception of Physical Causality. London: Routledge; 1999.

[21] Scott J. Acupuncture in the Treatment of Children. Seattle, WA: Eastland Press; 1991.

[22] Shaywitz BA, Fletcher JM, Shaywitz SE. Attention-deficit/hyperactivity disorder. Adv Pediatr 1997;44:331–67.

[23] Veith I. Translator. Nei Ching: The Yellow Emperor's classic of internal medicine. Berkeley, CA: University of California Press; 1949.

[24] Zhang ZJ. Shang Han Lun: Wellspring of Chinese Medicine. Long Beach, CA: Keats Publishing; 1981.

[25] Zhang ZJ. Treatise on Febrile Diseases Caused by Cold with 500 Cases. Beijing: New World Press; 1993.

21. *QIGONG, TAIJI QUAN (TAI CHI)* AND HIV: THE PSYCHONEUROIMMUNOLOGY CONNECTION

[1] Kirksey KM, Goodroad BK, Kemppainen JK, et al. Complementary therapy use in persons with HIV/AIDS. J Holist Nurs 2002;20(3):264–78.

[2] Schroecksnadel K, Sarcletti M, Winkler C, et al. Quality of life and immune activation in patients with HIV-infection. Brain Behav Immun 2008;22(6):881–9.

[3] Vogl D, Rosenfeld B, Breitbard W, et al. Symptom prevalence, characteristics, and distress in AIDS outpatients. J Pain Symptom Manage 1999;18(4):253–62.

[4] Nachega JB, Trotta MP, Nelson M, et al. Impact of metabolic complications on antiretroviral treatment adherence: clinical and public health implications. Curr HIV/AIDS Rep 2009;6(3):121–9.

[5] Tsao JC, Dobalian JD, Myers CD, et al. Pain and use of complementary and alternative medicine in a national sample of persons living with HIV. J Pain Symptom Manage 2005;30(5):418–32.

[6] Gore-Felton C, Vosvick M, Power R, et al. Alternative therapies: a common practice among men and women

living with HIV. J Assoc Nurses AIDS Care 2003;14(3):17–27.

[7] Ozsoy M, Ernst E. How effective are complementary therapies for HIV and AIDS? A systematic review. Int J STD AIDS 1999;10(10):629–35.

[8] Power R, Gore-Felton C, Vosvick M, et al. HIV: effectiveness of complementary and alternative medicine. Primary Care: Clinics in Office Practice 2002;29(2):361–78.

[9] Wiwanitkit V. The use of CAM by HIV-positive patients in Thailand. Complement Ther Med 2003;11(1):39–41.

[10] Mutimura E, Stewart A, Crowther NJ, et al. The effects of exercise training on quality of life in HAART-treated HIV-positive Rwandan subjects with body fat redistribution. Qual Life Res 2008;17(3):377–85.

[11] Calabrese C, Wenner CA, Reeves C, et al. Treatment of human immunodeficiency virus-positive patients with complementary and alternative medicine: a survey of practitioners. J Altern Complement Med 1998;4(3):281–7.

[12] Nixon S, O'Brien K, Glazier RH, et al. Aerobic exercise interventions for adults living with HIV/AIDS. Cochrane Database Syst Rev 2005;18(2) CD001796.

[13] Malita FM, Karelis AD, Toma E, et al. Effects of different types of exercise on body composition and fat distribution in HIV-infected patients: a brief review. Can J Appl Physiol 2005;30(2):233–45.

[14] O'Brien K, Tynan AM, Nixon S, et al. Effects of progressive resistive exercise in adults living with HIV/AIDS: Systematic review and meta-analysis of randomized trials. AIDS Care 2008;20(6):631–53.

[15] Aberg JA. Cardiovascular complications in HIV management: past, present, and future. J Acquir Immune Defic Syndr 2009;50(1):54–64.

[16] What is CAM? 2007. NCCAM Publication No. D347 Online. Available: http://nccam.nih.gov/health/whatiscam/overview.htm 7 Mar 2010.

[17] Chu DA. Tai chi, qi gong, and reiki. Phys Med Rehabil Clin N Am 2004;15(4):773–81.

[18] Hankey A. Qigong: life energy and a new science of life. J Altern Complement Med 2006;12(9):841–2.

[19] Sun GC. Qigong: bio-energy medicine. J Altern Complement Med 2008;14(8):893.

[20] Hanna L. Chinese medicine for HIV positive women. BETA 1997;(3)39–44.

[21] Ng BH, Tsang HW. Psychophysiological outcomes of health qigong for chronic conditions: a systematic review. Psychophysiology 2009;46(2):257–69.

[22] Lee MS, Huh HJ, Hong SS, et al. Psychoneuroimmunological effects of Qi-therapy: preliminary study on the changes of level of anxiety, mood, cortisol and melatonin and cellular function of neutrophil and natural killer cells. Stress and Health 2001;17(1):17–24.

[23] Manzaneque JM, Vera FM, Rodriguez FM, et al. Serum cytokines, mood and sleep after a qigong program: is qigong an effective psychobiological tool? J Health Psychol 2009;14(1):60–7.

[24] Shinnick P. Qigong: where did it come from? Where does it fit in science? What are the advances? J Altern Complement Med 2006;12(4):351–43.

[25] Wang PS, Chen GH. Relaxing and Calming Qigong. Beijing: New World Press; 1987.

[26] Cohen KS. The Way of Qigong. London: Bantam; 1997.

[27] Lee MS, Kim MK. Qi-training (qigong) enhanced immune functions: what is the underlying mechanism? Int J Neurosci 2005;115(8):1099–104.

[28] McCain NL, Elswick RK, Gray DP, et al. Tai chi training enhances well-being and alters cytokine levels in persons with HIV disease. Brain Behav Immun 2005;19(4 Suppl. 1):e50–1.

[29] Robins JL, McCain NL, Gray DP, et al. Research on psychoneuroimmunology: tai chi as a stress management approach for individuals with HIV disease. Appl Nurs Res 2006;19(1):2–9.

[30] Cheng M-C. Tai Chi: The supreme ultimate exercise for health, sport, and self-defense. Upper Saddle River, NJ: Prentice Hall; 1986.

[31] Galantino ML, Shepard K, Krafft L, et al. The effect of group aerobic exercise and t'ai chi on functional outcomes and quality of life for persons living with acquired immunodeficiency syndrome. J Altern Complement Med 2005;11(6):1085–92.

[32] Robins JL, McCain NL, Gray DP, et al. Tai chi as a stress management approach for individuals with HIV. Journal of Sport and Exercise Psychology 2007;29(4):545–6.

[33] Qu M. Taijiquan: a medical assessment. In: Chinese Sports Editorial Board. Simplified Taijiquan. Beijing: China International Book Trading Corporation; 1986. p. 6–9.

[34] Han A, Judd M, Welch V, et al. Tai chi for treating rheumatoid arthritis. Cochrane Database Syst Rev 2004;(3) CD004849.

[35] Tse SK, Bailey DM. Tai Chi and postural control in the well elderly. Am J Occup Ther 1992;46(4):295–300.

[36] Wolf SL, Coogler CE, Green RC, et al. Novel interventions to prevent falls in the elderly. Perry HM, Morley JE, Coe RM, editors. Aging and Musculoskeletal Disorders: Concepts, diagnosis, and treatment. 1993. p. 178–95.

[37] Province MA, Hadley EC, Hornbrook MC, et al. The effects of exercise on falls in elderly patients. J Am Med Assoc 1995;273(17):1341–7.

[38] Lai JS, Wong MK, Lan C, et al. Cardiorespiratory responses of T'ai Chi Chuan practitioners and sedentary subjects during cycle ergometer. J Formos Med Assoc 1993;92(10):894–9.

[39] Jin P. Efficacy of Tai Chi, brisk walking, meditation, and reading in reducing mental and emotional stress. J Psychosom Res 1992;36(4):361–70.

[40] Jahnke R. Physiological mechanisms operating in the human system during the practice of Qigong and Pranayama. Jahnke R, editor. The Most Profound Medicine. Santa Barbara, CA: Health Action Press; 1996. p. 126.

[41] Benson H. The Relaxation Response. New York: William Morrow; 1975.

[42] Krippner S, Villoldo A. The Realms of Healing. Santa Barbara, CA: Celestial Arts; 1976.

[43] Green E, Green A. Beyond Biofeedback. New York: Delacorte Press; 1977.

[44] Burr HS, Northrop FSC. The electrodynamic theory of life. Q Rev Biol 1935;10(3):322–33.

[45] Burr HS. Fields of Life. New York: Ballantine Books; 1973.

[46] Becker RO, Selden G. The Body Electric: Electromagnetism and the foundation of life. New York: William Morrow; 1985.

[47] Nordenström BEW. Biologically Closed Electrical Circuits: Clinical, experimental, and theoretical evidence for an additional circulatory system. Stockholm: Nordic Medical Publications; 1983.

[48] Lee MS, Huh HJ, Jeong SM, et al. Effects of qigong on immune cells. Am J Chin Med 2003;31(2):327–35.

[49] McCune JM. The dynamics of CD4+ T-cell depletion in HIV disease. Nature 2001;410(6831):974–9.

[50] Creswell JD, Myers HF, Cole SW, et al. Mindfulness meditation training effects on CD4+ T lymphocytes in HIV-1 infected adults: a small randomized controlled trial. Brain Behav Immun 2009;23(2):184–8.

[51] Jones BM. Changes in cytokine production in healthy subjects practicing Guolin Qigong: a pilot study. BMC Complement Altern Med 2001;1:8.

[52] McKinnon W, Baum A, Morokoff P. Neuroendocrine measures in stress. Wagner HL, editor. Social Psychophysiology and Emotion: Theory and clinical application. Chichester, Sussex: John Wiley; 1988. p. 43–64.

[53] Dobbin JP, Harth M, McCain GA. Cytokine production and lymphocyte transformation during stress. Brain Behav Immun 1991;5(4):339–48.

[54] Selye H. The Stress of Life. New York: McGraw-Hill; 1956.

[55] Tsang HW, Fung KM. Neurobiological and psychological mechanisms underlying the anti-depressive effect of qigong exercise. J Health Psychol 2008;13(7):857–63.

[56] Esch T, Fricchione GL, Stefano GB. The therapeutic use of relaxation response in stress-related diseases. Med Sci Monit 2003;9(2):RA23–34.

[57] Ironson G, O'Cleirigh C, Fletcher MA, et al. Psychosocial factors predict CD4 and viral load change in men and women with human immunodeficiency virus in the era of highly active antiretroviral treatment. Psychosom Med 2005;67(6):1013–21.

[58] Vera FM, Manzaneque JM, Maldonado EF, et al. Biochemical changes after a qigong program: lipids, serum enzymes, urea, and creatine in

healthy subjects. Med Sci Monit 2007;10(6):CR264–70.

[59] Evans DL, Leserman J, Perkins DO. Severe life stress as a predictor of early disease progression in HIV infection. Am J Psychiatry 1997;154(5):630–4.

[60] Neidig JL, Smith BA, Brashers DE. Aerobic Exercise Training for Depressive Symptom Management in Adults Living With HIV Infection. J Assoc Nurses AIDS Care 2003;14(2):30–40.

[61] Lyons S, Pope M. Constructs in motion. Kirkcaldy B, editor. Normalities and Abnormalities in Human Movement, vol. 26. New York: Karger; 1989. p. 147–65.

[62] Mackinnon LT. Clinical implications of exercise. Mackinnon LT, editor. Exercise and Immunology. Current Issues in Exercise Science 2. Champaign, IL: Human Kinetics; 1992. p. 77–84.

[63] Doyne EJ, Ossip-Klein DJ, Bowman ED, et al. Running versus weight training in the treatment of depression. J Consult Clin Psychol 1987;55(5):748–54.

[64] American Psychiatric Association (APA). Diagnostic and Statistical Manual of Mental Disorders. 3rd rev ed. Washington DC: APA; 1987.

[65] Duncombe LW, Howe MC. Group treatment: goals, tasks, and economic implications. Am J Occup Ther 1995;49(3):199–205.

[66] Trahey PJ. A comparison of the cost-effectiveness of two types of occupational therapy services. Am J Occup Ther 1991;45(5):397–400.

[67] Targ EF, Karasic DH, Diefenbach PN, et al. Structured group therapy and fluoxetine to treat depression in HIV-positive persons. Psychosomatics 1994;35(2):132–7.

[68] Kelly JA, Murphy DA, Bahr GR, et al. Outcome of cognitive–behavioral and support group brief therapies for depressed, HIV-infected persons. Am J Psychiatry 1993;150(11):1679–86.

[69] Kendall J. Promoting wellness in HIV-support groups. J Assoc Nurses AIDS Care 1992;3(1):28–38.

[70] Lutgendorf S, Antoni MH, Schneiderman N, et al. Psychosocial counseling to improve quality of life in HIV infection. Patient Educ Couns 1994;24(3):217–35.

[71] Nunes JA, Raymond SJ, Nicholas PK, et al. Social support, quality of life, immune function, and health in persons living with HIV. J Holist Nurs 1995;12(2):174–98.

[72] Belcher AE, Dettmore D, Holzemer SP. Spirituality and sense of well-being in persons with AIDS. Holistic Nurse Practitioner 1989;3(4):16–25.

[73] Kendall J. Wellness spirituality in homosexual men with HIV infection. J Assoc Nurses AIDS Care 1994;5(4):28–34.

[74] Carson VB. Prayer, meditation, exercise, and special diets: behaviors of the hardy person with HIV/AIDS. J Assoc Nurses AIDS Care 1993;4(3):18–28.

[75] Buchacz K, Rangel M, Blacher R, et al. Changes in the clinical epidemiology of HIV infection in the United States: Implications for the clinician. Current Infectious Disease Report 2009;11(1):75–83.

22. ENERGY-BASED THERAPIES IN NEUROLOGY: THE EXAMPLE OF THERAPEUTIC TOUCH

[1] Byrd RC. Positive therapeutic effects of intercessory prayer in a coronary care unit population. South Med J 1988;81(7):826–9.

[2] Wirth D. The effect of noncontact therapeutic touch on the rate of healing of full thickness dermal wounds. Subtle Energies 1990;1(1):1–21.

[3] Ellenberger H. The Discovery of the Unconscious. New York: Basic Books; 1970.

[4] Becker R. Cross Currents: The promise of electromedicine, the perils of electropollution. Los Angeles: J Tarcher; 1990.

[5] Green E, Parks PA, Guyer PM, et al. Anomalous electrostatic phenomena in exceptional subjects. Subtle Energies 1991;2(3):69–81.

[6] Wager S. A Doctor's Guide to Therapeutic Touch. New York: Perigee Books; 1996.

[7] Mulloney SS, Wells-Federman C. Therapeutic touch: a healing modality. J Cardiovasc Nurs 1996;10(3):27–49.

[8] Rosa L, Rosa E, Sarner L, et al. A close look at Therapeutic Touch. J Am Med Assoc 1998;279(13):1005–10.

[9] Leskowitz E. Un-debunking Therapeutic Touch. Altern Ther Health Med 1998;4(4):101–2.

[10] Kiecolt-Glaser JK, Marucha PT, Malarkey WB, et al. Slowing of wound healing by psychological stress. Lancet 1995;346(8984):1194–6.

[11] Solfvin J, Benor DJ, Leskowitz E. Concerning the work of Daniel P. Wirth (letter). J Altern Complement Med 2006;11(6):949–50.

[12] Gronowicz GA, Jhaveri A, Clarke LW, et al. Therapeutic touch stimulates the proliferation of human cells in culture. J Altern Complement Med 2008;14(3):233–9.

[13] Olson M, Sneed N, LaVie M, et al. Stress-induced immunosuppression and therapeutic touch. Altern Ther Health Med 1997;3(2):68–74.

[14] Payne MB. The use of therapeutic touch with rehabilitation clients. Rehabil Nurs 1989;14(2):69–72.

[15] Fawcett J, Sidney JS, Hanson MJ, et al. Use of alternative health therapies by people with multiple sclerosis: an exploratory study. Holist Nurs Pract 1994;8(2):36–42.

[16] Snyder M, Egan EC, Burns KR. Interventions for decreasing agitation behaviors in persons with dementia. J Gerontol Nurs 1995;21(7):34–40.

[17] Keller E, Bzdek VM. Effects of therapeutic touch on tension headache pain. Nurs Res 1986;35(2):101–6.

[18] Meehan TC. Therapeutic touch and postoperative pain: a Rogerian research study. Nurs Sci Q 1993;6(2):69–78.

[19] Turner JG, Clark AJ, Gauthier DK, et al. The effect of therapeutic touch on pain and anxiety in burn patients. J Adv Nurs 1998;28(1):10–20.

[20] Leskowitz E. Phantom limb pain treated with Therapeutic Touch: a case report. Arch Phys Med Rehabil 2000;81(4):522–4.

23. QI IN CHRONIC FATIGUE SYNDROME AND FIBROMYALGIA

[1] Hakariya Y, Kuratsune H. Chronic fatigue syndrome: biochemical examination of the blood. Nippon Rinsho 2007;65(6):1071–6.

[2] Fukuda K, Strauss SE, Hickie I, et al. The chronic fatigue syndrome: a comprehensive approach to its definition and study. Ann Intern Med 1994;121(12):953–9.

[3] Meeus M, Nijs J. Central sensitization: a biopsychosocial explanation for chronic widespread pain in patients with fibromyalgia and chronic fatigue syndrome. Clin Rheumatol 2007;26(4):465–73.

[4] Devaneur LD, Kerr JR. Chronic fatigue syndrome. J Clin Virol 2006;37(3):139–50.

[5] Fark AR. Infectious mononucleosis, Epstein–Barr virus, and chronic fatigue syndrome: a prospective case series. J Fam Pract 1991;32(2):202–6, 205, 209.

[6] Lerner AM, Beqaj SH, Deeter RG, et al. Valacyclovir treatment in Epstein–Barr virus subset chronic fatigue syndrome: thirty six months follow-up. In Vivo 2007;21(5):707–13.

[7] Bellmann-Weller R, Schoecksnadel K, Holzer C, et al. IFN-gamma mediated pathways in patients with fatigue and chronic active Epstein–Barr virus infection. J Affect Disord 2008;108(1–2):171–6.

[8] Evengard B, Nilsson CG, Lindh G, et al. Chronic fatigue syndrome differs from fibromyalgia. No evidence for elevated substance P levels in cerebrospinal fluid of patients with chronic fatigue syndrome. Pain 1998;78(2):153–5.

[9] McMakin C, Gregory W, Phillips T. Cytokine changes with microcurrent treatment of fibromyalgia associated with cervical spine trauma. J Bodyw Mov Ther 2005;9(3):169–76.

[10] Juhl J. Fibromyalgia and the serotonin pathway. Altern Med Rev 1998;3(5):367–75.

[11] Crofford LJ. Neuroendocrine abnormalities in fibromyalgia. Am J Med Sci 1998;315(6):359–66.

[12] Crofford LJ. The hypothalamic–pituitary–adrenal stress axis in fibromyalgia and chronic fatigue syndrome. J Rheumatol 1998;57(Suppl. 2):67–71.

[13] Crofford LJ, Engleberg NC, Demitrack MA. Neurohormonal perturbations in fibromyalgia. Rheum Dis Clin North Am 1996;22(2):267–84.

[14] Crofford LJ, Pillemer SR, Kalogeras KT, et al. Hypothalamic–pituitary–adrenal axis perturbations in patients with fibromyalgia. Arthritis Rheum 1994;37(11):1583–92.

[15] Neeck G, Riedel W. Hormonal perturbations in fibromyalgia

syndrome. Ann N Y Acad Sci 1999;876:325–38.

[16] Bennett RM, Cook DM, Clark SR, et al. Hypothalamic–pituitary–insulin-like growth factor-I axis dysfunction in patients with fibromyalgia. J Rheumatol 1997;24(7):1384–9.

[17] Cleare AJ. The HPA axis and the genesis of chronic fatigue syndrome. Trends in Endocrine Metabolism 2004;15(2):55–9.

[18] Physicians' Desk Reference 2010. 64th ed. Montvale, NJ: PDR Network; 2009. p. 2731–40.

[19] Physicians Desk Reference 2010. 64th ed. Montvale: PDR Network; 2009. p. 1871–81.

[20] Sarzi Puttini P, Caruso I. Primary fibromyalgia syndrome and 5-hydroxy-L-tryptophan: a 90-day open study. J Int Med Res 1992;20(2):182–9.

[21] Nichols DS, Glenn TM. Effects of aerobic exercise on pain perception, affect, and level of disability in individuals with fibromyalgia. Phys Ther 1994;74(4):327–32.

[22] Jaeschke R, Adachi J, Guyatt G, et al. Clinical usefulness of amitriptyline in fibromyalgia: the results of 23 N-of-1 randomized controlled trials. J Rheumatol 1991;18(3):447–51.

[23] Goodnick PJ, Sandoval R. Psychotropic treatment of chronic fatigue syndrome and related disorders. J Clin Psychiatry 1993;54(1):13–20.

[24] Fortin PR, Lew RA, Liang MH, et al. Validation of meta-analysis: the effects of fish oil in rheumatoid arthritis. J Clin Epidemiol 1995;48(11):1379–90.

[25] Kremer JM, Bigauotte J, Michalek AV, et al. Effects of manipulation of dietary fatty acids on clinical manifestations of rheumatoid arthritis. Lancet 1985;1(8422):184–7.

[26] Van de Rest O, Geleijnse JM, Kok FJ, et al. Efect of fish oil on cognitive performance in older subjects. Neurology 2008;71(6):430–8.

[27] Klenner F. Significance of high daily intake of ascorbic acid in preventive medicine. Journal of the International Academy of Preventive Medicine 1974;1(1):45–69.

[28] Dalton WL. Massive doses of vitamin C in the treatment of viral disease. Indiana Med 1962;55:1151–4.

[29] Wannamethee SG, Lowe GDO, Rumley A, et al. Associations of vitamin C status, fruit and vegetable intakes, and markers of inflammation and hemostasis. Am J Clin Nutr 2006;83(3):567–74.

[30] Cheng N. The effects of electric currents on ATP generation, protein synthesis and membrane transport of rat skin. J Clin Orthop Relat Res 1982;(171)264–72.

[31] Reilly W, Reeve VE, Quinn C. Anti-inflammatory effects of interferential, frequency-specific applied microcurrent. Sydney: Australian Health and Medical Research Congress; 2004.

[32] McMakin C. Microcurrent treatment of myofascial pain in the head, neck and face. Topics in Clinical Chiropractic 1998;5(1):29–35.

[33] McMakin C. Microcurrent therapy: a novel treatment method for chronic low back myofascial pain. J Bodyw Mov Ther 2004;8(2):143–53.

[34] McMakin C. Frequency Specific Microcurrent in Pain Management. Edinburgh: Churchill Livingstone; 2010.

[35] Craske M, Turner W, Zammit-Maempe J, et al. Qigong ameliorates symptoms of chronic fatigue: a pilot uncontrolled study. Evidence-based Complementary and Alternative Medicine: eCAM 2009;6(2):265–70.

[36] Ryu H, Jun CD, Lee BS, et al. Effect of qigong training on proportions of T lymphocyte subsets in human peripheral blood. Am J Chin Med 1995;23(1):27–36.

[37] Lee MS, Jeong SM, Oh SW, et al. Effects of chundosunbup Qi-training on psychological adjustments: a cross-sectional study. Am J Chin Med 1998;26(2):223–30.

[38] Lee MS, Hong SS, Lim HJ, et al. Retrospective survey on therapeutic efficacy of Qigong in Korea. Am J Chin Med 2003;31(5):809–15.

[39] Deluze C, Bosia L, Zirbs A, et al. Electroacupuncture in fibromyalgia: results of a controlled trial. Br Med J 1992;305(6864):1249–52.

[40] Melzack R, Stillwell DM, Fox EJ. Trigger points and acupuncture points for pain: correlation and implications. Pain 1977;3(1):3–23.

[41] Fraser P, Massey H, Wilcox JP. Decoding the Human Body Field:

The new science of information as medicine. Rochester, VT: Healing Arts; 2008.

[42] Nutri-Energetics Systems. Online. Available: http://www.neshealth.com (formerly http://www.nutrienergetics.com).

[43] Oschman JL. Energy Medicine: The scientific basis. Edinburgh: Churchill Livingstone; 2000.

[44] Riordan J, Zhang XC. Sampling of free-space magnetic pulses. Opt Quant Electron 2000;32(4–5):489–502.

[45] Wolff M. Exploring the Physics of the Unknown Universe: An adventurer's guide. Manhattan Beach, CA: Technotran Press; 1990.

[46] Wolff M. Schrödinger's Universe: Einstein, waves and the origin of the natural laws. Parker, CO: Outskirts Press; 2008.

[47] Haselhurst G. Howie K. On truth and reality: the spherical standing wave structure of matter (WSM) in space Online. Available: http://www.spaceandmotion.com 17 Nov 2010.

[48] Buchanan M. Beyond reality: watching information at play in the quantum world is throwing physics into a flat spin. New Sci 1998;(2125)26.

[49] Bjorken JD. Asymptotic sum rules at infinite momentum. Phys Rev 1969;179(5):1547–53.

[50] Chislenko LL. Struktura fauny i flory v svyazi s razmerami organizmov [Structure of Fauna and Flora in Connection with Organism Size]. Moscow: Moscow University Press; 1981 [in Russian].

[51] Zhirmunsky AV, Kuzmin VI. Critical Levels in Developmental Processes of Biological Systems. Moscow: Nauka; 1982 [in Russian].

[52] Original papers Online. Available: Global scaling website http://www.info.global-scaling-verein.de/Global-Scaling/Global-Scaling-Publications-Original.htm.

[53] Suchergebnis für 'Hartmut Müller' Online. Available: Raum und Zeit website http://www.raum-und-zeit.com.

24. THE ELECTRICAL HEART: ENERGY IN CARDIAC HEALTH AND DISEASE

[1] Graham H. Time, Energy and the Psychology of Healing. London: Jessica Kingsley; 1990.

[2] Birse RM (rev Knowlden PE). Muirhead, Alexander (1848–1920). In: Oxford Dictionary of National Biography. Oxford: Oxford University Press; 2004. Online. Available: http://www.oxforddnb.com/view/article/37794 3 Feb 2010.

[3] Sanderson JB, Page FJM. Experimental results relating to the rhythmical and excitatory motions of the ventricle of the heart of the frog, and of the electrical phenomena which accompany them. Proceedings of the Royal Society of London 1878;27:410–4.

[4] Waller AD. A demonstration on man of electromotive changes accompanying the heart's beat. J Physiol 1887;8(5):229–34.

[5] Wilber K. The Marriage of Sense and Soul: Integrating science and religion. New York: Random House; 1998.

[6] Watkins AD. Medicine and the heart's energy. Advances 1996;13(2):70–4.

[7] Jankowski M, Hajjar F, Al Kawas S, et al. Rat heart: a site of oxytocin production and action. Proc Natl Acad Sci U S A 1998;95(24):14558–63.

[8] Strogatz S. Sync: The emerging science of spontaneous order. New York: Hyperion (HarperCollins;); 2003.

[9] Beauregard M, Paquette V. Neural correlates of a mystical experience in Carmelite nuns. Neurosci Lett 2006;405(3):186–90.

[10] Hon EH, Lee ST. Electronic evaluation of the fetal heart rate. VIII. Patterns preceeding fetal death, further observations. Am J Obstet Gynecol 1965;87:814–26.

[11] Wolf MM, Varigos GA, Hunt D, et al. Sinus arrhythmia in acute mycardial infarction. Med J Aust 1978;2(2):52–3.

[12] Tsuji H, Larson M, Venditti F, et al. Impact of reduced heart rate variability on risk for cardiac events: the Framingham heart study. Circulation 1996;94(11):2850–5.

[13] Tsuji H, Venditti F, Manders E, et al. Reduced heart rate variability and mortality risk in an elderly cohort: the Framingham heart study. Circulation 1994;90(2):878–83.

[14] Kleiger RE, Miller JP, Bigger Jr JT, et al. Decreased heart rate variability and its association with increased mortality after acute myocardial infarction. Am J Cardiol 1987;59(4):256–62.

[15] Voss A, Hnatkova K, Wessel N, et al. Multiparametric analysis of heart rate variability used for risk stratification among survivors of acute myocardial infarction. Pacing Clin Electrophysiol 1998;21(1 pt 2):186–92.

[16] American College of Cardiology Cardiovascular Technology Assessment Committee. Heart rate variability for risk stratification of life-threatening arrhythmias. J Am Coll Cardiol 1993;22(3):948–50.

[17] Dekker JM, Schouten EG, Klootwijk P, et al. Heart rate variability from short electrocardiographic recordings predicts mortality from all causes in middle-aged and elderly men: the Zutphen Study. Am J Epidemiol 1997;145(10):899–908.

[18] Gerritsen J, Dekker JM, TenVoorde BJ, et al. Impaired autonomic function is associated with increased mortality, especially in subjects with diabetes, hypertension, or a history of cardiovascular disease: the Hoorn Study. Diabetes Care 2001;24(10):1793–8.

[19] Whang W, Bigger Jr JT. Comparison of the prognostic value of RR-interval variability after acute myocardial infarction in patients with versus those without diabetes mellitus. Am J Cardiol 2003;92(3):247–51.

[20] Umetani K, Singer DH, McCraty R, et al. Twenty-four hour time domain heart rate variability and heart rate: relations to age and gender over nine decades. J Am Coll Cardiol 1998;31(3):593–601.

[21] Rennie KL, Hemingway H, Kumari M, et al. Effects of moderate and vigorous physical activity on heart rate variability in a British study of civil servants. Am J Epidemiol 2003;158(2):135–43.

[22] Christensen JH, Schmidt EB. n-3 fatty acids and the risk of sudden cardiac death. Lipids 2001;36(Suppl.):S115–8.

[23] Sakuragi S, Sugiyama Y, Takeuchi K. Effects of laughing and weeping on mood and heart rate variability. J Physiol Anthropol Appl Human Sci 2002;21(3):159–65.

[24] Raghuraj P, Ramakrishnan AG, Nagendra HR, et al. Effects of two selected yogic breathing techniques of heart rate variability. Indian J Physiol Pharmacol 1998;42(4):467–72.

[25] Jovanov E. On spectral analysis of heart rate variability during very slow yogic breathing. Conf Proc IEEE Eng Med Biol Soc 2005;3:2467–70.

[26] Khattab K, Khattab AA, Ortak J, et al. Iyengar yoga increases cardiac parasympathetic nervous modulation among healthy yoga practitioners. Evidence-Based Complementary and Alternative Medicine 2007;4(4):511–7.

[27] Lee MS, Kim MK, Lee YH. Effects of qi-therapy (external qigong) on cardiac autonomic tone: a randomized placebo controlled study. Int J Neurosci 2005;115(9):1345–50.

[28] Lee MS, Rim YH, Jeong DM, et al. Nonlinear analysis of heart rate variability during qi therapy (external qigong). Am J Chin Med 2005;33(4):579–88.

[29] Bäcker M, Grossman P, Schneider J, et al. Acupuncture in migraine: investigation of autonomic effects. Clin J Pain 2008;24(2):106–15.

[30] Napadow V, Dhond RP, Purdon P, et al. Correlating acupuncture fMRI in the human brainstem with heart rate variability. Conf Proc IEEE Eng Med Biol Soc 2005;5:4496–9.

[31] Kline JP. Heart rate variability does not tap putative efficacy of Thought Field Therapy. J Clin Psychol 2001;57(10):1187–92 1251,1260 (discussion).

[32] Losada M, Heaphy E. The role of positivity and connectivity in the performance of business teams. Am Behav Sci 2004;47(6):740–65.

[33] Boneva RS, Decker MJ, Maloney EM, et al. Higher heart rate and reduced heart rate variability persist during sleep in chronic fatigue syndrome: a population-based study. Auton Neurosci 2007;137(1–2):94–101.

[34] Richert KA, Carrion VG, Karchemskiy A, et al. Regional differences of the prefrontal cortex in pediatric PTSD: an MRI study. Depress Anxiety 2006;23(1):17–25.

[35] Zucker TL, Samuelson KW, Muench F, et al. The effects of respiratory sinus arrhythmia biofeedback on heart rate variability and posttraumatic stress disorder symptoms: a pilot study. Appl Psychophysiol Biofeedback 2009;34(2):135–43.

[36] Keary TA, Hughes JW, Palmieri PA. Women with posttraumatic stress disorder have larger decreases in heart

rate variability during stress tasks. Int J Psychophysiol 2009;73(3):257–64.

[37] McCraty R, Atkinson M, Tiller WA, et al. The effects of emotions on short-term power spectrum analysis of heart rate variability. Am J Cardiol 1995;76(14):1089–93.

[38] Siepmann M, Aykac V, Unterdörfer J, et al. A pilot study on the effects of heart rate variability biofeedback in patients with depression and in healthy subjects. Appl Psychophysiol Biofeedback 2008;33(4):195–201.

[39] Karavidas MK, Lehrer PM, Vaschillo E, et al. Preliminary results of an open label study of heart rate variability biofeedback for the treatment of major depression. Appl Psychophysiol Biofeedback 2007;32(1):19–30.

[40] Hassett AL, Radvanski DC, Vaschillo EG, et al. A pilot study of the efficacy of heart rate variability (HRV) biofeedback in patients with fibromyalgia. Appl Psychophysiol Biofeedback 2007;32(1):1–10.

[41] Nolan RP, Kamath MV, Floras JS, et al. Heart rate variability biofeedback as a behavioral neurocardiac intervention to enhance vagal heart rate control. Am Heart J 2005;149(6):1137.

[42] Lehrer PM, Vaschillo E, Vaschillo B, et al. Biofeedback treatment for asthma. Chest 2004;126(2):352–61.

[43] Yucha CB, Clark L, Smith M, et al. The effect of biofeedback in hypertension. Appl Nurs Res 2001;14(1):29–35.

[44] Nakao M, Nomura S, Shimosawa T, et al. Clinical effects of blood pressure biofeedback treatment on hypertension by auto-shaping. Psychosom Med 1997;59(3):331–8.

[45] Giardino ND, Chan L, Borson S. Combined heart rate variability and pulse oximetry biofeedback for chronic obstructive pulmonary disease: preliminary findings. Appl Psychophysiol Biofeedback 2004;29(2):121–33.

[46] Raymond J, Sajid I, Parkinson LA, et al. Biofeedback and dance performance: a preliminary investigation. Appl Psychophysiol Biofeedback 2005;30(1):64–73.

25. THEMES OF *QI* AND A DOZEN DEFINITIONS: CONTENT ANALYSIS AND DISCUSSION

[1] Kaptchuk TJ. Vitalism. Micozzi MS, editor. Fundamentals of Complementary and Integrative Medicine. St Louis: Saunders Elsevier; 2006. p. 53.

[2] Stemler S. An overview of content analysis. Practical Assessment, Research & Evaluation 2001;7(17). Online. Available: http://PAREonline .net/getvn.asp?v=7&n=17 23 Mar 2010.

[3] Ergil KV. Diagnosis in Chinese medicine. Ergil MC, Ergil KV, editors. Pocket Atlas of Chinese Medicine. New York: Thieme; 2009. p. 132.

[4] Raknes O. The orgonomic concept of health and its social consequences. Orgonomic Medicine 1955;1(2):106–20.

[5] Mayor DF. Vitalism: flow, connection, and the awareness of being alive. Micozzi MS, editor. Fundamentals of Complementary and Alternative Medicine. 4th ed. St Louis, MO: Saunders; 2011. p. 61–80.

[6] Bergson HL. Matière et Mémoire: Essai sur la relation du corps à l'ésprit. Paris: Félix Alcan; 1896.

[7] Sheets-Johnstone M. The Primacy of Movement. Amsterdam: John Benjamins; 1999.

[8] Cairns D, editor. Conversations with Husserl and Fink. The Hague, Netherlands: Nijhoff; 1976. p. 78.

[9] Davis CM. Introduction. In: Davis CM, editor. Complementary Therapies in Rehabilitation. Thorofare, NJ: SLACK; 2004. p. xvii–xxv.

[10] Battaglia D. On the Bones of the Serpent: Person, memory, and mortality in Sabarl Island society. Chicago, IL: University of Chicago Press; 1990.

[11] Bisilliat J. Village diseases and bush diseases in Songhay: an essay in description and classification with a view to a typology. Loudon JB, editor. Social Anthropology and Medicine. London: Academic Press; 1976. p. 553–93.

[12] Devisch R. Weaving the Threads of Life: The Khita gyn-eco-logical healing cult among the Yaka. Chicago, IL: University of Chicago Press; 1993.

[13] Lewis-Williams D, Thomas Dowson T. Images of Power: Understanding San rock art. 2nd ed. Johannesburg, S Africa: Southern; 1999.

[14] Hall S. Images of interaction. Dowson TA, David Lewis-Williams D, editors. Contested Images: Diversity in Southern African rock art research.

Johannesburg, S Africa: Witwatersrand University Press; 1994. p. 61–82.

[15] Lewis-Williams JD, Pearce DG. San Spirituality: Roots, expression, and social consequences. Walnut Creek, CA: AltaMira Press; 2004.

[16] Grant C. Rock Art of the American Indian. New York: Thomas Y Crowell; 1967.

[17] Grim JA. The Shaman: Patterns of Siberian and Ojibway healing. Norman, OK: University of Oklahoma Press; 1983.

[18] Uher J. Zigzag rock art. Dowson TA, David Lewis-Williams D, editors. Contested Images: Diversity in Southern African rock art research. Johannesburg, S Africa: Witwatersrand University Press; 1994. p. 293–313.

[19] Kaku K. The Mysterious Power of Ki – the force within. Folkestone, Kent: Global Oriental; 2000. p. 5, 144.

[20] Partridge CH. In: The Re-enchantment of the West: Alternative spiritualities, sacralization, popular culture, and occulture, vol. 2. London: T & T Clark; 2005. p. 34.

[21] Sachs J. Aristotle (384–322 BCE): Motion and its place in nature. Internet Encyclopedia of Philosophy 2006;. Online. Available: http://www.utm.edu/research/iep/a/aris-mot.htm 21 Mar 2010.

[22] Martin RE. American Literature and the Universe of Force. Durham, NC: Duke University Press; 1981.

[23] Tait PG. Lectures on Some Recent Advances in Physical Science. With a special lecture on force. 2nd ed. London: Macmillan; 1876.

[24] Rabinbach A. The Human Motor: Energy, fatigue, and the origins of modernity. Berkeley, CA: University of California Press; 1992. p. 50.

[25] Brown G. The Energy of Life. London: HarperCollins; 1999.

[26] Needham J, Wang L. History of Scientific Thought. Science and Civilisation in China, vol. 2. Cambridge: Cambridge University Press; 1956.

[27] Soulié de Morant G. L'Acuponcture Chinoise. Paris: Maloine; 1985.

[28] Bergson H. L'Évolution Créatrice. Paris: Félix Alcan; 1914.

[29] Motoyama H. Theories of the Chakras: Bridge to higher consciousness. Wheaton, IL: Theosophical Publishing House; 1981.

[30] Motoyama H, Brown R. Science and the Evolution of Consciousness: Chakras, ki, and psi. Brookline, MA: Autumn Press; 1978.

[31] Wiseman N, Ellis A. Fundamentals of Chinese Medicine (Zhong Yi Xue Ji Chu). Revised ed. Brookline, MA: Paradigm; 1995.

[32] Schwartz BI. The World of Thought in Ancient China. Cambridge, MA: Harvard University Press; 1985.

[33] Birch SJ, Felt RL. Understanding Acupuncture. Edinburgh: Churchill Livingstone; 1999. p. 105, 108.

[34] Sivin N. Traditional Medicine in Contemporary China. A partial translation of Revised Outline of Chinese Medicine (1972) with an introductory study on change in present-day and early medicine. Ann Arbor, MI: Center for Chinese Studies, University of Michigan; 1987.

[35] Robinet I. Taoism: Growth of a religion. Stanford, CA: Stanford University Press; 1997.

[36] Bivins RE. Alternative Medicine? A history. Oxford: Oxford University Press; 2007.

[37] Wiseman N, Feng Y. A Practical Dictionary of Chinese Medicine. 2nd ed. Brookline, MA: Paradigm; 1998.

[38] Smith NW. An Analysis of Ice Age Art: Its psychology and belief system. New York: Peter Lang; 1992.

[39] Unschuld PU. Nan-Ching: The classic of difficult issues. With commentaries by Chinese and Japanese authors from the third through the twentieth century. Berkeley, CA: University of California Press; 1986.

[40] Bastien JW. Qollahuaya-Andean body concepts: a topographical-hydraulic model of physiology. American Anthropologist n.s. 1985;87(3):595–611.

[41] Maciocia G. The Channels of Acupuncture: Clinical use of the secondary channels and eight extraordinary vessels. Edinburgh: Churchill Livingstone; 2006.

[42] Lévy-Bruhl L. The 'Soul' of the Primitive. London: Allen & Unwin; 1965.

[43] Laughlin Jr CD. Psychic energy and transpersonal experience: a biogenetic structural account of the Tibetan dumo yoga practice. Young DE, Goulet JG, editors. Being Changed by Cross-Cultural Encounters. Peterborough, ONT: Broadview Press; 1994. p. 99–134.

[44] Peat FD. Towards a process theory of healing: energy, activity and global form. Subtle Energies 1992;3(2):1–40.

[45] Montagu A. Touching: The human significance of the skin. New York: Columbia University Press; 1971.

[46] Nussbaum MC. Aristotle's 'De Motu Animalium': Text; with translation, commentary and interpretive essays. Princeton, NJ: Princeton University Press; 1978. p. 36, 38.

[47] Sheets-Johnstone M. The Corporeal Turn: An interdisciplinary reader. Devon: Imprint Academic, Exeter; 2009. p. 380.

[48] Liu ZW. Philosophical aspects of Chinese medicine from a Chinese medicine academician. Chan K, Lee H, editors. The Way Forward for Chinese Medicine. London: Taylor & Francis; 2002. p. 23–49.

[49] Eddington AS. The Nature of the Physical World. Ann Arbor, MI: University of Michigan Press; 1974. p. 276.

[50] Pfeiffer T, Mack JE, editors. Mind Before Matter: Visions of a new science of consciousness. Winchester, Hants: O Books; 2007.

[51] Harman WW. The postmodern heresy: consciousness as causal. Griffin DR, editor. The Reenchantment of Science: Postmodern proposals. Albany, NY: State University of New York Press; 1988. p. 115–28.

[52] Micozzi MS. Vital Healing: Energy, mind and spirit in Indian, Tibetan and Middle Eastern medicine. London: Singing Dragon Press; 2010.

[53] Turner E. The Hands Feel It: Healing and spirit presence among a northern Alaskan people. DeKalb, IL: Northern Illinois University Press; 1996.

[54] Benor DJ. Healing Research: Holistic energy medicine and spirituality, vol 1. Research in healing. Deddington, Oxon: Helix; 1993. p. 55.

[55] Southgate 5. Traditional Chinese Medicine and Reichian Theory. Aberystwyth: Northern College of Acupuncture, York, and University of Wales; 2002. MSc thesis Online. Available (summary): Orgone Discovery website http://org.ieasysite.com/website1_007.htm 2 Apr 2010.

[56] Fuller R. Alternative Medicine and American Religious Life. New York: Oxford University Press; 1989.

[57] Palmer DA. La fièvre du Qigong: Guérison, religion et politique en Chine, 1949–1999. Paris: École des Hautes Études en Sciences Sociales; 2005.

[58] McClean S. An Ethnography of Crystal and Spiritual Healers in Northern England: Marginal medicine and mainstream concerns. Lewiston, NY: Edwin Mellen; 2006.

[59] Chace C. The shape of qi: enhancing the vocabulary of contact in acupuncture. The Lantern: A Journal of Traditional Chinese Medicine 2008;5(1). 2 Online. Available: www.thelantern.com.au/resource:detail.php?id=198 21 Mar 2010.

[60] Clottes J, Lewis-Williams D. The Shamans of Prehistory: Trance and magic in the painted caves. New York: Harry N Abrams; 1998. p. 95.

[61] Guthrie RD. The Nature of Paleolithic Art. Chicago, IL: University of Chicago Press; 2005.

[62] Reich W. Selected Writings: An introduction to orgonomy. Revised ed. London: Vision Press; 1973. p. 29, 37, 111, 147, 293, 517.

[63] Jawer MA, Micozzi MS. The Spiritual Anatomy of Emotion: How feelings link the brain, the body, and the sixth sense. Rochester, VT: Park Street Press; 2009. p. 307, 330, 440.

[64] Yuasa Y. The Body: Toward an Eastern mind-body theory. Albany, NY: State University of New York Press; 1987. p. 111, 220.

[65] James W. What is an emotion? Mind 1884;9(34):188–205.

[66] de Quincey C. Radical Nature: Rediscovering the soul of matter. Montpelier, VT: Invisible Cities Press; 2002. p. 61, 145.

[67] Bloom K. Articulating preverbal experience. Totton N, editor. New Dimensions in Body Psychotherapy. Maidenhead, Berks: Open University Press; 2005. p. 65.

[68] Thalbourne MA, Fox B. Paranormal and mystical experience: the role of panic attacks and kundalini. Journal of the American Society for Psychical Research 1999;93(1):99–115.

[69] White DG. Yoga in early Hindu tantra. Whicher I, Carpenter D, editors. Yoga: The Indian tradition. London: RoutledgeCurzon; 2003. p. 143–61.

[70] Hayes GA. Metaphoric worlds and yoga in the Vaisnava Sahajiyā

tantric traditions of medieval Bengal. In: Whicher I, Carpenter D, editors. Yoga: The Indian tradition. London: RoutledgeCurzon; 2003. p. 162–84.

[71] Findly EB. Breath and breathing. Eliade M, editor. The Encyclopedia of Religion, vol. 2. New York: Macmillan; 1987. p. 302–8.

[72] Eliade M. Yoga: Immortality and freedom. London: Routledge & Kegan Paul; 1958.

[73] Gerber R. Vibrational Medicine for the 21st Century: A complete guide to energy healing and spiritual transformation. London: Judy Piatkus; 2000.

[74] Shamdasani S, editor. The Psychology of Kundalini Yoga: Notes of the seminar given in 1932 by C G Jung. London: Routledge; 1996.

[75] Judith A. Eastern Body, Western Mind: Psychology and the chakra system as a path to the self. Berkeley, CA: Celestial Arts; 2004.

[76] Myss C. Anatomy of the Spirit: The seven stages of power and healing. London: Bantam; 1997.

[77] Reich W. Character Analysis. 3rd ed. New York: Farrar, Straus and Giroux; 1972.

[78] Boadella D. Lifestreams: An introduction to biosynthesis. London: Routledge & Kegan Paul; 1987. p. 89.

[79] Zhuangzi Ch 4 Pt II. Translated by DM on the basis of:
 (a) Robinet. 1997 (ref 29 above);
 (b) Correa N. translator Zhuangzi Chapter 4 Relating to the Human World. 2009. Online. Available: http://www.daoisopen.com/ZZ4 .html 6 April 2010; (c) Legge J. translator Zhuangzi: Man in the world, associated with other men. 1891. Online. Available: Chinese Text Project website http://chinese.dsturgeon.net/text. pl?node=2713&if=en 6 April 2010.

[80] Tokitsu K. Ki and the Way of the Martial Arts. Boston, MA: Shambhala; 2003.

[81] Seel M. On the scope of aesthetic esperience. Shusterman R, Tomlin A, editors. Aesthetic Experience. New York: Routledge; 2008. p. 98–105.

[82] Rickett WA. Guanzi. Political, economic, and philosophical essays from early China. A study and translation, vol. 2. Princeton, NJ: Princeton University Press; 1998. p. 31.

[83] Ots T. The segmental structure of the body – appraisal of classical Chinese phenomenology and destruction of its theoretical framework. British Medical Acupuncture Society Spring Meeting, University of Warwick; 2006 26 March 2006.

[84] Schachtel EG. Metamorphosis. New York: Basic Books; 1959.

[85] Sun GC. Qigong: bio-energy medicine. J Altern Complement Med 2008;14(8):893–7.

[86] Hankey A. CAM and the phenomenology of pain. Evidence-based Complementary and Alternative Medicine 2006;3(1):139–41.

[87] Thompson EA, Geraghty J. The vital sensation of the minerals: reducing uncertainty in homeopathic prescribing. Homeopathy 2007;96(2):102–7.

[88] McCown D, Reibel D, Micozzi M. Teaching Mindfulness. New York: Springer; 2011.

[89] Williams C. Traditions, paradigms and perspectives: Chinese med treading a path in the West. European Journal of Oriental Medicine 2009;6(2):4–11.

[90] Reynolds DK. The Quiet Therapies: Japanese pathways to personal growth. Honolulu: University Press of Hawaii; 1982.

[91] Ferguson M. The Aquarian Conspiracy: Personal and social transformation in the 1980s. London: Granada; 1982. p. 274.

[92] Barfield O. Poetic Diction: A study in meaning. London: Faber & Gwyer; 1928. p. 157.

[93] Ohnishi ST, Ohnishi T. How far can ki-energy reach? A hypothetical mechanism for the generation and transmission of ki-energy. Evidence-based Complementary and Alternative Medicine 2009;6(3):379–91.

[94] Keleman S. Emotional Anatomy. Berkeley, CA: Center Press; 1985. p. 12.

[95] Oschman JL. Energy Medicine: The scientific basis. Edinburgh: Churchill Livingstone; 2000.

[96] Oschman JL. Energy Medicine in Therapeutics and Human Performance. Philadelphia, PA: Butterworth-Heinemann; 2003.

[97] Marcel G. Metaphysical journal and a metaphysical diary. Spicker SF, editor. The Philosophy of the Body: Rejections of Cartesian dualism. Chicago, IL: Quadrangle Books; 1970. p. 202.

[98] Dutton D. The lived body: changing conceptions of embodiment and their challenge to modern Chinese medicine. European Journal of Oriental Medicine 2009;6(4):43–51.

[99] Scott A. The knowledge in our bones: standpoint theory, alternative health and the quantum model of the body. Maynard M, editor. Science and the Construction of Women. London: UCL Press; 1997. p. 12, 109.

[100] Humphrey N. A History of the Mind. London: Chatto & Windus; 1992.

[101] Capra F. The Tao of Physics: An exploration of the parallels between modern physics and Eastern mysticism. London: Wildwood House; 1975.

[102] Chopra D. Quantum Healing: Exploring the frontiers of mind/body medicine. New York: Bantam Books; 1989.

[103] Jackson M. Paths Toward a Clearing: Radical empiricism and ethnographical inquiry. Bloomington, IN: Indiana University Press; 1989.

[104] Stalker D, Glymour C, editors. Examining Holistic Medicine. Buffalo, NY: Prometheus; 1985.

[105] Pert CB. Molecules of Emotion: Why you feel the way you feel. New York: Charles Scribner's Sons; 1997. p 766.

[106] Coward R. The Whole Truth: The myth of alternative health. London: Faber & Faber; 1989.

[107] Siahpush M. Postmodern values, dissatisfaction with conventional medicine and popularity of alternative therapies. Journal of Sociology 1998;34(1):58–70.

[108] Fadlon J. Meridians, chakras and psycho-neuro-immunology: the dematerializing body and the domestication of alternative medicine. Body and Society 2004;10(4):69–86.

[109] Bishop LM. Words, Stones, and Herbs: The healing word in medieval and early modern England. Syracuse, NY: Syracuse University Press; 2007.

[110] Kinsbourne M, editor. Cerebral Hemisphere Function in Depression. Washington DC: American Psychiatric Press; 1988.

[111] Onians RB. The Origins of European Thought about the Body, the Mind, the Soul, the World, Time, and Fate. New interpretations of Greek, Roman and kindred evidence also of some basic Jewish and Christian beliefs. New York: Arno Press; 1973.

[112] Gordon AH, Schwabe CW. The Quick and the Dead: Biomedical theory in ancient Egypt. Leiden: Brill; 2004.

[113] Heritier-Auge F. Semen and blood: some ancient theories concerning their genesis and relationship. Feher M, with Naddaff R, Tazi N, editors. Fragments for a History of the Human Body. Part Three. New York: Zone; 1989. p. 158–75.

[114] Hugh-Jones C. From the Milk River: Spatial and temporal processes in Northwest Amazonia. Cambridge, Cambs: Cambridge University Press; 1979.

[115] Meigs AS. Food, Sex and Pollution: A New Guinea religion. New Brunswick, NJ: Rutgers University Press; 1984.

[116] Strathern AJ. Body Thoughts. Ann Arbor, MI: University of Michigan Press; 1996.

[117] Hall TS. History of General Physiology, 600 BC to AD 1900. I. From Pre-Socratic times to the Enlightenment. Chicago: University of Chicago Press; 1975.

[118] Claus DB. Toward the Soul: An inquiry into the meaning of ψυχή before Plato. New Haven, CT: Yale University Press; 1981.

[119] Williams EA. A Cultural History of Medical Vitalism in Enlightenment Montpellier. Burlington, VT: Ashgate; 2003.

[120] Skultans V. Intimacy and Ritual: A study of spiritualism, mediums and groups. London: Routledge & Kegan Paul; 1974.

[121] Frohock FM. Lives of the Psychics: The shared worlds of science and mysticism. Chicago, IL: University of Chicago Press; 2000.

[122] Reed H. Close encounters in the liminal zone: experiments in imaginal communication Part I. J Anal Psychol 1996;41(1):81–116.

[123] Totton N. Introduction. Totton N, editor. New Dimensions in Body Psychotherapy. Maidenhead, Berks: Open University Press; 2005. p. 1–10.

[124] (Mayor D, Trans.) Senf B. Wilhelm Reich: discoverer of acupuncture energy? Am J Acupunct 1979;7(2):109–18.

[125] Reinard A, Réquéna Y. Qi gong. Ergil MC, Ergil KV, editors. Pocket Atlas of Chinese Medicine. New York: Thieme; 2009. p. 319–43.

[126] Ruggieri V, Milizia M, Sabatini N, et al. Body perception in relation to muscular tone at rest and tactile sensitivity to tickle. Percept Mot Skills 1983;56(3):799–806.

[127] Sabatini N, Ruggieri V, Milizia M. Barrier and penetration scores in relation to some objective and subjective somesthetic measures. Percept Mot Skills 1984;59(1):195–202.

[128] Kinsbourne M. Awareness of one's own body: an attentional theory of its nature, development, and brain basis. Bermúdez JL, Marcel A, Eilan N, editors. The Body and the Self. Cambridge, MA: MIT Press; 1995.

[129] Castaneda C. The Wheel of Time. The shamans of ancient Mexico, their thoughts about life, death and the universe. London: Allen Lane/ Penguin Press; 1998.

[130] Tunneshende M. Medicine Dream: A woman's encounter with the healing realms of Don Juan. London: Thorsons; 1997.

[131] Lewis-Williams D. The Mind in the Cave: Consciousness and the origins of art. London: Thames & Hudson; 2002. p. 121.

[132] Glik DC. Symbolic, ritual and social dynamics of spiritual healing. Soc Sci Med 1988;27(11):1197–206.

[133] Csordas T. The Sacred Self: A cultural phenomenology of charismatic healing. Berkeley, CA: University of California Press; 1994.

[134] Voss RW. Native American healing. Micozzi MS, editor. Fundamentals of Complementary and Alternative Medicine. St Louis, MO: Saunders; 2011. p. 531–50.

[135] Merkur D. The Ecstatic Imagination: Psychedelic experiences and the psychoanalysis of self-actualization. Albany, NY: State University of New York Press; 1998.

[136] Braden W. The Private Sea: LSD and the search for God. London: Pall Mall; 1967.

[137] Siegel RK. Fire in the Brain: Clinical tales of hallucination. New York: Dutton; 1992.

[138] Davis A. Exploring Inner Space: Personal experiences under LSD-25. London: Scientific Book Club; 1961.

[139] Nagatomo S. Attunement Through the Body. Albany, NY: State University of New York Press; 1992.

[140] Mayor DM, editor. Electroacupuncture: A practical manual and resource. Edinburgh: Churchill Livingstone; 2007.

[141] Snow CP. The Two Cultures; and A second look. An expanded version of The Two Cultures and the Scientific Revolution. Cambridge, Cambs: Cambridge University Press; 1964. p. 9.

[142] Spicker SF. Introduction. Spicker SF, editor. The Philosophy of the Body: Rejections of Cartesian dualism. Chicago, IL: Quadrangle Books; 1970. p. 3–23.

[143] Hoeller SA. The Gnostic Jung and the Seven Sermons to the Dead. Wheaton, IL: Quest; 1982.

[144] Yuasa Y. Contemporary science and an Eastern mind-body theory. Shaner DE, Nagatomo S, Yuasa Y, editors. Science and Comparative Philosophy. Introducing Yuasa Yasuo. Leiden: E J Brill; 1989. p. 193–240.

[145] Motoyama H, Yuasa Y. How to Measure and Diagnose the Functions of Meridians. Research for Religion and Parapsychology 1975;1(2) International Association for Religion and Parapsychology, Tokyo.

[146] Nagatomo S. The Japanese concept of self: another analysis of a culturally reinforced attitude. Shaner DE, Nagatomo S, Yuasa Y, editors. Science and Comparative Philosophy. Introducing Yuasa Yasuo. Leiden: E J Brill; 1989. p. 126–192.

[147] Yuasa Y. The Body, Self-cultivation, and Ki-energy. Albany, NY: State University of New York Press; 1993.

[148] Yuasa Y. A cultural background for traditional Japanese self-cultivation philosophy and a theoretical examination of this philosophy. Shaner DE, Nagatomo S, Yuasa Y, editors. Science and Comparative Philosophy. Introducing Yuasa Yasuo. Leiden: E J Brill; 1989. p. 241–77.

[149] Kidel M, Rowe-Leete S. Mapping the body. Feher M, with Naddaff R, Tazi N, editors. Fragments for a History of the Human Body. Part Three. New York: Zone; 1989. p. 448–69.

[150] Johnson M. The Meaning of the Body: Aesthetics of human understanding. Chicago, IL: University of Chicago Press; 2007.

[151] Langer SK. Mind: An essay on human feeling, abridged edn. Baltimore, MD: Johns Hopkins University Press; 1988.

[152] James W. Does consciousness exist? Journal of Philosophy, Psychology and Scientific Method 1904;1(18):477–91.

[153] Schilpp PA, editor. The Philosophy of Alfred North Whitehead. New York: Tudor Publishing; 1999. p. 169.

[154] Lakoff G, Johnson M. Metaphors We Live By. Chicago, IL: University of Chicago Press; 1980. p. 193.

[155] Tu WM. Confucian Thought: Selfhood as creative transformation. Albany, NY: State University of New York Press; 1985.

[156] Leskowitz E. Energy-based therapies for chronic pain. Audette JF, Bailey A, editors. Integrative Pain Medicine: The science and practice of complementary and alternative medicine in pain management. New York: Springer; 2008. p. 225–41.

[157] Rothschild B. Making trauma therapy safer: the psychophysiology of trauma and pTSD. London: Chiron Centre; 2010 22/23 May 2010 (leaflet advertising 2-day training).

[158] Leder D. The Absent Body. Chicago, IL: University of Chicago Press; 1990.

[159] Thalbourne MA, Bartemucci L, Delin PS, et al. Transliminality: its nature and correlates. Journal of the American Society for Psychical Research 1997;91(4):305–31.

[160] Sannella L. Kundalini: Psychosis or transcendence? San Francisco, CA: Lee Sannella; 1976.

[161] Sacerdoti G. On a case of hysterical psychosis in a subject adhering to 'Subud'. Arch Psicol Neurol Psichiatr 1965;26(4):412–25.

[162] Krishna G. Kundalini: The evolutionary energy in man. Boulder, CO: Shambhala; 1971.

[163] Ots T. The silenced body – the expressive Leib: on the dialectic of mind and life in Chinese cathartic healing. Csordas TJ, editor. Embodiment and Experience: The existential ground of culture and self. Cambridge, Cambs: Cambridge University Press; 1994. p. 116–36.

[164] Xu SH. Psychophysiological reactions associated with qigong therapy. Chin Med J 1994;107(3):230–3.

[165] Ng BY. Qigong-induced mental disorders: a review. Aust N Z J Psychiatry 1999;33(2):197–206.

[166] Mills N. The experience of fragmentation in psychosis: can mindfulness help? Clarke I, editor. Psychosis and Spirituality: Exploring the new frontier. London: Whurr; 2001. p. 211–21.

[167] Schneider A, Löwe B, Streitberger K. Perception of bodily sensation as a predictor of treatment response to acupuncture for postoperative nausea and vomiting prophylaxis. J Altern Complement Med 2005;11(1):119–25.

[168] Banissy MJ, Walsh V, Ward J. Enhanced sensory perception in synaesthesia. Exp Brain Res 2009;196(4):565–71.

[169] Hickey E. The Painted Kiss. London: Pocket; 2006.

[170] Gardner F. Self-Harm: A psychotherapeutic approach. Hove, East Sussex: Brunner-Routledge; 2001.

[171] Hall H. Sufism and rapid healing. Micozzi MS, editor. Fundamentals of Complementary and Alternative Medicine. St Louis, MO: Saunders; 2011. p. 509–21.

[172] Crick F. Of Molecules and Men. Seattle, WA: University of Washington Press; 1966. p. 172.

[173] Rubik B. Can Western science provide a foundation for acupuncture? Altern Ther Health Med 1995;1(4):41–7.

[174] Bensing J. Bridging the gap: the separate worlds of evidence-based medicine and patient-centered medicine. Patient Educ Couns 2000;39(1):17–25.

[175] Hahn RA. Sickness and Healing: An anthropological perspective. New Haven, CT: Yale University Press; 1995.

[176] Stöckenius S, Brugger P. Perceived electrosensitivity and magical ideation. Percept Mot Skills 2000;90(3 part 1):899–900.

[177] Swartz L. Being changed by cross-cultural encounters. Young DE, Goulet JG, editors. Being Changed by Cross-Cultural Encounters. Peterborough, ONT: Broadview Press; 1994. p. 209–36.

INDEX

Note: Page numbers followed by *b* indicate boxes; *f* figures; *t* tables.
Some major terms (eg. Flow, Meridians, Channels, *Li* etc.) are only represented by a few references.

INDEX

Medical *qigong* 81–82
Medicinal foods 78
Medicinal herbs 78
Meditation 5, 7–8, 9, 54–55, 68,
    85, 93, 123, 156, 159–160,
    186–187, 197–209, 218,
    273–274, 275, 276, 277,
    277t, 278, 279, 328–329
  acupuncture 199–201
  qigong 200–201
Melatonin 278
Mental health, *qigong* 94–95
Mental therapeutics 238
Meridian(s)
  Thought Field Theraphy
    (TFT) 240
  nutri-energetics systems
    theory 297–300
  Applied Kinesiology 239
  hado shiatsu 221
  shiatsu 214, 216–217
  see also specific meridians
Merrell-Wolf, Franklin 34
Mesmer, Franz Anton 32, 155,
    284
  animal magnetism 284
Meta-analysis 91–92
Metabolic syndrome, *qigong*
    92–93
Metal element (Air quality)
    203–204
Metaparadigms 179–182, 181t,
    183
  see also specific models
Metaphors
  language use 103
  qi 40
*Methods at the Heart of Medicine
    see Ishimpo (Methods at
    the Heart of Medicine)*
Metw (vessel) 32
Meyrink, Gustav 36
Microcurrent therapy 223–236
  accommodation 229
  applications 227
  branch treatment 234–235
  chronic low back pain 235b
  'circling the dragon' 232
  conductance 228–229
  electromassage 234, 234f
  interferential techniques
    231f, 233
  kinetic electrotherapy 233
  law of specificity 229, 230
  'less is more' 229
  microcurrent *mu–shu*
    technique 232, 233f
  microcurrent probes 231,
    231f, 232–233
  pad electrodes 231–232, 231f
  polarization 228, 230
  proprioception 229–230
  qi 230
  resistance 228–229
  resonance 228, 230

Microcurrent therapy
    (Continued)
  reverse body image/'great
    loops' 233
  root treatment 234–235
  sequence therapy 234–235
Microlight therapy™ 227
Middendorf, Ilse 329
Middle *dantian (zhong dantian)*
    77f
Mid Tide
  craniosacral biodynamics
    256
Miller Technique 110
Mindfulness 329
Mitochondria 145, 146–147,
    148f
Modern literature, *qi* 35–41, 36t,
    37t, 38t
Moggach, Deborah 38t
Monro, Jean 114
Mood, movement therapies
    281–282
Mostert, Natasha 38t
'Mother–Child law'
Motoyama, Hiroshi 225
Movement 326
Movement therapies
  depression 281–282
  endocrine system 278
  immune system 279
  mood 281–282
  *see also specific movement
    therapies*
Moxibustion *(jiu)* 61–62, 81–82
Muirhead, Alexander 305–306
Mukama, Rwandan
    medicine 15
Muladhara (first/base) *chakra*
    198f, 207
  neurophysiological/endocrine
    associations 57t
Müller, Hartmut 299–300
Multidimensional model
    of human function
    283–284
Multiple sclerosis, Therapeutic
    Touch 286
Mu (alarm/collecting) points
    (qian mu xue) 232, 233f
Muscle changing *see Yi jin
    jing* (muscle/tendon
    changing)
Muscle testing 239, 244
Music therapy 224
Mutations, cancer 145

N

Nadi 7–8, 45, 56, 336
Naess, Arne 43–44
Namikoshi, Tokujiro 213
Nan Jing (Canon of 81 Difficulties)
    26
Naoqi (brain *qi*) 26

National Center for
    Complementary and
    Alternative Medicine
    (NCCAM) 153
Natural killer (NK) cells 279
Needle sensing, Acuperceptions
    Project 169–178
Neidan 9–10
Neijing Suwen, qi 24
Neo-Confucianism 25, 88–89,
    143–144
Nervous system 278
Ñes-pa 9
Network 130, 136, 138, 161,
    214, 218, 226, 227,
    298, 322
Neurasthenia *see Shen jing shuai
    ruo* (neurasthenia)
Neurologic disorganization 242
New Age movement 42
Newtonian physics 52, 102
  metaparadigms 179
Nicotinamide adenine
    dinucleotide (NAD) 146
Niggli, Hugo 218
Nirvana 82
N/om (n/um) 26, 27f
Non-being (non-existence *wu*)
    86–87
Noncontact *daoyin* 130
  heart rate 132
  studies in 132–135
  treatment characteristics 136
Nonlinear 132–133, 136
Nonlinear fractal analysis, heart
    rate variability 132–133
Nonlocality 103
Nordenström, Bjørn 225
Norepinephrine 94
North American Nursing
    Diagnosis Association
    (NANDA) 158–159
Nourishing 81
Novalis 32
Novels, reading of 41
Nutri-energetics systems theory
    296–297
  bioinformation 299–300
  cavity dynamics 298
  connective tissue matrix
    298–300
  energetic driver fields
    297
  energetic integrator fields
    297, 301
  energetic terrain information
    sequences 297
  global scaling 300–301
  interactional fields 297
  meridian system 297–300
  quantum electrodynamics 299
  reverse transcriptase 301–302,
    302f
  scaling drop-out 301
Nutritive *qi (ying qi)* 68t

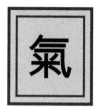

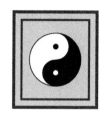

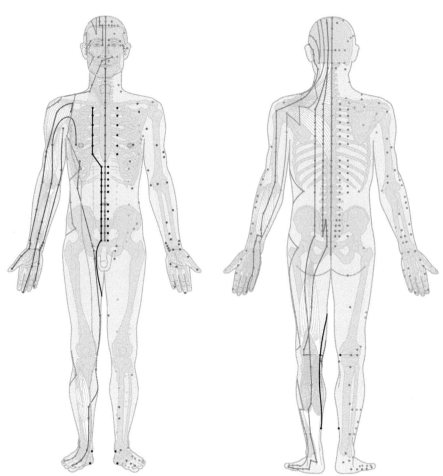

Front view of the 12 principal acupuncture meridians.

(After Kubiena G, Sommer B 2010 Practice Handbook of Acupuncture. Churchill Livingstone, Edinburgh, with permission.)

Back view of the 12 principal acupuncture meridians.

(After Kubiena G, Sommer B 2010 Practice Handbook of Acupuncture. Churchill Livingstone, Edinburgh, with permission.)

A vocabulary of *qi*

Glossary for the book *Energy Medicine East and West: A natural history of Qi*, edited by David Mayor and Marc S Micozzi (Edinburgh: Churchill Livingstone, 2011)

Qi is in essence indescribable, if not ineffable. Somewhat paradoxically, the vocabulary of *qi* is therefore large, as each person who wrestles with trying to grasp it conceptually creates their own vocabulary or adapts terms from other fields. Although some of the definitions in this glossary are context dependent, most will be of help not only in reading this book, but also in understanding other writings on the topics covered.

Glossary terms appear in the form that is generally used in the text – e.g. Blood (*xue* 血), not *xue* (Blood 血).

Absolute chance The notion that, at the quantum level, nature is fundamentally unpredictable

Accommodation The 'tuning out' of repetitive, intrusive stimuli

Acetyl coenzyme A Molecule involved in many important metabolic reactions such as passing on carbon atoms from glycolysis to the Krebs cycle to be oxidized for energy production

Acetylcholine A biogenic amine and neurotransmitter

Action potential Brief increase in positive potential within a nerve relative to that outside it, when initial stimulus exceeds a certain threshold

Active information Information contained within Bohm's quantum potential. Such information has its own activity

Acupuncture From the Latin words *acus* and *pungere*, the insertion of needles into the body at specific points for therapeutic purposes

Adenosine triphosphate The main transport molecule of intracellular energy, carrying the chemical energy used in cell metabolism; adenine diphosphate and a free phosphate ion

Agni Spirit of light or fire, one of a trilogy of forces in Ayurveda

AIDS-related dementia complex Metabolic brain disorder associated with chronic HIV infection

Aikido (合気道) Japanese martial art, literally 'the way of unifying (with) life energy'

Ajna Literally, 'command'; the sixth *chakra*, between the eyebrows

Alexander technique Bodily education practice to improve posture and movement, created by F Matthias Alexander (1869–1955)

Algorithm Term used by Roger Callahan to refer to commonly occurring meridian (channel) sequences underpinning particular states of distress; different states of distress are associated with different algorithms

Allodynia Hyperesthesia to normally innocuous temperature or touch stimuli

Allometric (1) Structural elements, such as branching networks of tubes found across various species, that appear to obey the same geometrical rules and therefore share common features in their spatial organization; (2) growth of different parts within an organism at different rates, or the relations between these parts

Allopathic Refers to orthodox medicine (Western medicine or biomedicine), where the therapeutic approach is to treat the symptoms of a disease with medication whose effect on the body is the opposite of that of the disease; term coined by Samuel Hahnemann (1755–1843), originator of homeopathy

Allostasis Process of achieving stability (homeostasis) through physiological or behavioral change

Alpha scaling A nonlinear measure that quantifies the 'landscape' of a complex fluctuation in terms of the correlation properties of successive values which make up its variation: an Alpha value of 0.5 equates to a completely random fluctuation (white noise); a value of 1.5 signifies a random walk fluctuation (Brownian noise) where successive values within the variability series are correlated only with the preceding value; a value of 1 is indicative of a broad bandwidth spectrum (1/f noise) that has scale-invariant or fractal properties with correlated behavior on multiple timescales – the higher the value of Alpha, the smoother the 'landscape'

Alpha wave Cortical electromagnetic oscillations in the 8–12 Hz range

Anahata Literally, 'unbeaten'; the fourth *chakra*, in the center of the chest

Anandamide N-arachidonoylethanolamine, an endogenous cannabinoid neurotransmitter

Anima Breath, soul

Animal magnetism (1) Mesmer's name for the universal fluid (*fluidum*) responsible for the properties of both organic and inorganic matter; (2) the techniques of 'Mesmerism'

Animal spirits *Pneuma physicon* (πνεύμα φύσικων), material spirits in Galenic medicine, occupying brain and nerves and mediating between and connecting Will and muscle

Animus Rational soul, consciousness

Anma (按摩) Traditional form of Japanese massage (from Chinese *anmo*, 'pressing and rubbing')

Antibody A gamma globulin protein used by the immune system to identify and neutralize foreign objects (bacteria, viruses)

Antigen Molecule that binds specifically to an antibody

Apolipoprotein A-I Major protein component of high-density lipoprotein (HDL)

Apoptosis Programmed cell death, a natural orderly death mechanism that is initiated to terminate a cell

Applied Kinesiology Term developed by chiropractor George Goodheart (1918-2008) to refer to the investigation of health and sickness using muscle testing (weaknesses in specific muscles reflect imbalances within the body)

Arrhythmia Loss of synchronized contraction of the upper and lower chambers of the heart

Asana Posture in yoga

Ashi (啊是) point Acupoint that may be spontaneously tender or sensitive to pressure

Asthenia Weakness

Atrium An upper chamber of the heart

Attractor A dynamic behavior pattern under the influence of two or more variables; attractors can be depicted graphically in two- or three-dimensional space in the form of phase space plots, which may be used to map the genesis and evolution of complex dynamic processes over time; a 'strange attractor' exhibits nonlinear behavior

Autocentric Referring to oneself as the centre of things

Autopoiesis Literally, 'self-creation': the capacity of an organism for self-renewal or self-organization on structural, functional and cognitive levels

Aura Energy field

Ayurveda 'Science of life', one of the main traditional medical systems of India, dating back to the second millennium BCE

Ba gua (八卦) The eight trigrams that represent the fundamental principles of the *Yi Jing* (易經), or *Book of Changes*

Balanced salts solution Solution with physiological pH and concentrations of salts

Bandwidth Frequency range spanning a resonance, a measure of how precise a resonance is

Bias The amount of a steady signal or quantity superimposed on an alternating one

Bifurcation An abrupt change in the behavior and evolution of a complex system or process, deriving from relatively small changes in one or more parameters governing its behavior

Binary thinking Simple yes/no thinking governed by the stress response

Bioelectromagnetic-based therapy A therapy that involves unconventional use of known electromagnetic fields

Bioenergy Biological energy, such as *qi, ki* or *prana*

Biofield Hypothetical energy field of the living organism; in craniosacral biodynamics, the total interactive field of the physical body (its anatomy, physiology and tissue forms), with the fluid body (the unified and holistic field of body fluid), and the tidal body (the bioenergy field of potency within and around the human body)

Bioinformation Information that is relevant for biological systems, capable of inducing a change in the system that is receiving or sending such information

Biological age Actual age of your system rather than your chronological age in years

Biomedicine Usually considered to encompass the knowledge and research underpinning the practice of medicine; loosely also covers the practice of Western medicine

Biomolecule backbone A linear biomolecule made up of linking simpler molecules (monomers)

Biophilia Edward O Wilson's term for the innate tendency to focus on life and lifelike processes

Biophoton Photon produced by cellular activity

Biphasic stimulation Treatment using (probes of) alternating polarity

Bipolar leads The simplest way of obtaining an ECG using two electrodes, with one positive and one negative lead

Black Bile (*saudā*) One of the four humors in *Unani*, along with Blood, Phlegm, and Yellow Bile

Blood (*dam*) One of the four humors in *Unani*, along with Black Bile, Phlegm, and Yellow Bile

Blood (*xue* 血) A *yin*/dense form of *qi*

B lymphocyte Type of lymphocyte important in humoral immunity

Bodyfulness Paying careful attention to the body and its messages

Body-soul Soul that remains with the body during life (and in some cases after death)

Bonghan ducts and nuclei Threadlike, almost microscopic structures found to overlay the internal organs, blood and lymph vessels in the 1960s by North Korean Kim Bonghan, making up what he called the *kyungrak* system; in more recent Korean research these almost translucent tubules have been found to conduct coherent light

Borderline personality Personality with prolonged instability of mood and sense of self

Bowing Imparting a bending or microflexion movement to a limb or bone

Brain synchronization State in which cortical oscillations show similar amplitude, frequency and phase in different regions, usually for a relatively short period

Breath of Life A mysterious and sacred presence that connects the created to the Source of the creative intention, and which generates primary respiration and its ordering potencies in craniosacral biodynamics

Breath work Therapeutic method devised by Ilse Middendorf (1910–2009)

Buqi (布氣) Literally, 'spreading *qi*'; an ancient Chinese practice akin to proximal healing with external *qigong* in which *qi* is 'spread' or 'infused' by the healer to the recipient

Capsid Protein shell around the virus particle

Cardiac coherence Heart rate that varies in a stable, orderly and harmonious manner rather than chaotically

Cartesian split The division between mind and body prevalent in Western thought, particularly since Descartes

Catabolism Process of (molecular) breakdown

Causal diagnostic procedure Muscle testing procedure developed by Roger Callahan to discern the precise meridian (channel) sequence underpinning a particular state of distress experienced by a particular person

Causative factor Principle used within a branch of Five Element Acupuncture developed by J R Worsley, which categorizes individuals into five constitutional or 'CF' Types: Fire, Earth, Metal, Water and Wood

Cell-field Energetic field of the cell

Cell-mediated immunity Immune response involving T lymphocytes

Centering action Term coined by Rollin Becker to describe the action of potency or life force in centering and compensating for unresolved conditional forces within the human system (forces generated by trauma, pathogens, etc.)

Chakra Literally, 'wheel', a constantly moving current (vortex) of energy where *prana* is received, assimilated and transformed; the seven main *chakras* are located along the spine, from the perineum in the lower pelvis to the top of the head

Chaos theory A body of theory applied to the study of complex systems whose behavior is neither random nor explicable in terms of linear dynamics

Character armor Term created by Wilhelm Reich to indicate a habitual pattern of organized characterological defenses against anxiety or other unwanted emotional excitation

Chemiosmosis Diffusion of ions across a selectively permeable membrane

Chongmai (衝脈): 'Penetrating' vessel, one of the eight extraordinary channels (*qi jing ba mai*) in Chinese medicine, running from the pelvic cavity up the front of the body to the lips

Chronic fatigue syndrome Severe fatigue for 6 months or longer characterized by a constellation of symptoms involving low viral immunity, such as muscle ache, tender lymph nodes, impaired short-term memory or concentration, headache, malaise after exertion, and unrefreshing sleep

Chun-do-sun-bup A Korean form of *qigong*

Cinnabar A red mercury ore

Citrate Intermediate substance in the Krebs cycle, formed from the fusion of acetyl coenzyme A with oxaloacetate

Clear visceral *qi*, *qing zang qi* (清臟氣) Pure and strong *qi* uncontaminated by improper diet or emotions

Cognitive behavioral therapy Technique-driven, time-limited counseling method using goal-oriented, systematic procedures to modify emotion, behavior, or cognition

Coherence A coherent signal consists of waves with identical parameters of frequency and amplitude that are also in phase (occurring at the same time); for example, particle oscillation in unison

Coherency wave Term coined by Peter Levine PhD to describe his experience of the Long Tide as a coherent waveform which emerges as traumatic forces are resolved in the healing process

Collar bone breathing Technique originally developed by Roger Callahan, involving a breathing sequence and tapping, carried out whilst the fingers are placed on the KI-27 acupoints below the medial ends of the collar bones; used to help correct states of neurologic and energetic disorganization

Complement C3 An immune system protein

Confluence Cell growth such that the maximum number of cells is present in a single layer in a given area without them starting to overlap

Connective tissue matrix High-speed, superconductive network for transmitting information throughout the body

Conversion symptom Symptom (usually neurological) without a discernible etiology; conversion disorder (formerly 'hysteria') involves such symptoms

Copenhagen interpretation A particular interpretation of quantum mechanics encompassing wave-particle complementarity and the uncertainty principle

Cortical inhibition Inhibition of the frontal cortex when the person is under pressure to perform

Corticotropin releasing hormone Hormone secreted in the hypothalamus that controls release of corticotropin (adrenocorticotropic hormone) from the pituitary

Cortisol Major corticosteroid synthesized in the adrenal cortex; a stress hormone

Counter-culture Cultural group whose values run counter to the mainstream values of the day, as in early nineteenth century Romanticism or the anti-war, anti-technocracy youth movement of the 1960s

Couplet Pair of *yin* and *yang* organs associated with a particular Element

C pain fiber Unmyelinated nerve fiber involved in pain perception

C peptide Connecting peptide, often high in type-2 diabetics

Cranial field Denotes the scope of work developed by many teachers and practitioners in osteopathic and craniosacral practice

Cranial rhythmic impulse (CRI)/cranial rhythm A superficial rhythm that resembles the waveforms of experience, autonomic activation and unresolved history, manifesting as a relatively fast rhythmic impulse (8–14 cycles a minute)

Craniosacral motion Involuntary tissue motion at a CRI level

Creative Intelligence The mysterious intelligence from which all creation emerges and all things arise, and to which they return

Cupping Method of applying suction to the skin, used in many traditional medical systems

Cybernetics The study of regulatory (control) systems

Cyclooxygenase Enzyme that catalyzes formation of several inflammatory mediators

Cytokine Immunomodulating agent involved in local intercellular signaling; effector glycoprotein that modulates both pro-inflammatory and anti-inflammatory regulators; type 1 cytokines promote cell-mediated responses, type 2 favor humoral responses

Cytotoxicity Toxicity to cells (e.g. of a chemical, or an immune cell)

Damp, *shi* (濕) In Chinese medicine, a *yin* pathogenic factor, heavy (flowing downward), sticky, and dirty

Dantian (丹田) Elixir field (or 'cinnabar field'), where one substance is transformed into another; in craniosacral biodynamics, term for an energetic, primary ordering and organizing fulcrum; divided into upper (*shang*), middle (*zhong*) and lower (*xia*) *dantians*.

Dao (道) Literally, 'Way' or 'path'; responsible for the creation and support of the universe, like *qi* it has many interpretations

Daoyin (導引): Therapeutic healing and self-healing practice from the Chinese medical tradition, with non-contact variants; literally, the way of 'quiding and pulling' *qi*

Da Yu (大禹) Son of Gun, and one of the forefathers of Daoism

Deep ecology Philosophy in which humans are considered as interdependent with their living environment

Deficiency, *xu* (虛) One of the three main imbalances in Chinese medicine (also translated as 'vacuity'): *yin xu* means insufficiency of *yin* constituents – Essence (*jing*), Blood (*xue*), Fluid (*jin ye*) – or of function in the *yin* organs; *qi xu* is an insufficiency of all its physiological functions, or in an organ, e.g. Spleen *qi* deficiency (*pi qi xu*, 脾气虚), which manifests as insufficiency of one or several of the Spleen's functions

Deqi (得氣) Literally, 'get *qi*'; patient's or practitioner's feeling of *qi* during acupuncture needling

Differentiation Process by which a cell specializes in a specific function or functions

Diuresis (Therapy to) increase the quantity of urine passed

Divergent/Distinct meridians, *jingbie* (經別) Vertical branches of the 12 primary acupuncture meridians, sometimes known as the 'distinct' meridians

Dopamine 3-hydroxytyramine, a monoamine neurotransmitter

Doshas The three regulator principles (humors) of Ayurveda: *vata*, *pitta*, and *kapha*

Dumai (督脈): Governing/Governor Vessel, one of the eight extraordinary channels (*qi jing ba mai*) in Chinese medicine, running up from the coccyx to the frenulum inside the upper lip

Dumo (gtum-mo) Tibetan meditation practice associated with sensation of intense inner heat

Dynamic Stillness The ground of dynamic and alive stillness that holds the potential for all form and from which the Breath of Life and primary respiration emerge; similar perhaps to the concept of the zero point field in physics, an implicate field of infinite energy from which all subatomic particles arise, take their form, and to which they return

Dysmorphia Excessive preoccupation with a negative body self-image

Dysphoric Anxious, depressed or otherwise uneasy

Echocardiogram Cardiac ultrasound imaging method

Ectopic beat Heart beat generated by cells outside the normal location for heart beat generation

Edge of chaos Qualitative term describing the dynamic state of coexistence between contrasting states of order and chaos within a complex system; frequently applied to living systems which are at, or near, a critical point

Effector Molecule that binds to a protein, altering its activity

Eight Extraordinary Channels/Vessels, *qi jing ba mai* (奇經八脈) A set of meridians that are the first to develop during the formation of the fetus and the first to be influenced by the practice of *qigong*

'Eight Techniques of the Magic Turtle', *Ling gui ba fa* (灵龟八法) Acupuncture treatment using the opening points of the extraordinary channels (*qi jing ba mai*) according to the Chinese calendar

Élan vital Henri Bergson's term for vital force

Electrical potential The potential energy per unit charge of an electrically charged particle placed in an electrical field

Electroacupuncture according to Voll (EAV) Influential system developed by Reinhold Voll (1909–1989) from the 1950s onwards, involving both measurement and treatment at acupoints, as well as remedy testing

Electrocardiogram The electric signal recorded from the heart via surface skin electrodes, representing the sequence of electrophysiological events occurring during a heart beat or continuous series of heartbeats

Electrodermal Concerning the electrical properties of the skin

Electrodynamic field Field determined by the atomic physiochemical components of a biological system and which in part determines the behavior and orientation of those components, as proposed by Harold Saxton Burr (1889–1973)

Electroencephalogram Recording of skin potentials on the scalp, the sum of many different electrical events in the cortex

Electromassage A method of massage in which the practitioner's hands are used as electrodes

Electromyogram Recording of extracellular electrical activity in skeletal muscle

Electron acceptor A chemical compound that accepts electrons transferred to it from another compound, the donor; by accepting electrons, it is defined as an oxidizing agent that itself becomes reduced upon taking the electrons

Electron donor A chemical compound that donates its electrons to another compound, the acceptor; by donating electrons, it is defined as a reducing agent that itself becomes oxidized upon losing its electrons

Emotional Freedom Techniques Simplified derivative of Thought Field Therapy

Endogenous frequency Frequency with no external cause or source

Endothermic Describes a reaction that requires heat input in order to take place, as opposed to exothermic that produces heat when it occurs

Energetic Driver Subfields correlated to the organs that arise during fetal development and that 'power' them

Energetic Integrator Nonlinear energy and information pathways in the body-field similar to meridians in that they regulate many disparate aspects of the body

Energetic Terrain Complex energetic and information structures representing emotional states and other energy configurations

Energy (1) Physical energy, the capacity to do work; (2) For other forms of energy, see *subtle energy*

Energy medicine Method of treatment usually considered to involve subtle energy rather than physically measurable energy; in Chinese, translates as *de nengliang yixue*, 的能量醫學

Energy psychology Term originally proposed by Fred Gallo to denote the range of methods that explore the interface between psyche and the body's informational energy fields

Energy toxin Concept developed by Roger Callahan, to describe foods, environmental pollutants or other factors (e.g. electromagnetic disturbance, or 'geopathic stress') that disrupt a person's energy system, causing disorganization or psychological reversal, and blocking the TFT procedure

Enterovirus RNA virus sometimes implicated in CFS

Entoptic phenomenon Visual effect without an external source; specifically, one of a small family of geometric patterns ('form constants') observed during trance

Entropy Measure of a system's disorder or tendency toward spontaneous change

Eosinophil Type of granular leukocyte

Epidermis Outermost, nonvascular layer of the skin

Epinephrine Monoamine neurotransmitter in the ANS, secreted by the adrenal medulla and associated with stress; adrenaline

Epistemology Theory of knowledge

Ergometer Exercise machine that also measures work performed

Ergotropic Pertaining to sympathetic nervous activity

Essence, *jing* (精) One of the three fundamental substances in the human body, and the densest (*yin*) form of *qi*

Ethnography Study of a culture or society based on observation

Ethnology Comparative study of different cultures or societies

Eukaryotic A term describing organisms which are made of cells that contain a membrane-bound nucleus containing the genetic material (the DNA)

Excess, *Shi* (實) Excess, fullness, repletion; one of the three main imbalances in Chinese medicine, the opposite of *xu* (deficiency), resulting in signs and symptoms that correlate to excessive, imbalanced functions; a Western disease correlation would be hyperthyroidism (excessive thyroid hormone levels) as opposed to hypothyroidism (insufficient thyroid hormone)

Explicate Order The order of objects that are well defined in space and time

External *qi*, *kong qi* (空氣) (*Qi* in) air/oxygen; the basis for Lung *qi*

Eye Movement Desensitization and Reprocessing Structured integrative psychotherapy approach using eye movements to desensitize and reprocess memory-related emotional distress

Falun gong (法輪功) Literally, 'practice of the wheel of the law', a politicized *qigong* movement that started in China in 1992

Faraday cage Enclosure that blocks static electric fields and, depending on design, some other electromagnetic fields

Feldenkrais method Somatic educational system designed to improve use of the self through awareness, in order to enhance movement, reduce pain, and promote general wellbeing

Felt sense A subtle perception of feeling or sensation, frequently unfamiliar to the subject and therefore difficult to name or categorize

Fengshui (風水) Literally, 'wind water'; geomancy, a method of positioning things in harmonious relationships for beneficial effect

Fibroblast Most common type of connective tissue cell; synthesizes collagen

Fibromyalgia Syndrome characterized by widespread muscle pains, tactile hypersensitivity, and fatigue; may also involve sleep disturbance

Field (1) Physical fields (electric, gravitational, etc.) contain energy and exert force; they are present wherever their effects (electric, gravitational, etc.) are evident; (2) mathematical fields are regions of space containing objects

Five Elements/Phases, Wuxing (五行) The fundamental Phases, or Elements, in Chinese medicine and cosmology: Wood, Fire, Earth, Metal, Water

Fluctuation A recorded variation of output from a system such as the RR interval time series which may be characterized statistically according to its dynamic pattern; hence, random f. (white noise), random walk f. (Brownian noise), fractal f. (1/f) and multifractal f.

Fluid body The body's holistic fluid field, which manifests a unified field of action; it is primordial in origin as all life depends on its presence, from the humblest single-celled entity to the complex human form

Fluid tide The tidal motion within the fluid body generated by the action of potency or life force

Fluid–tissue (matrix) Fluids and tissues form a unified field of action, manifesting in a matrix-like fashion

Fluidum The universal fluid responsible for the properties of both organic and inorganic matter; health results from harmony with the cosmic fluid, all disease being due to an unequal distribution of or 'obstacles' to its flow

Food qi, gu qi (穀氣) *Qi* formed by digestion of food in the stomach and the transformation of food into *qi* by the Spleen; also often called Postnatal Essence

Force gestalt Irreducible experiential metaphor (an organized, unified whole) based on early childhood experience of force and movement

Form of feeling Suzanne K Langer's term for a fundamental metaphor or other trope expressing an inner feeling

Fractal Quantity with no absolute scale of value; applied to an object or process whose structure or temporal elements exhibit the property of self-similarity (defined mathematically as 'scale invariance') on different scales of magnitude

Free radical(s) A class of atoms, molecules or ions that can carry an extra high-energy unpaired electron which can easily be given away to induce a chemical reaction; excess of free radicals may lead to undesired side reactions resulting in cell damage

Free-soul Soul that leaves the body in dreams and at death

Frenulum Small fold of membrane restricting movement, e.g. between gum and upper lip

Frequency Number of cycles or direction changes of a wavelike signal (current or radiation) per second; inversely proportional to wavelength

Frontal lobe shutdown Cortical inhibition in its extreme form

Fulcrum (1) The point on which a lever turns (mechanical). (2) A complex geometric form, created with the hands, around which, when held stable, a person can reorganize themselves or reorient (dynamic)

Fu Xi (伏羲) Ox Tamer, legendary emperor of China, c. 2953 BCE

Gabapentin Antiseizure medication used for severe chronic inflammatory or functional pain

Gaia hypothesis James Lovelock's hypothesis that the earth's biosphere, atmosphere, oceans and soil form one single self-preserving system

Galenic medicine Preeminent form of medicine practiced in Europe until the Renaissance, based on the work of the Greco-Roman physician Galen

Gathering/Ancestral qi, zong qi (宗氣) *Qi* formed from the interaction of Food *qi* (*gu qi*) with air/oxygen (*kong qi*)

Geopathic stress Subtle energy disturbances inherent in the earth and local physical environment; sometimes used to refer to the stress on the body due to these

Glial cells (neuroglia) Connective tissue cells forming a supportive perineural network and probably modulating neurotransmission

Global scaling theory Mathematical theory that describes and predicts the arrangement of nature using logarithmic, fractal nonlinear scales

Glucocorticoid Corticosteroid that regulates carbohydrate, lipid and protein metabolism and inhibits release of corticotropin

Glucose A 6-carbon molecule that is the basic building block of complex sugars like starch and glycogen

Glycolysis Breakdown of glucose to two 3-carbon molecules called phosphoglycerate in the cell cytoplasm

Glycoprotein Proteins that also contain sugar chains; glycoproteins have many different functions in the body

Golgi tendon organ A tendon mechanoreceptor that monitors muscle tension

Ground state Physical state unable to lose energy and so change to a lower state

Growth hormone Hormone stimulating growth, secreted in the anterior pituitary

Guanzi (管子) Compilation of Chinese philosophical texts, including the *Neiye* (內業, *Inner Training*)

Gun (鯀) A demigod, grandson of Huangdi

Hado (波動 はどう) 'Wave-like movement', or innate transforming power (Japanese)

Han yixue (韩医学) Korean medicine

Hara (腹) Abdomen, lower *dantian* (Japanese)

Hatha yoga Form of *yoga* traditionally practiced as a precursor to spiritual practices; used widely in the West for mental and physical health purposes

Healing Touch Method of healing developed by US nurse Janet Mentgen (1938–2005) and taught as an energy medicine program from 1989

Heart rate variability Relates to the dynamic properties of the heart rate; characterized by a variety of geometrical, time or frequency domain, and nonlinear measures with differing degrees of clinical utility

Heat, *re* (熱) In Chinese medicine, a *yang* pathogenic factor, often associated with feeling hot, thirst, insomnia, and a rapid pulse

Hemagglutination inhibition Method of measuring influenza specific antibody levels in blood serum

Hematopoiesis Formation of cellular blood components from stem cells

Hemoglobin A1c Glycoprotein increased by prolonged high glucose plasma levels

He (合) **points** Literally, 'sea' points; the most proximal of the five transporting points (*shu xue*, 輸穴) on the limbs, located at elbows or knees in Chinese medicine

'Hidden' information In the context of the ECG, this refers to information embedded within an RR time series that becomes available only through nonlinear analytic methods

Hidden variables Term used by Louis de Broglie (1892–1987) in the 1920s, an attempt to avoid the acausality of conventional quantum theory by proposing that the electron is guided by a 'pilot wave'. Independently proposed in the 1950s by David Bohm (1917–1992) as a hypothesis in which the electron's path is causally determined, and later elaborated by him as a precursor to his theory of the quantum potential

Histamine Biogenic amine involved in the inflammatory response; also a neurotransmitter

Holistic shift A primary stage in the unfolding of the inherent treatment plan where the client's system settles out of conditions, forms, tension patterns and the CRI level of rhythm and reorients to primary respiration and wholeness in craniosacral biodynamics

Holograph Using two laser or coherent light beams (one direct and one reflected), a two-dimensional image ('hologram') of an object can be created. Laser light can then be used again to recreate the wave pattern originally recorded, appearing now as a *three*-dimensional image. The entire image can be reconstructed from only a part of the hologram. This is an instance of the *holographic paradigm*, which states that the whole is represented in each of its parts

Holomovement Bohm's notion of the movement of the whole

Homeodynamis Property of a system whereby it maintains a *dynamic* but stable condition

Homeopathy Method of treatment using 'potentized' remedies – usually prepared from serial dilutions of substances using 'succussion' – whose effects are similar to the patient's presenting symptoms

Homeostasis Property of a living organism whereby its body and cells maintain a stable constant condition

Huainanzi (淮南子) Collection of philosophical essays dating from c. 140 BCE

Huang Di (黃帝) Yellow emperor, legendary emperor of China 2698–2598 BCE and author of the *Huangdi Neijing* (黃帝內經), *Yellow Emperor's Canon of Internal Medicine*, a key text in Chinese medicine

Humor, ye (液) Thick form of body fluid, responsible for example for lubricating the joints in Chinese medicine

Humoral immunity Immunity mediated by antibodies secreted from cells of the B lymphocyte lineage

Hun (魂) Ethereal soul, residing in the Liver, in contrast to the corporeal soul (*po*) associated with the Lung

Hydrogen peroxide (H₂O₂) A natural byproduct of oxidative metabolism in all organisms, made from water and oxygen, which possesses a strong oxidizing capacity and is considered a highly reactive oxygen species

5-hydroxytryptophan Amino acid precursor to the neurotransmitter serotonin and a metabolite of tryptophan

Hyle (ύλη) Matter or substance

Hyperesthesia Abnormally increased sensitivity to sensory stimulation

Hypothalamic–pituitary–adrenal axis Part of the neuroendocrine system that controls reactions to stress and also regulates many body processes

Hypothalamic–pituitary–immune axis Term emphasizing the linkage between an up-regulated HPA axis and an over-vigilant immune system that eventually becomes exhausted along with HPA depletion

Hypothalamo-pituitary axis Unit formed by the hypothalamus and pituitary gland, which exerts control over many parts of the endocrine system

Ida *Nadi* on the left (lunar) side of the body parallel to the spine

Ignition Term coined by William G Sutherland (1873–1954) to denote the process whereby potency manifests within the fluid body via transmutation or a change in state from field energies to embodied ordering forces

'Immortal embracing the post' (cheng bao zhuang, 撐抱桩) Standing posture in *qigong*, practiced to integrate the bones, joints, and muscles, also called 'holding the balloon'

Immortality The ability in Daoist practice to fully gather one's consciousness and identity and launch it away from the physical human form at will

Immortalized cells Cells which continue to grow and divide indefinitely in favorable conditions, so avoiding apoptosis

Immunoglobulin A An antibody particularly important in mucosal immunity

Implicate Order An *enfolded* order that lies beneath the surface manifestations of the 'Explicate Order'. The explicate can enfold into the implicate and the implicate can unfold into the explicate

Infoceutical A liquid remedy of purified water and a minute quantity of plant-derived minerals, imprinted with information that is correlated to the body-field and its substructures

Informational field Alternative term for the body's energy field, based on Roger Callahan's emphasis that it contains information, encoded as meridian (channel) sequences

Inherent treatment plan Term coined by Rollin Becker to orient practitioners to the fact that the healing needs of a client are already present in the conditions manifesting within their system; the practitioner cannot know what needs to happen in its unfolding, but must facilitate and be able to orient to its unfolding

Innate intelligence Vitalistic term coined by Daniel David Palmer (1845–1913), founder of chiropractic, for the innate force in all life that is responsible for the organization, maintenance and healing of the body

Insulin resistance Condition in which the body produces insulin normally but is unable to use it properly

Integral practice A new approach to development of consciousness that seeks to make best use of the full spectrum of insights, methods, and teachings, both Western and non-Western, available for cultivating a more open, balanced, and integrated life; the term derives from the writings of Ken Wilber

Integrative medicine Approach in which CAM is integrated into mainstream medical practice

Intelligence William G Sutherland oriented practitioners to a mysterious ordering and healing presence that he called 'Intelligence with a capital "I" '; this denotes the innate intelligence present even in the direst conditions

Intentionality The use of intention, as a volitional aspect of the mind, to invoke a response; in the context of *daoyin* healing, 'intention' refers to volitional aspects of imagination, controlled respiration and posture directed to achieving healing

Interactional field Field relating to the body-field's interaction with the natural fields of the Earth and cosmos, and its orientation to them

Inter-beat interval Time interval between successive R-wave peaks of the ECG, expressed in seconds (s) or milliseconds (ms)

Interferential therapy Treatment using interference between two currents of different frequency to produce low-frequency stimulation in the region where they interfere

Interferon gamma Type of cytokine important for immunity against infection and tumor control

Interleukin There are many interleukins, most synthesized by CD4+ T lymphocytes and having important immune functions

Interoceptive Concerning the perception of inner sensations or feelings

Inverse square law Law that a force decreases in proportion to the inverse square of the distance from its source

Iokai (医王会) School of *shiatsu* founded by Shizuto Masunaga, literally 'Association of the King of Medicines'

Ion-pumping cord A wire with a diode in it, only allowing unidirectional flow of current

'Iron shirt', tieshan (鐵衫) A 'hard' or external style of martial *qigong* practiced to increase the body's resistance to blows from hands or weapons

Ishimpo (医心方) *Methods at the Heart of Medicine*, a premodern Japanese medical text based largely on Chinese sources

Jin (津) Thin form of Body Fluid, responsible for moistening surface areas of the body in Chinese medicine

Jing (精) Essence, one of the three fundamental substances in the human body, and the densest (*yin*) form of *qi*

Jingluo (經絡) Channels and collaterals in Chinese medicine; the deeper vertical main and divergent channels (literally, 'paths') and their connecting, more superficial collaterals (literally, 'network')

Jing (Well, 井) points The end points of the meridians (channels) on the fingers and toes

Jurkat cells An immortalized line of T lymphocyte cells

Kampo (漢方) Japanese adaption of Chinese medicine

Kapha Phlegm, one of the three main Ayurvedic *doshas* (humors)

!Kia Trance state experienced in the rhythmic dance of the San people

Kinetic electrotherapy Electrical treatment with simultaneous active or passive movement of the affected area

Kiryoku (氣力) 'Energy' in modern Japanese

Krebs cycle Series of enzyme-catalyzed chemical reactions that take place within the mitochondria of the cells, a process essential to the production of metabolic energy; also called the citric acid cycle or tricarboxylic acid cycle

Kundalini Psychospiritual energy that lies dormant at the base of the spine (symbolized as a coiled serpent); may be activated through yoga or other practices, and channeled upward through the *chakras*

Kunlun shan (崑崙山) *Kunlun* mountain range in China; mythical *axis mundi* and Daoist paradise, also associated with some martial arts

Large heavenly cycle (da zhou tian, 大周天) Circulation exercise taught in most *qigong* systems, involving the circulation of *qi* along the *dumai, renmai* vessels plus the *yin* and *yang* heel and stepping vessels

Law of specificity The more specific the treatment sites, the less stimulus is needed

Leukocyte White blood cell, either granular or nongranular

Leukopoiesis Formation of white blood cells (leukocytes)

Li (理) Principle; the natural patterning of things

Libido First defined by Freud as instinctual energy, later as a drive toward any form of pleasurable bodily sensation; Jung considered it more as psychic energy, while for Reich it became a real energy ('orgone' or 'bio-energy')

Liminal Intermediate or transitional (as in 'liminal state')

Linger effect Lasting effect following an intervention

Lingshu (靈樞), Spiritual Pivot Second part of the *Huangdi Neijing*

Lipodystrophy Abnormal condition of fatty tissue (local or generalized)

Lipoxygenase Family of enzymes involved in inflammatory processes

Liquid crystal State of matter with properties between those of a conventional liquid and those of a solid crystal, for instance flowing like a liquid, but with molecules oriented in a crystal-like way

Living matrix A continuous and dynamic connective tissue 'webwork', extending throughout the body

Local Correlated behavior of systems within a restricted region that involves a signal or force (as opposed to 'nonlocal')

Logical Atomism The philosophical theory that the world consists of ultimate logical, unambiguous 'facts' (or 'atoms') that cannot be broken down any further

Long Tide Term coined by Rollin Becker to denote the primary ordering force generated by the creative intention of the Breath of Life, which manifests as primary respiration in slow and stable respiratory cycles of 50-second inhalation and 50-second exhalation within a vast field of action; it seems to move from the horizon to the midline of the human system, generating the ordering matrix within which embryological differentiation occurred, and through which cellular order is maintained throughout life

Lower *dantian*, *xia dantian* (下丹田) Energy center located in the abdominal region responsible for transforming *jing* into *qi*

Luo (絡) Collaterals, connecting channels (literally, 'network') in Chinese medicine

Lymphocyte Mononuclear, nonphagocytic nongranular leukocyte

McGill Pain Questionnaire Rating Index Method of rating pain using sensory, affective, and evaluative terms, developed by Melzack and Torgerson in 1971

Magnetic flux Amount of magnetism passing (flowing) through a given area; measured in Wb (quantized in units of $h/2e$)

Magnetic resonance A spinning particle in a magnetic field absorbs energy from the field and can then reradiate it at a specific resonance frequency

Magnetic resonance imaging Method for obtaining images of soft tissue changes using the principle of nuclear magnetic resonance

Magnetic vector potential $\underline{A}$-field, mathematically ('curl') related to the magnetic field but in the direction of the associated electric current; measured in Wb/m

Mai (脈) Vessels, undifferentiated precursors to the *jingluo*

Maishu (脈書) *Book of Pulses*, of which different versions were found at Mawangdui and Zhangjiashan

Mana Impersonal sacred power that may be possessed by objects and places as well as people, so distinct from 'soul'

Manipura Literally, 'city of jewels'; the third *chakra*, at the solar plexus

Mantra A word or vocal sound considered to have a particular transformative effect

Matter wave Wave aspect of matter in the wave-particle duality

Mechanoreceptor Sensory receptor that is sensitive and receptive to mechanical pressure or distortion

Medical acupuncture Adaptation of Chinese acupuncture based on biomedical principles and rejecting traditional Chinese theories such as *yinyang* and the circulation of *qi*

Melatonin Hormone secreted by the pineal gland

Membrane potential Voltage across the membrane of a biological cell (1/10 V across a 1/100 μm distance results in a large electric field of the order of 10 MV/m)

Meridian brushing Exercise to cleanse the acupuncture meridians

Meridian-like channel In biological systems information does not propagate uniformly in space but along lines of almost a single dimension. These lines closely resemble those of the 12 main meridians (channels) of Chinese medicine and *shiatsu*

Meta-analysis Statistical method in which the results of several studies addressing related research hypotheses are combined

Metabolism Sum of all chemical reactions that take place within an organism

Metw Vessel; undifferentiated conduits (12 in some medical papyri) which transport air and various types of fluid around the body in ancient Egyptian medicine

Microsystem System of acupoints in a local area that represents a map of the whole body; sometimes considered an application of the holographic principle

Middle *dantian*, *zhong dantian* (中丹田) Energy center located in the chest that is responsible for transforming *qi* into *shen*

Mid Tide A tidal phenomenon generated by the action of tidal potency, the embodied life force manifesting within the fluid body; it manifests in relatively stable rhythms from 1 to 3 cycles per minute

Miller Technique Technique of using successive serial dilutions of an allergen (or their frequency equivalents) to provoke or neutralize an allergic reaction (named after Dr Joseph Miller of Mobile, AL)

Mingmen (命門) Gate of Vitality (destiny), located at the point in the spine directly behind the navel, and source of both *qi* and *jing* within the body

Miscellaneous qi, za qi (杂氣) For all intents and purposes synonymous with Pestilential *qi* (*li qi*)

Mitochondrial matrix Inner compartment of the mitochondria where many metabolic reactions related to ATP production take place

Mitochondrion (pl. mitochondria) Cellular organelles where almost all energy is produced as ATP

Modulation Changing patterns of stimulation to reduce accommodation

Monocyte Mononuclear, phagocytic nongranular leukocyte

Morphic field Holistic organizing field at the whole body level

Morphogenesis Generation of biological form and structure, often applied to the differentiation and growth of tissues and organs during development, but applicable to adult as well as embryonic tissues as it encompasses the maintenance, degeneration, and regeneration of tissues and organs as well as their formation; may concern the structure of individual cells, formation of multicellular arrays and tissues, or the higher order assembly of tissues into organs and whole organisms

Mother–Child cycle, xiang sheng (相生) *Sheng* cycle: the creative, nutritive cycle of the Five Elements: Wood feeds Fire; Fire creates Earth (ash); Earth contains Metal; Water condenses on Metal; Water nourishes Wood

Moxibustion, jiu (灸) Method of treatment in which the herb wormwood or mugwort (もぐさ, mokusa, in Japanese; 艾, ai, in Chinese) is burnt on or over acupoints

Muladhara Literally, 'root place'; the first *chakra*, at the perineum

Mu (Alarm/Collecting) points, Qian mu xue Frontal acupuncture meridian (channel) points that, when tender, indicate that the associated organ is out of balance; used together with muscle testing to detect the sequence of meridians underpinning a particular state of distress in Energy Psychology

Muscle testing Use of light pressure on a muscle, in order to allow the body to communicate a response to a question through subtle variations in muscle tone; the basis of Applied Kinesiology and the causal diagnostic procedure of TFT

Nadi Channels through which *prana* flows in Ayurveda and yoga

Naoqi (腦氣) Brain *qi*, electrical *qi* posited by Tai Sitong

Naturalistic study Observational study of subjects (or phenomena) in their natural setting, with minimal interference

Natural killer cell Small lymphocyte called into action as a first nonspecific defense against invading cells

Neidan (內丹) Inner alchemy, source for many internal and meditative forms of *qigong* with a more spiritual focus

Neigong (內功) Internal *qigong*, self-practice to harmonize healthy *qi* flow

Neijin (內勁) *Qi*-like 'internal power'

Ñes-pa The three regulatory principles (humors) of Tibetan medicine

Network In neural and biological systems, linked elements in a relationship which confers structural and functional integrity

Neurologic disorganization Term developed by Applied Kinesiologists, referring to subtle forms of disorganization, as in clumsiness, dyslexia, etc., and usually characterized as problems with contralateral synchronization

Neuropathic pain Pain arising from damage to neurons, although sustained by changes in the central nervous system

Neutral Osteopathic term which denotes a state where all of the factors present have come into a dynamic state of equilibrium

Neutrophil Most abundant type of leukocyte in humans; a subtype of granulocytes

New Age Social and spiritual movement, predominantly Anglo-American in origin, characterized by a *subjective-life* rather than *live-as* approach; developed in the mid-1970s out of the counter-culture of the 1960s (with earlier roots in Romanticism and various esoteric groups); associated with the growth of alternative and holistic medicine in the 1980s

Newtonian physics Physics dealing with the motions of bodies distributed within a certain boundary ('locally') under the action of a system of forces; classical physics

Nicotinamide adenine dinucleotide A coenzyme that functions in all living cells, carrying electrons from one reactant to another in reduction–oxidation reactions

Nilpotency Of two quantities that multiplied together give zero

Nirvana A state in which the underlying unity of all things is realized

Nitric oxide Gaseous neurotransmitter

Node Point of minimum amplitude on a standing wave

N/om or n/um Fiery power or force experienced as rising up the body in *San* trance dance

Nonlinear Property of a system in which output bears a disproportional relationship to input (in contrast to a linear system, where this relationship is proportional)

Nonlocality Used to describe two quantum systems that were originally entangled but are now separated in space, yet still remain correlated without the exchange of signals or forces

Norepinephrine Monoamine neurotransmitter in the ANS; noradrenaline

Nourishing *see Tonifying*

Nucleotide Cellular molecule that forms the structural units of the genetic material (nucleic acids); is also involved in many important metabolic reactions, serving as a source of chemical energy (adenosine triphosphate and guanosine triphosphate), participant in cellular signaling (cyclic guanosine monophosphate and cyclic adenosine monophosphate), and a component incorporated in important cofactors of enzymatic reactions (e.g. coenzyme A)

Nutri-Energetics Systems (theory) Comprehensive theory of the human body-field originated by Peter Fraser

Nutritive qi, ying qi (營氣): *Qi* formed by the combination of Lung *qi* and *gu qi*, which flows within the meridians and blood vessels in Chinese medicine (also known as *rong qi*)

Occulture Wide range of beliefs and practices characterized by an interest in the paranormal and forming the basis for the new spiritual atmosphere in the West

Odic energy or force (Od) Vital energy or life force (from Odin the Norse god), a term invented by Karl von Reichenbach (1788–1869) in 1845

'Offensive precipitation sect', gong xia pai (攻下派) Chinese Ming dynasty sect of physicians

Ojas Term in Ayurvedic medicine referring to the 'energy', 'vigor', or 'power' that is said to manifest at the core of every cell in the human body

Ontogeny Origin and development of the individual organism from embryo to adult

Ontology Study of the nature of reality or existence

Ordering field/matrix The quantum level ordering field laid down by the action of the Long Tide at conception; the underlying matrix from which potency manifests in the fluid of the body via transmutation and which maintains the body's order throughout life

Organelle Specialized intracellular structure

Organ-field Energetic field of the organ

Organ flow meditation A method of strengthening the five *zang* organs by directing the breath to each of them in turn, in the order of the Mother–Child cycle

Orgone Primordial cosmic energy developed theoretically by Wilhelm Reich (1897–1957) on the basis of Freud's *libido* and with experimentally measurable effects; both universally present and associated with the living organism (as 'bioenergy')

Orgone-acupuncture Method of acupuncture using orgone devices, first developed by Bernd Senf

Original Motion Term coined by Victor Schauberger (1885–1958) to denote his experience of the Long Tide as a primary ordering field of action

Osteopenia Low bone mineral density, often a precursor to osteoporosis

Oxaloacetate Cellular organic compound also referred to as oxaloacetic acid; in the Krebs cycle, this forms from the oxidation of malate, catalyzed by malate dehydrogenase, and reacts with acetyl-CoA to form citrate, catalyzed by citrate synthase

Oxidative phosphorylation Metabolic process within the cell's mitochondria that uses energy released by the oxidation of nutrients to produce adenosine triphosphate, a high-energy compound

Oxytocin The 'bonding hormone', produced in the brain (hypothalamus), heart and ovarian *corpus luteum*

Parasympathetic nervous system Division of the nervous system that controls functions not requiring immediate reaction ('rest and digest'), so conserves energy to promote homeostasis

Paraventricular nucleus A nucleus within the hypothalamus, next to the third ventricle of the brain

Pathogenic evils, *xie* (邪氣) Disease-causing factors in Chinese medicine, such as Wind, Heat, Cold (*han*, 寒), Damp, Dryness (*zao*, 燥) and so forth

Peptide Short chain of amino acids

Pestilential *qi*, *li qi* (疠氣) A wide range of *qi* or influences that could have a role in disease causation; this idea, emerging out of the Warm Disease school, was intended to broaden the concept of evil *qi*, which were theoretically limited to six distinct excesses

Phase (1) Fraction of a complete cycle of oscillation; coherent oscillations will be 'in phase', but oscillations of identical frequency and with a phase difference between them will be 'out of phase'; (2) state of matter

Phase coherence Maintenance of precise phase relationships of a constant frequency oscillation in different regions of its domain

Phase locked Two signals are phase locked if the phase of one has a fixed relation to the phase of the other; coherent systems have the ability to phase lock to specific signals and to one another, and also to shift the frequency of signals received from their environment

Phase space plot A two- or three-dimensional display of data showing the relationship between two or three variables. In this context, the 'phase space' is the two- or three-dimensional space defined by the axes of the variables

Phase transition Transition from one 'phase' (state) of matter to another

Phase wave Wave that moves in a fixed rhythm as measured against a fixed point; in bioenergetics, a matter wave that encodes the information specific to that unique entity

Phlegm (*balgham*) One of the four humors in *Unani*, along with Black Bile, Blood, and Yellow Bile

Phonon 'Particle' of acoustic energy equivalent to the 'photon' for light

Photon Smallest particle of electromagnetic radiation such as light

Piezoelectricity Charge or voltage that appears following mechanical pressure on a nonlinear material, e.g. quartz or bone

Pingala *Nadi* on the right (solar) side of the body parallel to the spine

Pitta Bile, one of the three main Ayurvedic *doshas* (humors)

Placebo effect Measurable, observable, or felt improvement in health not attributable to active treatment, possibly associated with expectation or a 'meaning response'

Pneuma (πνεύμα) The cosmic breath-soul of ancient Greece, for Aristotle the intermediary between psyche (ψυχή) and soma (σομα)

Polarity agent Any device that applies subtle (minimal) polarized signals to the body; used by Yoshio Manaka (1911–1989) to activate only the X-system, in contrast to the physiological effects of acupuncture

Polarity reversal Within the body, reversal of normal electrical polarity is associated with pathology; appropriate therapeutic interventions may renormalize such reversals

Polarization (1) Separation of positive and negative electrical charges, on either side of a cell membrane, for instance; (2) application of fixed polarity positive and negative probes to different zones on the body; (3) balance of positive and negative bioelectrical charge found in the healthy human body energy system

Post-Heaven (postnatal) *qi*, *hou tian zhi qi* (後天之氣) Acquired *qi*, derived from food and air

Posttraumatic stress disorder Illness that develops following a traumatic incident, often involving re-experiencing the event, or extreme sensitivity to normal life experiences

Potency (1) Effective strength of a homeopathic preparation, increasing with potentization; (2) William G Sutherland's term for the embodied ordering and healing force present within the fluids of the body (the fluid body)

Potentization Process of preparation of a homeopathic remedy involving serial dilution and succussion that increases its potency

Power law Mathematical relationship between two parameters (aspects) of a system that describes its structural organization or behavior

Prana Sanskrit for 'vital life'; in Vedantic philosophy, it is the vital, life-sustaining force of living beings, and vital energy, comparable to the Chinese notion of *qi*; in Ayurveda, as 'breath of life', it is one of a trilogy of forces

Pranayama Practice of nurturing *prana* initially through breathwork and control techniques

Pregabalin Anticonvulsant also used for chronic inflammatory or functional pain

Pre-Heaven (prenatal) Essence, *Xian tian zhi jing* **(先天之精)** Congenital Essence inherited from the ancestors, present at conception; determines basic constitution, stored in the Kidney and essential for children's growth and development

Presence A state of wide, soft and receptive awareness that practitioners enter as they orient to a client's system; this is a natural state present at the core of our being

Primary respiration Term coined by William G Sutherland to denote the enlivening and ordering principle at work within and around the human system

Processual Metaparadigm emphasizing persons, movement, and interrelation (in contrast to *reductionist*)

Proprioception Feedback system between peripheral muscles and nerves and the central nervous system, allowing (unconscious) perception of movement and spatial orientation on the basis of stimuli from within the body itself

Proto-mind A non-conceptual precursor of mind present in all organisms, and possibly from the beginning of the universe. Phenomenologically, proto-mind experience is thus based more in body than mind

Psyche (*ψυχή*) Mind, consciousness, rational soul, or free-soul

Psychoanalytic Energy Psychotherapy Method developed by Phil Mollon using Thought Field Therapy often together with free association

Psychological reversal Term developed by Roger Callahan referring to conditions in which a person's energy system is organized against health or recovery; indicated by reversed muscle responses (testing weak in response to positive self-statements, and vice versa)

Psychoneuroimmunology Study of the interaction between psychological processes and the nervous and immune systems of the human body

'Pulling down the heavens/sky' (*yinxia tian*, 引下天) Preliminary exercise used in *qigong* to cleanse and root the *qi*

Punch biopsy Form of full thickness skin biopsy

Pure *yang, chun yang* (純陽) *Yang* at its maximal potential, in children

Purifying *qigong Qigong* exercises to cleanse the physical, energy and/or spiritual body

Pyruvate Cellular organic molecule that is a key component in several metabolic pathways; produced from glucose through glycolysis, it is involved in energy production through the Krebs cycle; it can also be converted to carbohydrates via gluconeogenesis, to fatty acids through acetyl-CoA, to the amino acid alanine, to lactic acid, and to ethanol

Qi (氣) Chinese version of the vitalist concept of an immanent life force in the world (part agency, part image or form, part metaphor), of key importance in health promotion and therapeutics; also a metaphor for interconnectedness in many aspects of Chinese culture; one of the three fundamental substances in the human body

Qi cultivation The process whereby one accumulates and refines one's life energy

Qi deficiency, *qi xu* (氣虛) A pattern of disharmony in Chinese medicine in which *qi* is insufficient to perform one or more of its functions

Qigong (氣功) Literally, '*qi* practice' or '*qi* mastery', to develop the skill of (labor at, *gong*, 工) *qi* force or strength (*li*, 力); a formalized set of movements involving deep breathing and meditation with *daoyin* as their generic core; used for healing, preventing diseases, and improving quality of life

Qili (氣力) 'Energy' in modern Chinese

Qi stagnation, *qi zhi* (氣滯) *Qi* stagnation, or *qi* that is 'stuck', not moving

Quantum Indivisible unit of energy; for electromagnetic radiation its value is the frequency multiplied by Planck's constant

Quantum electrodynamics A theory describing how light and matter interact

Quantum entanglement Nonlocal connection of two or more spatially separated objects that can no longer be adequately described without full mention of the other/s

Quantum level A level of reality where organization is based upon quantum effects and quantum order; recent research has shown that multicellular organisms can be considered as such organized quantum fields

Quantum potential Unlike the classical notion of potential (of an electron for example), this is a complex pattern of encoded information about the electron's physical environment

Quantum reality Reality at the atomic and subatomic level

Quantum touch State described by Rollin Becker, where the practitioner's perceptual field can sense and perceive a quantum level of organization

Quantum wholeness The unanalyzable nature of quantum systems, such as the observer and observed at the moment of an observation

Radical 'Root' part of a Chinese character; conventionally, there are 214 radicals

Radionics Method of diagnosis and treatment at a distance using specially designed instruments whose settings ('rates') correspond to different organs, diseases and remedies (different radionic systems use different rates)

Rational emotive therapy Forerunner of cognitive behavioral therapy

Reactive oxygen species Small reactive molecules containing oxygen

Rebellious *qi*, *niqi* (逆 氣) *Qi* reversal – the flow of *qi* in the opposite direction to normal, resulting in specific signs and symptoms; for example, digestive *qi* should move downward; when there is reversal of digestive *qi*, the person may belch or vomit; reversal of Lung *qi* results in cough or wheezing

Reductionist (1) Standpoint seeking to describe a phenomenon in terms of its component parts, without reference or respect to the whole; (2) metaparadigm emphasizing order and disorder (in contrast to *processual*)

Reed Eye-movement Acupressure Psychotherapy Combination of Eye Movement Desensitization and Reprocessing, Thought Field Therapy and Emotional Freedom Techniques with self-administered acupressure

Reiki Japanese method of hands-on healing developed in the 1920s

Relaxation response A physical state of deep rest that changes the physical and emotional responses to stress and the opposite of the fight or flight response

Renmai (任脈), Conception/Directing Vessel One of the eight extraordinary channels (*qi jing ba mai*) in Chinese medicine, running up the front of the body from the perineum to the lower lip

Renshen (人神) Human spirit; also, a system of acupuncture in which treatment is based on the position of the *renshen* in the body, determined according to a calendrical method

Repolarization Relaxation of the heart between contractions

Res cogitans Thinking thing or mind, a 'substance' in Descartes' ontology

Res extensa Extended thing, extension being the primary attribute of material/corporeal substance in Descartes' ontology

Resonance (1) Matching of an applied signal frequency with the natural vibratory frequency of an object that allows for greater interaction; this increased interaction is often referred to as entrainment; (2) process whereby the state of the practitioner, and his or her orientation, resonates within the client's body-mind system; it is through resonance with the practitioner's state of presence and orientation to primary respiration that the holistic shift emerges in craniosacral biodynamics

Respiration (oxidative metabolism) Set of chemical reactions and processes that take place at the cellular level to convert biochemical energy from nutrients into adenosine triphosphate

Retroid Class of virus; may also refer to bacterial elements

Reverse transcriptase DNA enzyme that transcribes single-stranded RNA into double-stranded DNA

Rgyud-bzhi *Four Tantras*, the main Tibetan medical treatise

Rheomode Verb-based, flowing language developed by David Bohm

Rong qi (營氣), Nutritive *qi* *Qi* formed by the combination of Lung *qi* and *gu qi*, which flows within the meridians and blood vessels in Chinese medicine (more often known as *ying qi*)

Ruach/ruah (רוּחַ) Hebrew for 'spirit', associated with breath or wind, sometimes interpreted as 'vital energy' (in Arabic, *rouh*)

Sahasrara Literally, 'thousand-petalled lotus'; the seventh, or crown *chakra*, at the vertex of the cranium

Salutogenic Focused on health and wellbeing rather than disease factors

San The original inhabitants of southern Africa ('Bushmen')

Scalar wave Hypothetical type of immaterial waves lacking directionality

Scale invariance A mathematical property (an exact form of self-similarity) of a fractal object or process; for example, in a scale-invariant time series, the appearance of fluctuations may be precisely similar at widely different timescales

Scaling drop-out Pattern in which certain bands of scaling frequencies of a system disappear and cease to transfer vital information

Scintillation counter Instrument for quantifying ionizing radiation such as gamma rays

Sedation A culturally resonant, but misleading biomedical term sometimes used to translate the concept of *xie* (泻), more properly 'draining'; supplementing (补, *bu*) and draining are two fundamental approaches in acupuncture, *tuina*, and Chinese medicine treatment, and are applied to 'vacuous' or 'replete' conditions respectively; supplementing reinforces and boosts the correct *qi* while draining is used to eliminate, disperse, or clear a replete evil (*note*: use of the expression 'sedate' to convey the idea of draining is entirely misleading and suggests an analogy to pharmacological sedation that is entirely absent from the concept of draining)

Sei (井) **points** Japanese equivalent to *jing* (Well) points

Self-organization Process of attraction and repulsion whereby the internal organization of a (usually open) system increases in complexity without guidance or management from an external source

Self-similarity Property of an object whereby it is exactly or approximately similar to a part of itself

Serial dilution Dilution in some ratio of solution to solvent which is then repeated using the product as a new solution

Serotonin 5-hydroxy-tryptamine (5-HT), a monoamine neurotransmitter

Serotonin reuptake inhibitor (SSRI) Antidepressant that increases the amount of serotonin available

Shamanism Wide range of beliefs and practices concerning communication with the different levels of the spirit worlds and often involving healing

Shangqing (上清) Supreme Clarity, a school of Daoism

Shen (神), **Spirit** One of the three fundamental substances in the human body; also translated as mind, or character

Shen jing shuai ruo (神经衰弱) Neurasthenia – vague fatigue thought to be caused by psychological factors

Shen Nong (神農) Divine Husbandman, legendary emperor of China, 2838 to 2698 BCE

Shen Nong Bencaojing (神農本草經) *Divine Farmer's Materia Medica*, an early Chinese compilation on agriculture and medicinal plants (c. 220 CE)

Shiatsu (指圧) Literally, 'finger pressure'; Japanese method of massage in which pressure exerted from different parts of the practitioner's body is applied along the channels

Shin (神) Spirit (Japanese equivalent of *shen*)

Shinto (神道) Way of the spirit (or of the Gods); traditional Japanese religion

Shuowen Jiezi (說文解字 说文解字) *Explanation of Characters*, a text written by Xu Shen c. 100 CE

Shu (Associated/Transporting) points, Bei shu xue (背俞穴) Back points on both sides of the spine that directly connect with associated *zangfu* organs and can be used both diagnostically and for treatment in acupuncture or *tuina* practice

Shuxin pingxue gong (舒心平血功) Form of *qigong* developed by Zhang Guangde

Singular point A point of abrupt transition from one state to another, for example in an electromagnetic field

Sink Node in a network or system with more incoming than outgoing flow

Sinus rhythm Normal beating of the heart at rest

Sinus tachycardia Rapid heart beat caused by dysfunction of the pacemaker in the right atrium of the heart

Small heavenly cycle (xiao zhou tian, 小周天) The first circulation exercise taught in most *qigong* systems, involving the circulation of *qi* along the *dumai* and *renmai* vessels

Soliton Localized wave packet that does not dissipate energy in its movement and so preserves its shape and velocity

Soma (1) Harmony and love, one of a trilogy of forces in Ayurveda; (2) Body (Greek, σομα)

Sotai (操体) Twentieth-century Japanese form of breath and movement therapy

Spectrofluorometry Method of electromagnetic spectroscopy used to analyze fluorescence (emission of light)

Spectroscopy Study and measurement of a physical quantity over a range of values of frequency/wavelength

Spirit, shen (神) One of the three fundamental substances in the human body; also translated as mind, or character

Standing wave A stationary wave through which energy moves

Status asthmaticus Severe, prolonged and progressive asthma attack unresponsive to standard treatment; can lead to pulmonary insufficiency and be life threatening

Step-down Term coined by Randolph Stone (1890–1981) to denote a shift in state from one level of life force to another; similar in concept to William G Sutherland's term 'transmutation'

Stillness Many expressions of stillness arise in session work, from a dynamic equilibrium of forces, to tensile equilibrium, to an expression of Dynamic Stillness, which maintains balance and equilibrium within the human system and which is present at the core of every organizing fulcrum

Stillpoint A process wherein a gateway opens as the system deepens into stillness and session work orients to the Long Tide or to the Dynamic Stillness itself; the Stillpoint commonly manifests as a relative state of deepening stillness in which healing processes emerge and potency within the fluids augments in intensity and action

Streaming sensations Sensations of flow within the body often accessible to those in a state of interoceptive awareness

Stress The body's nonspecific response to a demand placed on it and the consequences of the failure to respond appropriately to emotional or physical threats

Student's t-test A particular statistical method of hypothesis testing, originally devised to monitor the quality of Guinness beer

Substance P Neurotransmitter important in pain perception

Subtle body The body as open, extensive, interconnected, inherently intersubjective and processural

Subtle energy (1) A putative form of energy used when the intention of a healer is to cause healing; (2) Energy effect arising out of 'form' or 'information'; it is this information that is accessed in Energy Psychology ideas of 'morphic fields' [1] postulate subtle energetic patterning that regulates the form of biological organisms; different authors and traditions have used various terms for subtle energy, including *qi*, orgone, animal magnetism and bioelectrical energy [2]; whilst possessing some characteristics akin to electromagnetic energies, subtle energy also seems somewhat different [3]

Subud Indonesian spiritual movement founded in the 1920s, its central practice being *latihan*, which involves following what arises from within

Succussion Originally a repeated mechanical shock applied to a serial dilution, but can be effected in other ways

Superimplicate Order An order that *observes* the space-time manifestations of the Explicate Order and feeds back into the Implicate Order

Superoxide The reduction of dioxygen (O_2) by an unpaired electron, a widely occurring reaction in nature, produces a superoxide ion (O_2^-) that is also a free radical

Susumna Central *nadi* running from the base to the crown *chakra*

Suwen (素問) *Basic Questions*, the first part of the *Yellow Emperor's Canon of Internal Medicine, Huangdi Neijing*

Svadisthana Literally, 'one's own abode'; the second *chakra*, at the pelvis

Sympathetic nervous system Thoracolumbar division of the nervous system, mobilizing body systems during 'fight or flight'; contributes to homeostasis through its complementary opposition to the parasympathetic division

Synesthesia Condition in which two or more of the five senses normally experienced separately are involuntarily and automatically conjoined (e.g. feeling tactile sensations as colored)

Systematic review Literature review to identify, appraise, select and synthesize all high-quality research evidence relevant to a specific question

Tachogram Recording of changes in heart rate over time

Tachypnea Rapid breathing

Taiji quan (太極拳) Literally 'Supreme ultimate fist', a 'soft' or internal form of Chinese martial art that specializes in techniques of 'sticking' and 'yielding' and utilizing internal *qi* rather than external force

Taijitu (太極圖) Classic Daoist symbol for *yin* and *yang*

Tantric medicine Medical system associated with the Indian psychospiritual methods of *tantra*: a body of beliefs and practices based on the view that the universe is a manifestation of (divine) energy, and that seeks to channel that energy, within the human microcosm, in a creative and emancipatory manner

Tapas Acupressure Technique Application of light pressure to specific areas on the face and head while mentally addressing issues of concern

T cell, T lymphocyte Type of lymphocyte essential to cell-mediated immunity

Tendinomuscular meridians Meridians (channels) in Chinese medicine taking their names from the 12 primary meridians whose external courses they generally follow, each comprising a musculokinetic chain of muscle, tendon, ligaments and other connective tissue and having a primary impact on the postural alignment and energetic balance of body structures; in contrast to the primary meridians, the tendinomuscular meridians originate in the extremities and ascend to the trunk and head; they may be considered as much structural as energetic pathways

Tendon changing qigong A *qigong* practice involving a systematic softening and energizing of the fascia, tendons, and ligaments

Tensile field Field of action that holds a natural tension, such as the reciprocal tension membrane in the cranium, and the connective tissue field as a whole

Therapeutic potency Meaningful consequences (usually, causal efficacy) arising from application of a therapeutic agent (a force or activity that restores health)

Therapeutic Touch Standardized healing method developed for use by nurses by Dolores Krieger and Dora Kunz; may or may not involve body contact

Third Eye The seat of insight, the sixth *chakra*

Thought field Term developed by Roger Callahan to denote the expression of a person's thought as information in their body's energy field; hence Thought Field Therapy (TFT)

Three treasures, sanbao (三宝) In Chinese philosophy and medicine, the three fundamental substances in the human body: *jing*, Essence, *qi*, Life Force, and *shen*, Spirit

Tian qi (天氣) Literally, 'heavenly *qi*', or the universal rules that *qi* follows

Tidal potency The ordering force that manifests within the fluids of the body as a tidal motion generating the fluid tide and tissue motility

Tide William G Sutherland's term for the deepest expression of primary respiration, the Long Tide

Time series Series in which a sequence of values reveals a dynamic pattern over time, as in the RR inter-beat interval time series

Time structure Rhythmic order embedded within a time series

Tissue field The tissues of the body as a unified tensile field of action

Tissue motility An inherent primary respiratory motion within cells and tissues driven by the action of the tidal

potency; it has embryological origins and is an expression of the ordering intentions of the Breath of Life

Tonifying The action of adding energy to the body (sometimes understood as from outside it)

Transliminality Susceptibility for psychological (affective or ideational) material to cross thresholds into or out of consciousness

Transmutation Term coined by William G Sutherland to denote a change in state of the ordering forces of life from the field phenomenon of the Tide, to the 'potency', the embodied forces within the fluids

Transparency State of being in which one is so coherent with regard to one's body-person that one simply lives well, feeling 'healthy' and not continually assessing one's self, but simply 'getting on with' one's life and occupation; an outsider looking in might say 'that person is well'

Treasure points (12 light points of the soul) Twelve acupuncture points surrounding *baihui* (百會, Du-20) in three concentric circles

Triad of health The chiropractic concept of three interacting areas of health or sickness, deriving from the chemical, the physical or structural, and the mental

Tricyclic antidepressant Type of antidepressant inhibiting reuptake of serotonin, norepinephrine (noradrenaline), and dopamine (to a lesser extent)

Trigger point Tender point where sustained pressure reproduces pain in areas where it occurs spontaneously

Trophotropic Pertaining to parasympathetic activity

Tryptophan Essential amino acid precursor of serotonin

Tryptophan 2.3-dioxygenase Enzyme catalyzing the breakdown of tryptophan

Tsubo (壺 or ツボ) *Shiatsu* equivalent of an acupuncture point

Tuina (推拿) Literally 'pushing and grasping', Chinese system of massage, manual acupuncture point stimulation and manipulation

Tumor necrosis factor Protein important in regulating immune function; can also trigger cell death (apoptosis); sometimes refers to TNF-α only

Ubiquinone Coenzyme present primarily in mitochondria, particularly important for generating energy in the form of adenosine triphosphate

Ubuvuzi bwa Gihanga Traditional Rwandan medicine (after the legendary king Gihanga)

Unani 'Greek', or Greco-Islamic, humoral medicine

Uncertainty principle Heisenberg's principle that certain pairs of physical properties, such as position and momentum, cannot both be known precisely at the same time

Unified field theory Term coined by Albert Einstein for a theory that allows all of the fundamental forces of physics to be described in terms of a single field

Upanishads Hindu texts, the earliest of which date from the first millennium BCE

Upper dantian, shang dantian (上丹田) Energy center located in the head responsible for transforming *shen* into *wuji*

Vata Wind, one of the three main Ayurvedic *doshas* (humors)

Vayu Literally, 'air'; name of the Hindu deity of the Winds

Vector A quantity, such as a magnetic line of force, with both magnitude and direction (in contrast to a scalar such as temperature, which has dimension only)

Vector potential In a vector field, such as a magnetic field, there is an associated vector at every point. These thus have a vector potential (as contrasted with the scalar potential at points around a source of heat, for example)

Ventricle Lower chamber of the heart

Vishuddha Literally, 'purification'; the throat *chakra*

Visual analog scale Psychometric instrument for subjective characteristics or attitudes that cannot be directly measured

Vital force Proposed in 1907 by Henri Bergson (1859–1941) as a special property of life; the force that allows life and keeps living things alive; further, this force is like electricity but, unlike electricity, is unique to living things

Vitalism Doctrine that the origin and phenomenon of life are due to or produced by a vital principle, as distinct from a purely chemical or physical force

Vitality affect Daniel Stern's term for a fundamental metaphor expressing an inner feeling of aliveness, often of movement

Waidan (外丹) Outer alchemy, *qigong* emphasizing 'hard' *qi* and a 'hard' body

Waigong (外功) External *qigong*; manipulation of *qi* by a master with healing power

Wave function Equation describing the probability of a particle being in a given state

Wave packet Short burst of wave action that travels as a unit

Weak nuclear force One of four fundamental interactions in nature, weaker than electromagnetic force and the strong nuclear force, but stronger than the gravitational force

Wei qi (衛氣) Protective *qi* that flows outside the vessels and superficially in the body

Whorf–Sapir hypothesis Hypothesis that there is a link between the cultural concepts enfolded within a language and the worldview of the native speakers of that language

Witness state A broad relaxed attention to the flow of the present moment

Working field of influence Active and maintained application of different vectors or directions of pressure (traction/stretching, rotation) which are then held, combined, and directed into or through or across an area of tightness, congestion … or absence

Wuji (無極) Infinite space or ether

Xisui (洗髓) Marrow washing, an advanced *qigong* practice involving the circulation and compression of *qi* through the bones

X-signal system Primitive (deep-level) biological information system at the heart of acupuncture theory that ultimately regulates all life processes but is unexplainable by current neurophysiology

Yang (陽) The relatively *yang* constituents of the body are *qi* and the body's physiological function. The 'hollow' Organs (*fu*, 腑), which primarily function for storage and transport, are *yang*: Large Intestine, Urinary Bladder, Gall Bladder, Small Intestine, *sanjiao* and Stomach

Yangsheng (養生) Self-cultivation, as in *daoyin* or *neidan*

Yang deficiency, yang xu (陽虛) Condition similar to *qi* deficiency, but with symptoms of Cold (*han*, 寒) in addition

Yellow Bile (*safrā*) One of the four humors in *Unani*, along with Black Bile, Blood and Phlegm

Yi jin jing (易筋經) Muscle/tendon changing, a traditional form of *qigong*

Yin (陰) The relatively *yin* constituents of the body are the Essence (*jing*), Blood (*xue*) and Fluids (*jin ye*), its more material/structive aspects. The 'solid' Organs (*zang*, 臟), which carry out the physiological processes of *qi* production, transformation and metabolism, are *yin*: Lung, Kidney, Liver, Heart, Pericardium, and Spleen/Pancreas

Ying (營) Nutrients, which when absorbed are distributed throughout the body via the vascular system

Yinggong (硬功) Hard form of *qigong*, more external and physical than some 'softer' versions

Yin deficiency, yin xu (陰虛) Insufficiency of *yin* constituents (Essence, Blood, Body Fluids) or insufficiency of function in the *yin* Organs (*zang*); may lead to symptoms of apparent excess of *yang*

Yinyang (陰陽) The opposite but complementary qualities of all things in nature (literally, 'shady hillside' and 'sunny hillside'): female–male; Earth–Heaven; night–day; soft–hard; emotional–rational; cold–hot; etc.; *yin* and *yang* are not absolute opposites but exist in dynamic equilibrium

Young yang and young yin Yang and *yin* in children, not yet fully developed (年轻 陽, *nianqing yang*, and 年轻陰, *nianqing yin*, respectively)

Zangfu (臟腑) Composite term, extensively used in Chinese medicine and Daoist health promotion practices, referring to the main Internal Organs of the body categorized as six 'solid' (*zang*) and six 'hollow' (*fu*) Organs

Zhenjiu (針灸) Acupuncture and moxibustion

Zhenqi (真氣) True or genuine *qi*, equated by Kendall with the basic dynamic process responsible for all vital bodily functions

Zhenxue (針穴) Acupuncture point (literally, 'needle pit')

Zhishi (指事) Ideograph, Chinese character representing an abstract notion

Zouhuo lümo (作火魯莫) Roughly equivalent to '*qigong*-induced psychosis'

Zuo Zhuan (左轉) *Zuo's Annals*, a chronicle of earlier times by the blind historian Zuo (c. 310 BCE)

Zygote Single cell formed by the union of sperm and ovum before cell division occurs and it develops into the embryo

REFERENCES AND FURTHER READING

[1] Sheldrake AR. A New Science of Life: The hypothesis of formative causation. London: Blond; 1985.

[2] Oschman JL. Energy Medicine: The scientific basis. Edinburgh: Churchill Livingstone; 2000.

[3] Tiller WA. Science and Human Transformation: Subtle energies, intentionality and consciousness. Walnut Creek, CA: Pavior Publishing; 1997.

Printed and bound by CPI Group (UK) Ltd, Croydon, CR0 4YY

03/10/2024

01040848-0014